Regional Anatomy Illustrated

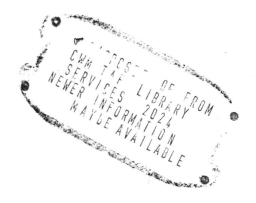

Regional Anatomy Illustrated

J. W. SMITH MD(St Andrews)
Professor of Regional Anatomy,
University of St Andrews, UK

T. R. MURPHY MSc(Adelaide), MDS(Edinburgh), LRCP&S
Formerly Senior Lecturer in Anatomy,
University of St Andrews, UK

J. S. G. BLAIR OBE, BA, ChM(St Andrews), FRCS
Consultant Surgeon, Perth Royal Infirmary,
Perth; Honorary Senior Lecturer in Surgery,
University of Dundee, UK

K. G. LOWE CVO, MD(St Andrews), FRCP
Emeritus Professor of Medicine,
University of Dundee, UK

CHURCHILL LIVINGSTONE
EDINBURGH LONDON MELBOURNE AND NEW YORK 1983

CHURCHILL LIVINGSTONE
Medical Division of Longman Group Limited

Distributed in the United States of America by Churchill Livingstone
Inc., 1560 Broadway, New York, N.Y. 10036, and by associated
companies, branches and representatives throughout the world.

First published 1983

ISBN 0 443 01615 1

British Library Cataloguing in Publication Data
Regional anatomy illustrated
  1. Anatomy, Human—Atlases
  I. Smith, J. W.
  611′.0022′2   QM25

Library of Congress Cataloging in Publication Data
Main entry under title:

Regional anatomy illustrated.

  Includes index.
  1. Anatomy, Surgical and topographical
I. Smith, J. W. (James William) [DNLM:
1. Anatomy, Regional. QS 4 R335]
QM531.R425 1983   611′.9   82-19799

Printed in Great Britain by B.A.S. Printers Limited, Stockbridge, Hampshire.

Preface

Regional anatomy is the study of the gross morphology and spatial interrelations of the structures of the body and the changes which occur in these features in various circumstances. It also customarily includes consideration of the functions of some body structures, particularly those functions which are highly dependent on morphology. Thus the nature of the movements of which the knee joint is capable is dictated by the morphology of the articulating bones, the articular surfaces and the joint ligaments, and the subject is therefore appropriately considered in textbooks of regional anatomy. In contrast, most would regard the inclusion of the functions of the thyroid gland as inappropriate, as these are influenced in no way by the shape of the gland or its relationship to surrounding structures.

Despite its abiding importance as a basis of clinical practice, the subject matter of regional anatomy does not grow or undergo rapid change as it does in many other areas of biology. Consequently the production of a new account of regional anatomy at this time cannot be justified on the grounds that it presents a large volume of new knowledge. Such a production can only be justified if it presents the existing subject matter to medical students in a format which is more relevant than others to present day medical practice and to the present day medical curriculum.

The text of this book is therefore short, amounting to some two hundred and eighty pages. It is also selective. It emphasises those aspects of the subject which clinicians believe from their professional experience to be essential knowledge, and those aspects which the teaching experience of anatomists shows a significant number of students find difficult to understand. These emphases have been achieved at the expense, or even to the exclusion, of aspects of the subject which have always been, or through clinical advances have now become, largely of academic interest.

Because the visualisation of complex structural interrelationships is achieved more readily by many students through the visual sense, we have tried (as the name of our book indicates) to illustrate every relationship mentioned in the text by diagrams. In order to facilitate and encourage the use of these diagrams, the manner in which they have been arranged and the methods which have been used to refer to them are unusual, though not unique. As far as possible, diagrams are placed on the page facing the text to which they refer and each is labelled by a capital letter. Thus (**C**) in the text directs the reader to diagram **C** on the apposing page, and (**A**, **B**) to diagrams **A** and **B** on the apposing page. Although this simple arrangement is maintained as far as possible, it is obviously necessary at some points to refer to distant text or diagrams. A distant textual reference is given by quoting the relevant page number, e.g. (**238**), while a distant diagram reference is given by quoting the relevant page number and diagram letter, e.g. (**239D**). Thus, to take an extreme example, reference on page 122 to (**B, 356, 443B**) directs the reader to diagram **B** on page 123, to the text on page 356 and to diagram **B** on page 443.

We are grateful to a number of colleagues for the help they have given us in the production of this book. Dr D. Emslie-Smith, Department of Medicine, University of Dundee, Dr F. Fletcher, Department of Diagnostic Radiology, Ninewells Hospital, Dundee, Dr J. A. K. Meikle, Department of Diagnostic Radiology, Perth Royal Infirmary and Dr R. N. Johnston, Department of Respiratory Diseases, King's Cross Hospital, Dundee have kindly allowed us to use several of their X-rays. We are indebted to the technical staffs of the Department of Medical Photography, Bridge of Earn Hospital and of the Department of Anatomy and Experimental Pathology, University of St Andrews for their technical assistance. The expert secretarial services of Mrs Wilma Pogorzelec have been invaluable. The staff of Churchill Livingstone, particularly Mr Andrew Stevenson, have guided our work with a patience and understanding for which we have been very grateful.

St Andrews, Perth and Dundee 1983

J.W.S.
T.R.M.
J.S.G.B.
K.G.L.

v

Contents

THE ANATOMICAL POSITION

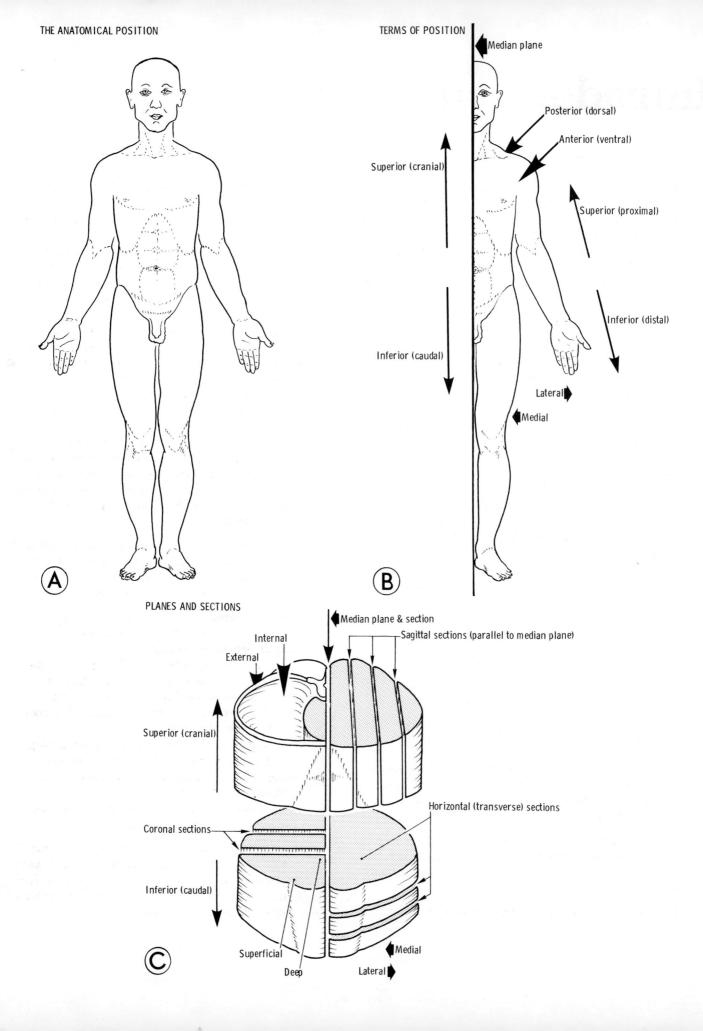

A

TERMS OF POSITION

Median plane

Posterior (dorsal)

Anterior (ventral)

Superior (cranial)

Superior (proximal)

Inferior (caudal)

Inferior (distal)

Lateral

Medial

B

PLANES AND SECTIONS

Median plane & section

Sagittal sections (parallel to median plane)

Internal

External

Superior (cranial)

Horizontal (transverse) sections

Coronal sections

Inferior (caudal)

Medial

Superficial

Lateral

Deep

C

Introduction

The interpretations of the structures of the body are described in the context of a standard position of the body which is called the *anatomical position* (**A**). In this position the body is standing upright, the upper limbs hang downwards and the palms of the hands and the eyes are directed forwards. The body so orientated is divided into right and left halves by the *median plane* (**B**). As far as the body surface is concerned, the two halves are symmetrical, but the same symmetry does not apply to all internal structures. Thus the normal spleen is entirely in the left half of the body.

The body in the anatomical position is also regarded as being traversed by three orthogonally intersecting sets of planes which form a reference grid (**C**). *A sagittal plane* is any vertical plane which is parallel to the median plane. *A coronal plane* is any vertical plane at right angles to the median plane. *A horizontal plane* is any plane at right angles to both sagittal and coronal planes. As defined above, sagittal, coronal and horizontal planes are all multiple, but it should be noted that there is an alternative usage of the term sagittal plane. Some authors regard the term as synonymous with median plane. For them, therefore, there is only one sagittal plane and all planes parallel to it are described as parasagittal.

Aspects of the surface of the body as a whole or of the surfaces of individual structures are named in the following manner.

1. The terms *anterior* or *ventral*, which are synonymous in human anatomy, are applied to aspects which face forwards. Aspects which face backwards are described by one of the synonymous terms *posterior* or *dorsal*. Note, however, that the anterior or ventral aspect of the hand is customarily designated *palmar*.
2. Aspects which face away from the median plane are called *lateral* and those which face towards the median plane *medial*.
3. Aspects which face upwards are described as *superior* and those which face downwards as *inferior*. Note however that these aspects of the foot are customarily designated *dorsal* and *plantar* respectively.

The spatial relationship of separate structures are described on the basis of their relative proximity to aspects or parts of the body in the anatomical position and to the median plane.

1. Thus, of two structures, one is *anterior* to the other (an anterior relation of the other) if it is the closer to the anterior aspect of the body, and *posterior* to the other (a posterior relation of the other) if it is closer to the posterior aspect of the body. Similarly, one is *medial* to the other if it is closer to the median plane and *lateral* to the other if it is farther from that plane. Again, one is *superior* to the other if it is at a higher level and *inferior* to the other if it is at a lower level.
2. Some relationships are best described by compound terms. Thus one structure is *anterolateral* to another if it is both closer to the anterior aspect of the body and farther from the median plane.
3. The terms *superficial* and *deep* refer to the comparative distances of structures from the skin surface.
4. In the limbs, the term *proximal* indicates relative proximity to the root of the limb, and *distal* relative separation. The same terms are sometimes used to indicate relative distances along the course of a nerve or vessel (e.g. one branch of a nerve is given off proximal to another).

The six cardinal movements which occur at the joints of the body are called flexion, extension, adduction, abduction, rotation and circumduction. These can be defined in the following very general terms.

1. *Flexion* is the movement which makes the angle between the articulating bones more acute and thus reduces the length of the part.
2. *Extension* tends to bring the articulating bones into alignment and thus lengthens (extends) the part.
3. *Adduction* displaces the distal articulating bone towards the median plane, while *abduction* displaces it away from the median plane.
4. *Rotation* occurs around the long axis of the moving bone and is designated *medial* or *lateral rotation* according to the direction of displacement of the anterior aspect of the bone.
5. In *circumduction* the moving bone describes a cone with its apex at the joint concerned.

Many movements do not conform to these simple definitions and several are indeed given individual names not included in the above list. Consequently, joint movements will be discussed throughout the text with the descriptions of the joints at which they occur.

CHAPTER 1

The vertebral column and skull

THE VERTEBRAL COLUMN

The vertebral column consists of a large number of ring-like bones united in series by joints and ligaments. These bones, joints and ligaments enclose the longitudinal vertebral canal (**A**).

In the neck there are seven cervical vertebrae, in the thorax twelve thoracic, in the abdominal region five lumbar, and in the pelvic region five sacral and a variable number of vestigial coccygeal vertebrae (**A**).

In the foetus and newborn infant the vertebral column has a continuous primary curvature which is concave forwards (**B**). Throughout postnatal life the thoracic, sacral and coccygeal parts of the column retain this form (**A**), but secondary curves which are convex forwards appear, first in the cervical region when the child learns to sit up at about 6 months, and later in the lumbar region when standing is accomplished at about 18 months (**A**). The primary and secondary curvatures merge smoothly into one another except at the lumbosacral junction where the change in direction is abrupt (lumbosacral angle). These curvatures may be altered by disease of the vertebrae or by spasm of the vertebral muscles.

The first cervical vertebra supports the skull, while the thoracic vertebrae articulate with the ribs which enlose the thorax. The sacral part of the column articulates laterally with the hip bones which join anteriorly to complete the bony pelvis. The outer aspects of the hip bones articulate with the bones of the lower limbs.

The vertebral column has three main functions.

1. It supports the weight of the head and neck, upper limbs, and trunk and transmits this force through the hip bones to the lower limbs.
2. It contains and protects the spinal cord and the spinal nerve roots within the vertebral canal.
3. It allows considerable changes in the form of the trunk and neck by virtue of the summation of small movements between the cervical, thoracic and lumbar vertebrae. These movements are flexion (forward bending), extension (backward bending), lateral flexion (bending to one side) and rotation.

The general features of vertebrae

Most vertebrae exhibit the same basic features and these can be examined from above in **C** and in a median section in **D**.

Note the approximately cylindrical body anteriorly and the approximately semilunar vertebral arch attached to its posterior aspect. The vertebral foramen is enclosed by these two parts. The arch consists of two pedicles and two laminae which converge posteriorly to unite in a single spinous process. On both sides a transverse process and superior and inferior articular processes arise from the junction of pedicle and lamina. The transverse and spinous processes are strong struts which give attachment to many of the vertebral muscles and their associated fascial layers.

Intervertebral articulations

These articulations, which involve a number of joints and ligaments, are similar throughout the vertebral column except in the upper cervical, sacral and coccygeal regions.

The intervertebral disc

On the apposed surfaces of adjacent vertebral bodies a circular strip of dense bone surrounds a plate of hyaline cartilage which lies directly over cancellous bone (**C, D, E**). These surfaces are joined by a thick ring of fibrocartilage, the anulus fibrosus, which encloses the nucleus pulposus (**E, F**). The anulus fibrosus, the nucleus pulposus and the two hyaline cartilage plates constitute a secondary cartilaginous joint (symphysis) called an intervertebral disc.

When an intervertebral disc is compressed by the longitudinal stress caused by body weight, radial forces in the incompressible nucleus pulposus are directed against the elastic cartilage plates and anulus fibrosus so that the whole complex acts as a shock absorber (**F**).

In youth an intervertebral disc is as strong as the vertebrae it unites and the nucleus pulposus is opalescent and gelatinous. However from early adulthood the nucleus becomes more rigid and fibrosed while the anulus often undergoes degenerative changes.

An excessive stress, particularly acting on a degenerate disc, may rupture either one of the cartilage plates or the anulus fibrosus and allow herniation (prolapse) of the nucleus pulposus. Although herniations may occur in any direction, those which protrude through the anulus in a posterolateral direction are of particular clinical interest (see below).

VERTEBRAL COLUMN:
MEDIAN SECTION

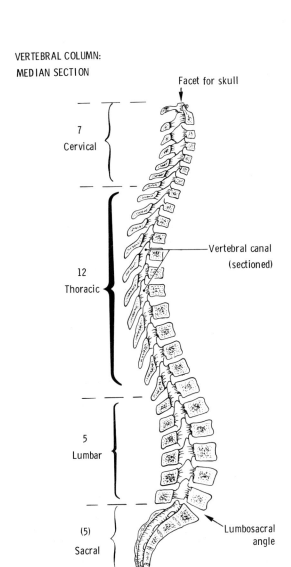

Facet for skull

7 Cervical

12 Thoracic

Vertebral canal
(sectioned)

5 Lumbar

(5) Sacral

Lumbosacral
angle

Coccygeal

(A)

VERTEBRAL COLUMN IN FOETUS

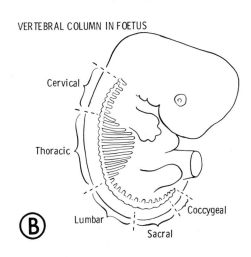

Cervical

Thoracic

Lumbar

Coccygeal

Sacral

(B)

GENERAL STRUCTURE OF VERTEBRA: SUPERIOR ASPECT

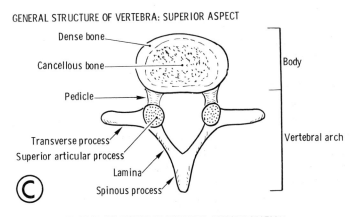

Dense bone

Cancellous bone

Pedicle

Transverse process
Superior articular process
Lamina
Spinous process

Body

Vertebral arch

(C)

GENERAL STRUCTURE OF VERTEBRA: MEDIAN SECTION

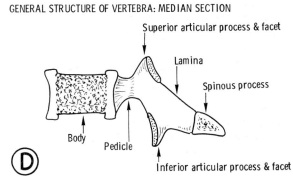

Superior articular process & facet

Lamina

Spinous process

Body

Pedicle

Inferior articular process & facet

(D)

INTERVERTEBRAL DISC: MEDIAN SECTION

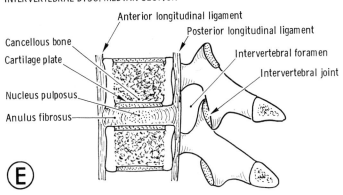

Anterior longitudinal ligament
Posterior longitudinal ligament

Cancellous bone
Cartilage plate

Intervertebral foramen
Intervertebral joint

Nucleus pulposus
Anulus fibrosus

(E)

DISC COMPRESSION

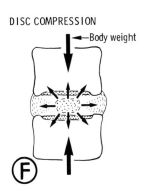

Body weight

(F)

3

The longitudinal ligaments

The strength of the intervertebral discs is augmented by two powerful ligaments. The broad, strap-like anterior longitudinal ligament is attached to the anterior aspects of the vertebral bodies and the discs, and extends from the base of the skull to the upper end of the sacrum (**A**). The posterior longitudinal ligament lies on the anterior wall of the vertebral canal, from skull to sacrum. Note its pectinate margins (**B**). Each wide segment of the ligament is firmly attached to the back of an intervertebral disc, but the narrow segments are separated from the vertebral bodies by the large basi-vertebral veins which issue from them.

The intervertebral joints

The superior and inferior articular processes of adjacent vertebral arches articulate by small synovial intervertebral joints. Each is enclosed by a fibrous capsule (**3E**) (**C**).

The intervertebral joints are strengthened by a series of ligaments which lie between adjacent transverse processes (intertransverse ligaments), between adjacent spinous processes (interspinous and supraspinous ligaments), and between adjacent laminae (ligamenta flava) (**C**). The supraspinous ligament becomes wider in the median plane as it is followed upwards into the cervical region, and is attached above to a median ridge on the base of the skull. This part is known as the ligamentum nuchae. In large quadrupeds such as the ox, in which a large force is necessary to support the head, it is a thick structure containing a very high proportion of elastic fibres. In man it is much thinner and almost purely fibrous. The ligamenta flava are so called because of their content of yellow elastic fibres.

The intervertebral foramina

Paired intervertebral foramina lead laterally from the vertebral canal between adjacent vertebrae (**3E**) (**C**). Observe that a typical foramen is bounded above and below by pedicles, in front by a vertebral body and an intervertebral disc and behind by the fibrous capsule of an intervertebral joint.

Each foramen is largely occupied by a spinal nerve, artery and vein. These contents may be compressed by pathological expansion of any of the boundaries.

Compression may be caused by arthritic changes in intervertebral joints or, more commonly, by posterolateral herniation of a nucleus pulposus (**C**). The latter usually occurs in the lumbosacral region where it gives rise to the symptoms of sciatica (**9D**) or in the cervical region where it causes neuritis in the arm.

Regional differences in the vertebrae and intervertebral articulations

The typical cervical vertebrae

Apart from the first and second (the atlas and axis) the cervical vertebrae are similar though not identical in form and have features which readily distinguish them from vertebrae of other regions (**D, E**).

1. The spinous processes are bifid.
2. The facets on the superior and inferior articular processes are flat and face upwards and backwards, and downwards and forwards, respectively.
3. The most lateral parts of the upper surfaces of the vertebral bodies and to a less marked degree the same parts of the lower surfaces incline upwards and are separated by small synovial joints on either side of each intervertebral disc. These are the joints of Lushka, which may become arthritic in later life and give rise to chronic pain.
4. The transverse processes arise from the lateral aspects of the bodies and pedicles (**D**). Their upper surfaces are in continuity with the lower boundary of intervertebral foramina and are deeply grooved in a mediolateral direction (**E**). Each process is pierced by a large foramen transversarium. The bar of bone forming the anterior boundary of the foramen represents a vestigial rib, and in a few individuals the costal element of the seventh transverse process is abnormally long and projects laterally into the root of the neck as a cervical rib.
5. The seventh cervical vertebra differs from the others in this group in a few minor respects. The spinous process is long, palpable and ends in a single tubercle. The transverse processes are longer and contain foramina transversaria which are comparatively small and sometimes double.
6. Because of the orientation of the articular facets, intervertebral movements in this region are relatively free in all directions.

ANTERIOR LONGITUDINAL LIGAMENT

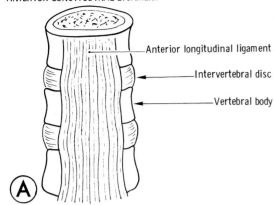

— Anterior longitudinal ligament

— Intervertebral disc

— Vertebral body

Ⓐ

POSTERIOR LONGITUDINAL LIGAMENT: VERTEBRAL ARCHES REMOVED

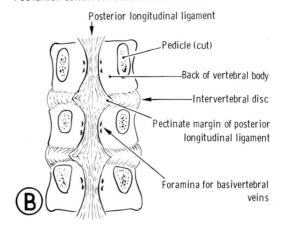

Posterior longitudinal ligament

— Pedicle (cut)

— Back of vertebral body

— Intervertebral disc

— Pectinate margin of posterior longitudinal ligament

— Foramina for basivertebral veins

Ⓑ

INTERVERTEBRAL ARTICULATION: MEDIAN SECTION

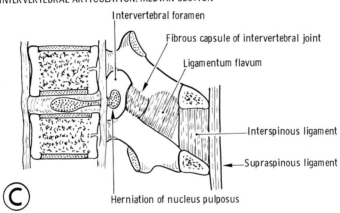

Intervertebral foramen

Fibrous capsule of intervertebral joint

Ligamentum flavum

— Interspinous ligament

— Supraspinous ligament

Herniation of nucleus pulposus

Ⓒ

TYPICAL CERVICAL VERTEBRA: SUPERIOR ASPECT

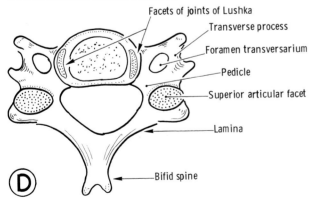

Facets of joints of Lushka

Transverse process

Foramen transversarium

Pedicle

Superior articular facet

Lamina

Bifid spine

Ⓓ

TYPICAL CERVICAL VERTEBRA: ANTERIOR ASPECT

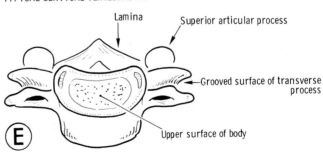

Lamina

Superior articular process

Grooved surface of transverse process

Upper surface of body

Ⓔ

The axis

The axis is the second cervical vertebra (**A**, **B**). Its inferior aspect is similar to those of the typical cervical vertebrae described above and its articulation with the superior aspect of the third cervical vertebra is of typical form (**E**). However its superior surface presents a number of atypical features (**A**, **B**).

1. A stout tooth-like process called the dens or the odontoid process extends vertically upwards from the anterior part of the body. Its posterior aspect is grooved transversely while its anterior aspect exhibits a small oval cartilaginous facet.
2. Two larger lateral facets, which are flat, oval and more or less horizontal, lie on the upper surface of the body and the anterior part of the pedicle on either side of the dens.
3. There are no superior articular processes at the junctions of the pedicles and the laminae.

The atlas

This is the first cervical vertebra and is of unique shape. It consists essentially of a ring of bone from which transverse processes extend laterally on either side (**C**).

1. The lateral masses carry articular facets on both upper and lower surfaces. The superior facets are elongated anteroposteriorly and concave upwards along their long axes. As will be seen later in this chapter, they articulate with the occipital condyles on the base of the skull forming the paired atlanto-occipital joints. The inferior facets are flat and articulate with the lateral facets on the upper surface of the axis (**A**) forming the paired lateral atlanto-axial joints (**E**).
2. The short anterior arch joins the anterior parts of the lateral masses. A small facet on the posterior aspect of its central part articulates with that on the anterior aspect of the dens of the axis forming the median atlanto-axial joint (**A**, **B**, **C**, **D**).
3. The longer posterior arch joins the posterior parts of the lateral masses. Immediately behind each lateral mass its upper surface is crossed by a wide transverse groove.
4. The transverse processes of the atlas are longer than others in the cervical region, so that their tips are usually palpable just behind the angle of the lower jaw.

The atlanto-axial articulation

This consists of three synovial joints, the median and the paired lateral atlanto-axial joints (**D**, **E**). The articulation is equipped with a number of stabilising accessory ligaments.

1. The strong transverse ligament of the atlas extends between the medial aspects of the lateral masses of the atlas and is separated from the grooved posterior aspect of the dens of the axis by a bursa (**D**). It prevents backward displacement of the dens from the anterior arch of the atlas.
2. The upper part of the anterior longitudinal ligament joins the anterior surface of the body of the axis to the anterior arch of the atlas (**E**).
3. The uppermost pair of ligamenta flava bridge the interval between the laminae of the axis and the posterior arch of the atlas. They are continuous in the midline with the ligamentum nuchae (**E**).
4. Notice in **E** the unusual boundaries of the atlanto-axial intervertebral foramen.

Movements at the atlanto-axial articulation involve rotations of the atlas and the skull, moving as one, around the dens together with anteroposterior sliding movements at the lateral atlanto-axial joints.

Injury of the articulation may be produced by hyperflexion or hyperextension of the region as when the head whiplashes during the rapid deceleration associated with many road accidents. The dens may be snapped off from the body of the axis or it may be displaced backwards relative to the atlas through tearing of the transverse ligament. Such injuries distort the upper part of the vertebral canal and may damage severely the related part of the spinal cord.

The thoracic vertebrae

1. The thoracic intervertebral discs are uniformly thick from before backwards and the normal thoracic curve (see above) is due to the vertebral bodies being slightly deeper behind than in front (**F**).
2. The spinous processes are long, sharp and angled acutely downwards (**F**). Thus palpation of a spine does not indicate directly the level of the corresponding vertebral body.
3. Nearly all the vertebrae carry characteristic facets on the upper and lower margins of the lateral aspects of their bodies and on the anterior aspects of their transverse processes (**F**) for articulation with the ribs (**129A**, **129B**).
4. At the thoracic intervertebral joints the superior facets face backwards and to a much lesser extent laterally and upwards (**F**). The inferior have the opposite orientation.
5. The attachment of the thoracic cage to this part of the vertebral column considerably restricts its movements in all directions.

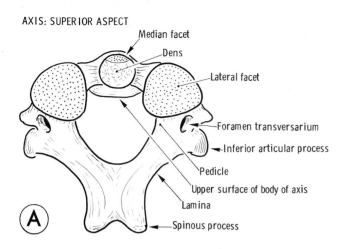

AXIS: SUPERIOR ASPECT

- Median facet
- Dens
- Lateral facet
- Foramen transversarium
- Inferior articular process
- Pedicle
- Upper surface of body of axis
- Lamina
- Spinous process

(A)

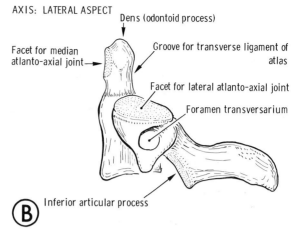

AXIS: LATERAL ASPECT

- Dens (odontoid process)
- Facet for median atlanto-axial joint
- Groove for transverse ligament of atlas
- Facet for lateral atlanto-axial joint
- Foramen transversarium
- Inferior articular process

(B)

ATLAS: SUPERIOR ASPECT

- Anterior median tubercle
- Anterior arch
- Lateral mass
- Transverse process
- Foramen transversarium
- Groove for vertebral artery
- Median facet for dens
- Vertebral foramen
- Facet for occipital condyle

(C)

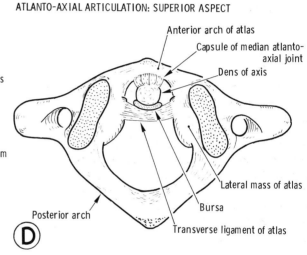

ATLANTO-AXIAL ARTICULATION: SUPERIOR ASPECT

- Anterior arch of atlas
- Capsule of median atlanto-axial joint
- Dens of axis
- Lateral mass of atlas
- Bursa
- Transverse ligament of atlas
- Posterior arch

(D)

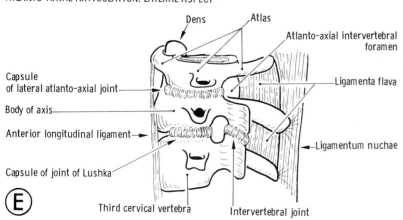

ATLANTO-AXIAL ARTICULATION: LATERAL ASPECT

- Dens
- Atlas
- Atlanto-axial intervertebral foramen
- Capsule of lateral atlanto-axial joint
- Ligamenta flava
- Body of axis
- Anterior longitudinal ligament
- Ligamentum nuchae
- Capsule of joint of Lushka
- Third cervical vertebra
- Intervertebral joint

(E)

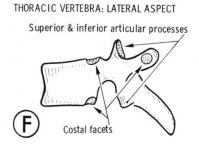

THORACIC VERTEBRA: LATERAL ASPECT

- Superior & inferior articular processes
- Costal facets

(F)

The lumbar vertebrae

1. The bodies are large, deep and kidney-shaped in the transverse plane. Unlike thoracic vertebral bodies they have equal anterior and posterior depths (**A**), and the normal lumbar curve is due to wedging of the intervertebral discs.
2. The spinous processes are massive and square (**A**).
3. The intervertebral joints are distinct from those in other regions. The facets on the superior articular processes face backwards and medially and are concave, while those of the inferior processes face forwards and laterally and are convex (**A**).
4. As a result of the orientations of the paired facets at the intervertebral joints, they interlock and almost entirely prevent rotation in the lumbar region. On the other hand flexion and extension are quite free.

The sacrum and coccyx

In the lower part of the vertebral column five originally separate vertebrae fuse at about 20 years to form the single consolidated sacrum of the adult. The fusion process converts the vertebral foramina of the five original vertebrae into a continuous central bony canal called the sacral canal (**C**). The sacrum is concave forwards from above down and approximately triangular in shape. Observe the following features of the bone.

1. On the anterior or pelvic surface (**B**) four transverse ridges indicate the lines along which the bodies of the sacral vertebrae have fused. On either side of these ridges lie four large pelvic sacral foramina.
2. The posterior or dorsal surface (**C**) presents four comparatively small dorsal sacral foramina on either side of the median plane. In the lower part of the surface the posterior wall of the bony sacral canal is deficient and this sacral hiatus is filled in by a fibrous membrane.
3. Openings on each lateral wall of the sacral canal lead into the stems of four T-shaped canals which run through the substance of the sacrum to open at the pelvic and dorsal sacral foramina (**F**). The canals transmit the upper four sacral spinal nerves and the ventral and dorsal rami (**27A**).
4. Around the upper end of the sacral canal the upper surface of the sacrum has features similar to those of a lumbar vertebra and it is joined to the fifth lumbar vertebra by typical lumbar intervertebral joints and ligaments and the lumbosacral intervertebral disc (**C**, **D**). The sharpness of the lumbosacral angle is due to the pronounced wedge shape of the intervertebral disc (**D**). The upper surfaces of the lateral parts of the sacrum (the alae) are smooth (**E**).
5. The upper half or so of each lateral surface of the sacrum carries the auricular articular facet (**G**) which articulates with the hip bone at the sacro-iliac joint. Note the orientation of this ear-shaped facet.
6. The narrower lower end of the sacrum is joined by fibrous tissue to a small number of bony nodules. These are the vestigial coccygeal vertebrae which collectively constitute the coccyx (**C**, **G**).

LUMBAR VERTEBRA: MEDIAN SECTION

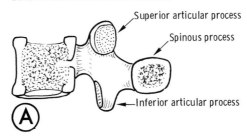

Superior articular process

Spinous process

Inferior articular process

(A)

SACRUM: ANTERIOR ASPECT

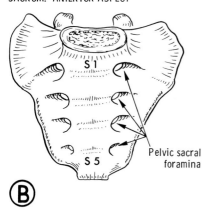

S 1

S 5

Pelvic sacral foramina

(B)

SACRUM: POSTERIOR ASPECT

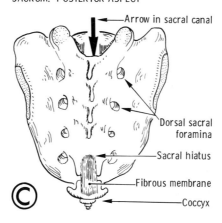

Arrow in sacral canal

Dorsal sacral foramina

Sacral hiatus

Fibrous membrane

Coccyx

(C)

SACRUM: MEDIAN SECTION

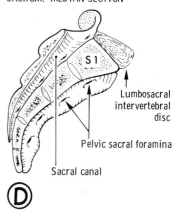

S 1

Lumbosacral intervertebral disc

Pelvic sacral foramina

Sacral canal

(D)

SACRUM:

SUPERIOR ASPECT

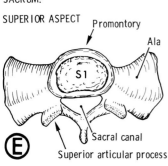

Promontory

Ala

S 1

Sacral canal

Superior articular process

(E)

SACRUM: TRANSVERSE SECTION

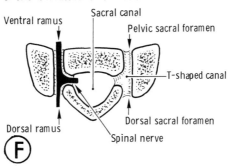

Ventral ramus

Sacral canal

Pelvic sacral foramen

T-shaped canal

Dorsal ramus

Dorsal sacral foramen

Spinal nerve

(F)

SACRUM & COCCYX:
LATERAL ASPECT

Articular facet for hip bone

Coccyx

(G)

Ossification of a typical vertebra

After two months or so of intrauterine life three primary centres of ossification appear in the cartilage model of the vertebra (**A**). Although that in the body is nearly always central, it occasionally forms in the right or left half and produces a half vertebral body (hemivertebra). During the first year the two halves of the vertebral arch unite behind, while at about 4 or 5 years of age the pedicles unite with the vertebral body (**A**).

At puberty the upper and lower surfaces of the vertebral body and the extremities of the transverse processes and the spinous process are still cartilaginous. At about 14 years secondary ossification occurs in these sites (**B**). On the vertebral bodies this process produces upper and lower anular bony epiphyses, surrounding persistent cartilage plates (**B, C**). All secondary centres fuse with the rest of the vertebra in early adult life (**D, E**).

Abnormalities of the vertebral column

1. Variations in the fusion process which normally affects the five sacral segments of the vertebral column may produce either a separate first sacral vertebra (lumbarisation of the first sacral vertebra) or incorporation of the fifth lumbar vertebra in the sacrum (sacralisation of the fifth lumbar vertebra).
2. In spina bifida the two primary centres of ossification in the vertebral arch fail to fuse. The defect usually occurs in the lumbar region. The bony abnormality of itself is of little importance and may indeed be accidentally discovered on radiological examination. Frequently, however, this bony defect is associated with gross abnormalities of the spinal cord, the meninges and the overlying skin which give rise to very serious symptoms and are extremely difficult to treat.
3. Permanent lateral flexion of part of the vertebral column is called scoliosis. It is usually observed in the thoracic region. In the majority of cases the cause is obscure but in a few instances the condition is due to a hemivertebra.
4. Spondylolisthesis is a condition in which there is bilateral discontinuity of the fifth lumbar vertebral arch between the superior and inferior articular process which is probably of developmental origin (**F**). This allows backward displacement of the sacrum and the posterior part of the fifth lumbar vertebral arch on the rest of the vertebral column.

THE SKULL

Parts of the skull

The skull may be divided into three parts (**13A**).

1. The cranium encloses the cranial cavity which contains the brain and its associated membranes and blood vessels. It consists of the vault above and the base below.
2. The facial skeleton, which is stippled in (**13A**), consists of light and irregular bones. It is attached to the antero-inferior aspect of the brain box and 'tied' to its lateral aspects by slender bony bridges called the zygomatic arches. This part contains the paired orbital cavities which are occupied by the eyeballs and their associated structures, and the bony parts of the nasal cavity which open both forwards and backwards. The inferior margins of the maxillae, which are the longest components of the facial skeleton, carry the upper teeth and are often described as the upper jaw.
3. The mandible which carries the lower teeth is the lower jaw. It articulates with the base of the skull by the paired synovial temporomandibular joints and is thus freely movable on the other two parts.

During the first half of life the cranium and facial skeleton consist of a number of separate bones. Some of these are paired while others are single.

OSSIFICATION OF VERTEBRA: Primary centres (black)
Cartilage model (stipple)

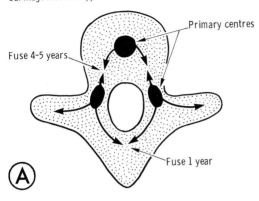

Primary centres

Fuse 4-5 years

Fuse 1 year

A

OSSIFICATION OF VERTEBRA
Secondary centres (black) Appear 14 years, fuse 25 years
Cartilaginous epiphyses (stipple)

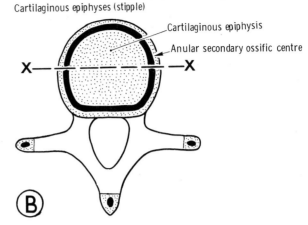

Cartilaginous epiphysis

Anular secondary ossific centre

X———X

B

CORONAL SECTION OF (B) ALONG PLANE X-X

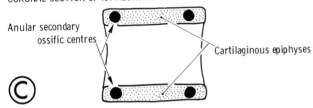

Anular secondary
ossific centres

Cartilaginous epiphyses

C

OSSIFICATION OF VERTEBRA: SECONDARY CENTRES FUSED

Ring of dense bone

Persistent part of cartilaginous epiphysis

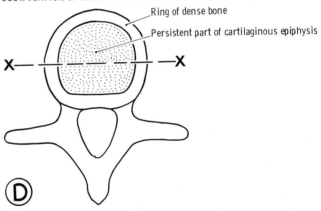

X———X

D

CORONAL SECTION OF (D) ALONG PLANE X-X

Dense bony ring

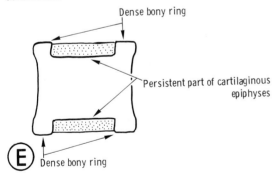

Persistent part of cartilaginous
epiphyses

Dense bony ring

E

SPONDYLOLISTHESIS

Discontinuity of arch→
of L 5

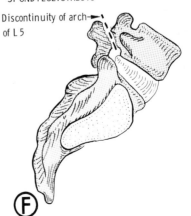

F

Structure of the skull bones

The free surfaces of the skull bones are formed by compact bone. After childhood, in many of the bones the region between the two compact tables is occupied by trabecular bone, which contains bone marrow and is known as the diplœ. In some bones, particularly those of the facial skeleton and the adjacent part of the brain, the interval between the compact tables contains one or more air-containing spaces which communicate with the nasal cavity and are called paranasal air sinuses.

In many situations in the skull, foramina or canals pass through or between the individual bones and allow the passage of vessels and nerves between the various skull compartments (e.g. cranial cavity and orbit), or between one of these compartments and the exterior.

The joints of the skull

Besides the temporomandibular joint already mentioned three other types of joints separate the bones of the skull although none of these persists throughout life.

1. The most common are sutures where the frequently serrated edges, or in some cases the surfaces of adjacent bones, are joined by a narrow zone of fibrous tissue. Beyond the age of about 30 years these joints are progressively obliterated by ossification, the process extending in a centrifugal direction.

2. Two bones in the central part of the base of the cranium (occipital and sphenoid) ossify in the anterior and posterior parts of the same mass of cartilage. Throughout childhood and adolescence the bones remain separated by a transverse strip of radiolucent cartilage constituting a synchondrosis. At about 20 years ossification spreads through the cartilage so that in adults the two bones are directly continuous.

3. At birth the two halves of the mandible are separated in the midline by the symphysis menti which consists of paired cartilage plates united by fibrous tissue. The symphysis is obliterated during the first year of life, but, although the mandible is thereafter a single bone, its median part traditionally retains its original name.

THE CRANIUM

The rest of this section will deal with the form of the cranium and certain additional features which are relevant to that part. Detailed consideration of the facial skeleton and the mandible will be postponed until the sections dealing with the orbit, nose and mouth.

Although detailed knowledge of the individual cranial bones is not in itself of great importance, it is helpful to observe some of their features and relationships at this stage.

The sphenoid (**B, C**) is a single bone which extends across the base of the brain box from one side to the other and contributes to the posterior part of the facial skeleton. In the adult, as has been noted, it is in bony continuity behind with the occipital bone. The sphenoid consists of the following parts.

1. The central part called the body exhibits many features on its upper surface which will be described later.

2. On both sides slender lesser wings and more massive greater wings extend laterally from the upper and lower parts of the body respectively. The greater wing has lateral and inferior surfaces (**B**), an orbital surface (**B**) which faces into the orbit and an intracranial surface (**C**) which faces into the cranial cavity. The medial end of the lesser wing projects backwards and a little medially as the anterior clinoid process.

3. On either side the border of the greater wing between its orbital and intracranial surfaces is separated from the under surface of the lesser wing by a pear-shaped gap called the superior orbital fissure.

4. On both sides a narrow medial pterygoid plate and a broader lateral pterygoid plate descend from the junction between the body and greater wing. Each pair of plates diverges posteriorly (**C**) but their anterior margins are fused to form a coronal surface of appreciable width (**B**).

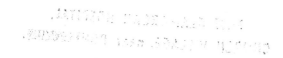

THE MAJOR PARTS OF THE ADULT SKULL

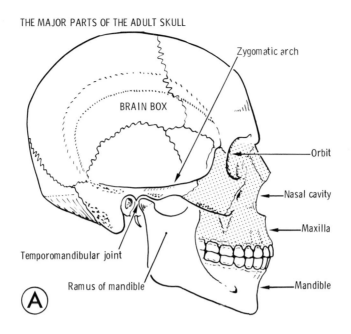

Zygomatic arch

BRAIN BOX

Orbit

Nasal cavity

Maxilla

Temporomandibular joint

Ramus of mandible

Mandible

Ⓐ

SPHENOID: FROM IN FRONT

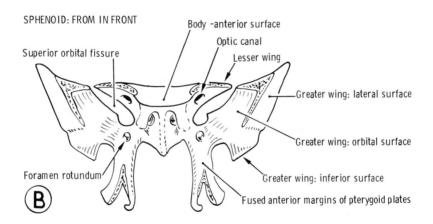

Body -anterior surface

Optic canal

Lesser wing

Superior orbital fissure

Greater wing: lateral surface

Greater wing: orbital surface

Greater wing: inferior surface

Foramen rotundum

Fused anterior margins of pterygoid plates

Ⓑ

SPHENOID: FROM BEHIND

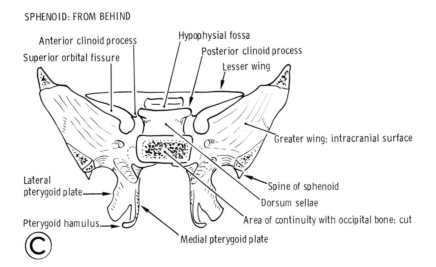

Anterior clinoid process

Hypophysial fossa

Superior orbital fissure

Posterior clinoid process

Lesser wing

Greater wing: intracranial surface

Lateral pterygoid plate

Spine of sphenoid

Dorsum sellae

Pterygoid hamulus

Area of continuity with occipital bone: cut

Medial pterygoid plate

Ⓒ

The single occipital bone forms the postero-inferior aspect of the cranium (**A**). Its major feature is the large foramen magnum through which the brain stem and the spinal cord are continuous. The foramen is used to divide the bone into parts, the squamous part behind, the condylar parts on either side and the basilar part (basi-occiput) in front. In the adult, the basi-occiput is in bony continuity with the basisphenoid; their upper surfaces form the smooth surface known as the clivus.

The single ethmoid forms parts of the walls of the cranial cavity, the nasal cavity and the orbits. It consists of several parts (**B**).

1. The labyrinths, so named because they contain numerous intercommunicating air spaces (paranasal air sinuses), are rectangular and intervene between the orbital and nasal cavities.
2. The upper surfaces of the two labyrinths are joined by paired thin horizontal plates perforated by numerous small foramina and consequently known as the cribriform plates. These separate the upper parts of the nasal cavity from the cranial cavity.
3. From the junction of the two cribriform plates thin bony laminae project upwards and downwards in the median plane. The upper is fancifully named the crista galli while the lower, called the vertical plate, constitutes part of the nasal septum.

The paired maxillae are the major components of the facial skeleton (**C**). The bodies are approximately pyramidal and present anterior, posterolateral and superior (orbital) surfaces. These three meet laterally forming a blunt apex which articulates with the zygomatic bone. The base faces medially and downwards into the nasal cavity.

The frontal bone is usually a single entity in the adult. Although the median (metopic) suture, which separates the bone into two symmetrical halves at birth, is usually obliterated by 8 years, it is important to note that it may persist past middle age. The main part of the bone forms the anterior wall of the cranium but from its lower margin two separate thin plates extend backwards, one on either side of the median plane. Observe the relationship of these orbital plates to the ethmoid and the relationship of both to the cranial, orbital and nasal cavities in the coronal section in **E**.

The paired temporal bones form parts of the lateral aspects and the base of the brain box. The right bone is seen from below in **F** and from the lateral side in **17C**. Each temporal bone is developed from four originally separate units, the petromastoid (stippled), the tympanic (hatched), and the squamous and styloid parts (white). The independent origin of these parts is seldom evident in the adult bone, except between the anterior surface of the tympanic part and the squamous part of the mandibular fossa, which are demarcated by the well-marked squamotympanic suture. Note the following features.

1. The mastoid part of the petromastoid component lies posteriorly and exhibits the mastoid process and the occipital groove.
2. The petrous part of the same component extends forwards and medially in the base of the cranium but its blunt apex does not reach the midline. In sagittal section it is triangular with inferior, anterosuperior and posterosuperior surfaces and a superior border.
3. The tympanic part has a gutter-like upper surface which forms the deeply grooved floor of the bony external acoustic meatus, an inferior margin which ensheaths the root of the slender styloid process, and an anterior surface which forms the posterior wall of the mandibular fossa.
4. The squamous part forms the roof and medial wall of the mandibular fossa and the rounded ridge called the articular tubercle which marks the anterior limit of the fossa. It also forms the roof of the external acoustic meatus and extends upwards as a flat sheet in the lateral wall of the cranium.

INNER SURFACE OF OCCIPITAL BONE

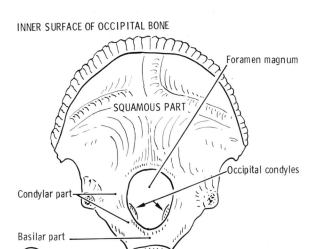

Foramen magnum

SQUAMOUS PART

Occipital condyles

Condylar part

Basilar part

Ⓐ

ETHMOID: FROM BEHIND

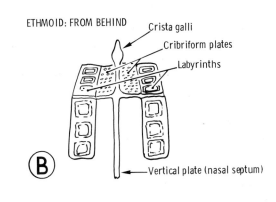

Crista galli

Cribriform plates

Labyrinths

Vertical plate (nasal septum)

Ⓑ

LATERAL VIEW OF RIGHT MAXILLA

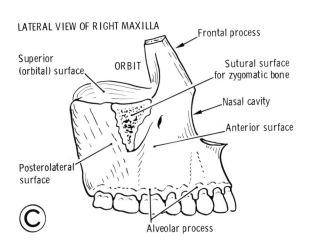

Frontal process

Superior (orbital) surface

ORBIT

Sutural surface for zygomatic bone

Nasal cavity

Anterior surface

Posterolateral surface

Alveolar process

Ⓒ

POSTERIOR VIEW OF FRONTAL BONE

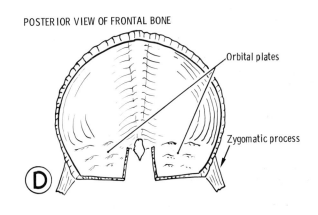

Orbital plates

Zygomatic process

Ⓓ

DIAGRAMMATIC CORONAL SECTION THROUGH CRANIAL CAVITY, ORBITS & NASAL CAVITIES

CRANIAL CAVITY

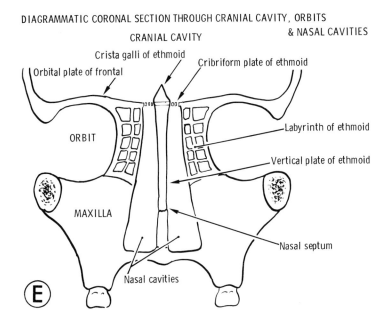

Crista galli of ethmoid

Cribriform plate of ethmoid

Orbital plate of frontal

ORBIT

Labyrinth of ethmoid

Vertical plate of ethmoid

MAXILLA

Nasal septum

Nasal cavities

Ⓔ

INFERIOR VIEW OF RIGHT TEMPORAL BONE

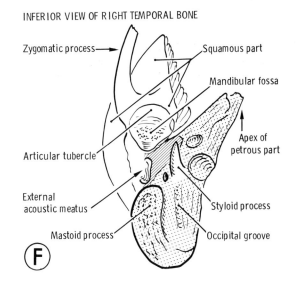

Zygomatic process

Squamous part

Mandibular fossa

Articular tubercle

Apex of petrous part

External acoustic meatus

Styloid process

Mastoid process

Occipital groove

Ⓕ

External surface of cranium

The superior and posterior aspects

These aspects of the cranium (**A, B**) are formed anteriorly by the single frontal bone, posteriorly by the squamous part of the single occipital bone (**15A**), and the mastoid parts of the paired temporal bones (**15F**) and centrally by the paired parietal bones.

Until middle age the two parietals articulate in the median plane at the sagittal suture (**A**). Recall that any vertical plane parallel to this feature is called a sagittal plane. The two parietals articulate anteriorly with the frontal at the coronal suture (**A, C,**). Both limbs of this suture have an anterior inclination as they descend onto the lateral aspect of the cranium (**C**). Consequently, although all vertical planes at right angles to the median plane are traditionally called coronal planes, none of them in fact conforms to the coronal suture unless the head is tilted sharply downwards. Behind, the two parietals articulate with the occipital at the two limbs of the Λ-shaped lambdoid suture (**B**), which extend downwards and forwards to the mastoid part of the temporal bone. The lambdoid suture frequently contains small separate ossicles known as sutural bones (**B**).

The superior nuchal line is a transverse ridge situated about the middle of the squamous part of the occipital (**B**). It demarcates the region of the scalp above from that of the back of the neck below. The external occipital protuberance, which is the prominent central part of the line, is usually palpable.

The mastoid part of the temporal presents two particular features. Below, the mastoid process descends for about 1 cm beyond the rest of the bone and is readily palpable. Behind, the mastoid foramen (**B**) contains a vein which connects the intracranial and extracranial venous systems (emissary vein).

The lateral aspect

Identify the features of the lateral aspect of the cranium labelled in (**C**) and correlate them with the accounts of the superior and posterior aspects of the cranium given in the preceding section and with the accounts of the isolated temporal and sphenoid bones given on the preceding pages.

Consider the following general features.

1. The temporal line arches from before backwards across the frontal, parietal and temporal bones and below becomes continuous with the anterior and posterior ends of the zyomatic arch. The area encicled in this way, and stippled in **C** is the temporal fossa.

2. In the anterior part of the temporal fossa the pterion is a circular area marked by an H-shaped formation of sutures separating four bones. It is sometimes necessary to remove this area of bone to reach an important intracranial artery (**103A**). The centre of the pterion is about 4 cm above the zygomatic arch and rather less behind the frontozygomatic suture, both of which are palpable landmarks.

3. The region below the level of the zygomatic arch and deep to the ramus of the mandible (**13A**) is the infratemporal fossa. Note the lateral pterygoid plate of the sphenoid (**13C**), the posterior surface of the maxilla (**15C**) and the pterygopalatine fossa extending medially between these parts to the lateral wall of the nose. These features will be considered in detail in the sections on the orbit and nasal cavity.

4. Compare the lateral view of the temporal bone in **C**, where the tympanic part is stippled and the petrous part is obscured, with the inferior aspect of the bone shown in **15F**. The suprameatal triangle marks the bone which forms the lateral wall of the mastoid antrum, a cavity in the temporal bone continuous anteriorly with the cavity of the middle ear. Access to these cavities may be gained by removing the bone in the region of the triangle.

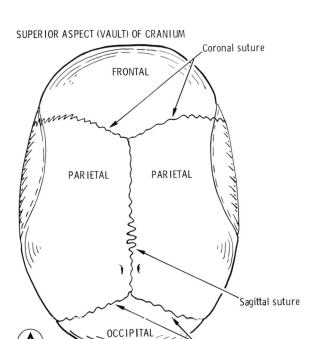

SUPERIOR ASPECT (VAULT) OF CRANIUM

Coronal suture

FRONTAL

PARIETAL   PARIETAL

Sagittal suture

OCCIPITAL

Lambdoid suture

(A)

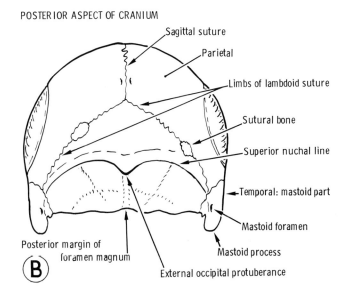

POSTERIOR ASPECT OF CRANIUM

Sagittal suture

Parietal

Limbs of lambdoid suture

Sutural bone

Superior nuchal line

Temporal: mastoid part

Mastoid foramen

Mastoid process

Posterior margin of foramen magnum

External occipital protuberance

(B)

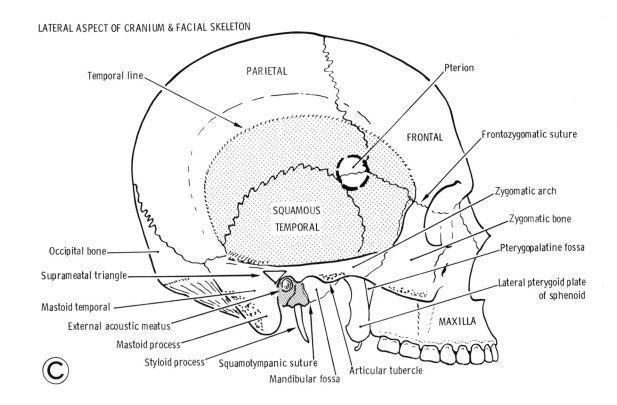

LATERAL ASPECT OF CRANIUM & FACIAL SKELETON

Temporal line

PARIETAL

Pterion

FRONTAL

Frontozygomatic suture

Zygomatic arch

Zygomatic bone

Pterygopalatine fossa

Lateral pterygoid plate of sphenoid

MAXILLA

SQUAMOUS TEMPORAL

Occipital bone

Suprameatal triangle

Mastoid temporal

External acoustic meatus

Mastoid process

Styloid process   Squamotympanic suture

Mandibular fossa

Articular tubercle

(C)

The inferior aspect

In the anterior third or so of **A** the central region is occupied by elements of the facial skeleton. These are shown in this diagram for the sake of completeness and will be considered later in the appropriate sections.

In the rest of the diagram (**A**) recognise the parts of the cranial base formed by the sphenoid, temporal and occipital bones.

1. The inferior surface of the greater wing of the sphenoid forms the greater part of the roof of the infratemporal fossa (**455B, 455D**). Near its medial margin is the foramen ovale and at its posterior corner the foramen spinosum and the small spine of the sphenoid.
2. Behind the greater wing lies the inferior aspect of the temporal bone. Observe the mandibular fossa, the external acoustic meatus, the mastoid process and the opening of the carotid canal. Revise the features which have been described already on the isolated bone (**15F**). Note also the stylomastoid foramen, the distal end of the facial canal which runs a complex course through bone (**409A, 415C**), and the lower opening of the carotid canal which passes first upwards and then forwards and medially to the foramen lacerum (interrupted line).
3. Behind and medial to the temporal bones is the occipital bone. As has been noted this contains the foramen magnum and is descriptively divided into the basilar, condylar and squamous parts (**15A**), the basilar part being in bony continuity with the body of the sphenoid. On either side of the anterior part of the foramen magnum is a cartilage-covered condyle which is convex along its long axis. The base of each condyle is traversed from medial to lateral side by a hypoglossal canal. Note the small pharyngeal tubercle on the basilar part of the bone.

A number of features are related to the sutures between these three bones.

1. Between the body and greater wing of the sphenoid and the apex of the petrous temporal is the foramen lacerum. In the dried skull this is a complete gap in the base of the cranium, with irregular margins of considerable depth. In life the lower half of the foramen is occluded by a plug of fibrocartilage (stippled) and the anterior end of the carotid canal opens into its patent upper half.
2. The adjacent parts of the greater wing of the sphenoid and the petrous temporal are grooved along the line of the intervening suture. In life the groove

lodges the cartilaginous part of the auditory tube. Anteriorly, this tube opens into the pharynx behind the upper part of the posterior margin of the medial pterygoid plate. Posteriorly, its lumen is in continuity through the bony part of the tube with the cavity of the middle ear .

3. The large jugular foramen interrupts the suture line between the condylar part of the occipital and the petrous part of the temporal. Anteriorly, it is separated from the opening of the carotid canal by a narrow transverse ridge of bone. Medially, it is closely related to the lateral end of the hypoglossal canal.

The atlanto-occipital joints

This is a convenient point at which to describe the paired synovial atlanto-occipital joints between the cranial base, which has been described on this page (**A**), and the atlas vertebra, which should be revised (**7C, 7D**).

At each joint the sagittally convex facet on the occipital condyle articulates with the sagittally concave facet on the upper surface of the lateral mass of the atlas, and the joint cavity is enclosed by a fibrous capsule attached close to both articular margins (**B, C**). The joints necessarily move simultaneously around a transverse axis through the condyles, allowing flexion and extension (nodding) of the head on the vertebral column. The joints are associated with three unpaired accessory ligaments.

The posterior atlanto-occipital membrane (**B**) fills the gap between the posterior margin of the foramen magnum, the posterior arch of the atlas and the capsules of the atlanto-occipital joints (**B**), and thus forms the uppermost part of the posterior wall of the vertebral canal. On either side it has a short, free margin which arches between the lateral mass and the posterior arch of the atlas. These three structures bound a triangular gap in the lateral wall of the vertebral canal which gives passage to the vertebral vessels and the first cervical spinal nerve.

The anterior atlanto-occipital membrane (**B**) is an upward continuation of the anterior longitudinal ligament which fills the interval between the anterior arch of the atlas, the capsules of the atlanto-occipital joints and the anterior margin of the foramen magnum.

The membrana tectoria is a broad strap-like band which lines the uppermost part of the anterior wall of the vertebral canal (**C**). It is continuous below with the posterior longitudinal ligament and ascends behind the body and dens of the axis and the transverse ligament of the atlas to be attached to the anterior margin of the foramen magnum.

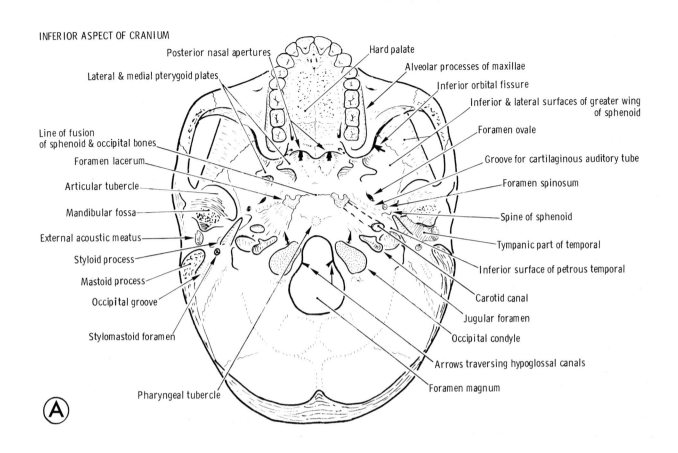

INFERIOR ASPECT OF CRANIUM

Posterior nasal apertures — Hard palate

Lateral & medial pterygoid plates — Alveolar processes of maxillae

Inferior orbital fissure

Inferior & lateral surfaces of greater wing of sphenoid

Line of fusion of sphenoid & occipital bones — Foramen ovale

Foramen lacerum — Groove for cartilaginous auditory tube

Articular tubercle — Foramen spinosum

Mandibular fossa — Spine of sphenoid

External acoustic meatus — Tympanic part of temporal

Styloid process — Inferior surface of petrous temporal

Mastoid process — Carotid canal

Occipital groove — Jugular foramen

Stylomastoid foramen — Occipital condyle

Arrows traversing hypoglossal canals

Pharyngeal tubercle — Foramen magnum

(A)

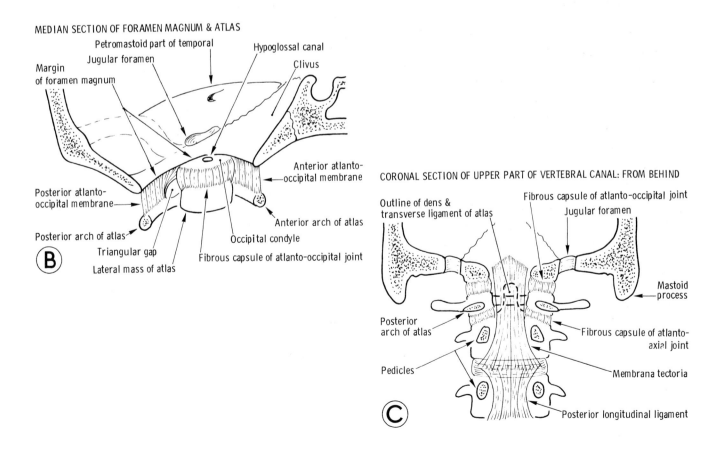

MEDIAN SECTION OF FORAMEN MAGNUM & ATLAS

Petromastoid part of temporal — Hypoglossal canal

Jugular foramen — Clivus

Margin of foramen magnum

Posterior atlanto-occipital membrane — Anterior atlanto-occipital membrane

Posterior arch of atlas — Anterior arch of atlas

Triangular gap — Occipital condyle

Lateral mass of atlas — Fibrous capsule of atlanto-occipital joint

(B)

CORONAL SECTION OF UPPER PART OF VERTEBRAL CANAL: FROM BEHIND

Outline of dens & transverse ligament of atlas — Fibrous capsule of atlanto-occipital joint

Jugular foramen

Mastoid process

Posterior arch of atlas — Fibrous capsule of atlanto-axial joint

Pedicles — Membrana tectoria

Posterior longitudinal ligament

(C)

The interior of the cranial cavity

The cranial base

Before considering the divisions of this region it is convenient to consider the shape of the upper surface of the body of the sphenoid (**A**).

1. Behind the flat anterior part of the surface it is crossed from side to side by the optic groove (sulcus chiasmatis). The ends of the groove lead into the optic canals, each of which passes through the root of the corresponding lesser wing of the sphenoid into the orbital cavity.
2. Immediately behind the posterior lip of the optic groove is the hypophysial fossa which is deeply concave sagittally.
3. Posteriorly the surface projects sharply upwards as the dorsum sellae which forms the posterior wall of the hypophysial fossa and exhibits a small posterior clinoid process at each end of its upper margin.
4. From the gently concave floor of the hypophysial fossa the surface slopes downwards and laterally on both sides to the levels of the greater wings of the sphenoid.

Examine the profiles of the upper surface of the body of the sphenoid in a median section (**B**) and in a coronal section through the floor of the hypophysial fossa (**C**). Because of the fanciful resemblance of the shape of the surface to that of a Turkish saddle it is often named as a whole the sella turcica.

The floor of the cranial cavity invites division into three parts called the anterior, middle and posterior cranial fossae (**A**).

The anterior cranial fossa

The anterior and lateral walls of this region are formed by the frontal bone. Its floor has the following components.

1. The paired orbital plates of the frontal which separate the fossa from the orbital cavities and the labyrinths of the ethmoid (**15B, 15D**).
2. The paired cribriform plates of the ethmoid lie between the orbital plates of the frontal and their numerous foramina lead from the fossa into the nasal cavity. From the junction between the two plates, the crista galli of the ethmoid projects upwards for about 1 cm in the median plane.
3. Behind these elements lie the body of the sphenoid as far back as the anterior lip of the optic groove and the anterior margin of the optic canal, and the lesser wing with its anterior clinoid process.

The middle cranial fossa

The central part of the fossa is formed by the upper surface of the body of the sphenoid from the anterior lip of the optic groove to the upper edge of the dorsum sellae (see above) and thus includes the openings of the optic canals.

On either side the fossa exhibits a wider and deeper lateral compartment. It extends from the posterior margin of the lesser wing of the sphenoid, including its anterior clinoid process, in front, to the superior margin of the petrous part of the temporal bone behind. In its floor note the intracranial surface of the greater wing of the sphenoid anteriorly, the anterosuperior surface of the petrous temporal posteriorly and the squamous part of the temporal laterally. Each lateral compartment presents a number of important foramina.

1. The pear shaped superior orbital fissure leads into the orbit between the greater and lesser wings of the sphenoid. It is obscured by the lesser wing in **A** but has already been visualised in the posterior view of the isolated sphenoid in **13B, 13C**.
2. Behind and below the wide medial part of the superior orbital fissure, the foramen rotundum leads downwards and forwards through the greater wing and the roots of the pterygoid plates (**13B**) into the upper part of the pterygopalatine fossa (**17C**).
3. Behind and lateral to the foramen rotundum, the foramen ovale leads downwards through the greater wing of the sphenoid into the infratemporal fossa (**19A**).
4. Posterolateral to the foramen ovale, in the posterior corner of the greater wing of the sphenoid, the small foramen spinosum leads downwards into the infratemporal fossa (**19A**). From the foramen, a bony groove passes forwards, laterally and upwards, and divides into anterior and posterior divisions. As the anterior ascends it passes deep to the pterion (**17C**) and in this region is frequently converted into a bony canal for a short distance.
5. Medial to the last two foramina the large foramen lacerum is situated between the body and greater wing of the sphenoid and the apex of the petrous temporal. As has been noted the lower half of the foramen is occluded in life by fibrocartilage and the horizontal part of the carotid canal opens into its upper half through its posterolateral wall. The bony roof of the terminal part of the carotid canal is very thin and is sometimes deficient.
6. About the middle of the anterosuperior surface of the petrous temporal are two minute foramina through which petrosal branches from the facial nerve emerge into the cranial cavity.

FLOOR OF CRANIAL CAVITY (dotted lines demarcate cranial fossae)

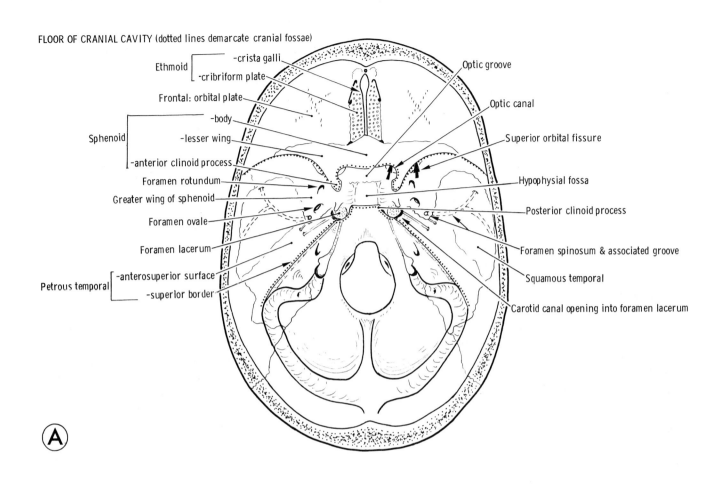

Ethmoid
- crista galli
- cribriform plate

Frontal: orbital plate

Sphenoid
- body
- lesser wing
- anterior clinoid process

Foramen rotundum

Greater wing of sphenoid

Foramen ovale

Foramen lacerum

Petrous temporal
- anterosuperior surface
- superior border

Optic groove

Optic canal

Superior orbital fissure

Hypophysial fossa

Posterior clinoid process

Foramen spinosum & associated groove

Squamous temporal

Carotid canal opening into foramen lacerum

(A)

PROFILE OF SELLA TURCICA IN MEDIAN PLANE

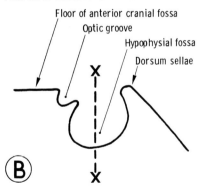

Floor of anterior cranial fossa

Optic groove

Hypophysial fossa

Dorsum sellae

X

X

(B)

PROFILE OF SELLA TURCICA ALONG CORONAL PLANE X-X IN (B)

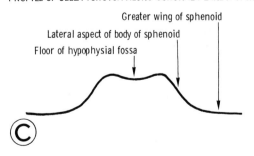

Greater wing of sphenoid

Lateral aspect of body of sphenoid

Floor of hypophysial fossa

(C)

The posterior cranial fossa

This is limited anteriorly by the superior margins of the petrous parts of the temporal bones and the superior edge of the dorsum sellae (**A**). In its deepest part is the foramen magnum through which the medial aspects of the occipital condyles are just visible. The smooth surface which slopes upwards and forwards from the foramen to the upper edge of the dorsum sellae is called the clivus. The median prominence above and behind the foramen is the internal occipital protuberance.

Recognise the parts of the fossa which are formed by the basilar, condylar and squamous parts of the occipital bone and the petrous and mastoid parts of the temporal bones. Observe on both sides of the midline the following features.

1. The orifice of the hypoglossal canal on the medial aspect of the occipital condyle.
2. The large jugular foramen which is situated between the petrous temporal and the occipital bone anterolateral to the occipital condyle.
3. The paired transverse sulci are bony grooves which begin on either side of the internal occipital protuberance. Each runs laterally and then forwards on to the upper part of the mastoid temporal. There it deepens and widens and, becoming known as the sigmoid sulcus, winds downwards along an S-shaped course to the posterior margin of the jugular foramen. The mastoid emissary foramen (**17B**) opens through the floor of the sigmoid part of the sulcus.
4. The internal acoustic meatus is a bony canal which runs laterally for about 1 cm in the substance of the petrous temporal. Its orifice is on the posterosuperior surface of that bone above and in front of the jugular foramen, while its lateral end lies close to the medial aspect of the internal ear.

The cranial vault

The vault as has been seen on the external aspect of the cranium (**17A**), is formed by the frontal, parietal and occipital bones joined at the coronal, sagittal and lambdoid sutures.

It is marked by numerous narrow grooves (**B**) which run towards the midline and stem below from the single groove which begins at the foramen spinosum in the cranial base (**21A**).

The sagittal sulcus is a shallow midline groove which begins just above the crista galli and widens as it is traced backwards. In the majority of individuals it becomes continuous behind with the transverse sulcus of the right side while in the rest of the population it joins that of the left side. The sagittal sulcus expands laterally in a number of situations and in these expansions, at some distance from the median plane, there are variable numbers of sharply outlined pits which usually become wider and deeper with increasing age.

Age changes in the cranial vault

The bones of the vault develop by intramembranous ossification in a dome-like fibrous sheet. At birth this process is incomplete so that the sagittal, coronal, lambdoid and metopic (**15D**) sutures are comparatively wide zones of fibrous tissue and their bony margins show no sign of the interdigitating processes characteristic of definitive sutures. At this time the sagittal, coronal and metopic sutures meet at a diamond-shaped fibrous region measuring 4 cm anteroposteriorly and 2.5 cm transversely and called the anterior fontanelle: the sagittal and lambdoid sutures meet at the appreciably smaller triangular posterior fontanelle (**C**). These features allow an appreciable degree of moulding of the cranium during birth of the child.

Both fontanelles can be palpated as soft areas in the otherwise bony cranial vault. The determination of their positions by vaginal examination during birth by vertex presentation (head first) indicates the orientation of the foetal head in relation to the maternal pelvis.

During the first two years after birth the bones of the vault grow mainly by accretion at their margins so that the sutures become narrower and their margins interlock. As part of this process the fontanelles become smaller, the posterior disappearing at 3 months and the anterior at about 18 months. Between the second and eighth year growth of the bones continues mainly by accretion on their outer surfaces and erosion on their inner surfaces. After that period there is little further growth of the vault and the metopic suture is quickly obliterated by ossification. The other sutures are more slowly obliterated from within outwards in middle adult life.

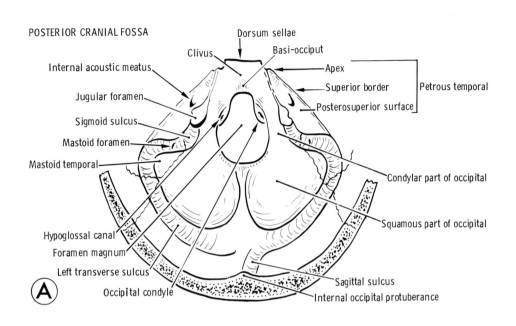

POSTERIOR CRANIAL FOSSA

Dorsum sellae
Clivus
Basi-occiput
Internal acoustic meatus
Apex
Jugular foramen
Superior border
Petrous temporal
Sigmoid sulcus
Posterosuperior surface
Mastoid foramen
Mastoid temporal
Condylar part of occipital
Squamous part of occipital
Hypoglossal canal
Foramen magnum
Left transverse sulcus
Sagittal sulcus
Occipital condyle
Internal occipital protuberance

(A)

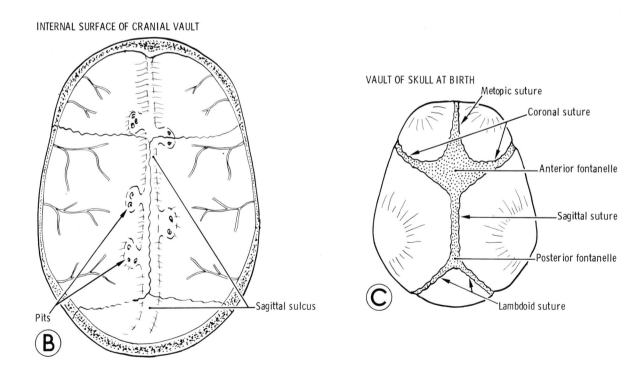

INTERNAL SURFACE OF CRANIAL VAULT

Sagittal sulcus

Pits

(B)

VAULT OF SKULL AT BIRTH

Metopic suture
Coronal suture
Anterior fontanelle
Sagittal suture
Posterior fontanelle
Lambdoid suture

(C)

CHAPTER 2

The nervous system

INTRODUCTION

Nervous tissue consists of two broad groups of cells. One group comprises the nerve cells or neurons, each of which consists of a cell body containing the nucleus and a variable number of slender processes which have the property of conducting an electrical impulse longitudinally. The other group consists of non-conducting supporting cells of various types which are known as neuroglial cells.

Divisions of the nervous system

The central nervous system consists of the brain, which lies in the cranial cavity, and the spinal cord which is contained within the vertebral canal (**A**). Both parts develop as a hollow tube, and although many elaborate changes in structure and shape subsequently occur, this hollow form persists throughout life. In the fully developed brain and spinal cord the lumen is lined by a layer of a particular kind of neuroglial cells, the ependyma, and varies greatly in diameter in different regions. In some, the lumen remains narrow and its ependymal lining is completely separated from the external surface of the part by nervous tissue (**B**). In other regions the lumen forms cavities of considerable size known as ventricles, and in such situations one part of the ventricular wall is very thin and consists only of the lining ependymal layer (**C**).

The brain and spinal cord are encapsulated and separated from their bony confines by three connective tissue layers called, from within outwards, the pia mater, the arachnoid mater and the dura mater. Between the inner two is the extensive trabeculated subarachnoid space (**B, C**).

The thin vascular pia mater is in immediate contact with the whole external surface of the central nervous system and it is evident that wherever the wall of a ventricle consists only of ependymal cells, those cells will be in immediate contact with pia mater (**C**).

In such regions of ependymal/pial contact, two particular arrangements of the twin tissue layers may occur.

1. The two layers may be invaginated into the ventricular cavity as a linear vascular fringe (**D**) known as a choroid plexus. The ependymal cells of such fringes continuously secrete a watery liquid called cerebrospinal fluid which completely fills the lumen of the central nervous system.
2. In other regions apertures interrupt the continuity of the two tissue layers and allow the escape of the continually produced cerebrospinal fluid from the lumen of the central nervous system into the subarachnoid space. The fluid is continually

transferred from that space to the venous blood stream by a mechanism described later (**105C**).

The peripheral nervous system consists essentially of neurons bound together by connective tissue into bundles known as nerves, which establish motor (efferent) and sensory (afferent) connections between the central nervous system and the other tissues of the body.

All functional classifications of these peripheral neurons are unsatisfactory in some respects, but it is nevertheless convenient to have some kind of nomenclature.

1. Special sensory neurons transmit certain unique sensations, vision, hearing, equilibration, olfaction and taste from highly specialised sensory receptors located in particular structures or regions.
2. Somatic sensory neurons carry information concerning the external environment (exteroceptive) from skin and some areas of mucous membrane, and information concerning the mechanical state of skeletal muscle and joints (proprioceptive).
3. Visceral sensory neurons transmit information from viscera and blood vessels which in most instances indicates the degree of distension of the structure or the tensile stress in its wall (interoceptive).
4. Somatic motor and branchial motor neurons innervate skeletal muscle developed from somites and branchial mesoderm respectively.
5. Visceral motor neurons control the activities of smooth and cardiac muscle and the secretory activities of exocrine glands. Since they are not under conscious control they are described collectively as the autonomic nervous system, but they may be distinguished as sympathetic and parasympathetic according to their different sites of connection with the central nervous system and their distinct peripheral effects.

All these peripheral neurons enter or leave the central nervous system through the spinal or cranial nerves.

Each of the series of 31 pairs of spinal nerves is attached to the spinal cord by a motor ventral root and a sensory dorsal root on which there is an ovoid swelling called a spinal ganglion (**A**). The roots unite just before they emerge through the appropriate intervertebral foramen as a definitive spinal nerve which thereafter divides into a ventral and a dorsal ramus.

Twelve pairs of cranial nerves are attached to the brain close to the midline and are numbered in craniocaudal order. A few of these are labelled in (**A**). Some exhibit one or two ganglia (**A**) which are similar in appearance and function to the spinal ganglia.

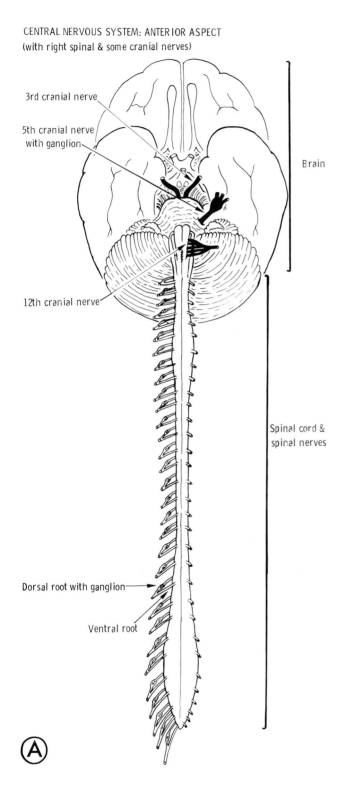

CENTRAL NERVOUS SYSTEM: ANTERIOR ASPECT
(with right spinal & some cranial nerves)

3rd cranial nerve

5th cranial nerve
with ganglion

Brain

12th cranial nerve

Spinal cord &
spinal nerves

Dorsal root with ganglion

Ventral root

(A)

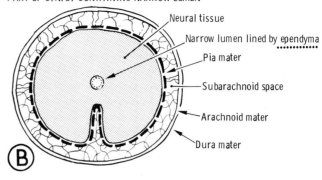

PART OF C.N.S. CONTAINING NARROW LUMEN

Neural tissue

Narrow lumen lined by ependyma ••••••••••••

Pia mater

Subarachnoid space

Arachnoid mater

Dura mater

(B)

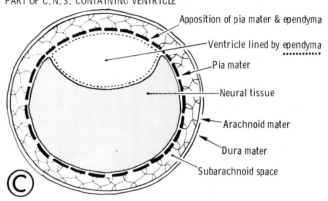

PART OF C.N.S. CONTAINING VENTRICLE

Apposition of pia mater & ependyma

Ventricle lined by ependyma ••••••••••

Pia mater

Neural tissue

Arachnoid mater

Dura mater

Subarachnoid space

(C)

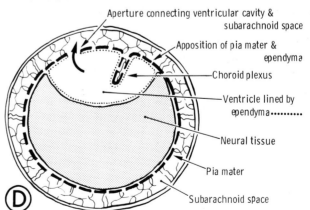

PART OF C.N.S. CONTAINING VENTRICLE

Aperture connecting ventricular cavity &
subarachnoid space

Apposition of pia mater &
ependyma

Choroid plexus

Ventricle lined by
ependyma ••••••••••

Neural tissue

Pia mater

Subarachnoid space

(D)

Special and somatic sensory, and somatic and branchial motor neurons run their whole courses in the peripheral nervous system within spinal or cranial nerves. On the other hand, although visceral sensory, sympathetic and parasympathetic neurons enter or leave the central nervous system through spinal or cranial nerves, the more peripheral parts of their courses lie in varying degree in distinct visceral pathways. Placed along these pathways are autonomic ganglia which will be seen later to be functionally distinct from spinal ganglia and the ganglia on the trunks of cranial nerves (**A, B**).

Features of neurons

Morphology

Neuron processes are of two types according to the direction in which they normally conduct electrical impulses. Those which conduct impulses towards, though not necessarily to, the cell body are designated as dendrites. They may be single or multiple and branched. On the other hand, impulses are always carried in a direction away from the cell body by a single process which is called an axon (**C, D**).

There are a number of distinct morphological types of neurons.

1. Some of the sensory neurons concerned with the transmission of special senses (apart from taste) to the central nervous system exhibit a single dendrite and a single axon arising from the opposite extremities of the cell body, and are consequently described as bipolar (**C**).

2. Multipolar neurons are by far the most common type in the brain and spinal cord and form a large component of the peripheral nervous system (**D**). Numerous branching dendrites arise directly from the cell body, and being short, tend to be confined to the region immediately around it. In contrast, the axon always arises as a single process from the cell body and is often comparatively very long, reaching in some instances a length of several feet. It gives off a series of orthogonal collateral branches along its length and finally divides into a number of comparatively short terminal branches.

3. The neurons which convey all sensations except those of smell, vision, hearing and equilibration (**26**) through the peripheral nervous system and for variable distances into the spinal cord and brain are called pseudo-unipolar (**E**). A single axon and a single dendrite are in structural and functional continuity. The point of continuity between axon and dendrite is joined by a single stem of variable length to a cell body which thus lies off the impulse-conducting channel of the neuron. Both axon and dendrite tend to branch near their terminations. The terminal branches of the dendrite may end freely in the tissue they serve, or they may end within specialised and often elaborate receptor organs which respond only to one specific type of stimulus.

EXAMPLE OF SYMPATHETIC PATHWAY
(indicated by arrows)

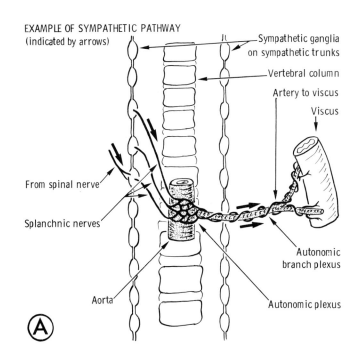

Sympathetic ganglia
on sympathetic trunks

Vertebral column

Artery to viscus

Viscus

From spinal nerve

Splanchnic nerves

Autonomic
branch plexus

Aorta

Autonomic plexus

Ⓐ

EXAMPLE OF PARASYMPATHETIC PATHWAY
(indicated by arrows)

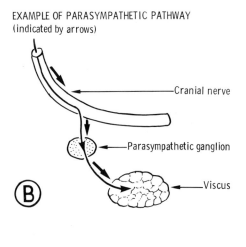

Cranial nerve

Parasympathetic ganglion

Viscus

Ⓑ

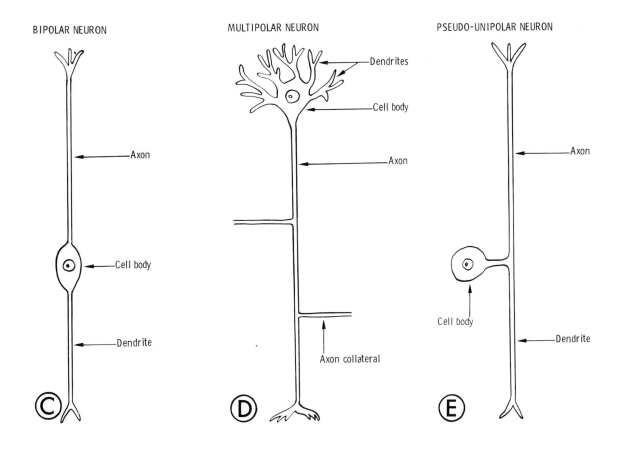

BIPOLAR NEURON

Axon

Cell body

Dendrite

Ⓒ

MULTIPOLAR NEURON

Dendrites

Cell body

Axon

Axon collateral

Ⓓ

PSEUDO-UNIPOLAR NEURON

Axon

Cell body

Dendrite

Ⓔ

Sheath cells of neuronal processes

The axons of all multipolar neurons and the continuous axon-dendrites of pseudo-unipolar neurons are ensheathed by special non-neuronal cells in all parts of the nervous system. These are neuroglial oligodendrocytes in the brain and spinal cord and the rather similar Schwann cells in the peripheral parts of the nervous system (**A, B**). These cells are disposed in longitudinal series along the neuron processes, which invaginate their cell membranes. One or more neuron process may be invaginated into each cell (**C**).

The cellular sheaths so formed may extend almost to the ends of the terminal branches of the neuron processes or stop a short distance from these ends, leaving terminal neuron segments of rather variable length bare of a specialised covering (**A, B**). Alternatively the neuron process may become evaginated out of the related Schwann cell or oligodendrocyte so that the terminal segment of the process is still related to one of these cells on one of its aspects but is bare on the opposite aspect.

Myelination of neurons

In some instances the invagination described above of neuron processes into Schwann cells or oligodendrocytes is simple and direct (**C**). In others the arrangement is considerably more complex so that the invaginated process becomes ensheathed by a variable number of directly apposed layers of plasma membrane. The mechanism presumably involves relative rotation of neuron and invaginated cell, but the details of the process are still obscure (**D**). Such an investment of multiple layers of plasma membranes is called a myelin or medullary sheath. A neuron process so invested has a bright white colour and is said to be myelinated. Processes which are simply invaginated without the formation of a myelin sheath are greyish in colour and are said to be unmyelinated (**C**). Generally a myelin sheath does not extend quite so close to the termination of the related neuron process as the Schwann cells or oligodendrocytes so that frequently a short unmyelinated segment intervenes between a myelinated neuron process and its bare extremity.

The occurrence and size of a myelin sheath is closely related to the size of the neuron process concerned and to the rate of conduction of impulses along it. Processes of large diameter are heavily myelinated and conduct impulses at rates of up to 100 m/sec, whereas narrower processes are usually unmyelinated and conduct at much slower rates of the order of 1 m/sec.

The process of myelination does not proceed simultaneously in all parts of the nervous system. It begins rather late in foetal development, at about the fourth month, and is not complete until some time after birth.

Synapses

All nerve pathways, carrying information either between different parts of the brain and spinal cord or between these parts and the tissues of the body, consist of a number of neurons arranged in series. The junctional complex by which an impulse passing along the axon of one neuron is able to influence activity in the next neuron in the chain is called a synapse. Usually such complexes are situated between the bare termination of the branch of an axon, and a dendrite or cell body of a multipolar neuron (**E**). Synapsing neurons are completely separated by a synaptic cleft of about 20 nm and the adjacent plasma membranes are thickened (**E**). The neighbouring cytoplasm stains densely and on the presynaptic side contains numerous vesicles.

Synapses always operate unidirectionally. The arrival of an impulse at a presynaptic axon terminal causes the release of one of a number of chemical substances from the synaptic vesicles into the synaptic cleft, which influences the plasma membrane of the postsynaptic neuron. It is known that acetylcholine, noradrenaline and dopamine act as such chemical neurotransmitters at some synapses, and there is evidence that other substances including a number of simple amino-acids act in the same way at others.

The influence which an impulse in a presynaptic axon may exert on a postsynaptic neuron may be of two kinds. On the one hand it may hyperpolarise the postsynaptic neuron and thus inhibit its firing, or it may cause depolarisation of the neuron and facilitate or excite firing.

It is important to note that in most instances the cell body and dendrites of one multipolar neuron are in synaptic relationship with hundreds or thousands of axon terminals, though usually by no means all the axons are operative at any one time. Some of these very numerous synapses may exert excitatory and others inhibitory influences upon the neuron. The actual effect upon the neuron at any one time may be regarded as the algebraic sum of the excitatory and inhibitory trans-synaptic influences which are brought to bear on it at that time.

It should be noted that the connections between the axons of motor neurons and muscle and those between some sensory dendrites and epithelial receptor cells are of a similar general nature to synapses, and operate in the same general way by the liberation of chemical transmitter substances. Although most of such junctions are excitatory, some associated with involuntary muscle may be inhibitory.

MULTIPOLAR NEURON

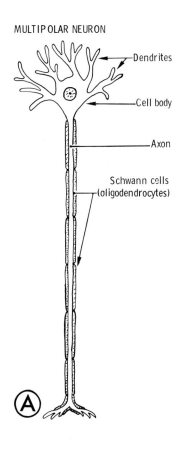

- Dendrites
- Cell body
- Axon
- Schwann cells (oligodendrocytes)

Ⓐ

PSEUDO-UNIPOLAR NEURON

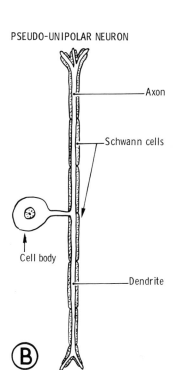

- Axon
- Schwann cells
- Cell body
- Dendrite

Ⓑ

SIMPLE INVAGINATION OF AXONS INTO SCHWANN CELLS OR OLIGODENDROCYTES
(unmyelinated fibre)

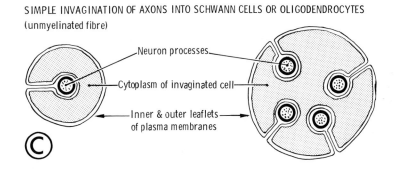

- Neuron processes
- Cytoplasm of invaginated cell
- Inner & outer leaflets of plasma membranes

Ⓒ

FORMATION OF MYELIN SHEATH (myelinated fibre)

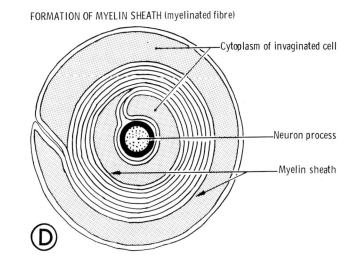

- Cytoplasm of invaginated cell
- Neuron process
- Myelin sheath

Ⓓ

STRUCTURE OF SYNAPSE

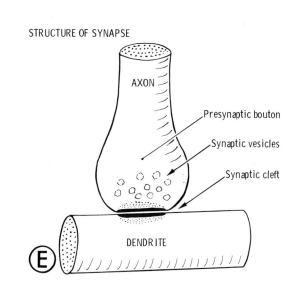

- AXON
- Presynaptic bouton
- Synaptic vesicles
- Synaptic cleft
- DENDRITE

Ⓔ

The siting of neuron bodies and synapses

In the central nervous system both the brain and the spinal cord consist of two tissues of distinct macroscopic appearances which are usually sharply demarcated from one another. One is pinkish grey in colour and is called grey matter whereas the other is white and is consequently called white matter. In some situations the grey matter forms continous longitudinal columns or isolated masses known as nuclei within surrounding white matter, while over the cerebral hemispheres and the cerebellum it forms a continuous surface layer enclosing central white matter.

These regions of grey matter contain all the neuron cell bodies and dendrites and consequently all the synapses in the central nervous system. The white matter contains the axons which arise from the neuron cell bodies in the grey matter, and also axons which have originated from neuron cell bodies in the peripheral nervous system (see below). Some of these axons are myelinated and others un-myelinated but the white colour of the myelinated axons is dominant. In the white matter it is usual for axons of like function to form compact tracts.

As has been seen, functional pathways in the central nervous system are formed by chains of several individual neurons linked by synapses. The general relationship of such a pathway to grey and white matter is shown very diagrammatically in **A**.

In the peripheral nervous system neurons of different functions are disposed in different fashions.

Excepting for future consideration the special senses, all other sensory impulses, whether they are derived from somatic tissues such as skin, or visceral tissues such as the intestine, are transmitted to the central nervous system along pathways which consist of only one neuron (**B**). These neurons are all of the pseudo-unipolar type but may be myelinated or unmyelinated. Irrespective of their association with somatic or visceral tissues, the cell bodies of these neurons are always situated outside the central nervous system, either in the spinal ganglia on the dorsal roots of spinal nerves or in the similar ganglia which lie on some cranial nerves.

Impulses concerned with the innervation of voluntary muscles are transmitted from the central nervous system to the muscles along one-neuron pathways (**C**). Two groups of neurons are involved, the alpha neurons which innervate the general muscle fibres and the gamma neurons which innervate the intrafusal muscle fibres of neuromuscular spindles. However, all are multipolar and myelinated. Their cell bodies lie in the grey nuclei or columns of the brain or spinal cord, but their axons quickly leave this region and run the rest of their course in the spinal or cranial nerves.

As has been seen (**26**) the autonomic system consists of those components of the nervous system which, together with other factors, control the activities of many exocrine glands and influence the strength and frequency of contraction of involuntary muscle. Both sympathetic and parasympathetic pathways in the autonomic system differ from other pathways in the peripheral nervous system in consisting of two neurons functionally linked by a synapse (**D**).

The first or preganglionic neuron is multipolar and its axon myelinated. Its cell body is in grey columns or nuclei in the spinal cord or brain stem, and its axon leaves these parts in a spinal or cranial nerve. Subsequently, the axon leaves this nerve and continues its course along a visceral nerve pathway. It synapses in an autonomic ganglion or in the wall of a viscus with the second or postganglionic neuron, which is also multipolar but unmyelinated, and which runs to the tissue to be innervated (**D**).

It is worth summarising the following features.

1. The cell bodies of both alpha and gamma somatic motor neurons and the cell bodies of preganglionic autonomic neurons are always within the central nervous system.
2. The cell bodies of all sensory neurons and postganglionic autonomic neurons are outside the central nervous system.
3. Autonomic ganglia contain synapses whereas the sensory ganglia on cranial nerves and the dorsal roots of spinal nerves do not.

NEURON CHAIN IN C.N.S.

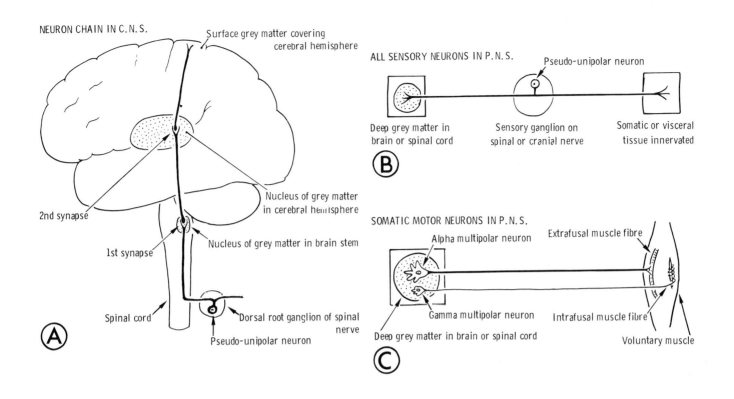

Surface grey matter covering cerebral hemisphere

2nd synapse

Nucleus of grey matter in cerebral hemisphere

1st synapse

Nucleus of grey matter in brain stem

Spinal cord

Dorsal root ganglion of spinal nerve

Pseudo-unipolar neuron

(A)

ALL SENSORY NEURONS IN P.N.S.

Pseudo-unipolar neuron

Deep grey matter in brain or spinal cord

Sensory ganglion on spinal or cranial nerve

Somatic or visceral tissue innervated

(B)

SOMATIC MOTOR NEURONS IN P.N.S.

Alpha multipolar neuron

Extrafusal muscle fibre

Gamma multipolar neuron

Intrafusal muscle fibre

Deep grey matter in brain or spinal cord

Voluntary muscle

(C)

AUTONOMIC PATHWAYS IN P.N.S.

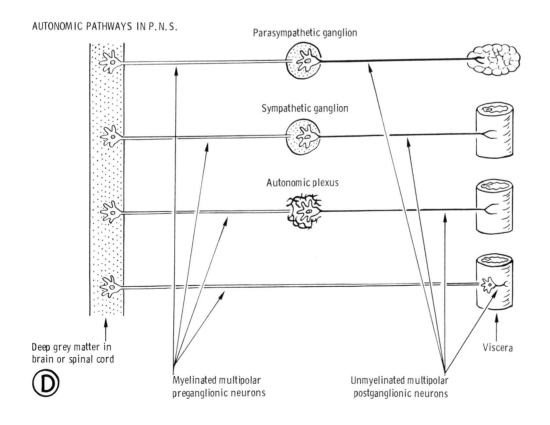

Parasympathetic ganglion

Sympathetic ganglion

Autonomic plexus

Deep grey matter in brain or spinal cord

(D)

Myelinated multipolar preganglionic neurons

Unmyelinated multipolar postganglionic neurons

Viscera

GENERAL FEATURES OF THE SPINAL CORD

External features

The spinal cord is continuous above with the medulla oblongata of the brain at the upper border of the atlas vertebra. In early development it extends to the lower end of the vertebral canal, but as prenatal development proceeds it elongates more slowly than the vertebral column, so that at birth its lower end is level with the third lumbar vertebra. The disparity in growth rates is very much less after birth and in the adult the lower end of the cord is at the level of L2 (**A**).

Two regions of the cord which are associated with the innervation of the upper and lower limbs are wider than the rest, particularly in the coronal plane (**A**). The cervical enlargement is situated in the lower half or so of the cervical part of the vertebral canal and the lumbar enlargement in the lower thoracic and upper lumbar part. Below the lumbar enlargement the cord tapers rapidly to a pointed extremity called the conus medullaris (**A**).

The surface of the cord is marked by a number of longitudinal grooves of different depths. Observe in the transverse section in **B** the deep anterior median fissure and the very much shallower posterior median sulcus and posterolateral sulci.

It has already been observed that each spinal nerve is formed by the union of ventral and dorsal roots just before it emerges from the vertebral canal and that a ganglion is present on the dorsal root just short of this union (**27A**).

The ventral and dorsal roots are each formed by the coalescence of a number of rootlets which arise from the lateral aspects of the cord. The dorsal rootlets emerge in line along the posterolateral sulci while the ventral rootlets appear as a more irregular longitudinal series from the anterolateral aspects of the cord (**C**). The length of the cord which gives rise to the rootlets of one pair of spinal nerves is often referred to as a spinal segment, which is numbered according to the nerve attached to it. This is a useful term even though there is no indication of segmentation in the internal structure of the cord.

The 31 pairs of spinal nerves are numbered sequentially from above down according to the primitive body segments with which their somatic fibres are predominantly associated. There are thus eight cervical, twelve thoracic, five lumbar, five sacral and a single coccygeal nerve on either side. It should be noted particularly that the number of cervical nerves is one greater than the number of cervical vertebrae, and that although the coccyx usually consists of a number of primitive vertebrae, there is only one coccygeal nerve. As a result, nerves C1–7 emerge from the vertebral canal above the vertebra of corresponding number, nerve C8 emerges between vertebrae C7 and T1, all the thoracic, lumbar and sacral nerves emerge below the vertebra of corresponding number, and the coccygeal nerve emerges below the first piece of the coccyx (**A**).

There are two consequences of the disparity between the lengths of the spinal cord and the vertebral canal.

From above downwards the successive segments of the cord lie more and more above the level of the numerically corresponding vertebra. Thus, as shown in **A**, the sixth cervical, fourth thoracic, tenth thoracic and twelfth thoracic vertebrae correspond in level with the seventh cervical, sixth thoracic, second lumbar and first sacral segments of the cord.

Because the roots of the spinal nerves always fuse just short of the exits of these nerves from the vertebral canal, the roots become progressively longer and more caudally inclined from above downwards (**A**). The nerve roots which descend for variable distances along the vertebral canal below the level of the conus medullaris constitute the cauda equina.

Groups of nerve rootlets additional to those of the spinal nerves emerge from both sides of the upper part of the cord in longitudinal series, between the dorsal and ventral rootlets of the upper four or five cervical nerves. Turning upwards, these join to form the spinal accessory nerves (**39B**) which pass into the cranial cavity.

Internal features

Although the internal features of the spinal cord are most frequently visualised in transverse sections, it is important to appreciate that many of these features are continuous through the whole length, or a large part of the length, of the cord and must therefore be thought of in a three-dimensional manner.

The posterior median septum, which is a thin lamina of neuroglial cells, the narrow central canal, which forms the caudal part of the lumen of the central nervous system, and the deep anterior median fissure, all extend along the whole length of the cord and almost divide it into symmetrical halves (**B**).

DIAGRAMMATIC REPRESENTATION OF SPINAL CORD, SPINAL
SEGMENTS & INTERVERTEBRAL FORAMINA

(Note for clarity, the spinal nerves are shown by single lines. In fact,
between the cord & the intervertebral foramina, each nerve
consists of separate ventral & dorsal roots)

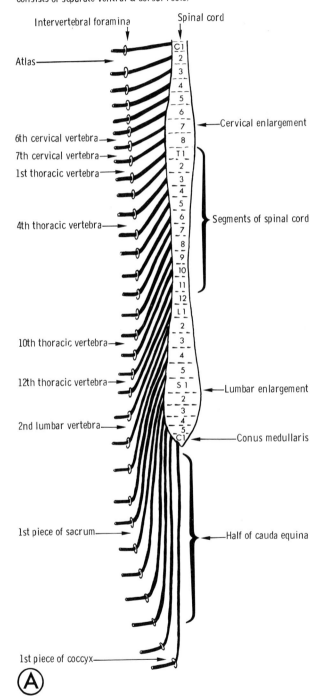

Intervertebral foramina
Spinal cord
Atlas
C1
2
3
4
5
6
7
8
Cervical enlargement
6th cervical vertebra
7th cervical vertebra
1st thoracic vertebra
T1
2
3
4
5
6
7
8
9
10
11
12
Segments of spinal cord
4th thoracic vertebra
L1
2
3
4
5
S1
2
3
4
5
Lumbar enlargement
10th thoracic vertebra
12th thoracic vertebra
2nd lumbar vertebra
C1
Conus medullaris
Half of cauda equina
1st piece of sacrum
1st piece of coccyx

Ⓐ

SPINAL CORD: TRANSVERSE SECTION

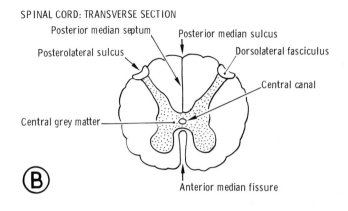

Posterior median septum   Posterior median sulcus
Posterolateral sulcus   Dorsolateral fasciculus
Central canal
Central grey matter
Ⓑ
Anterior median fissure

ATTACHMENT OF SPINAL NERVE TO SPINAL CORD: LATERAL VIEW

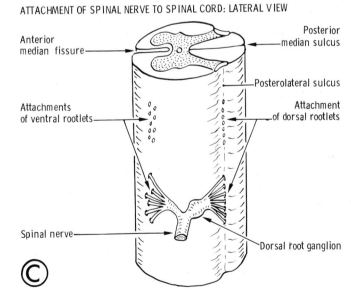

Anterior
median fissure
Posterior
median sulcus
Posterolateral sulcus
Attachments
of ventral rootlets
Attachment
of dorsal rootlets
Spinal nerve
Dorsal root ganglion
Ⓒ

35

The central grey matter is approximately H-shaped in transverse section (**A**). Although its exact shape and size vary at different levels, it is continuous along the length of the cord. The posterior parts of this formation constitute the posterior grey columns. Their posterior edges are narrow and are separated from the posterolateral sulci and the attachments of the posterior rootlets of the spinal nerves only by the slender dorsolateral fasciculus of white matter (**A**). The anterior parts form the anterior grey columns. Their anterolateral aspects are blunt and separated by some distance from the surface of the cord. On either side the anterior and posterior grey columns are joined by a zone known as the intermediate grey matter. From the T1 to the L2 segment of the cord, this tissue projects laterally for a short distance as the lateral grey column (**D**). In other segments of the cord it produces no such projection so that the lateral aspects of the anterior and posterior columns are smoothly continuous. The two intermediate zones of grey matter are joined across the midline by a narrow plate of grey matter which encloses the central canal and is known as the grey commissure (**A**).

All parts of the central grey matter contain large numbers of interneurons but different regions are characterised by groups of neuron cell bodies, or nuclei, with particular functional associations.

Thus the anterior grey columns contain the cell bodies of alpha and gamma motor neurons whose axons innervate respectively the extrafusal and intrafusal fibres of voluntary muscles. These cell bodies are aggregated into three longitudinal groups of nuclei (**B–F**).

1. The medial nuclear group supplies the muscles attached to the axial skeleton and is therefore particularly prominent in the thoracic segments of the cord (**D**).
2. The lateral nuclear group supplies the muscles of the limbs and is consequently prominent in the cervical and lumbar enlargements of the cord (**C, E**).
3. The central nuclear group is confined to the upper cervical segments (**B**) and sends axons into the phrenic nerve (to the diaphragm) and into the spinal accessory nerve (**39B**).

The intermediate grey matter contains an intermediomedial nucleus at all levels and an intermediolateral nucleus in two distinct regions. From the T1 segment to the L2 segment the latter nucleus bulges laterally forming the lateral grey column (**D**). It contains the cell bodies of all the preganglionic sympathetic neurons in the body. After a break in continuity the same nucleus reappears in the midsacral segments (**F**) but here does not bulge laterally to produce a lateral column. It contains the cell bodies of all sacral preganglionic parasympathetic neurons.

The posterior grey column is concerned with the reception of many of the sensory impulses reaching the cord through the posterior roots of the spinal nerves. Its neuronal cell bodies are aggregated into a number of nuclei. The connections of these will be dealt with later but their names and positions can be studied now in **B–F**. Most of these nuclei are continuous along the length of the cord but note the following exceptions.

1. The nucleus dorsalis (thoracic nucleus, Clarke's nucleus) is absent from the cervical segments (**B, C**).
2. The substantia gelatinosa becomes continuous with the spinal nucleus of the trigeminal nerve in the upper cervical segments (**B**).

The white matter which surrounds the central grey is customarily divided into a number of regions. In each half of the cord a posterior funiculus is situated between the posterior median septum and the posterior grey column, a lateral funiculus occupies the region between the posterior grey column and the narrow zone of attachment of the ventral rootlets of the spinal nerves, while an anterior funiculus lies between the attachment of these rootlets and the depth of the anterior median fissure (**A**). The two anterior funiculi are joined between the grey commissure and the floor of the anterior median fissure by a narrow zone of decussating fibres known as the white commissure (**A**).

A zone of white matter immediately adjacent to the central grey is occupied mainly by short longitudinal intersegmental fibres. The larger peripheral part is occupied mainly by long fibre tracts ascending to, or descending from, supraspinal levels. The positions of such individual tracts will be considered later (**77, 79, 81**).

The sizes of the white funiculi and the grey columns vary at different levels of the spinal cord. It is evident that, because most of the fibres of the white matter ascend or descend between the brain and the successive segments of the cord, the amount of white matter decreases rather evenly from above down. On the other hand, because the number of neuron cell bodies in any particular segment of the spinal cord is a function of the number of nerve fibres entering and leaving that segment through its paired spinal nerves (which, in turn, is a function of the volume of tissue the segment innervates), the amount of grey matter does not change in the same even manner along the cord. Rather, the volume of grey matter is large in the cervical and lumbar enlargements which innervate the limbs (**C, E**) and comparatively small in other regions of the cord (**B, D**).

The reticular formation is the term applied to the small isolated nodules and strands of grey matter which lie amongst the white matter of the lateral funiculi alongside the bases of the posterior grey columns. Although the formation is present to some degree at all levels, it is particularly noticeable in the cervical segments (**B**) and, as will be seen later, is continuous upwards into the brain stem.

SPINAL CORD: GENERAL TRANSVERSE SECTION

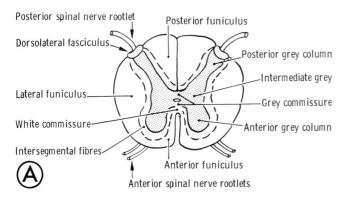

Posterior spinal nerve rootlet
Dorsolateral fasciculus
Posterior funiculus
Posterior grey column
Intermediate grey
Grey commissure
Lateral funiculus
White commissure
Anterior grey column
Intersegmental fibres
Anterior funiculus
Anterior spinal nerve rootlets

(A)

UPPER CERVICAL SEGMENT: TRANSVERSE SECTION

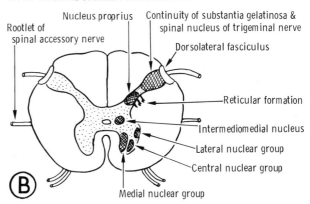

Nucleus proprius
Continuity of substantia gelatinosa & spinal nucleus of trigeminal nerve
Rootlet of spinal accessory nerve
Dorsolateral fasciculus
Reticular formation
Intermediomedial nucleus
Lateral nuclear group
Central nuclear group
Medial nuclear group

(B)

LOWER CERVICAL SEGMENT (CERVICAL ENLARGEMENT): TRANSVERSE SECTION

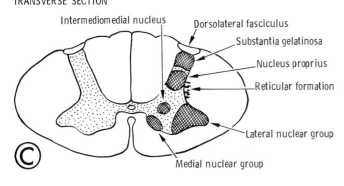

Intermediomedial nucleus
Dorsolateral fasciculus
Substantia gelatinosa
Nucleus proprius
Reticular formation
Lateral nuclear group
Medial nuclear group

(C)

THORACIC SEGMENT: TRANSVERSE SECTION

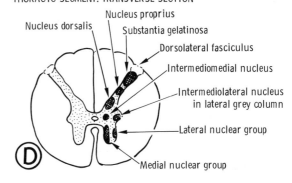

Nucleus dorsalis
Nucleus proprius
Substantia gelatinosa
Dorsolateral fasciculus
Intermediomedial nucleus
Intermediolateral nucleus in lateral grey column
Lateral nuclear group
Medial nuclear group

(D)

LOWER LUMBAR SEGMENT (LUMBAR ENLARGEMENT): TRANSVERSE SECTION

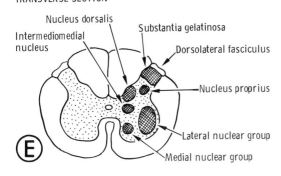

Nucleus dorsalis
Intermediomedial nucleus
Substantia gelatinosa
Dorsolateral fasciculus
Nucleus proprius
Lateral nuclear group
Medial nuclear group

(E)

SACRAL SEGMENT: TRANSVERSE SECTION

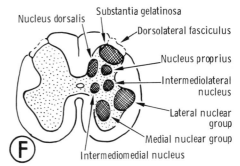

Nucleus dorsalis
Substantia gelatinosa
Dorsolateral fasciculus
Nucleus proprius
Intermediolateral nucleus
Lateral nuclear group
Medial nuclear group
Intermediomedial nucleus

(F)

GENERAL FEATURES OF BRAIN STEM AND CEREBELLUM

The brain stem connects the spinal cord with the cephalic part of the central nervous system, the forebrain. Its long axis is nearly aligned with that of the spinal cord but with a slight forward inclination, so that it has anterior or ventral and posterior or dorsal aspects. It consists from below upwards of the medulla oblongata (the medulla), the pons and the midbrain (**A**). Throughout the lower half of the medulla and in the midbrain the lumen of the brain is a narrow, more or less centrally situated canal, completely surrounded outside its ependymal lining by neural tissue. In the upper half of the medulla and in the pons, the lumen expands into a tent-like cavity with superior, inferior and lateral angles and an apex directed backwards. This is called the fourth ventricle and, as will be seen shortly, part of its posterior wall is devoid of neural tissue and consists of a layer of ependyma (**A**). A large additional division of the brain, the cerebellum, develops in the posteriorly directed roof of the fourth ventricle (**A**). It is connected to the three parts of the brain stem by thick paired bundles of white fibres known as the cerebellar peduncles, the superior peduncles passing to the midbrain, the middle peduncles to the pons and the inferior peduncles to the medulla. In **C** the peduncles have been cut and the cerebellum removed. Note the relationship of the three peduncles to one another.

The medulla, cerebellum and pons may be described collectively as the hindbrain.

External features of medulla oblongata

Examine the surfaces of this part in **B** and **C** and observe the following features.

1. The anterior aspect is smoothly continuous with that of the spinal cord but is sharply demarcated from that of the pons by a transverse groove (**B**). Along its length, an anterior median fissure, continuous with that of the spinal cord, separates paired, wide, longitudinal ridges composed of descending fibres. These ridges are called the pyramids, not because of their own shape, but because of the general shape of the cell bodies in the cerebral cortex from which some of their fibres arise. In the lowest part of the medulla the majority of the fibres of the pyramids decussate to the opposite side in the depths of the anterior median fissure. The decussating fibres are grouped as small oblique bundles which are readily visible when the lips of the fissure are separated.
2. On the anterolateral aspect of the upper half of the medulla is an oval swelling called the olive (**B**), which is separated from the corresponding pyramid by a longitudinal groove.

3. On the posterior aspect of the lower half of the medulla (**C**) a shallow posterior median sulcus continues upwards from the spinal cord to the lower angle of the fourth ventricle. On either side of its upper end are two small elevations, the gracile tubercle medially and the cuneate tubercle laterally.
4. On the posterolateral aspects of the upper half of the medulla (**C**) thick cylindrical ridges, the inferior cerebellar peduncles, extend upwards and somewhat laterally forming the lateral boundaries of the lower part of the fourth ventricle. Reaching the pons they turn sharply backwards into the cerebellum. In front, each peduncle is demarcated from the corresponding olive by a groove.

Between the inferior cerebellar peduncles, the posterior aspect of the upper half of the medulla forms the anterior wall or floor of the lower part of the fourth ventricle (**A, C**).

External features of pons

Examine the surfaces of this part in **B** and **C** and observe the following features.

1. The anterior surface (**B**) bulges forwards beyond the anterior surface of the medulla and midbrain, from both of which it is demarcated by transverse grooves. On either side of a shallow median (basilar) sulcus the surface is convex in the horizontal plane and marked by fine transverse ridges.
2. Traced laterally, the ventral tissues of the pons become collected into the thick cylindrical middle cerebellar peduncles (**B**) which turn backwards lateral to the terminal part of the inferior cerebellar peduncles before sinking into the substance of the cerebellum (**C**).
3. The paired superior cerebellar peduncles emerge from the cerebellum deep to the other two peduncles and turn upwards and medially on the posterolateral aspects of the pons before disappearing into the substance of the midbrain (**C**). The two superior peduncles form the converging lateral walls of the upper part of the fourth ventricle. They are connected across the midline by a thin lamina of white matter known as the superior medullary velum, which forms the roof of the upper part of the ventricle (**C**).
4. Between the superior cerebellar peduncles, the posterior surface of the pons forms the anterior wall or floor of the upper half of the fourth ventricle (**A**).

LUMEN OF BRAIN STEM: MEDIAN SECTION

Ependyma ·········

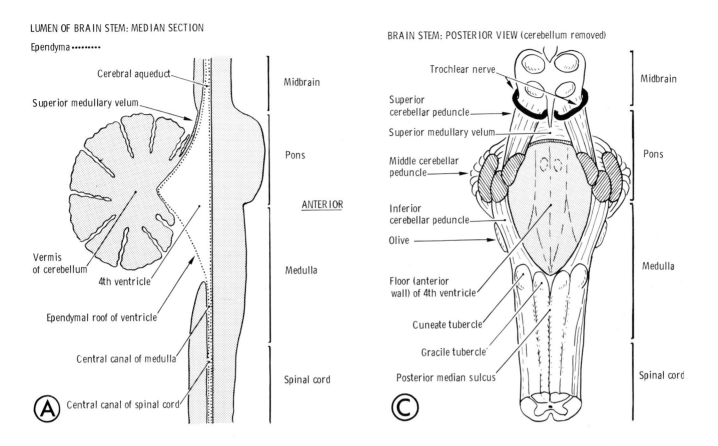

Cerebral aqueduct

Superior medullary velum

Midbrain

Pons

ANTERIOR

Vermis of cerebellum

4th ventricle

Medulla

Ependymal roof of ventricle

Central canal of medulla

Spinal cord

(A) Central canal of spinal cord

BRAIN STEM: POSTERIOR VIEW (cerebellum removed)

Trochlear nerve

Midbrain

Superior cerebellar peduncle

Superior medullary velum

Pons

Middle cerebellar peduncle

Inferior cerebellar peduncle

Olive

Floor (anterior wall) of 4th ventricle

Medulla

Cuneate tubercle

Gracile tubercle

Posterior median sulcus

Spinal cord

(C)

BRAIN STEM: ANTERIOR VIEW

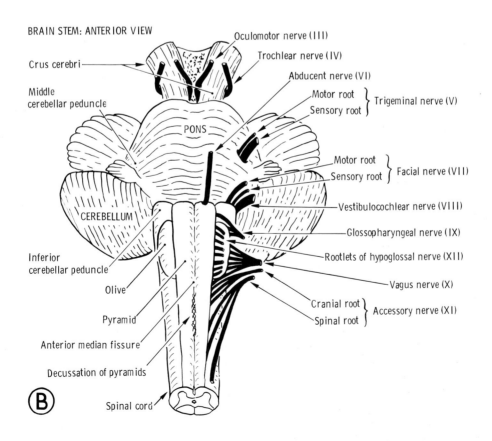

Crus cerebri

Oculomotor nerve (III)

Trochlear nerve (IV)

Abducent nerve (VI)

Middle cerebellar peduncle

Motor root
Sensory root } Trigeminal nerve (V)

PONS

Motor root
Sensory root } Facial nerve (VII)

CEREBELLUM

Vestibulocochlear nerve (VIII)

Glossopharyngeal nerve (IX)

Rootlets of hypoglossal nerve (XII)

Inferior cerebellar peduncle

Vagus nerve (X)

Olive

Pyramid

Cranial root
Spinal root } Accessory nerve (XI)

Anterior median fissure

Decussation of pyramids

(B) Spinal cord

External features of midbrain

This is a short segment of the brain stem which leads upwards from the pons to the forebrain.

Observe its surface features in **A**, **B**.

1. On the anterior surface (**A**) two broad rounded ridges, the crura cerebri, diverge upwards, forwards and laterally. As will be seen later, where they are crossed by the optic tracts they become continuous with the corresponding cerebral hemispheres. The crura are separated by a deep recess, the interpeduncular fossa, the floor of which is marked by numerous vascular apertures and is consequently known as the posterior perforated substance.

2. On the narrower posterior surface (**B**) two pairs of prominent elevations, the superior and inferior colliculi, are separated by a cruciform groove. The upper part of the region is overlapped in the midline by the pineal body, and on either side of the median plane by the blunt posterior end of a mass of grey matter called the thalamus. Hidden in the groove between the projecting thalamus and the posterior aspect of the midbrain are two elevations named the medial and lateral geniculate bodies. The lateral bodies receive the terminations of the optic tracts (**A, B**). All these structures mentioned above except the colliculi belong to the forebrain; but it is convenient, as will be evident below, to note their general position here.

From the colliculi, ridges produced by bundles of superficial fibres extend upwards and laterally to the geniculate bodies (**B**). On either side the inferior brachium arises from the inferior colliculus and passes lateral to the superior colliculus to reach the medial geniculate body, while the superior brachium joins the superior colliculus to the lateral geniculate body, passing between the medial geniculate body and the thalamus.

Attachment of the brain stem cranial nerves

It has been noted already that the twelve paired cranial nerves have individual names and are numbered in craniocaudal order. All but the first (olfactory) and the second (optic) are attached to the brain stem. The names and numbers of these nerves and their sites of attachment to the surface of the brain stem should be learned from **39B**. Observe the following facts.

1. The trochlear nerves are the only members of the group which are attached to the posterior aspect of the brain stem. They subsequently wind round the crura cerebri to reach the anterior aspect.

2. The oculomotor, trochlear and abducent which are motor, and vestibulocochlear which is sensory, are attached as single nerve trunks.

3. The trigeminal and facial nerves are attached as separate sensory and motor roots. In each case the sensory root is lateral to the motor. The sensory root of the facial is often known as the nervus intermedius.

4. The glossopharyngeal and vagus nerves are attached by a number of rootlets, each of which contains both sensory and motor fibres.

5. The hypoglossal nerve and the two roots of the accessory nerve both arise by a number of purely motor rootlets.

6. All the nerves which contain sensory fibres carry one or more sensory ganglia.

The cerebellum

This large division of the brain develops in the central part of the roof of the fourth ventricle (**C**). It expands from this small region so that what were originally the posterior surfaces of its upper and lower parts eventually face forwards towards the upper and lower parts of the brain stem (**C**). As growth proceeds, the surface of the cerebellum becomes demarcated into a narrow central region called the vermis, which is conveniently described as consisting of superior and inferior parts (**D**), and two cerebellar hemispheres, one on either side. The uppermost part of the superior vermis lies a little above the level of the hemispheres, whereas the inferior vermis lies in a deep recess between the hemispheres called the vallecula (**D**).

The vermis and hemispheres are divided by fissures, which are mainly transversely disposed, into narrow sheets of tissue called folia. Each of these consists of a slender branched lamina of white matter covered by a thin layer of grey matter which constitutes the cerebellar cortex (**E**). Traced centrally the white matter of the folia fuse in a central white core (**E**). Anteriorly, this central core is continuous on either side with the three cerebellar peduncles, considered earlier, while in the midline it is penetrated for a short distance by the apex of the fourth ventricle (**E**).

Some of the fissures between the folia form the basis of the division of the vermis into segments and the hemispheres into corresponding lobules. Two of the fissures, which appear early in development, are used to group these segments and lobules into three lobes. The several parts of the cerebellum so demarcated are most readily visualised in a diagram such as that in **F** in which the convex surface of the cerebellum is unrolled to form a flat surface. It is unnecessary to learn the names of all the parts but those which are labelled in **F** should be known.

MIDBRAIN: ANTERIOR ASPECT

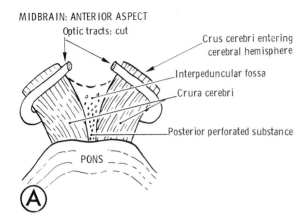

Optic tracts: cut

Crus cerebri entering cerebral hemisphere

Interpeduncular fossa

Crura cerebri

Posterior perforated substance

PONS

Ⓐ

DIAGRAMMATIC MEDIAN SECTION OF BRAIN STEM & CEREBELLUM SHOWING GROWTH OF CEREBELLUM

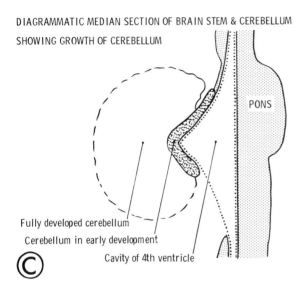

PONS

Fully developed cerebellum

Cerebellum in early development

Cavity of 4th ventricle

Ⓒ

PONS & CEREBELLUM: HORIZONTAL SECTION

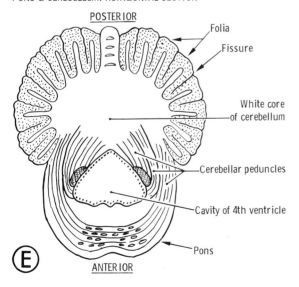

POSTERIOR

Folia

Fissure

White core of cerebellum

Cerebellar peduncles

Cavity of 4th ventricle

Pons

Ⓔ

ANTERIOR

MIDBRAIN AND ADJACENT STRUCTURES: POSTERIOR ASPECT

(posterior end of thalamus removed on left side)

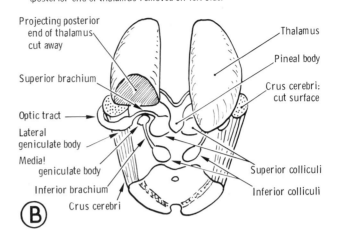

Projecting posterior end of thalamus cut away

Superior brachium

Optic tract

Lateral geniculate body

Medial geniculate body

Inferior brachium

Crus cerebri

Thalamus

Pineal body

Crus cerebri: cut surface

Superior colliculi

Inferior colliculi

Ⓑ

CEREBELLUM: FROM BEHIND

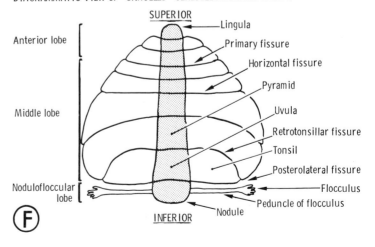

Midbrain

Superior vermis

Horizontal fissure

Inferior vermis

Retrotonsillar fissure

Tonsil

Part of ependymal roof of 4th ventricle

Vallecula

Medulla

Ⓓ

DIAGRAMMATIC VIEW OF "UNROLLED" CEREBELLUM (vermis shaded)

SUPERIOR

Anterior lobe

Middle lobe

Nodulofloccular lobe

Lingula

Primary fissure

Horizontal fissure

Pyramid

Uvula

Retrotonsillar fissure

Tonsil

Posterolateral fissure

Flocculus

Peduncle of flocculus

Nodule

Ⓕ

INFERIOR

Observe the following features of the cerebellum.

1. The lingula is the most anterior part of the superior vermis (**A, B**). Its transverse folia are poorly developed and its white matter is continuous with that of the superior medullary velum.

2. The primary fissure is V-shaped, open forwards and lies on the anterosuperior aspect of the cerebellum (**A**). It forms the posterior limit of the anterior lobe.

3. The nodule is the most anterior part of the inferior vermis (**B, C**). Its anterior aspect, which is fissured and coated with grey matter, is apposed to the ependymal roof of the fourth ventricle (**B**).

4. The tonsils are lobules on the inferior aspect of the hemispheres (**C**). The white matter of their folia is continuous with the central white core of the cerebellum and with the white matter of the folia of the uvula. They and the uvula are limited posteriorly by the deep retrotonsillar fissure and anteriorly by the shallow posterolateral fissure (**C, D**).

5. When a tonsil is separated from the rest of the cerebellum (**C**) a thin translucent crescentic lamina known as the inferior medullary velum, is exposed. Note in **D** that the superior margin of the velum is continuous with the central white core of the cerebellum, its anterior surface forms part of the roof of the fourth ventricle and is consequently lined by ependyma, its inferior margin gives attachment to the ependymal part of the roof of the ventricle, while its posterior surface is separated from the tonsil by the posterolateral fissure, and is consequently covered by pia mater. Note also in **C** that the velum is continuous medially with white matter on the lateral aspect of the nodule whereas laterally it is continuous with a slender strand of white matter called the peduncle of the flocculus.

6. This peduncle is attached above to the junction of the white cerebellar core and the inferior cerebellar peduncle, and below gives attachment to the ependymal roof of the fourth ventricle. Traced laterally, it joins a small, crenated, detached lobule of the cerebellum called the flocculus, which protrudes laterally (**C**) immediately behind the middle cerebellar peduncle (**45C**) in the anterior part of the horizontal fissure.

7. The major part of the cerebellum, which lies between the primary fissure (**A**) and the posterolateral fissure (**C**), is the middle lobe. The nodule, together with the flocculus, the floccular peduncle and the inferior medullary velum constitute the nodulofloccular lobe.

8. The tonsils have already been noted as paired, rather protuberant lobules on the inferior aspects of the cerebellar hemispheres (**C**). They bulge over, but are separate from, the posterior aspect of the medulla. With the medulla they form an irregular cone with its apex at the entrance into the vertebral canal. If the pressures in the cranial and spinal parts of the subarachnoid space (**105B**) are abnormally high, sudden decompression of the spinal part may forcibly displace the cone downwards so that it impacts in the foramen magnum, like a cork in a bottle, and causes death from sudden severe compression of the medulla.

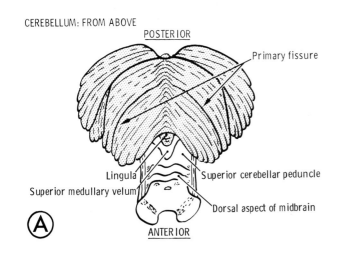

CEREBELLUM: FROM ABOVE

POSTERIOR

Primary fissure

Lingula
Superior medullary velum
Superior cerebellar peduncle
Dorsal aspect of midbrain

(A)

ANTERIOR

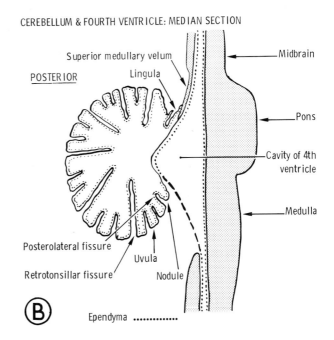

CEREBELLUM & FOURTH VENTRICLE: MEDIAN SECTION

Superior medullary velum
Lingula
POSTERIOR

Midbrain

Pons

Cavity of 4th ventricle

Medulla

Posterolateral fissure
Uvula
Retrotonsillar fissure
Nodule

(B)

Ependyma ....

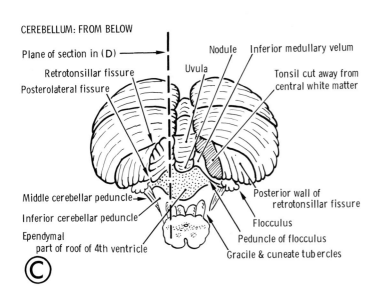

CEREBELLUM: FROM BELOW

Plane of section in (D)
Retrotonsillar fissure
Posterolateral fissure

Nodule
Uvula
Inferior medullary velum

Tonsil cut away from central white matter

Middle cerebellar peduncle
Inferior cerebellar peduncle
Ependymal part of roof of 4th ventricle

Posterior wall of retrotonsillar fissure
Flocculus
Peduncle of flocculus
Gracile & cuneate tubercles

(C)

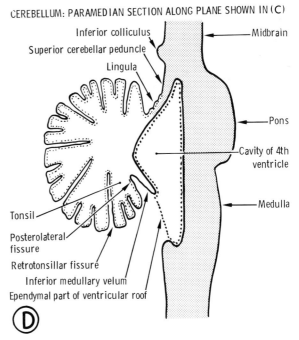

CEREBELLUM: PARAMEDIAN SECTION ALONG PLANE SHOWN IN (C)

Inferior colliculus
Superior cerebellar peduncle
Lingula

Midbrain

Pons

Cavity of 4th ventricle

Medulla

Tonsil
Posterolateral fissure
Retrotonsillar fissure
Inferior medullary velum
Ependymal part of ventricular roof

(D)

The fourth ventricle

In the lower half of the medulla and in the midbrain, the lumen of the central nervous system remains narrow during development and becomes completely surrounded by central grey matter (**A**). In contrast, in the upper half of the medulla and in the pons the lumen expands to form the fourth ventricle, so called because there are three other expanded regions in the forebrain. The mechanism of the expansion can be regarded as a transverse stretching of the posterior wall of the cavity particularly in its central part (**A**). This results in the originally posterior parts of the central grey matter becoming displaced laterally into the same plane as the originally anterior parts, so that, together, they form the anterior wall of the cavity. The development of the cavity is further influenced by the growth of the cerebellum in the central part of the roof and the formation of lateral walls by the establishment of cerebellar peduncles on either side. Despite these changes in shape the cavity of the fourth ventricle remains completely lined by a layer of ependyma like the rest of the lumen of the central nervous system.

The tent-like definitive cavity of the fourth ventricle has superior and inferior angles, and, on either side, just below the cerebellar peduncles as they pass backwards into the cerebellum, it extends laterally as a short cylindrical lateral recess.

The lateral walls of the cavity are formed by the superior and inferior cerebellar peduncles (**B**).

The floor or anterior wall of the cavity is rhomboidal and, as has been seen above, is formed by the central grey matter of the pons and upper half of the medulla covered by a layer of ependyma. Observe the named features of the floor in **B** and note particularly that the middle part of the vestibular area extends laterally across the postero-inferior aspect of the bend of the inferior cerebellar peduncle into the floor of the lateral recess.

The roof or posterior wall is in three parts (**C**).

1. The upper third or so is formed by the triangular superior medullary velum slung between the superior cerebellar peduncles (**C, D, E**).

2. The central third of the roof consists of the white core of the cerebellum which is continuous inferiorly with the upper part of the nodule, the inferior medullary vela and the floccular peduncles (**C, D, E**).

3. The lower third differs from other parts of the roof. It is devoid of neural tissue and is formed by a triangular sheet of ependymal cells (**C**). The base of this sheet, which is directed upwards, is 'attached' to neural tissue at the upper anterior extremity of the nodule (**D**), the inferior margins of the inferior medullary vela (**C, E**) and along the inferior margins of the floccular peduncles (**C**). The greater parts of the lateral margins of the sheet are attached to the vertical parts of the inferior cerebellar peduncles (**C**).

Between these two attachments there are two short free margins which are separated from the lateral parts of the vestibular areas by apertures at the lateral ends of the lateral recesses of the ventricle (**C**). A third, median aperture perforates the lower angle of the ependymal roof (**C, D**). These three apertures are the only openings in the walls of the whole ventricular system, and consequently form the only routes by which cerebrospinal fluid can pass from that system into the subarachnoid space (**105B**).

The tela choroidea of the fourth ventricle is a region of pia mater which covers the ependymal lower third of the roof, and thereafter sweeps downwards, backwards and then upwards over the surfaces of the inferior vermis and the tonsils (**D, E**).

The choroid plexus of the fourth ventricle is an invagination into that cavity of the ependymal roof and the pia mater which clothes its outer surface, that is, the anterior layer of the tela choroidea (**D, E**). The invagination occurs along a line which is shaped like a T with a double vertical limb, and hangs into the ventricular cavity (**C**). On either side the most lateral parts of the plexus are situated in the lateral recesses of the ventricle and usually protrude through the lateral apertures (**C**). The protruding parts can be seen in the intact brain as two nodules of vascular tissue lying behind the middle cerebellar peduncles and the flocculi.

DISPOSITION OF CENTRAL GREY MATTER (SHADED) IN DIFFERENT PARTS OF BRAIN STEM

:IN LOWER HALF OF MEDULLA & MIDBRAIN :IN REGION OF PONS & UPPER HALF OF MEDULLA

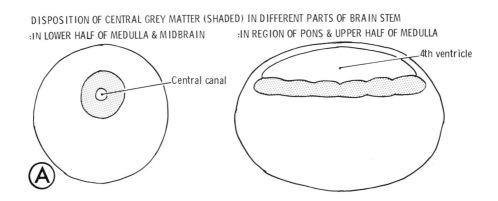

Central canal

4th ventricle

(A)

FLOOR (ANTERIOR WALL) OF FOURTH VENTRICLE

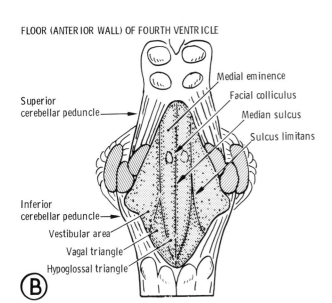

Superior cerebellar peduncle

Medial eminence
Facial colliculus
Median sulcus
Sulcus limitans

Inferior cerebellar peduncle

Vestibular area
Vagal triangle
Hypoglossal triangle

(B)

ROOF (POSTERIOR WALL) OF FOURTH VENTRICLE

Plane of (E)

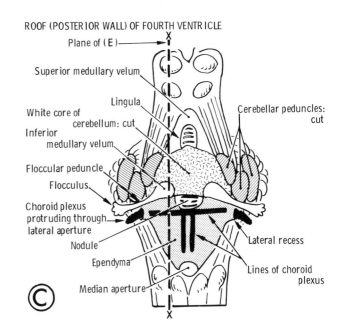

Superior medullary velum
Lingula
White core of cerebellum: cut
Inferior medullary velum
Floccular peduncle
Flocculus
Choroid plexus protruding through lateral aperture
Nodule
Ependyma
Median aperture

Cerebellar peduncles: cut
Lateral recess
Lines of choroid plexus

(C)

MEDIAN SECTION THROUGH FOURTH VENTRICLE

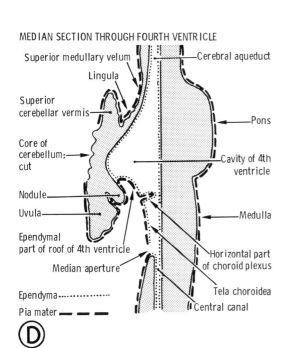

Superior medullary velum
Lingula
Superior cerebellar vermis
Core of cerebellum: cut
Nodule
Uvula
Ependymal part of roof of 4th ventricle
Median aperture
Ependyma............
Pia mater _ _ _ _

Cerebral aqueduct
Pons
Cavity of 4th ventricle
Medulla
Horizontal part of choroid plexus
Tela choroidea
Central canal

(D)

PARAMEDIAN SECTION THROUGH FOURTH VENTRICLE ALONG
PLANE X-X IN (C)

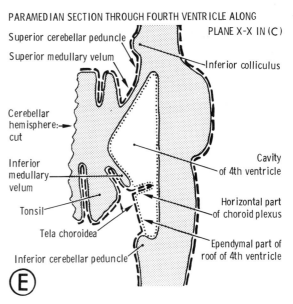

Superior cerebellar peduncle
Superior medullary velum
Cerebellar hemisphere: cut
Inferior medullary velum
Tonsil
Tela choroidea
Inferior cerebellar peduncle

Inferior colliculus
Cavity of 4th ventricle
Horizontal part of choroid plexus
Ependymal part of roof of 4th ventricle

(E)

The nuclei within the brain stem and cerebellum

The paired nuclei of grey matter which lie within the substance of the brain stem and cerebellum fall into two groups. On the one hand there are a number of nuclei which constitute relay stations on the course of tracts of fibres of like function, while on the other, there are the cranial nerve nuclei which send motor fibres into, or receive sensory fibres from, the individual cranial nerves which have already been seen to be attached to the surface of the brain stem (**39B**).

Tract nuclei

1. In the posterior part of the middle of the medulla three nuclei form relay stations on the fibre tracts which have ascended into the brain stem from the posterior funiculi of the spinal cord. The *nucleus gracilis* (**39C**), which is most medial, underlies the gracile tubercle (**B**) and the *nucleus cuneatus* (**B**), which is situated more laterally, underlies the cuneate tubercle. Both exhibit a degree of continuity with the central grey matter surrounding the central canal. The smaller *accessory cuneate nucleus* (**B**) lies posterolateral to the cuneate and is separate from both it and the central grey matter.

2. In the upper half of the medulla, deep to the olive on its lateral surface and posterior to the pyramid, are the *olivary and accessory olivary nuclei* (**C**). The olivary nucleus is an extensive crenated lamina of grey matter in the form of an oval sac open posteromedially. The accessory nuclei are smaller flat laminae which lie posterior and anteromedial to the main olivary nucleus.

3. For descriptive purposes it is usual to divide the substance of the pons into anterior or basal and posterior or tegmental parts (**D**). A large number of small masses of grey matter are scattered throughout the basal part: they are known as the pontine nuclei.

4. A prominent feature in transverse sections through both the upper and lower halves of the midbrain is a thick laminar nucleus of darkly pigmented grey matter which extends obliquely, on either side, from the lateral surface to the interpeduncular fossa. It is known as the *substantia nigra* (**E, F**). The whole midbrain is traversed longitudinally by the narrow cerebral aqueduct which is surrounded by central grey matter (**E, F**). These features are used to divide this segment of the brain stem into regions. The two crura cerebri are anterior to the substantia nigra, the tegmentum is the region between the substantia nigra and the plane of the cerebral aqueduct, while the tectum lies behind that plane (**E**).

   In the tectum the *nuclei of the superior and inferior colliculi* lie beneath the corresponding surface elevations (**E, F**). Just cranial to the nucleus of the superior colliculus, and consequently at the junction of the midbrain and the diencephalon, is a small collection of grey matter called the pretectal nucleus.

   The red nucleus (**F**) is a large oval mass of grey matter which lies close to the midline in the upper half of the tegmentum. Its pinkish colour in fresh preparations is due to the presence of a pigment within many of its cells.

5. *The reticular formation* is a long columnar zone containing numerous cell bodies of interneurons which are scattered diffusely amongst tract fibres running in many different directions and are nowhere aggregated into macroscopic nuclei. The formation extends the length of the brain stem and is situated in the cross-hatched regions in **B, C, D, E, F**. Caudally, it becomes continuous with the reticular formation already noted in the deep part of the lateral funiculus in the cervical part of the spinal cord (**37B, 37C**).

6. A number of paired nuclei lie in the white core of the cerebellum, close above the roof of the fourth ventricle (**G**). The largest and most lateral are the paired dentate nuclei which are crenated laminae of grey matter in the form of sacs open upwards and forwards. Three pairs of smaller round or oval accessory dentate nuclei lie between them.

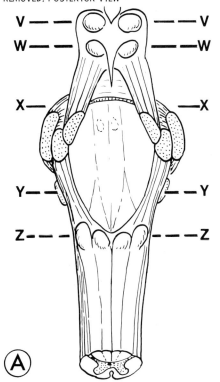

BRAIN STEM: CEREBELLUM & ROOF OF FOURTH VENTRICLE REMOVED: POSTERIOR VIEW

V — — — V
W — — — W
X — — — X
Y — — — Y
Z — — — Z

(A)

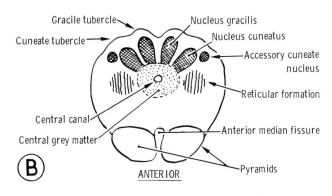

TRANSVERSE SECTION THROUGH MIDDLE OF MEDULLA:(PLANE Z-Z IN (A)

Gracile tubercle
Cuneate tubercle
Nucleus gracilis
Nucleus cuneatus
Accessory cuneate nucleus
Reticular formation
Central canal
Central grey matter
Anterior median fissure
Pyramids

(B)

ANTERIOR

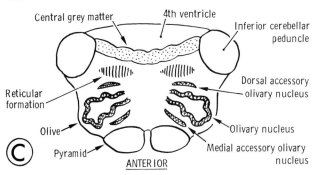

T.S. THROUGH UPPER PART OF MEDULLA: PLANE Y-Y IN (A)

Central grey matter
4th ventricle
Inferior cerebellar peduncle
Reticular formation
Dorsal accessory olivary nucleus
Olive
Olivary nucleus
Pyramid
Medial accessory olivary nucleus

(C)

ANTERIOR

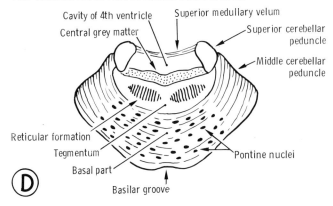

T.S. THROUGH UPPER PART OF PONS: PLANE X-X IN (A)

Cavity of 4th ventricle
Central grey matter
Superior medullary velum
Superior cerebellar peduncle
Middle cerebellar peduncle
Reticular formation
Tegmentum
Basal part
Basilar groove
Pontine nuclei

(D)

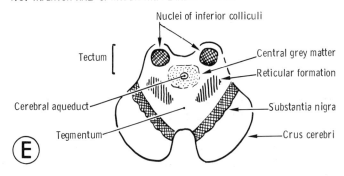

T.S. INFERIOR HALF OF MIDBRAIN: PLANE W-W IN (A)

Nuclei of inferior colliculi
Tectum
Cerebral aqueduct
Tegmentum
Central grey matter
Reticular formation
Substantia nigra
Crus cerebri

(E)

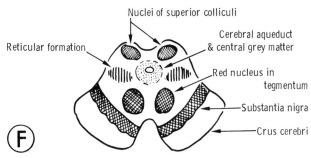

T.S. SUPERIOR HALF OF MIDBRAIN: PLANE V-V IN (A)

Nuclei of superior colliculi
Reticular formation
Cerebral aqueduct & central grey matter
Red nucleus in tegmentum
Substantia nigra
Crus cerebri

(F)

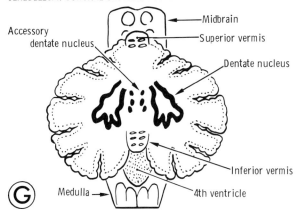

CEREBELLUM: CORONAL SECTION: POSTERIOR VIEW

Accessory dentate nucleus
Midbrain
Superior vermis
Dentate nucleus
Medulla
Inferior vermis
4th ventricle

(G)

The cranial nerves of the brain stem and their nuclei

The sites of attachment and the general form of the cranial nerves of the brain stem have been dealt with briefly already (**39B**). In this section these features are revised, and consideration is given to the positions of the motor nuclei which send axons into each of the nerves and the sensory nuclei which receive the central processes of the cells in the sensory ganglia which lie on some of the nerves.

With the exception of the vestibular and cochlear nuclei and the nucleus solitarius (solitary nucleus), these nuclei are arranged in a pattern in which those of similar function are aligned in the form of interrupted longitudinal grey columns (**A**). The nuclei which belong to the somatic motor and visceral motor columns, together with some sensory nuclei, lie within the central grey matter which surrounds the central canals in the lower half of the medulla and in the midbrain and forms the floor (anterior wall) of the fourth ventricle. On the other hand, those which belong to the branchial motor column and the rest of the sensory nuclei are separate to a greater or lesser degree from the central grey matter.

The oculomotor (3rd cranial) nerve arises from closely associated somatic motor and visceral motor nuclei in the anterior part of the central grey matter in the upper half of the midbrain (**B**). The fibres curve forwards through the substance of the red nucleus, and the definitive nerve emerges into the interpeduncular fossa at the medial edge of the substantia nigra. The nerve contains somatic motor fibres which innervate certain extrinsic muscles of the eye, and preganglionic parasympathetic fibres which form the proximal segment of the parasympathetic supply to the eye.

The trochlear (4th cranial) nerve arises from a single somatic motor nucleus placed in the anterior part of the central grey matter in the lower half of the midbrain (**C**) and supplies one extrinsic muscle of the eye. The fibres follow an unusual course. They pass round the lateral and posterior aspects of the central grey, and eventually decussate across the midline. Because at the same time they descend to a somewhat lower level the nerve emerges through the superior medullary velum just below the inferior colliculus (**39C**). The nerve, which contains only somatic motor fibres, is unique in two respects. It is the only cranial nerve to emerge on the posterior aspect of the brain stem and the only nerve to emerge on the opposite side of the median plane from its parent nucleus.

The trigeminal (5th cranial) nerve has been seen (**39B**) to be attached by a large lateral sensory root and a small medial motor root to the anterior aspect of the pons. The fibres of the sensory root are the central processes of pseudo-unipolar nerve cells in the trigeminal ganglion and transmit sensory information mainly derived from many of the tissues in the region of the face. Those of the motor root innervate the branchial muscles which move the jaw. In a section through the middle part of the pons, the fibres of both roots may be traced posteromedially to a region in the lateral part of the tegmentum just anterior to the vestibular area of the central grey matter and the superior cerebellar peduncle (**D**). Here the branchial motor nucleus gives rise to all the fibres in the motor root and the more laterally placed main sensory nucleus receives those fibres of the sensory root which are concerned with the sensation of touch. All the other fibres of the sensory root turn either upwards or downwards to reach other sensory trigeminal nuclei.

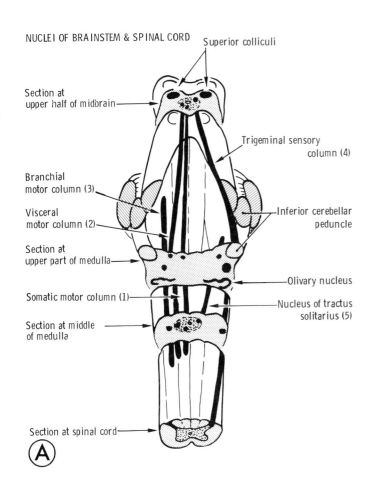

NUCLEI OF BRAINSTEM & SPINAL CORD

Superior colliculi

Section at
upper half of midbrain

Trigeminal sensory
column (4)

Branchial
motor column (3)

Visceral
motor column (2)

Inferior cerebellar
peduncle

Section at
upper part of medulla

Olivary nucleus

Somatic motor column (1)

Nucleus of tractus
solitarius (5)

Section at middle
of medulla

Section at spinal cord

(A)

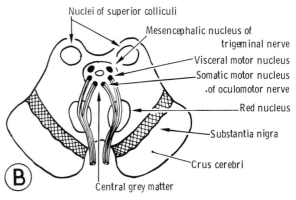

T.S. UPPER HALF OF MIDBRAIN

Nuclei of superior colliculi

Mesencephalic nucleus of
trigeminal nerve

Visceral motor nucleus

Somatic motor nucleus
.of oculomotor nerve

Red nucleus

Substantia nigra

Crus cerebri

Central grey matter

(B)

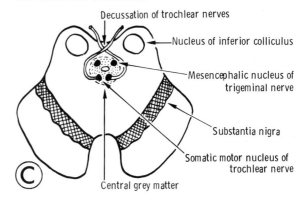

T.S. LOWER HALF OF MIDBRAIN

Decussation of trochlear nerves

Nucleus of inferior colliculus

Mesencephalic nucleus of
trigeminal nerve

Substantia nigra

Somatic motor nucleus of
trochlear nerve

Central grey matter

(C)

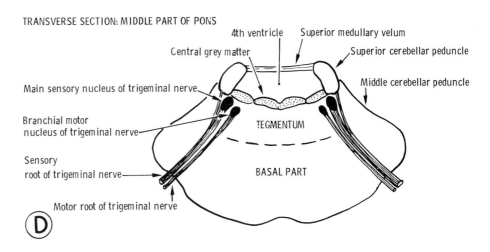

TRANSVERSE SECTION: MIDDLE PART OF PONS

4th ventricle

Superior medullary velum

Central grey matter

Superior cerebellar peduncle

Middle cerebellar peduncle

Main sensory nucleus of trigeminal nerve

Branchial motor
nucleus of trigeminal nerve

TEGMENTUM

Sensory
root of trigeminal nerve

BASAL PART

Motor root of trigeminal nerve

(D)

The ascending or mesencephalic tract carries proprioceptive information from muscles, joints and teeth. Its fibres pass upwards on the anteromedial aspect of the superior cerebellar peduncle (**A**) to reach the mesencephalic nucleus, which lies in the posterolateral part of the central grey matter throughout the midbrain (**49B, 49C**).

The descending or spinal tract contains fibres associated with pain and thermal sensations. It descends through the pons, medulla and the upper part of the spinal cord, lying lateral, in succession, to the motor nucleus of the facial nerve, the nucleus ambiguus, the cuneate nucleus and the posterior grey column of the spinal cord. However it is separated from these nuclei by a coextensive nucleus in which its fibres end, This spinal nucleus of the trigeminal nerve has an inverse relationship to the region of the face which most fibres of the tract innervate. Fibres from the upper part of the face terminate in the lowest part of the nucleus and vice versa.

The abducent (6th cranial) nerve arises from a single somatic motor nucleus in the central grey matter in the floor of the lower pontine part of the fourth ventricle (**B**) and supplies one extrinsic muscle of the eye. The nucleus is beneath the facial colliculus, an elevation at about the midpoint of the medial eminence. The apparent paradox in this terminology will be clarified when the facial nerve is considered. The purely somatic motor fibres pass anteriorly and slightly downwards, through the tegmentum and basal part of the pons, and emerge as a discrete nerve through the groove between the pons and the pyramid of the medulla (**39B**) a short distance from the median plane.

The facial (7th cranial) nerve has been seen to be attached to the brain stem at the lateral end of the groove demarcating the anterior aspects of the pons and medulla by a large medial motor root and a small lateral sensory root also known as the nervus intermedius (**39B**). The roots eventually unite as they pass through the skull, and just beyond this junction the nerve exhibits the sensory genicular ganglion.

A branchial motor facial nucleus lies deeply in the lateral part of the tegmentum of the pons, medial to the upper part of the spinal nucleus and tract of the trigeminal nerve (**45B**). The fibres arising in the nucleus innervate the muscles which control the expression of the face. They follow a peculiar course, illustrated in (**B**), passing posterior to the abducent nucleus where they give their name to the facial colliculus in the floor of the fourth ventricle. The visceral motor or preganglionic parasympathetic fibres arise from the superior salivary nucleus which lies in the central grey matter in the floor of the

fourth ventricle deep to the sulcus limitans and just above the vagal triangle (**45B**). Rather surprisingly, they leave the brain stem in the sensory root of the nerve. They innervate salivary glands in the mouth and the lacrimal gland which produces tears. The other fibres in the sensory root carry the sensation of taste from part of the tongue and palate and are the central processes of the pseudo-unipolar cells in the genicular ganglion. In the brain stem they turn downwards and end in the upper part of the solitary nucleus. This nucleus is confined to the medulla with its upper end just deep to the lower part of the vestibular area of central grey matter in the floor of the fourth ventricle and its lower end in the central grey matter posterior to the central canal (**49A**).

The vestibulocochlear (8th cranial) nerve is purely sensory. Its vestibular moiety transmits information regarding the posture and movements of the head from the vestibule and semicircular canals of the internal ear. Its cochlear part transmits impulses concerned with hearing from the cochlea of the internal ear. The fibres arise in two groups as the central processes of bipolar nerve cells in separate vestibular and cochlear ganglia. These groups join within the internal acoustic meatus and pass as a single nerve to reach the brain stem anterior to the inferior cerebellar peduncle, at the lateral end of the groove demarcating the medulla from the pons, and posterolateral to the emerging facial nerve (**39B**).

The cochlear fibres end in the dorsal and ventral cochlear nuclei placed respectively on the posterior and anterolateral aspects of the inferior cerebellar peduncle just before it bends backwards into the cerebellum (**A, C**).

The vestibular fibres penetrate into the upper part of the medulla anterior to the inferior cerebellar peduncle and then turn posteriorly to reach a number of distinguishable nuclei in the vestibular area of central grey matter in the floor of the fourth ventricle (**A, C**).

The glossopharyngeal (9th cranial) the *vagus (10th cranial)* and the *cranial root of the accessory nerve (11th cranial)* form a group of nerves which can be conveniently dealt with together. They are attached to the lateral aspect of the medulla by a longitudinal row of rootlets, those forming the glossopharyngeal and vagus along the groove between the olive and inferior cerebellar peduncle, and those of the cranial accessory at a slightly lower level (**39B**). They run laterally to leave the skull through the same foramen. As they do so the glossopharyngeal and vagus each exhibit superior and inferior sensory ganglia. The cranial accessory joins the vagus below its inferior ganglion and its fibres are subsequently distributed through the branches of that nerve (**53C**).

SOME BRAIN STEM NUCLEI

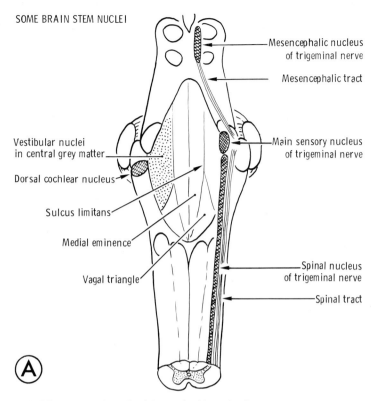

Mesencephalic nucleus of trigeminal nerve

Mesencephalic tract

Vestibular nuclei in central grey matter

Dorsal cochlear nucleus

Sulcus limitans

Medial eminence

Vagal triangle

Main sensory nucleus of trigeminal nerve

Spinal nucleus of trigeminal nerve

Spinal tract

(A)

T.S. LOWER PART OF PONS (sensory nucleus of facial nerve is at lower level)

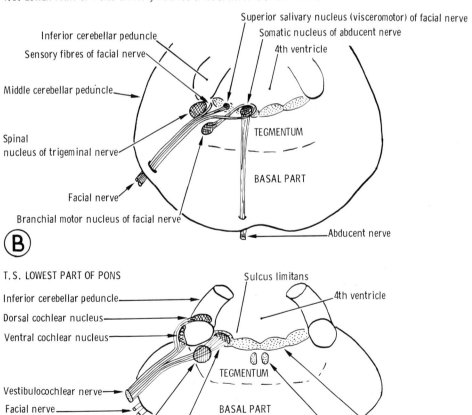

Superior salivary nucleus (visceromotor) of facial nerve
Somatic nucleus of abducent nerve
4th ventricle

Inferior cerebellar peduncle
Sensory fibres of facial nerve
Middle cerebellar peduncle

Spinal nucleus of trigeminal nerve

Facial nerve
Branchial motor nucleus of facial nerve

TEGMENTUM

BASAL PART

Abducent nerve

(B)

T.S. LOWEST PART OF PONS

Sulcus limitans
4th ventricle

Inferior cerebellar peduncle
Dorsal cochlear nucleus
Ventral cochlear nucleus

Vestibulocochlear nerve
Facial nerve
Spinal nucleus of trigeminal nerve

Vestibular fibres

TEGMENTUM

BASAL PART

Central grey matter

Medial longitudinal fasciculus

(C)

The three nerves all contain branchial motor fibres which supply striated muscle in the walls of the pharynx and larynx. These arise from the upper, middle and lower parts of the nucleus ambiguus (**A, B**) which is in linear series with the branchial motor nuclei of the trigeminal and facial nerves (see above). The nucleus lies deeply throughout the length of the medulla, medial to the spinal nucleus of the trigeminal nerve. Although branchial motor fibres are the sole component of the cranial root of the accessory nerve (**B**), the vagus and glossopharyngeal contain other moieties (**A**).

A large group of visceral motor (preganglionic para-sympathetic) fibres join the vagus from its dorsal nucleus, which is in the central grey matter forming the vagal triangle in the lower half of the floor of the fourth ventricle (**A, right**). They have a large distribution to thoracic and abdominal viscera. Fibres of the same type join the glossopharyngeal from the inferior salivary nucleus which lies in line with the dorsal vagal nucleus but at a slightly higher level (**A, left**). They supply the parotid salivary gland.

The sensory fibres which enter the brain stem in the vagus and glossopharyngeal nerves are all the central processes of pseudo-unipolar cells in the sensory ganglia which have been noted on the proximal parts of those nerves. Those which transmit the sensation of taste turn downwards and end, like the similar fibres in the facial nerve (see above), in the solitary nucleus (**A**). The destination of the more numerous fibres which convey general visceral sensation from many thoracic and abdominal viscera is uncertain but it is possible that they also end in the solitary nucleus.

It should be noted that all the fibres of the glossopharyngeal and vagus nerves, and the cranial root of the accessory nerve, pass through the spinal tract and nucleus of the trigeminal nerve between their nuclei and the surface of the brain stem.

The spinal root of the accessory nerve consists of motor fibres which arise from the central nuclear group in the anterior grey column in the upper five segments of the spinal cord (**C**). A series of rootlets emerges on the lateral aspect of the spinal cord between the ventral and dorsal roots of the upper cervical nerves and, turning upwards, coalesce to form a single nerve which enters the cranial cavity through the foramen magnum. It then becomes temporarily attached to the cranial root of the accessory, without interchange of fibres, and thereafter passes into the neck where it supplies two large muscles.

It is uncertain whether the motor fibres of this nerve are to be regarded as branchial or somatic in nature.

The hypoglossal (12th cranial) nerve arises from the lowest of the somatic motor cranial nuclei and innervates all but one of the muscles of the tongue. The upper half of the nucleus is in the central grey matter forming the hypoglossal triangle in the floor of the fourth ventricle (**A**) while the lower half lies in the anterior part of the central grey matter in the lower half of the medulla (**B**). The purely somatic motor fibres pass anteriorly, the upper traversing the olivary nucleus (**A**). The nerve emerges as a linear series of several rootlets through the sulcus which marks the lateral margin of the pyramid (**A**).

GENERAL FEATURES OF THE FOREBRAIN

The forebrain originates as the upper end of the neural tube which is known as the diencephalon (**D**). This contains an ependymal-lined cavity called the third ventricle which has a blind cephalic end and is continuous caudally with the cerebral aqueduct of the midbrain. During development the anterior part of the diencephalon expands to either side as the cerebral hemispheres, each of which contains an extension of the third ventricle known as a lateral ventricle (**D**). The communications between the lateral and third ventricles are the interventricular foramina. At first the connections between the diencephalon and the cerebral hemispheres are narrow, but once the hemispheres have enlarged, large parts of the lateral aspects of the diencephalon fuse with the central parts of the medial aspects of the hemispheres (**E**). The development of the definitive features of the diencephalon and cerebral hemispheres, and the fusion of these parts to one another, are to a certain extent contemporaneous processes, but it facilitates description and understanding if the major definitive features of diencephalon and hemispheres are considered separately and the three parts are then simply 'stuck' together.

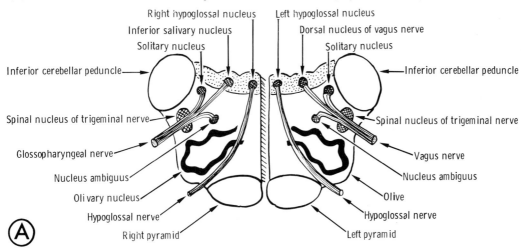

T.S. UPPER PART OF MEDULLA (note that the right half of the section is at a slightly lower level than the left)

Right hypoglossal nucleus
Inferior salivary nucleus
Solitary nucleus
Left hypoglossal nucleus
Dorsal nucleus of vagus nerve
Solitary nucleus
Inferior cerebellar peduncle
Inferior cerebellar peduncle
Spinal nucleus of trigeminal nerve
Spinal nucleus of trigeminal nerve
Glossopharyngeal nerve
Vagus nerve
Nucleus ambiguus
Nucleus ambiguus
Olivary nucleus
Olive
Hypoglossal nerve
Hypoglossal nerve
Right pyramid
Left pyramid

A

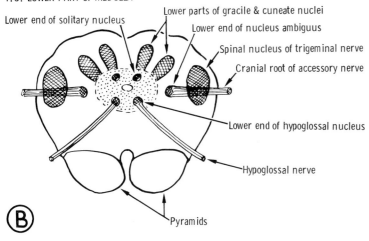

T.S. LOWER PART OF MEDULLA

Lower end of solitary nucleus
Lower parts of gracile & cuneate nuclei
Lower end of nucleus ambiguus
Spinal nucleus of trigeminal nerve
Cranial root of accessory nerve
Lower end of hypoglossal nucleus
Hypoglossal nerve
Pyramids

B

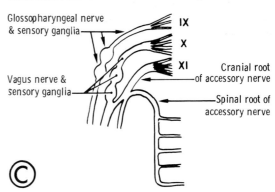

INTER-RELATIONSHIP OF CRANIAL NERVES IX, X & XI

Glossopharyngeal nerve & sensory ganglia
IX
X
XI
Cranial root of accessory nerve
Vagus nerve & sensory ganglia
Spinal root of accessory nerve

C

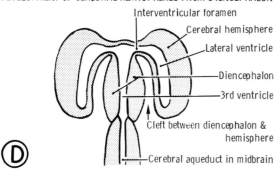

DEVELOPMENT OF CEREBRAL HEMISPHERES FROM DIENCEPHALON

Interventricular foramen
Cerebral hemisphere
Lateral ventricle
Diencephalon
3rd ventricle
Cleft between diencephalon & hemisphere
Cerebral aqueduct in midbrain

D

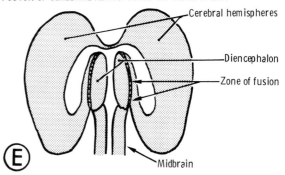

FUSION OF CEREBRAL HEMISPHERES & DIENCEPHALON

Cerebral hemispheres
Diencephalon
Zone of fusion
Midbrain

E

The diencephalon

The definitive diencephalon, isolated from the cerebral hemisphere but in continuity with the midbrain, is shown in **A, B, C, D, E.**

The third ventricle is a narrow, slit-like, median cavity whose long axis is angulated on that of the cerebral aqueduct of the brain stem so that it is more or less horizontal (**A**). Thus the ventricle has narrow anterior and posterior ends, floor and roof, and comparatively extensive lateral walls. The structural features of the diencephalon can be considered as forming the several walls of the ventricle.

1. The anterior wall consists of a lamina of grey matter called the lamina terminalis (**A**). This ends above and below in commissural bands of transverse white fibres. Above is the anterior commissure (**A**): it will be seen later that its fibres pass on either side into the cerebral hemispheres. Below is the optic chiasma (**A, B**): its lateral ends receive the optic nerves from the eyeballs and give rise to the optic tracts which continue backwards.

2. The floor is formed anteriorly by a median elevation called the tuber cinereum (**B**). From its centre the conical infundibulum passes downwards into continuity with the hypophysis cerebri (pituitary gland)(**A, B, D**). Behind this complex, twin elevations called the mamillary bodies lie on either side of the midline and contain the mamillary nuclei (**B**). Further posteriorly, the floor is formed by a short upwards and forward continuation of the tegmentum of the midbrain (**A**). Because, as will be seen shortly, this region lies below a large mass of grey matter called the thalamus, it is known as the subthalamus. Two of its features are shown in the section in (**C**). Close to the midline are the upper ends of the red nuclei, already noted in the midbrain, while between the red nuclei and the crura cerebri on either side are the subthalamic nuclei.

3. In the upper anterior corner of the lateral wall of the ventricle the interventricular foramen leads laterally (**A, E**). The ventricular aspect of the lateral wall (**A**) is crossed by the gently curved hypothalamic sulcus, which extends from the interventricular foramen to the cerebral aqueduct. Most of the lateral ventricular wall above this sulcus is formed by a large oval mass of grey matter called the thalamus (**A, D**). The anterior pole of the thalamus lies just behind the interventricular foramen (**A**). Its posterior pole, known as the pulvinar, projects backwards beyond the ventricle and overhangs the dorsal aspect of the uppermost part of the brain stem which is marked by the elevations of the medial and lateral geniculate bodies (**E**). The geniculate bodies and the nuclei of

grey matter they contain constitute collectively the metathalamus. The upper third or so of the thalamus rises above the level of the ventricular roof (**A, D**). The ventricular surfaces of the paired thalami are joined across the cavity of the ventricle by the interthalamic adhesion (**C**).

4. The region of the lateral walls below the hypothalamic sulci, together with those parts of the floor of the ventricle exhibiting the mamillary bodies and the tuber cinereum and hypophysis, constitute the hypothalamus. The hypothalamic part of the lateral wall contains a number of hypothalamic nuclei which are shown collectively in (**D**). Passing downwards and backwards amongst these hypothalamic nuclei, from the interval between the interventricular foramen and the anterior commissure to the mamillary nucleus is a thick bundle of white fibres called the column of the fornix. The rest of the fornix system will be seen later on the medial aspect of the cerebral hemisphere. Passing between the mamillary nucleus and the thalamus through the same region is the mamillothalamic tract.

5. Traced upwards, the crura cerebri of the midbrain diverge from one another into the lower parts of the lateral walls of the ventricle where they lie lateral to the subthalamus and inferior to the thalami (**C, D**). Here, in the developed forebrain, they become continuous with large fibre tracts in the cerebral hemispheres called the internal capsules and so in diagrams **C, D** and **E** their ends are shown as cut surfaces. It may be noted in **D, E** that the lateral geniculate bodies and their nuclei lie partly on the posterior surfaces of the corresponding crura.

6. From the lateral ends of the optic chiasma, thick bands of white fibres called the optic tracts extend backwards attached to the outer surfaces of the lateral walls of the hypothalamic part of the third ventricle (**D**). The tracts finally curl round the lateral and posterior aspects of the corresponding crura cerebri, at the level of the continuity of the crura with the internal capsule, to end in the nuclei of the lateral geniculate bodies.

7. The roof of the ventricle is formed by a narrow sheet of ependyma (**A, E**), which, as will be seen later, is in contact above with pia mater. The lateral margins of this sheet are attached to paired bundles of white fibres which run from before backwards across the medial surfaces of the thalami (**C**) and expand posteriorly into triangular zones of tissue called the habenular trigones (**E**). Anteriorly, the roof is attached to the columns of the fornix and the anterior commissure. Between the columns and the anterior poles of the thalami, the roof extends to either side to form also the roofs of the interventricular foramina.

MEDIAN SECTION THROUGH DIENCEPHALON & MIDBRAIN: X-X SHOWS PLANE OF (C)

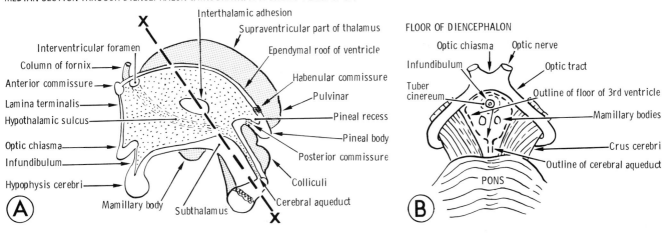

Interventricular foramen
Column of fornix
Anterior commissure
Lamina terminalis
Hypothalamic sulcus
Optic chiasma
Infundibulum
Hypophysis cerebri
Mamillary body
Subthalamus

Interthalamic adhesion
Supraventricular part of thalamus
Ependymal roof of ventricle
Habenular commissure
Pulvinar
Pineal recess
Pineal body
Posterior commissure
Colliculi
Cerebral aqueduct

(A)

FLOOR OF DIENCEPHALON

Optic chiasma
Optic nerve
Infundibulum
Optic tract
Tuber cinereum
Outline of floor of 3rd ventricle
Mamillary bodies
Crus cerebri
Outline of cerebral aqueduct
PONS

(B)

OBLIQUE SECTION OF DIENCEPHALON & MIDBRAIN:

ALONG PLANE X-X IN (A)

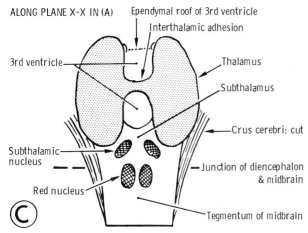

Ependymal roof of 3rd ventricle
Interthalamic adhesion
3rd ventricle
Thalamus
Subthalamus
Crus cerebri: cut
Subthalamic nucleus
Junction of diencephalon & midbrain
Red nucleus
Tegmentum of midbrain

(C)

DIENCEPHALON & MIDBRAIN: SUPERIOR ASPECT

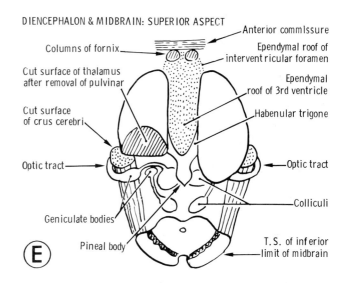

Columns of fornix
Anterior commissure
Ependymal roof of interventricular foramen
Cut surface of thalamus after removal of pulvinar
Ependymal roof of 3rd ventricle
Cut surface of crus cerebri
Habenular trigone
Optic tract
Optic tract
Geniculate bodies
Colliculi
Pineal body
T.S. of inferior limit of midbrain

(E)

DIENCEPHALON & MIDBRAIN: LATERAL ASPECT
(interrupted lines show outline of 3rd ventricle)

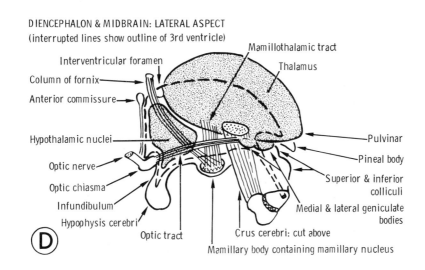

Interventricular foramen
Column of fornix
Anterior commissure
Mamillothalamic tract
Thalamus
Hypothalamic nuclei
Optic nerve
Optic chiasma
Infundibulum
Hypophysis cerebri
Optic tract
Pulvinar
Pineal body
Superior & inferior colliculi
Medial & lateral geniculate bodies
Crus cerebri: cut above
Mamillary body containing mamillary nucleus

(D)

55

8. The posterior limit of the ventricle is continuous below with the cerebral aqueduct, while above it is formed by a conical recess (the pineal recess) which penetrates backwards into the pineal body. The pineal body is a pear-shaped endocrine gland which projects backwards and rests on the groove which separates the superior colliculi of the midbrain (**55E**). Its stalk is separated centrally by the pineal recess into superior and inferior laminae (**55A**). The superior lamina is continuous on either side with the habenular trigones, and contains the transverse fibres of the habenular commissure. The inferior lamina contains the larger posterior commissure. The pineal body, its stalk and the habenular trigones are described collectively as the epithalamus.

The development and shape of the cerebral hemispheres

After the cerebral hemisphere has developed as a lateral outgrowth from the diencephalon, its central white matter, containing the cavity of the lateral ventricle , is at first covered by an unfolded layer of grey matter known as the cortex (**A**). At this time a mass of grey matter, forerunner of the corpus striatum, appears in the white matter close to the lower lateral part of the cortex, and below and lateral to the lateral ventricle (**A**).

The manner of enlargement of the hemisphere is strongly influenced by different growth rates in its upper and lower parts. The lower lateral part of the hemisphere, where the developing corpus striatum is close to the cortex, enlarges slowly, while the upper part of the hemisphere grows much more rapidly.

In an approximately sagittal plane the upper part of the hemisphere enlarges along a C-shaped axis around the more slowly growing lower part (**B**). The anterior region expands forwards and downwards establishing a frontal pole (**B, D**). The posterior region enlarges, backwards forming an occipital pole, and subsequently downwards and then forwards to establish a temporal pole (**B, D**). Subsequent to this C-shaped enlargement, the upper and posterior parts of the lateral surface bulge towards one another as thick folds over the lower part, which thus becomes buried and is known as the insula (**B,C**). Eventually, the expanding upper and posterior parts of the lateral surface come into close proximity, forming the deep lateral sulcus which extends from the inferior aspect of the hemisphere upwards and backwards across its lateral surface (**D**). Separation of the lips of the sulcus exposes the insular cortex (**C**).

Once the general form of the hemisphere has been established, the area of the cortex expands at a more rapid rate than the volume of the central white matter, so that it becomes elaborately folded into a large number of blunt ridges or gyri and intervening grooves or sulci (**C**).

The fully developed cerebral hemisphere presents frontal, occipital and temporal poles, and superolateral, inferior and medial surfaces.

The superolateral surface is convex from before backwards and from above down and is limited by superomedial and inferolateral borders (**D**). The downward concavity on the inferolateral border, a short distance in front of the occipital pole, is called the pre-occipital notch.

The shape of the inferior surface varies in its anterior, middle and posterior parts (**E**). Its anterior third (or orbital part since it lies above the orbit) is gently concave downwards. It is limited behind by the stem of the lateral sulcus, and medially extends to within a few millimetres of the median plane. In contrast, the middle third is comparatively widely separated from the corresponding region on the other hemisphere by the diencephalon and midbrain. It is distinctly convex from side to side (**E, 59B**). The posterior third of the inferior surface lies above the cerebellum but is separated from it by a thick partition of dura mater. It is gently concave in a downward and medial direction (**59D**) and its medial margin is again a few millimetres from the midline.

EARLY STAGE IN DEVELOPMENT OF CEREBRAL HEMISPHERE

CORONAL SECTION

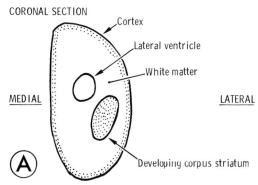

Cortex

Lateral ventricle

White matter

MEDIAL

LATERAL

Developing corpus striatum

Ⓐ

DIAGRAMMATIC CORONAL SECTION OF CEREBRAL HEMISPHERE

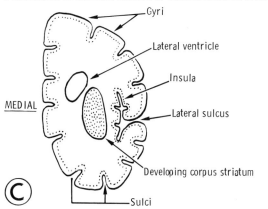

Gyri

Lateral ventricle

Insula

MEDIAL

Lateral sulcus

Developing corpus striatum

Ⓒ

Sulci

LATERAL ASPECT OF DEVELOPING RIGHT CEREBRAL HEMISPHERE

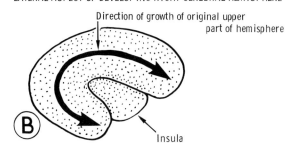

Direction of growth of original upper part of hemisphere

Ⓑ

Insula

INFERIOR SURFACES OF CEREBRAL HEMISPHERES

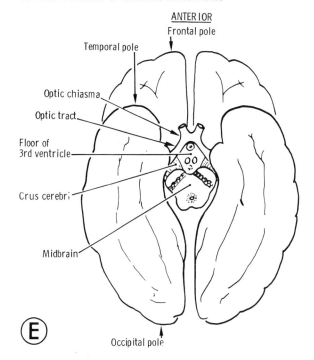

ANTERIOR

Frontal pole

Temporal pole

Optic chiasma

Optic tract

Floor of
3rd ventricle

Crus cerebri

Midbrain

Occipital pole

Ⓔ

SUPEROLATERAL SURFACE OF RIGHT CEREBRAL HEMISPHERE

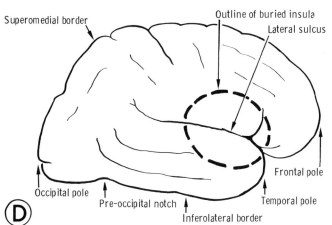

Superomedial border

Outline of buried insula

Lateral sulcus

Occipital pole

Pre-occipital notch

Inferolateral border

Temporal pole

Frontal pole

Ⓓ

When the hemisphere is viewed from the medial side after it has been separated from the diencephalon and brain stem (**A**), both its medial surface and the medial aspects of the middle and posterior thirds of its inferior surface are visible. The medial surface consists of a peripheral part and a central part (interrupted outline in **A**). The peripheral part is sagittal and very close to the median plane (**B, C, D**). The central part lies in an oblique plane facing medially and downwards (**B**), so that as has been seen already (**57E**) the medial aspect of the central third of the inferior surface of the hemisphere is some distance from the median plane. The greater part of this central part of the medial surface, that is, the shaded area in **A**, is the 'adhesion area' with which the lateral aspect of the diencephalon fuses during development.

The lateral ventricle

During development, the lateral ventricle enlarges from the interventricular foramen along the same axis as the cerebral hemisphere in which it lies, and eventually assumes the definitive shape shown in **E**. In **E** the ventricle is shown as if it lay within a transparent hemisphere. Note the names applied to its parts and observe that the inferior horn lies on a plane lateral to that of the central part (**B**).

The relationships of the several parts of the ventricle to the medial aspect of the cerebral hemisphere are indicated in **B, C, D**. The anterior horn extends for a short distance in front of the interventricular foramen while the posterior horn extends backwards, from the junction of the central part and the inferior horn, towards the occipital pole (**E**). Both are separated from the medial surface of the hemisphere by neural tissue (**C, D**). The central part and inferior horn of the ventricle lie very close to the superior, posterior and inferior margins of the adhesion area. The medial ventricular wall consists solely of a layer of ependymal cells (clear area in **E**). As will be seen later, this strip is invaginated into the body and inferior horn of the ventricle by pia mater on its outer surface to form a continuous choroid plexus, and is consequently known as the choroidal fissure (**E**). Note that anteriorly the ependyma of the choroidal fissure is continuous with the ependymal roof of the interventricular foramen (**E**).

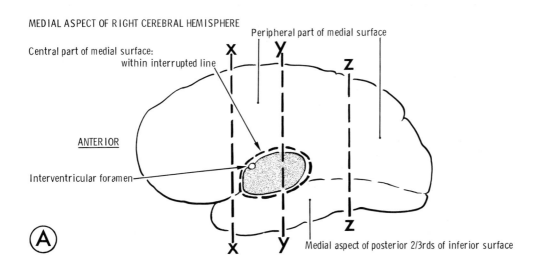

MEDIAL ASPECT OF RIGHT CEREBRAL HEMISPHERE

Central part of medial surface: within interrupted line

Peripheral part of medial surface

ANTERIOR

Interventricular foramen

Medial aspect of posterior 2/3rds of inferior surface

(A)

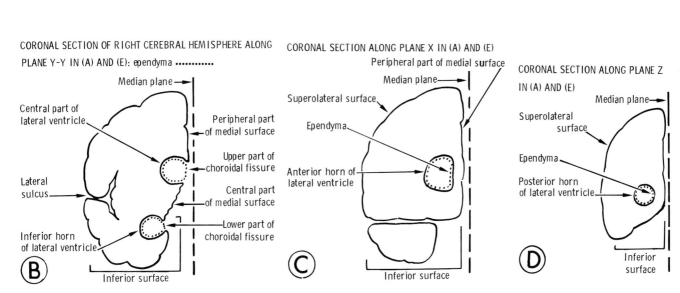

CORONAL SECTION OF RIGHT CEREBRAL HEMISPHERE ALONG PLANE Y-Y IN (A) AND (E): ependyma ············

Median plane

Central part of lateral ventricle

Peripheral part of medial surface

Upper part of choroidal fissure

Central part of medial surface

Lateral sulcus

Lower part of choroidal fissure

Inferior horn of lateral ventricle

Inferior surface

(B)

CORONAL SECTION ALONG PLANE X IN (A) AND (E)

Peripheral part of medial surface

Median plane

Superolateral surface

Ependyma

Anterior horn of lateral ventricle

Inferior surface

(C)

CORONAL SECTION ALONG PLANE Z IN (A) AND (E)

Median plane

Superolateral surface

Ependyma

Posterior horn of lateral ventricle

Inferior surface

(D)

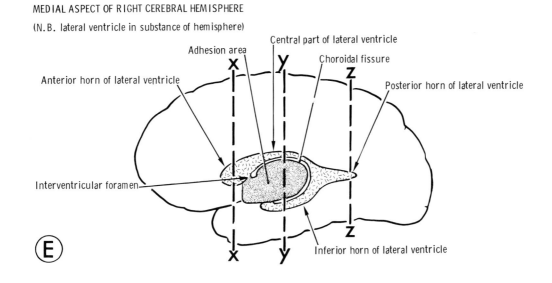

MEDIAL ASPECT OF RIGHT CEREBRAL HEMISPHERE

(N.B. lateral ventricle in substance of hemisphere)

Adhesion area

Central part of lateral ventricle

Choroidal fissure

Anterior horn of lateral ventricle

Posterior horn of lateral ventricle

Interventricular foramen

Inferior horn of lateral ventricle

(E)

The continuity of the cerebral hemispheres with the diencephalon

In early development the continuity between the cerebral hemisphere and the diencephalon is narrow and in the vicinity of the interventricular foramen. Later, however, as has been seen the area of continuity is enlarged by fusion of a large part of the medial aspect of the hemisphere which lies within the curve of the choroidal fissure, that is, the adhesion area (**59E**).

The region of the lateral aspect of the diencephalon which fuses with the adhesion area on the medial aspect of the cerebral hemisphere is vertically hatched in **A**. Identify the structures in that region and observe their positions on the hemisphere once adhesion has taken place (**B**). Note that the central margin of the ependymal choroidal fissure is then attached in continuity along the upper surface of the thalamus, along a line across the lateral aspect of the body of the thalamus at its junction with the pulvinar, and along the lower margin of the middle part of the optic tract. Observe also that the inferior part of the hypothalamus, the pulvinar of the thalamus, and the geniculate bodies remain separate from the hemispheres. In **B** the optic tract presents cut anterior and posterior ends at the extremities of the part fused to the adhesion area. Anteriorly, the tract diverges medially on the wall of the lower part of the hypothalamus to reach the lateral end of the optic chiasma (**55D**) while posteriorly it also turns medially to reach the lateral geniculate body which consequently lies just medially to the posterior part of the choroidal fissure (**55D**).

The fornix system

This consists of right and left C-shaped bundles of white fibres placed on the medial aspects of the corresponding cerebral hemispheres. Seen in isolation the whole system has the form shown in **C** and **D**.

Each fimbria lies on the medial aspect of the middle third of the inferior surface of one hemisphere (**E**) and is consequently at some distance from the median plane (**E**). Each crus ascends across the posterior part of the oblique central part of the medial surface of the hemisphere (**E**) so that the two crura approach one another as they ascend (**D**). As they approach, they are connected across the midline by a thin lamina of transverse fibres (**D, E**) which constitute the hippocampal commissure. Above, the two halves of the fornix fuse in the median plane forming the single body (**D, E**). Traced anteriorly the body divides into right and left columns (**C, D**). Each of these passes in front of the interventricular foramen (**E**) and then inclines downwards and backwards, through the zone of fusion of the diencephalon to the corresponding cerebral hemisphere, to reach the mamillary body (**55D**).

On either side, the fimbria, crus and body form that part of the medial wall of the inferior horn and central part of the lateral ventricle which is immediately peripheral to the choroidal fissure.

The choroidal fissure

It has been seen already that the choroidal fissure is a C-shaped strip of the medial wall of the central part and inferior horn of the lateral ventricle which consists of a single layer of ependymal cells. It is now convenient to revise the central and peripheral attachments of this layer of ependyma in **E**.

The corpus callosum and septum pellucidum

The corpus callosum is by far the largest of the several commissural collections of white fibres which extend transversely across the median plane and join the two cerebral hemispheres to each other.

Its general shape and the names of the parts into which it is customarily divided can be appreciated in **F**.

DIENCEPHALON AND MIDBRAIN: RIGHT LATERAL ASPECT
(area which fuses with cerebral hemisphere is hatched)

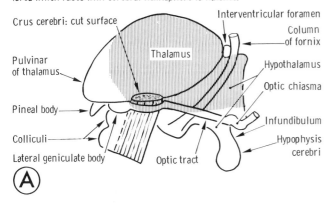

Crus cerebri: cut surface
Interventricular foramen
Column of fornix
Pulvinar of thalamus
Thalamus
Hypothalamus
Optic chiasma
Pineal body
Infundibulum
Colliculi
Hypophysis cerebri
Lateral geniculate body
Optic tract

(A)

ISOLATED FORNIX SYSTEM FROM LEFT SIDE

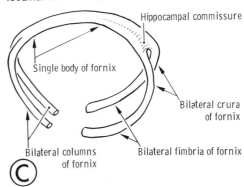

Hippocampal commissure
Single body of fornix
Bilateral crura of fornix
Bilateral columns of fornix
Bilateral fimbria of fornix

(C)

CENTRAL REGION OF MEDIAL SURFACE OF RIGHT CEREBRAL HEMISPHERE
WHICH ADHERES TO DIENCEPHALON & MIDBRAIN (hatched)

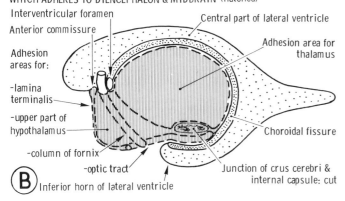

Interventricular foramen
Anterior commissure
Central part of lateral ventricle
Adhesion area for thalamus
Adhesion areas for:
-lamina terminalis
-upper part of hypothalamus
Choroidal fissure
-column of fornix
-optic tract
Junction of crus cerebri & internal capsule: cut
(B) Inferior horn of lateral ventricle

ISOLATED FORNIX SYSTEM FROM ABOVE

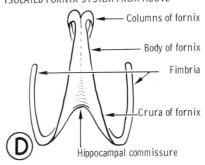

Columns of fornix
Body of fornix
Fimbria
Crura of fornix
(D) Hippocampal commissure

HALF OF FORNIX SYSTEM ON MEDIAL ASPECT OF RIGHT CEREBRAL HEMISPHERE
(Fine hatching indicates adhesion area, coarse hatching indicates area fused with opposite side)

Body of fornix: cut surface in median plane
Adhesion area for thalamus
Anterior horn of lateral ventricle
Hippocampal commissure: cut surface in median plane
Adhesion areas for:
-lamina terminalis
-upper part of hypothalamus
Crus of fornix
Choroidal fissure
-column of fornix
-optic tract
Fimbria of fornix
(E) Inferior horn of lateral ventricle

MEDIAN SECTION OF ISOLATED CORPUS CALLOSUM

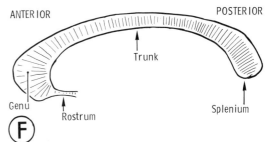

ANTERIOR
POSTERIOR
Trunk
Genu
Rostrum
Splenium
(F)

The relationship of the corpus callosum to the forebrain structures already described may be observed in the median section (**A**) and in the coronal sections (**B, C, D**).

1. The splenium, which is the somewhat expanded free posterior end, lies above and separate from the pineal body (**A**).
2. The posterior part of the trunk lies a small distance above the converging crura of the fornix and the hippocampal commissure (**A**).
3. The middle part of the trunk is firmly attached to the upper surface of the body of the fornix (**A, D**).
4. More anteriorly, the trunk, genu and rostrum become separated from the body of the fornix by a triangular interval (**A**). This is occupied on either side of the midline by a thin translucent sheet of neural tissue called the septum pellucidum (**B, C**). This forms the whole of the medial wall of the anterior horn and a variable part of the medial wall of the central part of the lateral ventricle (**B, C**).
5. The two septa are separated in the median plane by a slit-like cavity (**B, C**). It should be noted that this cavity is completely closed in all directions and is quite independent of the ventricular system.

The definitive relationship of the diencephalon and brain stem to the cerebral hemispheres

Study these relationships, many of which have already been alluded to, in **A, B, C, D, E**.

1. The greater part of the lateral surface of the thalamus is now incorporated into the substance of the medial part of the cerebral hemisphere (**C, D, E**).
2. On the other hand the posterior part of the thalamus, that is the pulvinar, projects backwards as a free structure above the upper part of the midbrain and the geniculate bodies (**A, E, 55E**). It is separate from the adjacent medial aspect of the cerebral hemisphere, and overlies and obscures most of the crus of the fornix and the adjacent part of the choroidal fissure in median sections (**A, E**).
3. The lower anterior two-thirds or so of the thalamus is covered by the ependymal lining of the third ventricle (**A, C, D, E**), but the upper third, between the attachments of the ependymal roof of the third ventricle and the upper part of the choroidal fissure, is a free surface (**A**). This free surface is separated from that of the other thalamus by a space which is indicated in solid black in **C** and **D**.
4. The upper anterior part of the hypothalamus fuses with the medial aspect of the cerebral hemisphere whereas the lower part including the tuber cinereum, the infundibulum, the optic chiasma and the anterior part of the optic tract has a free lateral surface (**C**).
5. The crus cerebri passes upwards forwards and laterally medial to, and separate from, the fimbria and choroidal fissure in the medial wall of the inferior horn of the lateral ventricle (**A, D**). As the crus enters the hemisphere below the thalamus (**55C**) the optic tract (**61B**) sweeps backwards in the angle between it and the choroidal fissure.
6. The midbrain overlies and obscures the lower part of the choroidal fissure and the fimbria in sagittal sections (**A, D**).

The tela choroidea of the forebrain

It has been noted earlier in this chapter that all free surfaces of the brain and spinal cord are covered by a continuous vascular connective tissue layer called the pia mater.

The pia mater which covers the upper and posterior aspects of the corpus callosum, and the upper surfaces of the midbrain and pineal body, is protruded forwards between the converging crura of the fornix as a conical recess. This has its blind apex immediately behind the columns of the fornix above the interventricular foramina. The recess is indicated in solid black in **C** and **D** and may be described as the tela choroidea of the forebrain. In those diagrams and in **A** it is evident that the pial roof of the recess rests on the under surfaces of the hippocampal commissure and the body of the fornix, while the floor is directly applied to the ependymal roofs of the third ventricle and the interventricular foramina. On either side, the lateral wall is in contact with the ependyma of the choroidal fissure in the medial wall of the central part of the lateral ventricle, and below that with the free surface of the thalamus.

MEDIAN SECTION OF FOREBRAIN AND MIDBRAIN

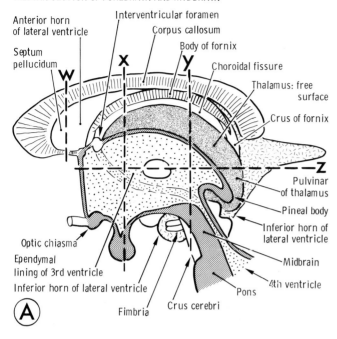

Anterior horn of lateral ventricle

Septum pellucidum

Interventricular foramen

Corpus callosum

Body of fornix

Choroidal fissure

Thalamus: free surface

Crus of fornix

Pulvinar of thalamus

Pineal body

Inferior horn of lateral ventricle

Midbrain

4th ventricle

Pons

Crus cerebri

Fimbria

Inferior horn of lateral ventricle

Ependymal lining of 3rd ventricle

Optic chiasma

W   X   Y

Z

(A)

CORONAL SECTION THROUGH W IN (A)

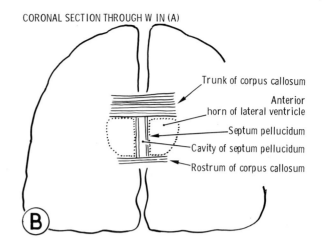

Trunk of corpus callosum

Anterior horn of lateral ventricle

Septum pellucidum

Cavity of septum pellucidum

Rostrum of corpus callosum

(B)

CORONAL SECTION THROUGH X IN (A)

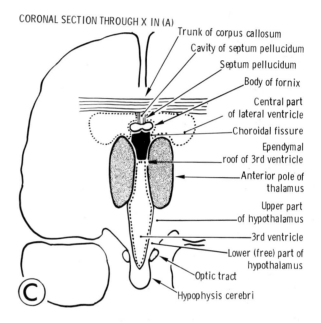

Trunk of corpus callosum

Cavity of septum pellucidum

Septum pellucidum

Body of fornix

Central part of lateral ventricle

Choroidal fissure

Ependymal roof of 3rd ventricle

Anterior pole of thalamus

Upper part of hypothalamus

3rd ventricle

Lower (free) part of hypothalamus

Optic tract

Hypophysis cerebri

(C)

CORONAL SECTION THROUGH Y IN (A)

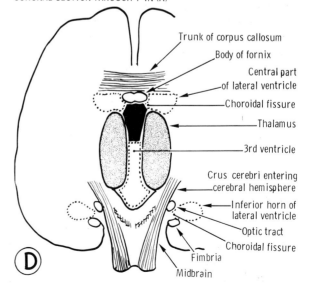

Trunk of corpus callosum

Body of fornix

Central part of lateral ventricle

Choroidal fissure

Thalamus

3rd ventricle

Crus cerebri entering cerebral hemisphere

Inferior horn of lateral ventricle

Optic tract

Choroidal fissure

Fimbria

Midbrain

(D)

HORIZONTAL SECTION THROUGH Z IN (A)

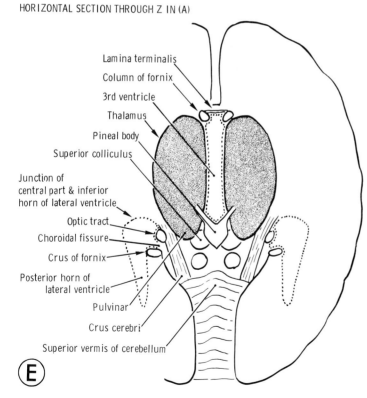

Lamina terminalis

Column of fornix

3rd ventricle

Thalamus

Pineal body

Superior colliculus

Junction of central part & inferior horn of lateral ventricle

Optic tract

Choroidal fissure

Crus of fornix

Posterior horn of lateral ventricle

Pulvinar

Crus cerebri

Superior vermis of cerebellum

(E)

Choroid plexuses of forebrain

The pia mater of the tela choroidea of the forebrain (**A**), together with that which is insinuated into the clefts between the midbrain and the medial aspects of the cerebral hemispheres, invaginates ependymal layers to form two long choroid plexuses, one on either side of the midline (**C**). Each plexus is suspended from the roof of the third ventricle (**A, C**), just to one side of the midline, turns laterally along the roof of the interventricular foramen (**C**), and thereafter is invaginated through the whole length of the choroidal fissure into the body and inferior horn of the lateral ventricle (**A, B**). Frequently the two choroid plexuses are continuous across the midline between the interventricular foramina.

EXTERNAL FEATURES OF THE CEREBRAL HEMISPHERES

As has been noted previously, the surface grey matter is folded during growth into a large number of ridges which are known as gyri and corresponding grooves which are known as sulci.

It is unnecessary to know the names of all these features but the positions of those which are labelled in the relevant diagrams should be memorised.

The superolateral surface of the right hemisphere is shown in **D**. Note particularly the following features, some of which are not evident in that diagram.

1. The lateral sulcus turns from the inferior surface on to the superolateral surface. Here it extends backwards and upwards, turning more sharply upwards at its posterior end. As has been noted previously, during growth the parts of the hemisphere above and below the sulcus form lids or opercula which cover a pear-shaped area of cortex, the insula. The extent of the insula is indicated by the interrupted line in **D**.
2. If the opercula are removed (**E**) the insula is seen to be marked by a number of short gyri and sulci and surrounded by a continuous circular sulcus. Antero-inferiorly, it narrows and turns medially on to the inferior surface of the hemisphere in the depths of the stem of the lateral sulcus. This narrow part is called the limen insulae.
3. The central sulcus begins below, a short distance above the lateral sulcus and extends upwards and backwards across the superolateral surface to a point on its superomedial border a little behind the midpoint between the frontal and occipital poles. Thereafter, as will be seen later, the sulcus turns on to the peripheral part of the medial surface for 1 cm or so.
4. Although the parieto-occipital and calcarine sulci are visible on the superolateral surface (**D**) the major parts of both sulci are on the medial surface of the hemisphere and will be considered later.
5. The four lobes into which each hemisphere is customarily divided are somewhat indefinite regions which are usually related to features on the superolateral surface only (**F**). The occipital lobe lies behind a line joining the parieto-occipital sulcus to the deepest part of the pre-occipital notch. The frontal lobe lies in front of the central sulcus, above the lateral sulcus and in front of a line joining the two sulci. The temporal lobe is situated below the lateral sulcus and below a line joining the terminal bend of that sulcus to the anterior limit of the occipital lobe. The region which occupies the interval between the frontal, temporal and occipital lobes is the parietal lobe.

It should be clearly understood that, although the cerebral lobes bear the same names as bones of the vault of the skull, the lobes and bones do not correspond in extent except in a general and very inexact fashion.

CORONAL SECTION THROUGH TELA CHOROIDEA OF FOREBRAIN & ASSOCIATED CHOROID PLEXUSES

Pia — — — Ependyma ·········

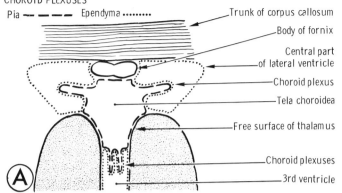

- Trunk of corpus callosum
- Body of fornix
- Central part of lateral ventricle
- Choroid plexus
- Tela choroidea
- Free surface of thalamus
- Choroid plexuses
- 3rd ventricle

DIAGRAMMATIC REPRESENTATION OF CONTINUITY OF CHOROID PLEXUSES OF THIRD & LATERAL VENTRICLES: FROM ABOVE

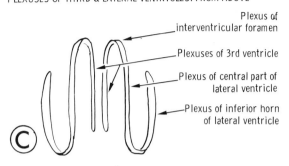

- Plexus of interventricular foramen
- Plexuses of 3rd ventricle
- Plexus of central part of lateral ventricle
- Plexus of inferior horn of lateral ventricle

CORONAL SECTION THROUGH CHOROID PLEXUSES IN INFERIOR HORNS OF LATERAL VENTRICLES

Pia — — — Ependyma ·········

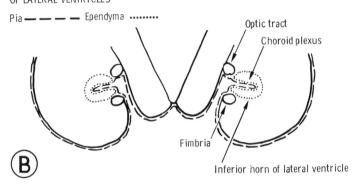

- Optic tract
- Choroid plexus
- Fimbria
- Inferior horn of lateral ventricle

GYRI & SULCI ON SUPEROLATERAL SURFACE OF RIGHT CEREBRAL HEMISPHERE (interrupted line indicates extent of insula)

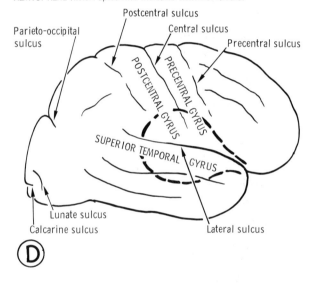

- Postcentral sulcus
- Central sulcus
- Precentral sulcus
- Parieto-occipital sulcus
- POSTCENTRAL GYRUS
- PRECENTRAL GYRUS
- SUPERIOR TEMPORAL GYRUS
- Lunate sulcus
- Calcarine sulcus
- Lateral sulcus

SUPEROLATERAL SURFACE OF RIGHT CEREBRAL HEMISPHERE: INSULA (SHADED) EXPOSED BY REMOVAL OF OPERCULA

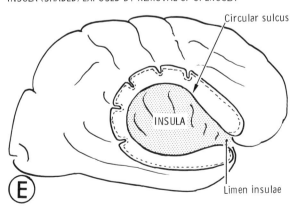

- Circular sulcus
- INSULA
- Limen insulae

LOBES OF RIGHT CEREBRAL HEMISPHERE: SUPEROLATERAL ASPECT

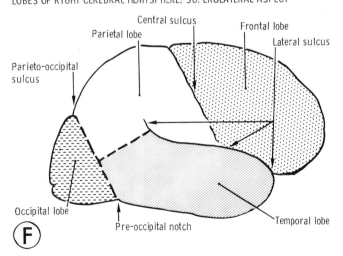

- Central sulcus
- Parietal lobe
- Frontal lobe
- Lateral sulcus
- Parieto-occipital sulcus
- Occipital lobe
- Pre-occipital notch
- Temporal lobe

The medial surface of the cerebral hemisphere is the region above the interrupted line in **A**. The area below the interrupted line in that diagram belongs to the middle and posterior thirds of the inferior surface (**57E**). The structures associated with the central part of the medial surface have been considered (**59A**). Now observe the features of the peripheral part of that surface.

1. As has been seen, although the greater part of the central sulcus is on the superolateral surface of the hemisphere, its upper part turns over the superomedial border and passes downwards for a short distance onto the medial surface. A quadrilateral area surrounds this termination of the central sulcus and is demarcated on three sides by the cingulate sulcus and its branches. This is the paracentral lobule.

2. The calcarine sulcus runs almost horizontally just above the border between the peripheral part of the medial surface and the posterior third of the inferior surface (**A**). It begins, anteriorly, a short distance below the posterior end of the corpus callosum. Posteriorly, in many individuals but not in all, it turns round the occipital pole for a short distance on to the superolateral surface (**65D**).

3. The parieto-occipital sulcus passes upwards and backwards from the anterior part of the calcarine sulcus (**A**). Reaching the upper border of the medial surface it turns a short distance on to the superolateral surface (**65D**).

The inferior surface, which is visible in both **A** and **B**, is divided into thirds. Observe the following features in these diagrams.

1. The anterior (orbital) third of the surface (**B**) is limited posteriorly by the limen insulae which, as has been seen above, is a strip of grey matter which forms the floor of the stem of the lateral sulcus and is continuous laterally with the insula.

2. Lying against, but not attached to, the olfactory sulcus on the anterior third of the inferior surface is a narrow white band which is an extension of the brain substance called the olfactory tract (**B**). The slightly expanded anterior end of the tract is the olfactory bulb. Posteriorly the tract becomes continuous with the brain substance and divides into divergent medial and lateral roots. The lateral root crosses the surface of the limen insulae and ends within the uncus (**B**). The medial root passes medially, and then upwards above the optic chiasma, and ends in the structures comprising the septal areas of the limbic system (**75A, 75B**).

3. A small area of the inferior surface is surrounded by the optic tract, the roots of the olfactory tract and the uncus. As the area is penetrated by a number of small but important arteries, it is known as the anterior perforated substance. It is continuous laterally with the limen insulae.

4. The continuous gyrus which extends along the medial margin of the middle and posterior thirds of the inferior surface (**A, B**) is named the lingual gyrus posteriorly and the parahippocampal gyrus anteriorly. It is limited below and laterally by the collateral sulcus. The anterior end of the parahippocampal gyrus is recurved backwards and medially and is known as the uncus.

5. Above the parahippocampal gyrus, the fimbria, which has already been described as part of the fornix system, runs from before backwards (**A**). It will be recalled that it lies in the medial wall of the inferior horn of the lateral ventricle immediately below the choroidal fissure (**65B**). A narrow gyrus passes from before backwards between the fimbria and the parahippocampal gyrus. It is usually obscured by these two structures but can be exposed by separating them gently from one another. Its surface is marked by very characteristic transverse grooves and it is consequently known as the dentate gyrus (**A**). Anteriorly the dentate gyrus ends in the uncus. Posteriorly it turns upwards, loses its dentate form, gradually separates from the fimbria and the crus of the fornix, and as the splenial gyrus (gyrus fasciolaris) passes round the splenium of the corpus callosum on to its upper surface. There the paired splenial gyri become continuous with a film of grey matter which covers the upper surface of the corpus callosum and is called the indusium griseum. On either side this grey matter becomes continuous with that of the cingulate gyrus, while anteriorly it merges on either side with the cortex of the paraterminal gyrus (**A**).

6. The hippocampal sulcus, which separates the dentate and parahippocampal gyri, bulges the cortical grey matter, covered by a thin lamina of white matter known as the alveus, into the inferior horn of the lateral ventricle as a rounded longitudinal elevation running from before backwards along its floor (**C**). This is known as the hippocampus, and it is the fibres of the alveus which stream backwards and laterally to form the fimbria.

RIGHT CEREBRAL HEMISPHERE: MEDIAL ASPECT

(Medial surface above interrupted line, inferior surface below)

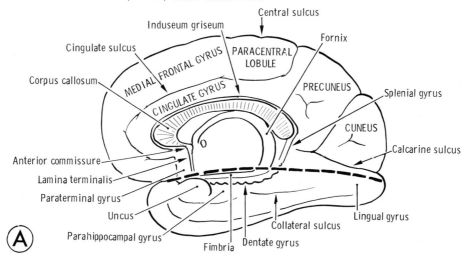

Central sulcus
Induseum griseum
Fornix
Cingulate sulcus
PARACENTRAL LOBULE
MEDIAL FRONTAL GYRUS
Corpus callosum
PRECUNEUS
CINGULATE GYRUS
Splenial gyrus
CUNEUS
Anterior commissure
Calcarine sulcus
Lamina terminalis
Paraterminal gyrus
Lingual gyrus
Uncus
Collateral sulcus
Parahippocampal gyrus
Fimbria
Dentate gyrus

(A)

RIGHT CEREBRAL HEMISPHERE: INFERIOR SURFACE

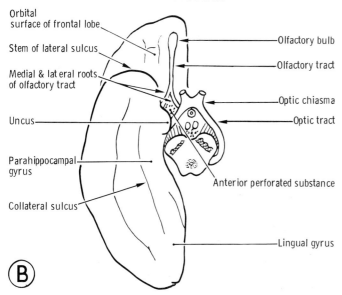

Orbital surface of frontal lobe
Olfactory bulb
Stem of lateral sulcus
Olfactory tract
Medial & lateral roots of olfactory tract
Optic chiasma
Uncus
Optic tract
Parahippocampal gyrus
Collateral sulcus
Anterior perforated substance
Lingual gyrus

(B)

CORONAL SECTION OF MIDDLE THIRD OF INFERIOR SURFACE OF HEMISPHERE

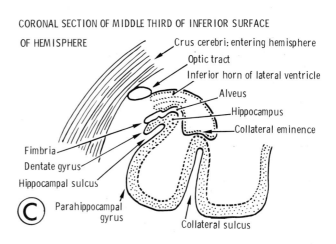

Crus cerebri: entering hemisphere
Optic tract
Inferior horn of lateral ventricle
Alveus
Hippocampus
Collateral eminence
Fimbria
Dentate gyrus
Hippocampal sulcus
Parahippocampal gyrus
Collateral sulcus

(C)

Cortical functional areas

The sensorimotor areas are four in number in each hemisphere, and they are described by this term because none of them is purely sensory or purely motor. On the contrary, each is concerned both in the appreciation of somatic sensation and in the initiation and integration of skeletal muscle activity. However because, in each, one of these two characteristics is dominant the areas are named accordingly as somatomotor or somatosensory

1. The primary somatomotor area is shown in **A** and **B**. Correlate its extent with the named surface features already considered in **65D, 67A** and note that, although it is not evident in **A**, the area includes the anterior wall of the central sulcus. The skeletal muscular activities of different parts of the body are represented in this cortical area in a more or less inverted order (**C**) although it will be noted that the eyeball is represented well above the tongue. The size of each representative cortical area is a function of the intricacy and delicacy of the movements involved in the normal function of the part of the body it represents, rather than the size of that part. Thus the cortical representation of the fingers is much larger than that of the trunk.
2. A supplementary somatomotor area is shown in **B**. It will be noted that it abuts on the primary somatomotor area both above and behind. However, within this area the somatotopic representation is horizontal, the muscles of the head region being associated with its anterior part and those of the leg and foot with its posterior part, adjacent to the leg and foot area of the primary somatomotor cortex.
3. The primary somatosensory area (**A, B**) occupies the posterior wall of the central sulcus, the postcentral gyrus and the postcentral part of the paracentral lobule. The representation of the parts of the body within this area is similar to that already noted in the primary somatomotor area (**D**). It is not, however, identical because the extent of a part's representation appears to be a function of the relative modalities of sensation, so that sensations derived from skin are appreciated in the anterior part of the area and proprioceptive sensations in the posterior part.
4. The supplementary somatosensory area is small and lies between the lower end of the primary area and the lateral sulcus (**A**). As in the supplementary somatomotor area the somatotopic representation is in a horizontal direction with the head anteriorly and the leg and foot posteriorly. There is some evidence that this area is particularly associated with the appreciation of pain.

The speech areas which are concerned with muscular activities inherent in speech, and with the understanding of language, are concentrated on one hemisphere in the majority of individuals. Usually, but not always, this is the left hemisphere in the right-handed and vice versa. There is evidence of a similar though lesser asymmetry in other cortical areas so that it is reasonable to use the term dominant hemisphere. The three speech areas which are usually present on the dominant hemisphere are shown in **A, B**. Note that the anterior area (Broca's area) is part of the primary somatomotor area, that the superior area is part of the supplementary motor area and that the posterior area is close to both the acoustic cortical area and visual area (III) (see below).

The visual areas are three adjacent cortical areas which are concerned with the reception and interpretation of impulses from the light sensitive layer of the eye called the retina. It seems reasonable to consider also in this section two motor eye fields which are concerned with movements of the eyes.

1. Visual area I is the primary receptive area for retinal impulses. It is shown in **B, A** but it should be noted that a large part of the area is hidden on the walls of the calcarine sulcus. It will be seen later that the area receives impulses from parts of both retinae and that these parts are represented within the area in a specific orderly manner.
2. Visual areas II and III (**A, B**) surround area I, except around its anterior extremity, so that part of area III is closely related to the posterior speech area (**A**). These areas appear to be involved in the integration and interpretation of the visual information reaching area I.
3. The occipital eye field lies within the visual areas I and II and is consequently sensorimotor in nature (**B**). It is concerned in reflex eye movements stimulated by visual impulses.
4. The frontal eye field is part of the primary somatomotor area (**A**) and motivates voluntary eye movements.

The acoustic area can be seen in part in **A** on the upper margin of the superior temporal gyrus but it should be appreciated that the greater part of the area is situated on the deep (insular) aspect of the gyrus and cannot be seen until the lips of the lateral sulcus are widely separated. It will be seen later that the acoustic area of one hemisphere receives and interprets impulses from the cochleae of both internal ears.

The olfactory area is small in man. It is situated over the anterior end of the uncus and parahippocampal gyrus and probably includes that part of the amygdaloid body which is structurally continuous with the cortex of the uncus and the anterior perforated substance (**B**). It differs from other sensory cortical areas in receiving its afferent fibres directly from the brain surface instead of from the interior of the hemisphere after relay in the thalamus or metathalamus.

SPECIAL FUNCTIONAL CORTICAL AREAS: SUPEROLATERAL SURFACE

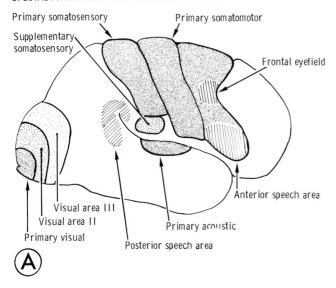

Primary somatosensory

Primary somatomotor

Supplementary somatosensory

Frontal eyefield

Anterior speech area

Visual area III

Visual area II

Primary acoustic

Primary visual

Posterior speech area

A

SPECIAL FUNCTIONAL CORTICAL AREAS: MEDIAL & INFERIOR SURFACES

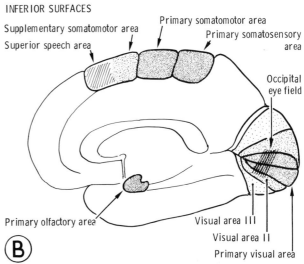

Supplementary somatomotor area

Primary somatomotor area

Superior speech area

Primary somatosensory area

Occipital eye field

Primary olfactory area

Visual area III

Visual area II

Primary visual area

B

REGIONAL REPRESENTATION IN PRIMARY SOMATOMOTOR CORTEX

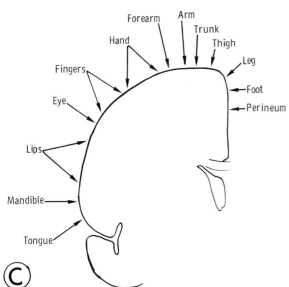

Forearm   Arm
Hand   Trunk
                        Thigh
Fingers   Leg
Eye   Foot
                          Perineum
Lips

Mandible

Tongue

C

REGIONAL REPRESENTATION IN PRIMARY SOMATOSENSORY CORTEX

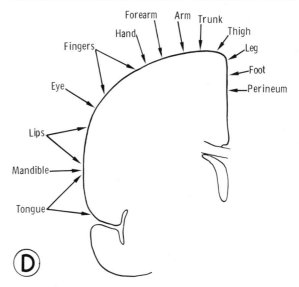

Forearm   Arm   Trunk
Hand   Thigh
Fingers   Leg
Eye   Foot
                         Perineum
Lips

Mandible

Tongue

D

69

INTERNAL FEATURES OF THE CEREBRAL HEMISPHERES

Within the white core of each hemisphere are a number of subcortical masses of grey matter. One is the thalamus and it has been seen already how its lateral surface, except in the region of the pulvinar, is incorporated into the medial aspect of the hemisphere during development. The other grey masses, known as the caudate and lentiform nuclei, the claustrum and the amygdaloid body, have varying degrees of individuality and are described collectively as the basal nuclei.

Passing through, between and around these grey masses, are tracts of white fibres of three types.

1. Projection fibres connect the cerebral cortex with the subcortical nuclei of the hemisphere and with grey matter in the brain stem and spinal cord.
2. Commissural fibres connect the two hemispheres across the midline.
3. Association fibres connect different cortical regions within one hemisphere.

The basal nuclei

The caudate nucleus is in the form of a **C**, convex forwards. Its shape and its relationship to the thalamus are shown diagrammatically in **A** and **B** and its relationships to other cerebral structures are evident in the sections (**D, E, 73B**).

The nucleus tapers in girth from its anterosuperior to its antero-inferior end and is customarily divided into named parts which have no exact limits (**A**). Observe the following features.

1. The thalamus is related anteriorly to the bulbous head (**A, B, C**) and above and somewhat laterally to the tapering body (**A, B, E**). The tail of the nucleus turns downwards and laterally, becoming gradually separated from the lateral surface of the thalmus (**B**), and thereafter turns forwards and laterally into the temporal lobe. Here it is separated from the lower part of the thalamus by a considerable interval, the importance of which will be seen later (**A, B, E**).
2. Most parts of the lateral ventricle are closely related to the nucleus. The head bulges massively into the inferolateral wall of the anterior horn and continues downwards for some distance below it (**D, 73B**). The body forms the lateral part of the inferolateral wall of the central part of the ventricle (**E**). The tail lies a short distance from the inferior horn, at first anterior to it (**73B**) and then above it (**E**).
3. As the fibres of the corpus callosum penetrate into the hemisphere many become closely related to parts of the nucleus. The rostral fibres descend below the

head (**D**) while those of the genu pass in front of it (**73B**). The fibres of the trunk pass above both the head and body (**D, E**).

The lentiform nucleus is seen from the lateral side lying on a plane lateral to that of the thalamus and the upper part of the caudate nucleus in the diagram (**C**) and in the sections (**D, E, 73B**). It is an oval mass (**C**) which is triangular in both coronal (**E**) and horizontal sections (**73B**), and consists of two distinct parts of different colour. The smaller medial part which is pale is called the globus pallidus while the larger and darker lateral part is the putamen.

The nucleus does not extend as high as the body or as low as the tail of the caudate and does not pass as far back as either the caudate or the thalamus (**C**). On the other hand, anteriorly the head of the caudate and the anterior part of the putamen are co-extensive (**C, 73B**).

Laterally the putamen is almost co-extensive with the insular cortex, with the claustrum intervening (**E, 73B**). On the medial side the lowest part of the bulging caudate head and the lower anterior part of the putamen are directly continuous just above the anterior perforated substance (**D**). Above and behind this zone of continuity the lentiform is separated from the head and body of the caudate and the thalamus by a wide interval occupied by projection fibres and known as the internal capsule (**E, 73B**).

The amygdaloid body is a smaller nucleus than the caudate or the lentiform. It lies in the temporal lobe above the extremity of the inferior horn of the lateral ventricle and continuous with both the anterior end of the tail of the caudate nucleus (**A, B, C**) and with the grey matter of the uncus and anterior perforated substance.

The claustrum is a thin sheet of grey matter which intervenes between, and is practically coextensive with, the insular cortex and the putamen. The white matter separating it from the putamen is called the external capsule (**E, 73B**).

The stria terminalis, although it is a bundle of white fibres, may be mentioned here because of its close topographical relationship with some of the basal nuclei. It arises from the amygdaloid body and runs backwards and then upwards on the medial side of the tail of the caudate nucleus (**B, E**). It then turns forwards in the groove between caudate nucleus and the upper aspect of the thalamus in the floor of the central part of the lateral ventricle (**B, E**). Below the interventricular foramen its fibres diverge, most reaching the ipsilateral septum pellucidum, paraterminal gyrus and anterior perforated substance while others join the opposite stria through the anterior commissure and pass through it to the opposite amygdaloid body.

THALAMUS & CAUDATE NUCLEUS: LATERAL VIEW

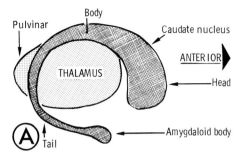

THALAMUS & CAUDATE NUCLEUS: FROM ABOVE

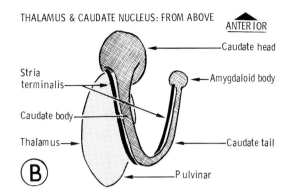

THALAMUS & CAUDATE & LENTIFORM NUCLEI:
LATERAL VIEW

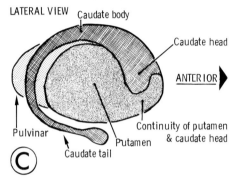

RIGHT HEMISPHERE: CORONAL SECTION

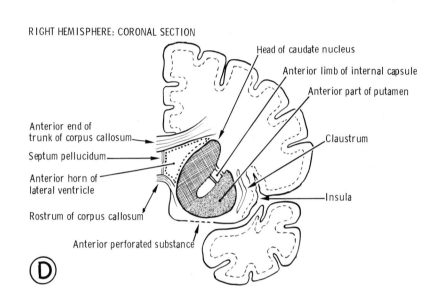

RIGHT HEMISPHERE: CORONAL SECTION

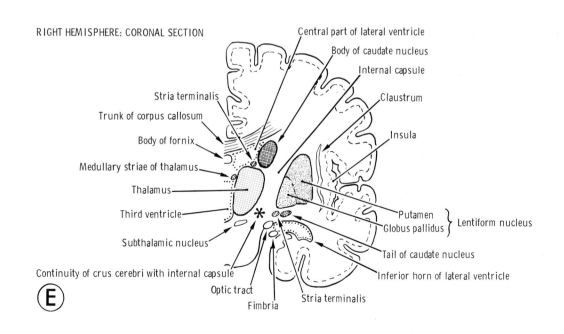

The internal capsule

Once continuity of the diencephalon and the midbrain with the central part of each cerebral hemisphere has been established during development, a large compact tract of ascending and descending fibres can be traced upwards from the crus cerebri and the geniculate bodies into the interval within the hemisphere between the inferior aspect of the thalamus and the horizontal part of the tail of the caudate nucleus (**A, 71E**). This is the lowest part of the internal capsule.

Just above this point some of the lateral fibres of the tract turn laterally above the tail of the caudate nucleus, and, passing below the posterior pole of the lentiform nucleus, the claustrum and the insula, reach the temporal lobe (**A, C**). These constitute the sublentiform part of the internal capsule.

A little further into the hemisphere the most posterior fibres of the capsule lie lateral to the thalamus but in a position posterior to the posterior pole of the putamen of the lentiform nucleus (**A, C**). This retrolentiform part of the capsule hooks backwards round the lateral side of the posterior parts of the caudate nucleus and passes into the occipital lobe (**C**) on the lateral side of the posterior horn of the lateral ventricle.

The rest of the fibres of the capsule diverge upwards and forwards through the interval between the medial aspect of the lentiform nucleus and the lateral aspects of the thalamus and the head and body of the caudate nucleus (**A, B, C, 71E**). Here they are joined by many additional fibres ascending and descending between the cortex of the frontal and parietal lobes and the thalamus and the basal nuclei. In horizontal section (**C**) this main part of the internal capsule is seen to be angled around the medial convexity of the lentiform nucleus, and it is described as consisting of an anterior limb, a genu and a posterior limb. The anterior limb lies between the lentiform and the caudate head and above and behind the region of continuity between the antero-inferior parts of these two nuclei (**A, 71D**). Indeed, a lesser degree of this continuity exists within the anterior limb itself as fine strands of grey matter (**C**) and the striated appearance caused by these strands is the origin of the term corpus striatum which is a collective name for the caudate and lentiform nuclei.

As the fibres of the internal capsule are traced above the level of the basal nuclei they fan out to all parts of the frontal and parietal lobes (**A**). This upward continuation of the capsule is called the corona radiata.

The cerebral commissures

The corpus callosum, as seen between the two cerebral hemispheres, has already been considered (**61F**). Entering the hemispheres its fibres diverge to connect nearly all corresponding right and left cortical areas, though it may be noted that there are some exceptions to this general pattern.

As the fibres diverge through the hemispheres they intersect with the projection fibres of the corona radiata and with numerous bundles of association fibres and have a particularly close relationship to most parts of the lateral ventricle. In the latter respect the rostral fibres form the narrow floor of the anterior horn (**71D**) and the fibres of the genu its anterior wall (**B**). The trunk fibres form the roof of the anterior horn and central part of the ventricle (**71D, 71E**) while the splenial fibres extend as a discrete sheet called the tapetum across the roof and lateral wall of the posterior horn (**C**).

The anterior commissure crosses the midline in the upper part of the lamina terminalis (**67A**). It penetrates into each hemisphere as a compact bundle which passes laterally through the region of fusion between the head of the caudate nucleus and the putamen (**D**) and subsequently spreads out to reach the cortex of the temporal lobe.

The hippocampal commissure has been seen as a thin lamina of transverse fibres joining the converging crura of the fornix (**61C, 61D**). Through the fimbria and crura of the fornix, it establishes communication between the right and left hippocampal formations.

The association fibres

One example of the very numerous sets of short association fibres and most of the main long association bundles are shown diagrammatically in **E**. Note the following features.

1. The cingulum runs in the white matter of the cingulate and parahippocampal gyri (**67A**).
2. The fronto-occipital fasciculus passes to the medial side of the lower part of the corona radiata.
3. The superior longitudinal fasciculus, which is not shown in **E**, passes on the lateral side of the lower part of the corona radiata and connects the frontal to the occipital and temporal regions of the cortex.
4. The uncinate fasciculus connects the anterior speech area which lies on the superolateral surface of the hemisphere (**69A**) with the cortex over the temporal pole.

INTERNAL CAPSULE, THALAMUS & CAUDATE NUCLEUS: LATERAL VIEW

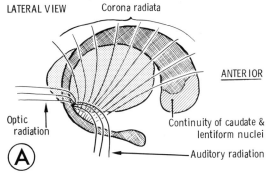

Corona radiata

ANTERIOR

Optic radiation

Continuity of caudate & lentiform nuclei

Auditory radiation

(A)

RIGHT HEMISPHERE: HORIZONTAL SECTION

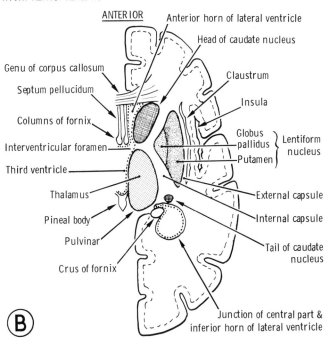

ANTERIOR

Genu of corpus callosum

Septum pellucidum

Columns of fornix

Interventricular foramen

Third ventricle

Thalamus

Pineal body

Pulvinar

Crus of fornix

Anterior horn of lateral ventricle

Head of caudate nucleus

Claustrum

Insula

Globus pallidus } Lentiform nucleus
Putamen }

External capsule

Internal capsule

Tail of caudate nucleus

Junction of central part & inferior horn of lateral ventricle

(B)

ANTERIOR COMMISSURE: CORONAL SECTION

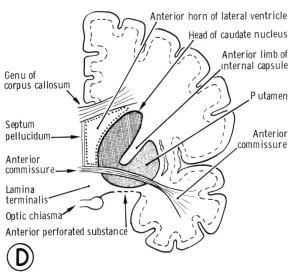

Anterior horn of lateral ventricle

Head of caudate nucleus

Anterior limb of internal capsule

Putamen

Anterior commissure

Genu of corpus callosum

Septum pellucidum

Anterior commissure

Lamina terminalis

Optic chiasma

Anterior perforated substance

(D)

INTERNAL CAPSULE: HORIZONTAL SECTION

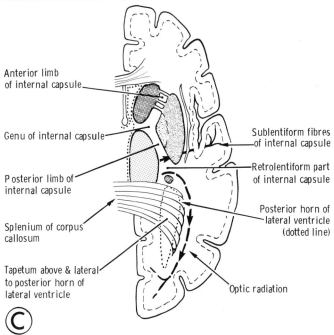

Anterior limb of internal capsule

Genu of internal capsule

Posterior limb of internal capsule

Splenium of corpus callosum

Tapetum above & lateral to posterior horn of lateral ventricle

Sublentiform fibres of internal capsule

Retrolentiform part of internal capsule

Posterior horn of lateral ventricle (dotted line)

Optic radiation

(C)

DIAGRAMMATIC PLAN OF ASSOCIATION FIBRES

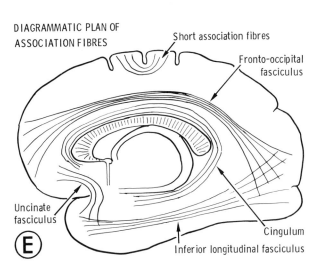

Short association fibres

Fronto-occipital fasciculus

Uncinate fasciculus

Cingulum

Inferior longitudinal fasciculus

(E)

The limbic lobe or system

This is a neurophysiological concept in which a large number of structures belonging to the cerebral hemispheres, the diencephalon and the midbrain are profusely and reciprocally interconnected. No less an authority than Brodal has stated 'It is difficult to see that the lumping together of these different regions under one anatomical heading, the limbic lobe, serves any purpose.' However, because of the interest the concept has for physiologists and psychiatrists it seems necessary to give a very brief account of its anatomical basis. And because nearly all the structures it includes have already been described elsewhere, the account can be highly diagrammatic. For the sake of simplicity two diagrams are used but it will be noted that they have common features.

Diagram **A** shows the connections of the olfactory bulb and tract with the septal areas, which include the septum pellucidum (**63A**) the paraterminal gyrus (**67A**) and the anterior perforated substance, and with the amygdaloid body, and the connection between these two entities through the stria terminalis (**71B, 71E**). The two entities in turn are connected in both directions with many of the hypothalamic nuclei (**55D**) and the midbrain reticular formation (**47E, 47F**) by fibres which run longitudinally through the diencephalon and are called the medial forebrain bundle. The other component shown stippled in this diagram is the medullary stria of the thalamus which draws fibres from the septal areas, the amygdaloid body and the hypothalamus, gives attachment to the ependymal roof of the third ventricle (**55A**) and ends in the habenular nucleus (**55E**). This small nucleus connects with the midbrain reticular formation.

Diagram **B** shows what may be described as the limbic areas of cortex. Note the following features.

1. The cingulate and parahippocampal gyri (**67A**) are interconnected by the association bundle called the cingulum (**73E**).
2. The dentate gyrus becomes continuous through the splenial gyrus with the induseum griseum (**67A**) which blends laterally with the grey matter of the cingulate gyrus.
3. The cingulate gyrus and induseum griseum are continuous anteriorly with the septal areas.
4. The hippocampus lies in the floor of the inferior horn of the lateral ventricle (**67C**). Its afferent connections are predominantly olfactory via the anterior part of the parahippocampal gyrus. Its efferent fibres pass almost wholly via the alveus, through the fimbria, crus, body and column of the fornix, to reach the hypothalamic nuclei, particularly that in the mamillary body (**55D**). The two hippocampi are interconnected through the hippocampal commissure (**61C, 61D**).
5. From the mamillary body the hippocampal outflow continues through the mamillothalamic tract (**55D**) and the profuse two-way thalamo-cingulate projection to the cingulate gyrus.
6. The limbic cortex is thus connected to the two-way medial forebrain bundle (**A**) at two sites, in the septal areas and in the hypothalamus.

ORDINARY SENSORY INPUT INTO THE CENTRAL NERVOUS SYSTEM

Impulses concerned with ordinary sensation of both somatic and visceral origin enter the central nervous system through the spinal nerves or through those cranial nerves having sensory ganglia, namely the trigeminal, glossopharyngeal and vagus nerves.

In the case of the spinal nerves, the impulses are conducted through the posterior nerve rootlets along the central processes of pseudo-unipolar cells in the dorsal root ganglia (**C**). Entering the spinal cord these fibres divide into ascending and descending divisions which run in the intersegmental tracts (**37A**) and give off collateral branches into the central grey matter in a variable number of spinal segments (**C**). These divisions and their collateral branches may terminate in three general ways.

1. Some ascending divisions, having given off collateral branches, continue upwards without interruption and form the first order fibres in an ascending spinal tract.
2. Some of the collaterals of ascending divisions synapse with cells in the posterior grey columns which give rise to second order fibres in an ascending spinal tract.
3. Most of the collaterals of both ascending and descending divisions form intrasegmental or intersegmental reflex circuits, either directly (monosynaptic) or indirectly (polysynaptic) with somatic motor cells in the anterior column of the central grey matter or with visceral motor cells in the intermediate grey column.

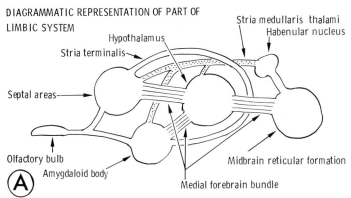

DIAGRAMMATIC REPRESENTATION OF PART OF
LIMBIC SYSTEM

Hypothalamus

Stria medullaris thalami
Habenular nucleus

Stria terminalis

Septal areas

Olfactory bulb

Amygdaloid body

Midbrain reticular formation

Medial forebrain bundle

(A)

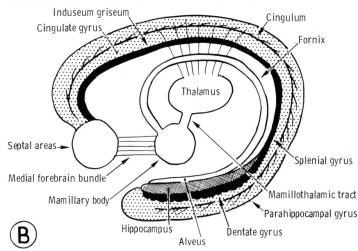

DIAGRAMMATIC REPRESENTATION OF PART OF LIMBIC SYSTEM

Induseum griseum

Cingulate gyrus

Cingulum

Fornix

Thalamus

Septal areas

Medial forebrain bundle

Mamillary body

Splenial gyrus

Mamillothalamic tract

Parahippocampal gyrus

Hippocampus

Alveus

Dentate gyrus

(B)

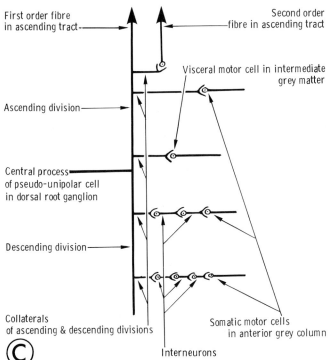

SCHEME OF SENSORY INPUT THROUGH SPINAL NERVES

First order fibre
in ascending tract

Second order
fibre in ascending tract

Visceral motor cell in intermediate
grey matter

Ascending division

Central process
of pseudo-unipolar cell
in dorsal root ganglion

Descending division

Collaterals
of ascending & descending divisions

Somatic motor cells
in anterior grey column

(C)

Interneurons

The gracile and cuneate fasciculi and medial lemniscus

These fasciculi occupy the posterior funiculus of the spinal cord and are demarcated by an incomplete septum (**A, B**). They consist of first order fibres which are the direct continuations of the ascending divisions of posterior rootlet fibres of the same side transmitting impulses concerned with proprioceptive sensations and fine tactile sensibility. Fibres from the lowest spinal nerves turn upwards adjacent to the posterior median septum, and those from successively higher nerves are added in progressively more lateral positions. Thus fibres entering below the mid-thoracic level of the cord form the medially-placed fasciculus gracilis which extends the whole length of the cord (**A, B**), while those entering above this level form the fasciculus cuneatus which is confined to the upper part of the cord (**B**).

The fibres of both fasciculi continue upwards into the brain stem and terminate about the middle of the medulla by synapsing with the cells of the nucleus gracilis or nucleus cuneatus (**B, C**). Throughout their spinal course the fibres of both fasciculi give off collateral branches which will be considered in the next section.

Second order fibres originating from the cells of the gracile and cuneate nuclei pass forwards and medially round the central grey matter (internal arcuate fibres) and after decussating across the midline (decussation of the lemnisci) turn upwards on the opposite side as the medial lemniscus (**C**).

In the upper half of the medulla the medial lemniscus occupies a sagittally elongated area adjacent to the midline and between the pyramid and the central grey matter in the floor of the fourth ventricle (**D**).

In the pons the lemniscus occupies a coronally elongated area in the anterior part of the tegmentum (**E**). At this level it is joined at its medial edge by fibres mediating tactile sensations from the head, which have arisen in the main sensory nucleus (**E**) of the opposite trigeminal nerve and have passed obliquely upwards and across the midline (**E**).

In the midbrain the appearance of centrally placed structures such as the red nuclei (**F**) displaces the lemniscus into the lateral part of the tegmentum and reorientates it once again.

As can be seen in the diagrammatic oblique section through a cerebral hemisphere and the corresponding half of the midbrain in **G**, the fibres of the lemniscus pass from the interval between the red nucleus and the substantia nigra in the tegmentum of the midbrain into the thalamus. They relay, and the third order fibres arising from the cells of the thalamus pass laterally into the posterior limb of the internal capsule. Passing upwards through that part, and then through the corona radiata, they end in the primary somatosensory cortex (**69A**) in the orderly pattern already described (**69D**).

The spinothalamic tract and spinal lemniscus

The fibres entering the spinal cord conveying impulses aroused by painful stimuli to both somatic and visceral structures, and by the thermal, tactile and pressure stimuli to somatic structures, give off collaterals which synapse with the cells of the nucleus proprius (**37B–F**) on the side of entry (**A**). The second order fibres arising from these cells decussate through the white commissure and turn upwards as a diffuse tract in the adjacent parts of the anterior and lateral funiculi of the opposite side of the cord (**A, B**). The fibres issuing into the anterior rootlets of the spinal nerves divide the tract (**A, B**) into an anterior part which is predominantly concerned with touch and pressure and a lateral part concerned mainly with pain and temperature.

The tract continues through the medulla in a superficial situation between the olive and the spinal trigeminal nucleus (**C**). Here it is joined by second order fibres arising in the opposite trigeminal spinal nucleus and mediating pain and temperature from the opposite side of the head region (**D**).

In the pons the tract becomes continuous with the lateral margin of the medial lemniscus and may be described thereafter as the spinal lemniscus (**E**).

Beyond this point the courses of the medial and spinal lemnisci are the same (**F**).

In the brain stem the spinothalamic tract becomes progressively smaller and this is probably due to the passage of groups of its fibres into the nuclei of the reticular formation, the olive and the superior colliculus. These offshoots constitute the spinoreticular, spino-olivary and spinotectal tracts.

It may be noted that, as in the case of the posterior funicular tracts, so in the spinothalamic tract sensation is projected to the contralateral cerebral cortex along three neuron pathways. The main differences between the medial and spinal lemnisci are the sites of the first synapse and the site of the decussation to the opposite side of the central nervous system.

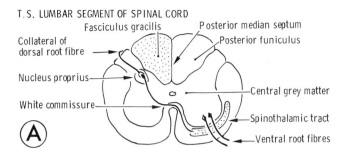

T.S. LUMBAR SEGMENT OF SPINAL CORD

Fasciculus gracilis
Posterior median septum
Posterior funiculus
Collateral of dorsal root fibre
Nucleus proprius
White commissure
Central grey matter
Spinothalamic tract
Ventral root fibres

(A)

T.S. CERVICAL SEGMENT OF SPINAL CORD

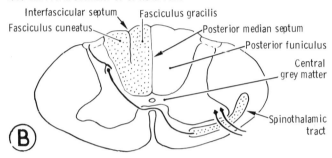

Interfascicular septum
Fasciculus gracilis
Fasciculus cuneatus
Posterior median septum
Posterior funiculus
Central grey matter
Spinothalamic tract

(B)

T.S. MID-MEDULLA

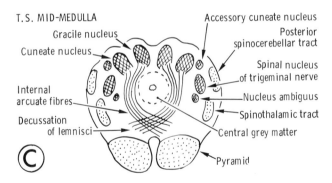

Gracile nucleus
Cuneate nucleus
Accessory cuneate nucleus
Posterior spinocerebellar tract
Spinal nucleus of trigeminal nerve
Nucleus ambiguus
Spinothalamic tract
Internal arcuate fibres
Decussation of lemnisci
Central grey matter
Pyramid

(C)

T.S. UPPER PART OF MEDULLA

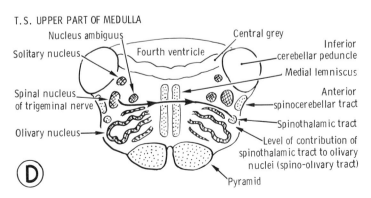

Nucleus ambiguus
Central grey
Solitary nucleus
Fourth ventricle
Inferior cerebellar peduncle
Medial lemniscus
Spinal nucleus of trigeminal nerve
Anterior spinocerebellar tract
Spinothalamic tract
Olivary nucleus
Level of contribution of spinothalamic tract to olivary nuclei (spino-olivary tract)
Pyramid

(D)

T.S. MID-PONS

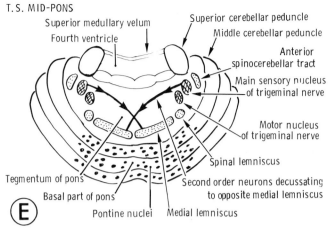

Superior medullary velum
Fourth ventricle
Superior cerebellar peduncle
Middle cerebellar peduncle
Anterior spinocerebellar tract
Main sensory nucleus of trigeminal nerve
Motor nucleus of trigeminal nerve
Spinal lemniscus
Second order neurons decussating to opposite medial lemniscus
Tegmentum of pons
Basal part of pons
Pontine nuclei
Medial lemniscus

(E)

T.S. UPPER PART OF MIDBRAIN

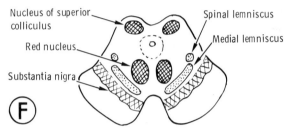

Nucleus of superior colliculus
Spinal lemniscus
Red nucleus
Medial lemniscus
Substantia nigra

(F)

OBLIQUE SECTION OF CEREBRAL HEMISPHERE & MIDBRAIN

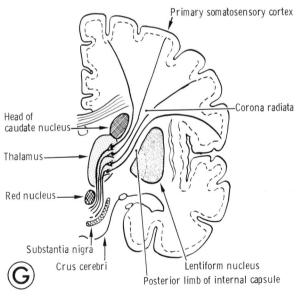

Primary somatosensory cortex
Corona radiata
Head of caudate nucleus
Thalamus
Red nucleus
Substantia nigra
Crus cerebri
Lentiform nucleus
Posterior limb of internal capsule

(G)

The spinocerebellar tracts

It has been noted above that fibres in the gracile and cuneate fasciculi give off collateral branches as they ascend the spinal cord. These end in two situations.

Those arising at lumbar and thoracic levels pass laterally and end by synapsing with the cells of the nucleus dorsalis in the base of the posterior grey column of the same side (**A**). The second order fibres coming from these cells pass into the lateral funiculus of the same side where they turn upwards as the posterior spinocerebellar tract (**A**). This occupies a surface position immediately in front of the dorsolateral fasciculus, and then ascends on the lateral surface of the lower half of the medulla (**77C**) before passing into the cerebellum through the ipsilateral inferior cerebellar peduncle (**B**).

The collaterals springing from the fibres of cervical origin in the lateral part of the fasciculus cuneatus ascend to synapse with the cells of the accessory cuneate nucleus of the same side (**77B, 77C**). Second order fibres arising from these cells form a cuneocerebellar tract which follows the posterior spinocerebellar tract into the cerebellum (**B**).

The pathway followed by the anterior spinocerebellar tract in the spinal cord and brain stem is shown in **A, B, 77D, 77E**. Note that, having passed through the pons, the tract bends acutely downwards and enters the cerebellum through the superior cerebellar peduncle (**B**). However the mode of formation of the tract, its function and the manner in which it ends are all somewhat uncertain.

It is probable that collaterals of posterior rootlet fibres transmitting proprioceptive impulses synapse in the basal part of the posterior grey column on the side of entry, and that the second order fibres originating in that region then cross the midline before turning upwards in the tract of the opposite side (**A**).

It also seems probable that, having passed through the superior cerebellar peduncle, these second order fibres cross the midline a second time before reaching the cerebellar cortex.

Thus it is likely that all spinocerebellar pathways consist of two neurons and transmit proprioceptive impulses from spinal nerves to the ipsilateral cerebellar cortex.

Ordinary sensation transmitted by the IX and X nerves

Although both these nerves transmit the sensation of taste which will be considered with other special sensations, both also transmit a number of types of ordinary sensation from a variety of situations. The neurons concerned are pseudo-unipolar and their cell bodies are in the sensory ganglia which lie on the upper parts of both nerves.

1. It is probable that impulses aroused by tactile and painful stimuli to the mucosa of the pharynx, which is innervated by the glossopharyngeal nerve, or to the small skin area supplied by the vagus, are relayed from the central processes of these nerves through the appropriate trigeminal sensory nucleus to the medial and spinal lemnisci.
2. Those general visceral sensations which are transmitted from thoracic and abdominal viscera through the vagus (and do not include pain) appear to reach either the nucleus solitarius (**49A**) or the dorsal vagal nucleus (**53A**). They are undoubtedly concerned in the formation of diverse reflex circuits, but the pathways involved in their projection to higher levels are not known.

SPECIAL SENSORY INPUT INTO THE CENTRAL NERVOUS SYSTEM

The auditory pathways

As has been seen earlier (**51C**) the central processes of the bipolar cells in the spiral ganglion of the cochlea (**407A**) reach the lowest part of the pons in the cochlear part of the vestibulocochlear nerve and synapse there in the dorsal and ventral cochlear nuclei. The second order fibres arising in these nuclei encircle the inferior cerebellar peduncle and pass into the anterior part of the tegmentum of the pons.

Here many decussate with corresponding fibres of the opposite side intersecting the spinal and medial lemnisci in the process. They form a thick transverse band of fibres called the trapezoid body which contains a number of nuclei in which the decussating fibres relay. Other fibres from the cochlear nuclei relay in the most lateral of the trapezoid nuclei but do not decussate.

Paired lateral lemnisci which lie lateral to, and in the same plane as, the spinal and medial lemnisci ascend from the lateral ends of the trapezoid body (**D**).

The lateral lemnisci thus consist of third order fibres and it is very important to note that each transmits impulses from both cochleae. Consequently, a lesion to one auditory pathway above the trapezoid body does not produce total deafness of either ear.

T.S. THORACOLUMBAR REGION OF SPINAL CORD

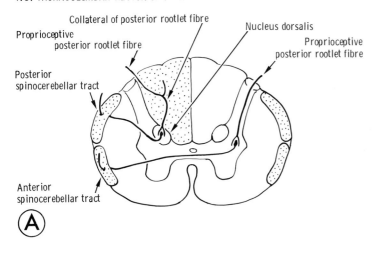

Collateral of posterior rootlet fibre

Proprioceptive posterior rootlet fibre

Nucleus dorsalis

Proprioceptive posterior rootlet fibre

Posterior spinocerebellar tract

Anterior spinocerebellar tract

(A)

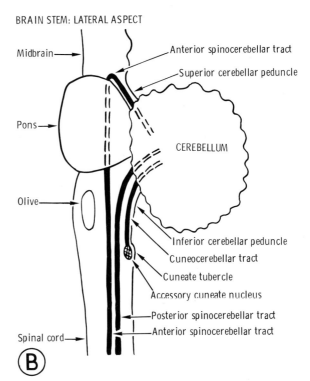

BRAIN STEM: LATERAL ASPECT

Midbrain

Anterior spinocerebellar tract

Superior cerebellar peduncle

Pons

CEREBELLUM

Olive

Inferior cerebellar peduncle

Cuneocerebellar tract

Cuneate tubercle

Accessory cuneate nucleus

Posterior spinocerebellar tract

Spinal cord

Anterior spinocerebellar tract

(B)

T.S. LOWEST PART OF PONS

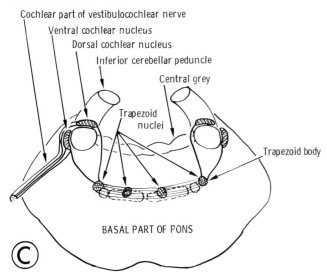

Cochlear part of vestibulocochlear nerve

Ventral cochlear nucleus

Dorsal cochlear nucleus

Inferior cerebellar peduncle

Central grey

Trapezoid nuclei

Trapezoid body

BASAL PART OF PONS

(C)

T.S. MIDDLE PART OF PONS

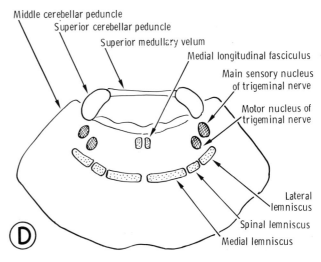

Middle cerebellar peduncle

Superior cerebellar peduncle

Superior medullary velum

Medial longitudinal fasciculus

Main sensory nucleus of trigeminal nerve

Motor nucleus of trigeminal nerve

Lateral lemniscus

Spinal lemniscus

Medial lemniscus

(D)

Reaching the tegmentum of the midbrain the three lemnisci are displaced laterally by the decussation of the superior cerebellar peduncles, and also become re-orientated so that the lateral is behind and the medial in front (**A**). Most of the fibres of the lateral lemniscus pass upwards and synapse in the nucleus of the inferior colliculus. The fibres arising in the colliculus, together with the remaining lemniscal fibres, pass through the inferior brachium to the medial geniculate body where they relay. The final fibres of the auditory pathway arise in the medial geniculate body and, passing laterally through the sublentiform part of the internal capsule as the auditory radiation (**73A**), pass below the insula to reach the acoustic area of the cerebral cortex (**69A**).

Vestibular pathways

The vestibular apparatus, which consists of parts of the internal ear (**403A–E**), gives rise to impulses which convey information concerning the position and movements of the head. Within the brain stem and spinal cord these impulses reflexly adapt body posture, and in particular the positions of the eyes, in conformity with this information.

The vestibular part of the vestibulocochlear nerve consists of the central processes of the bipolar cells in the vestibular ganglion on the proximal part of the nerve (**407A**). These fibres enter the lower part of the pons in front of the inferior cerebellar peduncle (**B**). Some pass directly into the cerebellum through that peduncle (**B**) but the majority synapse in the vestibular nuclei which lie in the vestibular area of central grey matter in the floor of the fourth ventricle (**B**)

Fibres arising in the vestibular nuclei follow four general courses.

1. The nuclei have connections in both directions with certain parts of the cerebellum through the inferior cerebellar peduncle (**B**). These will be considered together with the cerebellar fibre circuits.
2. Others descend on the same side as their nucleus of origin and constitute the vestibulospinal tract (**B, C**). This passes downwards through the medulla and thereafter through the whole length of the anterior funiculus of the spinal cord. Fibres leave the tract at all levels and, entering the anterior grey column of the same side, connect with motor neurons through short interneurons.
3. The nuclei send both ascending and descending fibres into the medial longitudinal fasciculi of both sides (**B**). These paired fasciculi lie close to one another on either side of the midline along the ventral aspect of the central grey matter of the midbrain, pons and medulla. They continue through the cervical and upper thoracic parts of the spinal cord as the anterior intersegmental fasciculi, which are situated between the anterior median fissure and the medial aspect of the anterior grey column (**C**)

These fasciculi interconnect motor nuclei in the central grey matter of the brain stem, particularly those concerned with movements of the eyes, and the motor cells in the anterior grey columns in the upper part of the spinal cord concerned with movements of the head, neck and upper limbs.
4. The fact that changes in the position of the head can be consciously appreciated shows that fibres from the vestibular nuclei reach the cerebral cortex, but their route is unknown.

The visual pathways

The retinae and the visual field

The light-sensitive tissue of the eyeball is the posterior half or so of the inner layer of the retina which is surrounded by concentric vascular and fibrous coats (**D**). In the outermost part of this tissue lie highly specialised photoreceptor cells called, from their shapes, rod cells (or rods) and cone cells (or cones). The two types of receptors are functionally as well as morphologically distinct. The rods have a low threshold to light but do not distinguish between colours, while the cones have a relatively higher threshold but distinguish by their response between one colour and another.

The centrally directed axons of the rods and cones synapse with the dendrites of bipolar cells, and the axons of the latter, continuing centrally, synapse with ganglion cells (**E**). The axons of these ganglion cells, running on the inner surface of the retina, converge on a circular area with a raised margin called the optic disc, which is a short distance medial to the visual axis of the eye. Here the ganglion cell axons pass through the three coats of the eyeball, become myelinated and form the optic nerve (**D**).

It should be noted that, because of the structure of most of the retina, light must traverse all its other layers before reaching that of the rods and cones.

MIDBRAIN & METATHALAMUS (pulvinar removed on left)

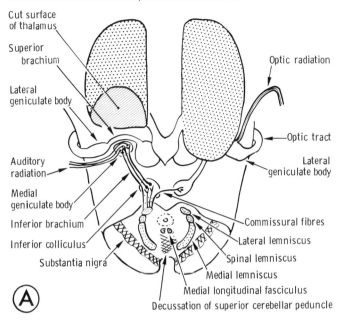

- Cut surface of thalamus
- Superior brachium
- Lateral geniculate body
- Auditory radiation
- Medial geniculate body
- Inferior brachium
- Inferior colliculus
- Substantia nigra
- Optic radiation
- Optic tract
- Lateral geniculate body
- Commissural fibres
- Lateral lemniscus
- Spinal lemniscus
- Medial lemniscus
- Medial longitudinal fasciculus
- Decussation of superior cerebellar peduncle

(A)

T.S. CERVICAL PART OF SPINAL CORD

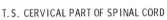

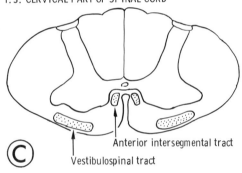

- Anterior intersegmental tract
- Vestibulospinal tract

(C)

BRAIN STEM: POSTERIOR ASPECT (cerebellum removed: floor of fourth ventricle stippled)

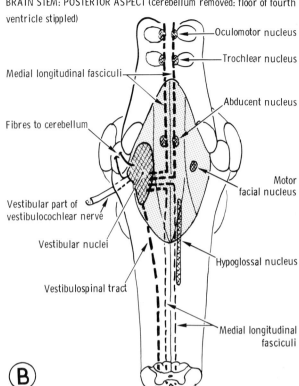

- Medial longitudinal fasciculi
- Fibres to cerebellum
- Vestibular part of vestibulocochlear nerve
- Vestibular nuclei
- Vestibulospinal tract
- Oculomotor nucleus
- Trochlear nucleus
- Abducent nucleus
- Motor facial nucleus
- Hypoglossal nucleus
- Medial longitudinal fasciculi

(B)

DIAGRAMMATIC HORIZONTAL SECTION OF EYEBALL

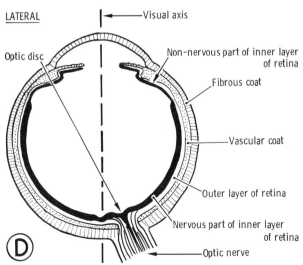

LATERAL

- Visual axis
- Optic disc
- Non-nervous part of inner layer of retina
- Fibrous coat
- Vascular coat
- Outer layer of retina
- Nervous part of inner layer of retina
- Optic nerve

(D)

DIAGRAM OF STRUCTURE OF RETINA

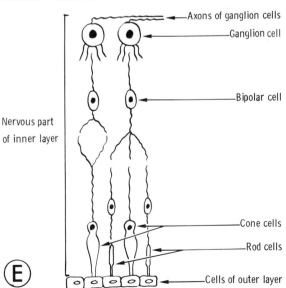

- Axons of ganglion cells
- Ganglion cell
- Bipolar cell
- Nervous part of inner layer
- Cone cells
- Rod cells
- Cells of outer layer

(E)

Over the posterior pole of the eye the retina exhibits a small yellow area called the macula lutea (**A**), which slopes from its periphery into a central depression named the fovea centralis. Because of the structural features listed below, the macula and particularly the fovea have a better resolving power than other parts of the retina.

1. It contains tightly packed cones and no rods.
2. It has a 1:1 relationship of cones to ganglion cells and their axons, whereas elsewhere each retinal fibre receives impulses from a number of photoreceptors.
3. The bipolar and ganglion cells of the macula radiate obliquely towards its margins, and fibres approaching the optic disc from the lateral side skirt round the macula and do not pass over it. Hence light falling on the macula has to traverse less retinal tissue than elsewhere before reaching the photoreceptors.

That part of the retina which is medial to the fovea centralis, including half of the macula, is called the nasal half because it is nearest to the nose. The rest of the retina is called the temporal half because it is nearest to the temporal region of the skull, i.e. the temple. Both halves may be further divided into upper and lower quadrants (**A**).

The visual field

When both eyes are in use and directed forwards, the area which can be seen, that is the visual field, may be divided into a large central part and a smaller peripheral part (**B**). Light from anywhere in the central part reaches both retinae, and it is therefore called the binocular field. On the other hand, largely because of the forward projection of the nose, light from the peripheral part reaches only one retina and is called the monocular field.

Because light must pass through the refractive media of the eye the image of an object in the visual field on the retina is reversed.

Observe in the diagram (**B**) the following facts which are essential for the diagnoses of lesions of the visual pathways.

1. Light from an object in the centre of the visual field falls on the maculae of both eyes.
2. Light from an object in the left half of the binocular visual field forms images on the nasal half of the left retina and the temporal half of the right retina and vice versa.
3. An image of an object in the left half of the monocular visual field is formed only on the nasal half of the left retina, whereas an image of an object in the right half of the monocular field is formed only on the nasal half of the right retina.
4. In each case, light from the lower half of the visual field falls on the upper retinal quadrants and light from the upper half of the visual field on the lower retinal quadrants.

The retinocortical visual pathways

As the retinal fibres pass backwards from the eyes, they are arranged in a particular pattern which is illustrated in a purely diagrammatic fashion in **C**.

1. The anatomy of the optic nerve will be considered later (**419A, 425C**). For the present it suffices to know that it begins at the optic disc and passes through the orbit into the cranial cavity where it joins the lateral end of the optic chiasma. Comparison of **B** and **C** shows that each nerve contains all the fibres from both the nasal and temporal halves of the corresponding retina.
2. The position of the optic chiasma in the brain has been considered previously. This should now be revised, particularly its relationship to the third ventricle (**55A, 55B**) and the hypophysis cerebri. Comparison of **B** and **C** shows that the chiasma contains fibres from the nasal halves of both retinae which are decussating across the midline from each optic nerve to the contralateral optic tract. Moreover it should be noted that the fibres from the lower nasal quadrants of the retinae cross in the lower part of the chiasma and vice versa.
3. The course and relations of the optic tracts have also been considered earlier. These should now be revised particularly their relationships to the hypothalamus (**63C**), the choroidal fissure (**63E**) and the crus cerebri (**67C**). Observe from **B** and **C** that each tract consists of fibres from the temporal half of the ipsilateral retina and the nasal half of the contralateral retina. Posteriorly the fibres of each tract end by synapsing with the cells of the corresponding lateral geniculate body. Some also send collateral branches into the superior brachium which will be considered later.
4. On each side, the fibres arising in the lateral geniculate body stream upwards and forwards (**81A**) and turn laterally in the concavities of the caudate nucleus and lateral ventricle (**73A**) into the retrolentiform part of the internal capsule (**73C**). The fibres then turn backwards as the optic radiation separated from the lateral wall of the posterior ventricular horn by the tapetum of the corpus callosum (**73C**). Finally the fibres of the radiation turn medially to reach and end in the primary visual cortex, the position of which has been noted already (**69A, 69B**).

RETINA: ANTERIOR VIEW

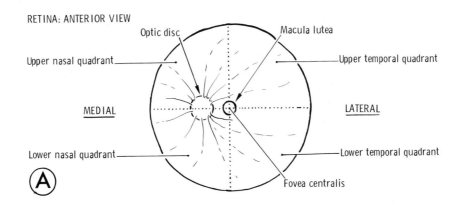

Optic disc   Macula lutea

Upper nasal quadrant   Upper temporal quadrant

MEDIAL   LATERAL

Lower nasal quadrant   Lower temporal quadrant

Fovea centralis

(A)

VISUAL FIELDS

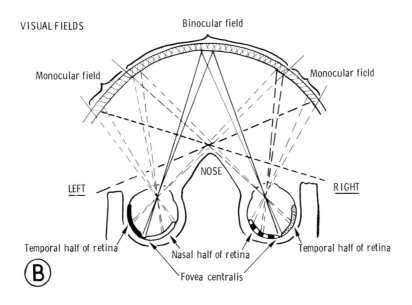

Binocular field

Monocular field   Monocular field

NOSE

LEFT   RIGHT

Temporal half of retina   Temporal half of retina

Nasal half of retina

Fovea centralis

(B)

VISUAL PATHWAYS

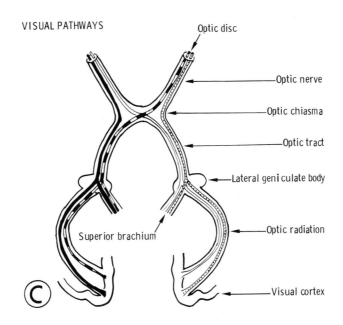

Optic disc

Optic nerve

Optic chiasma

Optic tract

Lateral geniculate body

Optic radiation

Superior brachium

Visual cortex

(C)

5. It will be evident from **83C** that each optic radiation and its visual cortex are associated with the same two half retinae as the ipsilateral optic tract. In the case of the visual cortical area it is important to note two other facts (**A**). First, the upper quadrants of the half retinae activate the upper half of the area and the lower quadrants the lower half. Secondly, the macular parts of the two half retinae are disproportionately represented, activating, despite their small size, about the posterior two-thirds of the visual area.

The effects of lesions of the visual pathways

It is a useful combined exercise in optics and anatomy to deduce from a consideration of **83** and **85A** the effects on the visual field of lesions of different parts of the visual pathways.

1. Division of one optic nerve obviously causes total blindness of the corresponding eye. However, it should be noted (**B**) that, provided the other eye is open, blindness is restricted to the monocular field on the side of the lesion.
2. Division of the optic chiasma isolates the nasal halves of both retinae from the visual cortex. Consequently, each eye is blind to the whole monocular visual field and to that part of the binocular field which is on the temporal side of its own visual axis (**B**). The condition is called bitemporal hemianopia. It may be caused by pressure on the lower aspect of the chiasma by enlargement of the hypophysis cerebri. In such circumstances the fibres from the lower nasal quadrants are affected before those from the upper quadrants–and consequently blindness appears in the upper parts of the visual field before the lower parts. Note in **B** that if a subject with bitemporal hemianopia keeps both eyes open blindness is restricted to both monocular visual fields and may of itself cause little disability.
3. Division of one optic tract isolates from the visual cortex the temporal half of the ipsilateral retina and the nasal half of the contralateral retina. When both eyes are open or when only the ipsilateral eye is open there is blindness over the whole of the contralateral half of the visual field (**B**). On the other hand, when only the contralateral eye is open there is blindness over both the contralateral half of the visual field and the ipsilateral monocular field (**B**). Thus the condition produced by division of the left optic tract is called a right homonymous hemianopia.

4. Lesions of the lateral geniculate body, the optic radiation and the visual cortex produce effects which are essentially similar to those associated with a lesion of the optic tract on the same side. But because such lesions are usually incomplete, blindness is usually restricted to only parts of the areas of the visual field which are affected in a complete homonymous hemianopia (**B**).

Pathways of visual reflexes

Visual reflexes are initiated by impulses from the retinae passing backwards along the visual pathways.

1. Collateral branches of fibres in an optic tract bypass the lateral geniculate body and pass through the superior brachium to end in the corresponding pretectal nucleus which lies immediately above the superior colliculus (**C**). The efferent fibres from this nucleus pass through the central grey matter to synapse in the visceral motor parts of the oculomotor nuclei of both sides (**49B**). Parasympathetic impulses pass from each of these nuclei to the corresponding eye, via a two neuron pathway, and these innervate the constrictor muscle of the pupil. When light is shone into one eye the pupils of both eyes constrict equally because of the connection of each pretectal nucleus to both oculomotor nuclei.
2. Other collaterals in the superior brachia end by synapsing with the cells of the corresponding superior colliculus (**C**). Efferent fibres from the colliculus form descending spinal pathways which will be considered later. This pathway forms the basis of some of the reflex activities of skeletal muscle which occur in response to light falling on the retinae.
3. The accommodation reflex, which occurs when a near object is viewed, involves convergence of the eyes by skeletal extra-ocular muscles innervated from the somatic motor part of the oculomotor nucleus (**49B**), and constriction of the pupil and alteration of the shape of the lens by parasympathetic impulses arising in the visceral motor part of the same nucleus. The pathway of this reflex carries visual impulses from the retinae to the visual cortical areas. Thereafter, impulses evoked in the occipital eye field (**69B**) pass through, via the optic radiation, the retrolentiform part of the internal capsule and the crus cerebri to both parts of the oculomotor nuclei.

In some diseases the pupils constrict during accommodation but not in response to light (Argyll Robertson pupil).

PRIMARY VISUAL CORTEX: REPRESENTATION OF HALF RETINAE

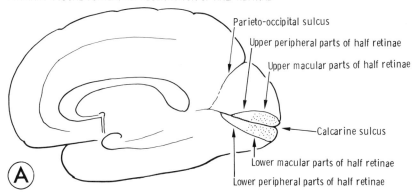

Parieto-occipital sulcus
Upper peripheral parts of half retinae
Upper macular parts of half retinae
Calcarine sulcus
Lower macular parts of half retinae
Lower peripheral parts of half retinae

(A)

THE VISUAL EFFECTS OF LESIONS OF THE VISUAL PATHWAYS

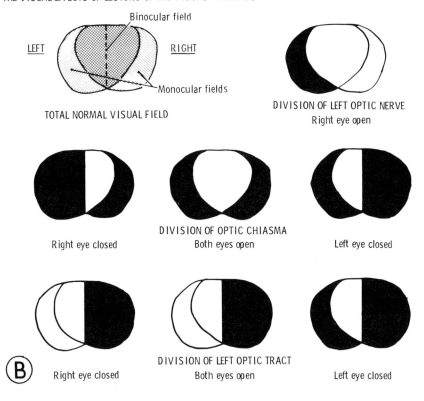

Binocular field
LEFT   RIGHT
Monocular fields

TOTAL NORMAL VISUAL FIELD

DIVISION OF LEFT OPTIC NERVE
Right eye open

DIVISION OF OPTIC CHIASMA

Right eye closed   Both eyes open   Left eye closed

DIVISION OF LEFT OPTIC TRACT

(B)   Right eye closed   Both eyes open   Left eye closed

PUPIL LIGHT REFLEX & RETINOSPINAL PATHWAY

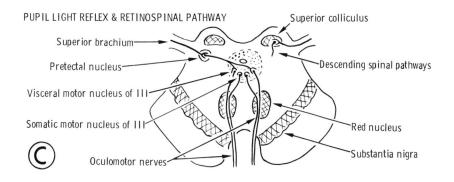

Superior brachium
Pretectal nucleus
Visceral motor nucleus of III
Somatic motor nucleus of III
Oculomotor nerves
Superior colliculus
Descending spinal pathways
Red nucleus
Substantia nigra

(C)

85

The olfactory pathway

The receptor cells of olfactory sensation are unique in that they lie in the surface epithelium lining the upper part of the nasal cavity (**A**).

These cells are bipolar. Their single dendrites have elaborate terminations which protrude beyond the general epithelial surface for a minute distance into the nasal cavity. Their single, very slender axons ascend and form some twenty or so separate bundles which constitute the olfactory nerve. These bundles pass through small foramina in a thin bone plate into the cranial cavity where they join the olfactory bulb (**A, B**).

The neuronal structure of the bulb is exceedingly complex. However, considering it in a very simplistic fashion, its essential components are the neurons known as mitral cells. The branched dendrites of these mitral cells synapse with numerous incoming fibres from the olfactory nerve and their axons stream backwards as the principal component of the olfactory tract (**A**).

As has been seen previously (**B**) the tract divides posteriorly in front of the anterior perforated substance into lateral and medial roots (olfactory striae). The lateral root, which contains the fibres concerned with the mediation of olfactory sensation to the conscious level, crosses the limen insulae (**65E**) and bends medially to reach the primary olfactory cortical area. This has already been seen (**69B**) to be situated over the uncus, the anterior part of the parahippocampal gyrus and part of the amygdaloid body (**B**). The medial root turns upwards above the optic chiasma and ends in the septal areas which are part of the limbic system (**75A, 75B**).

THE SOMATIC MOTOR SYSTEM

Voluntary muscles throughout the body are innervated by lower motor neurons. The cell bodies of these neurons lie in the spinal anterior grey column or in somatic or branchial motor nuclei in the brain stem, and their axons extend through spinal or cranial nerves to motor end plates in the muscles. The lower motor neurons are influenced by a large number of other neurons which either synapse with them directly or are connected to them through a surrounding pool of short interneurons. These influences may be either inhibitory or excitatory, so that in summation they select which lower motor neurons fire at any particular time and consequently the nature and strength of the movement which is produced.

A potent source of such influences are the somatic afferent fibres of spinal or cranial nerves which may inhibit or excite lower motor neurons at or near their own level of entry (**33B, 33C**). The effects of these influences on muscles and movement are reflex in that they do not necessarily involve impulses arising at higher levels.

Lower motor neurons may also be inhibited or excited, either directly or through internuncial neurons, by what may be called upper motor neurons which originate in masses of grey matter in the brain and pass downwards through long descending tracts.

The immediate sources of these descending tracts are the motor areas of the cerebral cortex (corticospinal tract), the vestibular nuclei in the floor of the fourth ventricle (vestibulospinal), the red nucleus (rubrospinal), the brain stem reticular formation (reticulospinal) and the superior colliculus (tectospinal). All of these sources are in turn strongly influenced by impulses from numerous areas of the cerebral cortex and from the cerebellum. We will consider this latter influence first.

The cerebellum

The afferent connections

The general anatomy of this part of the hindbrain has been considered already (**41, 43**).

The cerebellum receives information from a number of sources, the vestibular part of vestibulocochlear nerve, the spinal cord, the tectum of the midbrain and the cerebral cortex. These several sources project to different areas of the cerebellar cortex. It is important to note that vestibular, spinal and tectal afferents pass to the ipsilateral half of the cerebellum, while cerebral afferents pass to the contralateral half. The reception areas for fibres from different sources are shown in **C** although in fact there is some degree of overlap.

Consider the pathways followed by impulses from these sources.

1. Vestibular fibres carrying information concerning the position and the movements of the head enter the cerebellum through the inferior peduncle either directly or after relay in the vestibular nuclei (**D**).

DIAGRAMMATIC REPRESENTATION OF OLFACTORY NERVE, BULB & TRACT

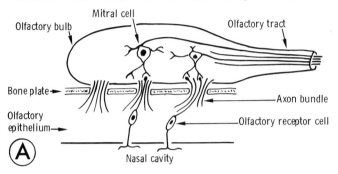

Olfactory bulb
Mitral cell
Olfactory tract
Bone plate
Axon bundle
Olfactory epithelium
Olfactory receptor cell
Nasal cavity

(A)

INFERIOR ASPECT OF CEREBRAL HEMISPHERE: OLFACTORY PATHWAY

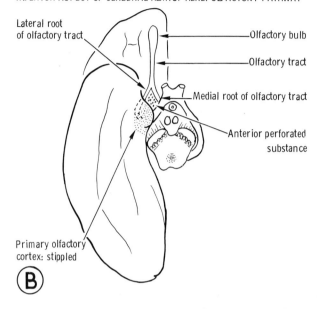

Lateral root of olfactory tract
Olfactory bulb
Olfactory tract
Medial root of olfactory tract
Anterior perforated substance
Primary olfactory cortex: stippled

(B)

RECEPTION AREAS OF CEREBELLAR CORTEX:

Vestibular areas black, spinal areas stippled, cerebral & tectal areas white

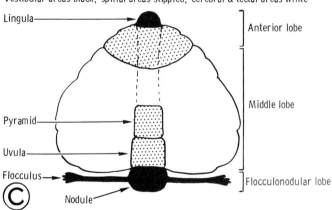

Lingula
Anterior lobe
Pyramid
Middle lobe
Uvula
Flocculus
Nodule
Flocculonodular lobe

(C)

VESTIBULAR AFFERENTS TO CEREBELLUM

Superior peduncle
Cerebellum
Middle peduncle
Inferior peduncle
Vestibular nuclei
Vestibular part of vestibulocochlear nerve

(D)

2. Spinal fibres (**A**), carrying proprioceptive information from the greater part of the body, reach the cerebellum in the posterior spinocerebellar and cuneocerebellar tracts (**79A**, **79B**) through the inferior peduncle.

3. The tectocerebellar tract carries impulses from the superior colliculus through the superior peduncle. That colliculus receives auditory information from both cochleae through the corresponding lateral lemniscus and inferior colliculus, and visual information from both retinae through the corresponding optic tract, superior brachium and occipital cortex (**B**).

4. The cortex of each cerebral hemisphere is connected with the opposite half of the cerebellum. The fibres descend through most parts of the internal capsule and become collected into two large bundles which continue through the lateral and medial parts of the crus cerebri (**C**). Entering the pons, they become dispersed amongst the fibres of the pyramidal tract and end by synapsing with the cells of the pontine nuclei (**47D**). Second order neurons arising in these nuclei run transversely to the opposite side of the midline and enter the cerebellum through the contralateral middle peduncle (**D**).

5. The efferent fibres of the olivary nuclei (**47C**, **53A**) stream transversely across the medulla and enter the cerebellum as one of the components of the opposite inferior peduncle (**A**). These nuclei receive afferents from the cerebral cortex, and others which carry cutaneous information from the spinal cord, but in neither case is the course of the fibres known with any certainty.

Efferent fibres

Fibres leave the cerebellum by two routes:

1. Some originate in the vestibular areas of the cerebellar cortex and pass directly, or after relay in the central cerebellar nuclei, through the inferior peduncle to the ipsilateral vestibular nuclei (**E**). This peduncle thus contains vestibulocerebellar and cerebellovestibular fibres.

2. From the greater part of the cerebellar cortex fibres converge on the dentate nucleus where they relay (**E**). The efferent fibres of that nucleus form the bulk of the superior peduncle through which they pass upwards into the tegmentum of the midbrain. Here they decussate across the midline and many end soon thereafter in contralateral brain stem nuclei, particularly the red nucleus, the reticular formation and the superior colliculus (**E**). The remaining fibres continue upwards around the red nucleus to synapse in the contralateral thalamus with thalamocortical fibres. These ascend through the lateral part of the internal capsule to reach the motor areas of the contralateral cerebral cortex.

SPINAL & OLIVARY AFFERENTS TO CEREBELLUM

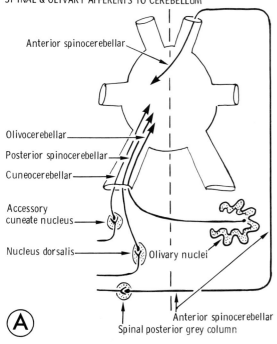

Anterior spinocerebellar

Olivocerebellar

Posterior spinocerebellar

Cuneocerebellar

Accessory cuneate nucleus

Nucleus dorsalis

Olivary nuclei

Anterior spinocerebellar

Spinal posterior grey column

(A)

TECTAL AFFERENTS TO CEREBELLUM

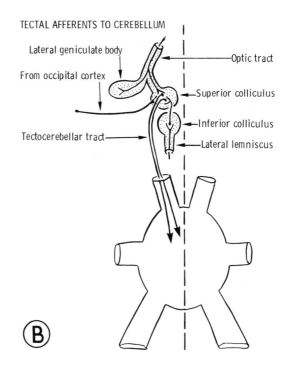

Lateral geniculate body

From occipital cortex

Optic tract

Superior colliculus

Inferior colliculus

Lateral lemniscus

Tectocerebellar tract

(B)

CORTICOPONTINE FIBRES IN CRURA CEREBRI

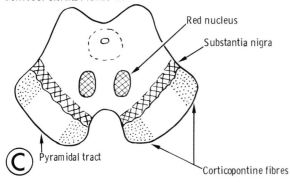

Red nucleus

Substantia nigra

Pyramidal tract

Corticopontine fibres

(C)

CEREBRAL AFFERENTS TO CEREBELLUM

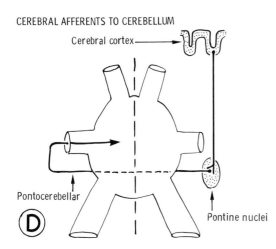

Cerebral cortex

Pontocerebellar

Pontine nuclei

(D)

EFFERENT FIBRES OF CEREBELLUM

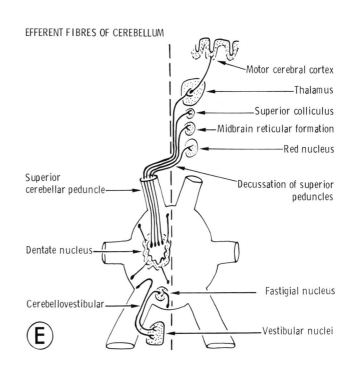

Motor cerebral cortex

Thalamus

Superior colliculus

Midbrain reticular formation

Red nucleus

Superior cerebellar peduncle

Decussation of superior peduncles

Dentate nucleus

Fastigial nucleus

Cerebellovestibular

Vestibular nuclei

(E)

Loop circuits to the motor cerebral cortex

The motor areas of each cerebral cortex receive information from other cerebral cortical areas of the same side through two loop-like pathways.

1. One of these is formed by afferent fibres to, and efferent fibres from, the contralateral half of the cerebellum which have been considered above. Beginning in wide areas of the cerebral cortex it passes successively to the ipsilateral pontine nuclei (**A**), the cortex, dentate nucleus and superior peduncle of the contralateral half of the cerebellum (**A**) through the decussation of the superior peduncles to the ipsilateral thalamus and so to the ipsilateral motor cerebral cortex (**A**).

   The pattern of activity in the motor cortex for the production of a movement, or a series of movements, can thus be made in conformity with the information received by the cerebellum concerning the state of the muscles and joints of the body, the position of the body in space and various aspects of the external environment.

2. The second circuit is also shown diagrammatically in **A**. The first fibres pass from all areas of the cerebral cortex to the corpus striatum (caudate nucleus and putamen) of the same side (**71D**). The second arise in the corpus striatum and converge on the corresponding globus pallidus (**71E**). The third pass to the thalamus, and the final fibres ascend, like those of the cerebellar loop, through the internal capsule to the ipsilateral motor cortex.

   Standing apart from the main circuit but reciprocally connected to the corpus striatum is the substantia nigra (**47E, 47F**). The nigrostriate fibres have become of particular interest. They appear to be essential to the normal functioning of the corpus striatum and are unusual in that their neurotransmitter is dopamine.

   The place of this loop in the production of motor activity is uncertain but it has been suggested that it may be concerned, in some way, in the conversion of an abstract intention to carry out a movement into the pattern of activity in the motor cortex necessary for its execution.

   The fact that the common neurological disorder known as Parkinson's disease appears to be associated with malfunction of this loop is of interest. The disease is characterised by degenerative changes in the cells of the substantia nigra and a gross reduction in the dopamine content of the corpus striatum. It can often be alleviated by the administration of L-Dopa which is a precursor of dopamine. And one of the first complaints of a patient suffering from the disease is often of difficulty in starting movements which he consciously wishes to perform.

Descending tracts

Of the several descending tracts which influence the activities of lower motor neurons, only one runs an uninterrupted course from the cerebral motor cortex to spinal levels. It is consequently called the corticospinal tract, but it is relevant to the rest of this paragraph to note that its older name, which is still quite frequently used, is the pyramidal tract. All the other descending tracts are associated with nuclei of grey matter between the cerebral cortex and the spinal cord, and it is sometimes convenient to refer to them collectively as the extrapyramidal tracts.

The corticospinal tract

Most of the fibres of each tract originate from cells in the regional areas of the primary and supplementary motor cortices which have been considered previously (**69A, 69B**). Converging downwards through the corona radiata and intersecting the fibres of the corpus callosum, they pass into the internal capsule. As is shown in **B** they occupy a comparatively small percentage of the total cross-sectional area of the capsule, the rest being composed of other corticofugal fibres and thalamocortical fibres. The corticospinal fibres are arranged in a number of groups in the genu and the anterior part of the posterior limb, the groups innervating the upper parts of the body in front and those innervating the lower parts behind.

The tract leaves the internal capsule by passing downwards through the middle three-fifths or so of the corresponding crus cerebri (**C**) with corticopontine fibres occupying the other two-fifths. The 'head-fibres' are now medial and the 'lower limb fibres' lateral, indicating a rotation of the tract through 90° from its orientation in the internal capsule.

Entering the basal part of the pons the tract becomes separated into numerous narrow longitudinal bundles which are dispersed amongst the pontine nuclei and intersect the transversely disposed pontocerebellar fibres (**D**).

LOOP CIRCUITS TO MOTOR CEREBRAL CORTEX

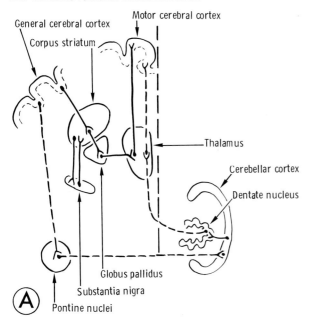

General cerebral cortex

Motor cerebral cortex

Corpus striatum

Thalamus

Cerebellar cortex

Dentate nucleus

Globus pallidus

Substantia nigra

Pontine nuclei

(A)

INTERNAL CAPSULE: HORIZONTAL SECTION

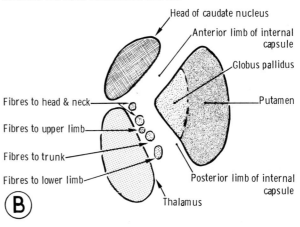

Head of caudate nucleus

Anterior limb of internal capsule

Globus pallidus

Putamen

Fibres to head & neck

Fibres to upper limb

Fibres to trunk

Fibres to lower limb

Posterior limb of internal capsule

Thalamus

(B)

MIDBRAIN: TRANSVERSE SECTION

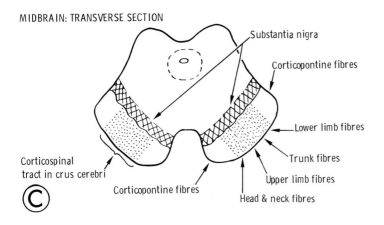

Substantia nigra

Corticopontine fibres

Lower limb fibres

Trunk fibres

Upper limb fibres

Head & neck fibres

Corticospinal tract in crus cerebri

Corticopontine fibres

(C)

PONS: TRANSVERSE SECTION

(Pontine nuclei black; bundles of corticospinal fibres stippled)

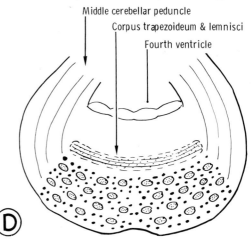

Middle cerebellar peduncle

Corpus trapezoideum & lemnisci

Fourth ventricle

(D)

As they leave the pons the separate bundles reaggregate to form the pyramid which, it will be recalled (**39B**), forms a prominent blunt ridge on the anterior aspect of the medulla alongside the anterior median fissure. Observe in **A**, **B** the relationship of the tract to the medial lemniscus and the olivary nuclei, and, at a somewhat lower level, to the decussation of the medial lemnisci.

In the lowest part of the medulla, and consequently some distance below the great sensory decussation, some 70–90% of the fibres of each pyramid decussate across the midline as coarse interdigitating bundles in the depths of the anterior median fissure (**C**). The decussated fibres pass backwards and laterally, separating the upper end of the spinal anterior grey column from the rest of the central grey matter (**C**), and then turn downwards in the posterior part of the lateral funiculus of the spinal cord as the lateral corticospinal tract (**D**, **E**). It extends to the lower end of the cord. The 20% of corticospinal fibres which do not decussate in the medulla continue into the spinal cord as the anterior corticospinal tract, which is situated in the anterior funiculus alongside the anterior median fissure (**D**). Unlike the previous tract it does not reach further than the midthoracic segments.

Branches of the undivided corticospinal tract arise in the brain stem and connect, either by direct synapses or through internuncial neurons, with the cells of the somatic motor nuclei of that region. They are consequently called corticonuclear (**A**). The great majority cross the midline and connect with nuclei of the opposite side. As an exception to this general rule, those cells of the facial nuclei of both sides which innervate the muscles of expression in the upper part of the face and the scalp are connected to both corticospinal tracts, so that the relevant muscles are bilaterally innervated and are not greatly affected by a lesion of one tract.

Branches arise in the spinal cord from both the lateral and anterior corticospinal tracts. The former have already crossed the midline in the medullary decussation. The latter cross in the white commissure at the level at which they arise (**D**). Thus the branches of both tracts reach the central grey matter on the side opposite to that of their cortical origin. Here they synapse with internuncial neurons in the basal part of the anterior grey column. These in turn synapse with lower motor neurons whose cell bodies lie predominantly in the lateral nuclear group in the anterior grey column.

It has been noted already that this nuclear group is largest in the cervical and lumbar enlargements of the spinal cord from which the muscles of the limbs are innervated (**37C**, **37E**). The spinal distribution of the corticospinal tract is thus in conformity with the fact that injury to that pathway at a supraspinal level (commonly in the internal capsule) is usually associated with a contralateral paralysis which particularly affects the delicate and intricate movements characteristic of the distal parts of the limbs, and is much less noticeable in the trunk and the proximal parts of the limbs.

UPPER PART OF MEDULLA: TRANSVERSE SECTION

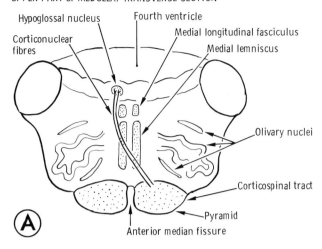

Hypoglossal nucleus
Corticonuclear fibres
Fourth ventricle
Medial longitudinal fasciculus
Medial lemniscus
Olivary nuclei
Corticospinal tract
Pyramid
Anterior median fissure

A

MIDDLE PART OF MEDULLA: TRANSVERSE SECTION

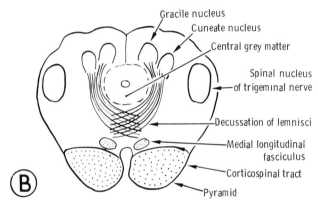

Gracile nucleus
Cuneate nucleus
Central grey matter
Spinal nucleus of trigeminal nerve
Decussation of lemnisci
Medial longitudinal fasciculus
Corticospinal tract
Pyramid

B

LOWER PART OF MEDULLA: TRANSVERSE SECTION

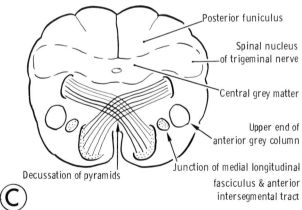

Posterior funiculus
Spinal nucleus of trigeminal nerve
Central grey matter
Upper end of anterior grey column
Junction of medial longitudinal fasciculus & anterior intersegmental tract
Decussation of pyramids

C

LOWER CERVICAL SPINAL CORD: TRANSVERSE SECTION

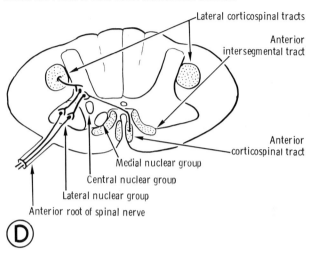

Lateral corticospinal tracts
Anterior intersegmental tract
Anterior corticospinal tract
Medial nuclear group
Central nuclear group
Lateral nuclear group
Anterior root of spinal nerve

D

LOWER THORACIC SPINAL CORD: TRANSVERSE SECTION

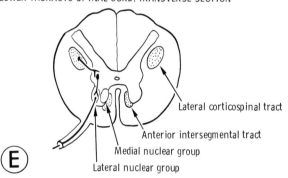

Lateral corticospinal tract
Anterior intersegmental tract
Medial nuclear group
Lateral nuclear group

E

The extrapyramidal tracts

The cortico-rubro-spinal tract arises from the motor areas of the cerebral cortex and descends as a discrete group of fibres into the middle of the posterior limb of the internal capsule (**91B**). Its fibres continue downwards into the tegmentum of the midbrain where they end in the red nucleus. As has been seen the other major input into the red nucleus is from the contralateral half of the cerebellum through the decussating superior peduncle (**89E**). The efferent fibres of the nucleus immediately cross to the opposite side of the midline, and descend as a diffuse formation through the reticular formations of the pons and branchial motor nuclei. Thereafter this crossed tract passes through the length of the spinal cord (**B**) lying just in front of, and partly intermingled with, the lateral corticospinal tract in the lateral funiculus. Its branches enter the central grey matter of the same side, and terminate in a manner essentially similar to those of the lateral corticospinal tract.

The reticulospinal tract begins in the continuous reticular formation of the midbrain, pons and medulla (**A**) which has three main afferent inputs. One consists of neuron chains which converge from wide areas of the ipsilateral cerebral cortex with relays in the corpus striatum and the globus pallidus (**71E**). Another reaches the reticulum from the contralateral cerebellar cortex and dentate nucleus and crosses the midline through the decussation of the superior cerebellar peduncles (**89E**). It is evident that both these pathways are closely related to the loop circuits to the motor cerebral cortex (**91A**). The third reaches the reticular formation from the hypothalamus and the other structures of the limbic system (**75A, 75B**) through the medial forebrain bundle.

Chains of neurons, synapsing frequently in the reticular formations of the brain stem and spinal cord, descend through the cord as diffuse crossed and uncrossed fibres in both the anterior and lateral funiculi (**C**). It appears probable that the fibres have two distinct modes of termination. First, they synapse with lower motor neurons in the medial nuclear group of the anterior grey column, mainly in the thoracic region, and consequently have a large effect on postural activity of the trunk muscles. Secondly, the fibres carrying impulses from the limbic system end in relation to preganglionic autonomic neurons in the intermediate grey matter in the thoracic and sacral regions, and thus exert control over numerous visceral activities in the body.

The vestibulospinal tract and the medial longitudinal fasciculus, which carry vestibular influences to the lower motor neurons of the brain stem and spinal cord, have been described previously (**81B, 81C**). It will be recalled that, whereas the vestibulospinal tract consists of uncrossed fibres, the medial longitudinal fasciculus and its continuation, the anterior intersegmental tract, contain fibres from both the ipsilateral and contralateral vestibular nuclei. The positions of the two tracts in the spinal cord are shown in **D**. Branches arise from both tracts mainly in the thoracic region and synapse directly with lower motor neurons in the ipsilateral anterior grey column, particularly in the medial nuclear group (**D**). Vestibular influences are thus predominantly concentrated on the postural trunk muscles.

The tectospinal tract arises from the superior colliculus. The afferent input into the colliculus has been discussed already (**85C**). The tectospinal tracts decussate across the midline immediately after their origin, and descend through the brain stem and the cervical segments of the spinal cord (**E**). The crossed tract sends branches to the lower motor neurons in the brain stem nuclei and the anterior grey column of the cervical spinal cord, and activate movements of the head and neck in response to visual and auditory sensations.

POSITIONS OF RETICULAR FORMATION (HATCHED) IN BRAIN STEM

(Identify other structures outlined)

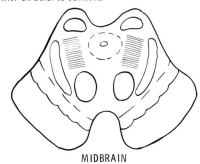

MIDBRAIN

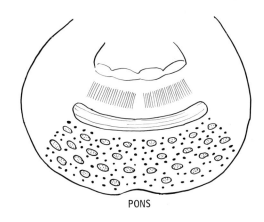

PONS

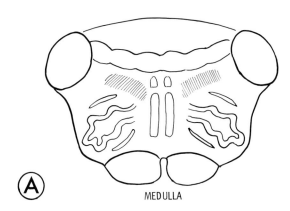

(A) MEDULLA

RUBROSPINAL TRACTS IN THORACIC SPINAL CORD

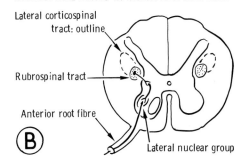

Lateral corticospinal tract: outline

Rubrospinal tract

Anterior root fibre

(B)

Lateral nuclear group

RETICULOSPINAL TRACT (STIPPLED) IN THORACIC SPINAL CORD

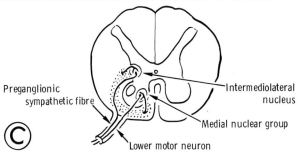

Preganglionic sympathetic fibre

Intermediolateral nucleus

Medial nuclear group

(C) Lower motor neuron

VESTIBULOSPINAL TRACTS IN THORACIC SPINAL CORD

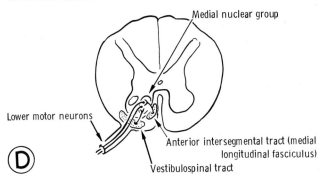

Medial nuclear group

Lower motor neurons

Anterior intersegmental tract (medial longitudinal fasciculus)

(D) Vestibulospinal tract

TECTOSPINAL TRACTS IN CERVICAL SPINAL CORD

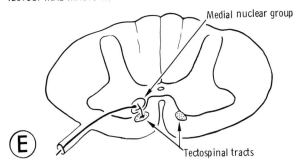

Medial nuclear group

(E) Tectospinal tracts

95

THE MENINGES

Except in one area, the brain and spinal cord are enclosed within the cranial cavity and vertebral canal by three concentric connective tissue layers. These are named from within outwards the pia mater, the arachnoid mater and the dura mater and referred to collectively as the meninges.

The exceptional area is the hypophysis cerebri. Neither pia nor arachnoid can be identified between it and its dural sac (see below).

With this exception, the pia mater covers closely and continuously the external surfaces of the brain and spinal cord, and the nerves or nerve roots which arise from these parts. Moreover, its involvement in the formation of the tela choroidea and the choroid plexuses of the brain has already been noted (**27B**, **45C**, **45E**, **63C**, **65A**). Consequently, its disposition does not require separate description or indication in this section.

The cerebral dura mater

Revise the form and features of the internal surface of the cranial cavity (**21A**, **23A**, **23B**). The internal periosteum of the cranial bones, or endocranium, follows every irregularity of this surface and coats the margins of the cranial foramina before becoming continuous with the external periosteum or pericranium (**B**).

The cerebral dura mater is a tough, opaque layer of interlacing collagen and elastic fibres which, throughout most of its extent, is in structural continuity with the endocranium. However, in relationship to many of the grooves and fossae which mark the internal surface of the cranium, the endocranium lines the irregularity while the dura bridges it, so that the two layers become temporarily separated (**A**). Several different arrangements of the dura occur in relationship to the cranial foramina and these will be noted individually when the structures passing through these foramina are considered later. For the moment it is worth noting that the dura bridges over many of these foramina so that their positions cannot be seen from within the intact dural envelope (**B**). Thus the dura obscures all the foramina in the lateral compartment of the middle cranial fossa, even the large superior orbital fissure (**21A**).

In certain situations, sheets of dura protrude from the cranial bones and their lining endocranium into the cranial cavity as partitions which partially separate adjacent parts of the brain. Each partition is sickle-shaped and has a convex attached margin and a concave free margin.

The dura of the sella turcica (**21B**, **21C**) exhibits an unusual and important disposition. The bone forming the region is completely and intimately lined by endocranium (**D, E**). On the other hand, traced backwards from the anterior cranial fossa (**D**), the dura parts company with the endocranium in the region of the hypophysial fossa and extends back as a flat sheet called the diaphragma sellae from the anterior clinoid process and the posterior lip of the optic groove to the posterior clinoid processes and dorsum sellae (**C**). A small opening in the centre of the diaphragm, which is traversed by the stalk of the hypophysis cerebri (**D**), leads downwards into a dural sac containing the hypophysis itself. This hypophysial dural sac occupies the greater part of the hypophysial fossa but is separate from the endocranium lining its anterior and posterior walls (**D**). From the lateral edges of the diaphragma sellae, between the anterior and posterior clinoid processes, the dura descends steeply a short distance lateral to the hypophysial sac and the body of the sphenoid (**E**) to reach and blend with the endocranium on the upper surface of the greater wing of the sphenoid. Note the triangular extradural spaces which are thus created on either side of the hypophysial sac.

The tentorium cerebelli is a dural partition which forms a partial roof over the posterior cranial fossa and intervenes between the cerebellum and the posterior parts of the cerebral hemisphere (**C**). Its attached margin blends with the dura lining the cranial cavity along the transverse sulci on the occipital bone and along the grooved superior margins of the petrous temporals (**C, F**). Its more acutely curved free margin is slung between the apices of the petrous temporals behind the clivus. It surrounds the communication between the posterior cranial fossa and the rest of the cranial cavity which is occupied by the midbrain.

RELATIONSHIP OF DURA TO INTRACRANIAL GROOVE

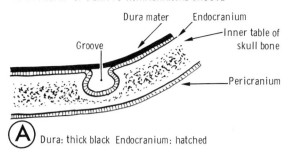

Dura mater
Endocranium
Inner table of skull bone
Groove
Pericranium
A Dura: thick black Endocranium: hatched

RELATIONSHIP OF DURA TO CRANIAL FORAMEN

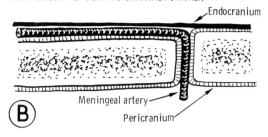

Endocranium
Meningeal artery
Pericranium
B

DIAPHRAGMA SELLAE & TENTORIUM CEREBELLI

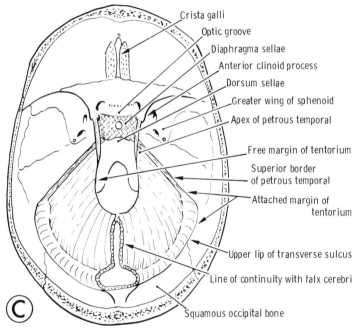

Crista galli
Optic groove
Diaphragma sellae
Anterior clinoid process
Dorsum sellae
Greater wing of sphenoid
Apex of petrous temporal
Free margin of tentorium
Superior border of petrous temporal
Attached margin of tentorium
Upper lip of transverse sulcus
Line of continuity with falx cerebri
Squamous occipital bone
C

SELLA TURCICA: MEDIAN SECTION

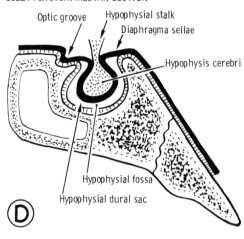

Optic groove
Hypophysial stalk
Diaphragma sellae
Hypophysis cerebri
Hypophysial fossa
Hypophysial dural sac
D

POSTERIOR CRANIAL FOSSA: SAGITTAL SECTION

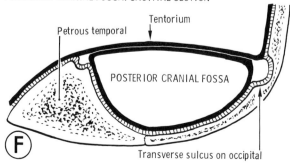

Tentorium
Petrous temporal
POSTERIOR CRANIAL FOSSA
Transverse sulcus on occipital
F

SELLA TURCICA: CORONAL SECTION

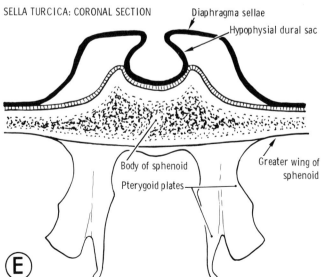

Diaphragma sellae
Hypophysial dural sac
Body of sphenoid
Pterygoid plates
Greater wing of sphenoid
E

As shown in **A**, the centre of the free margin lies at a considerably higher level than the approximately horizontal attached margin, so that the tentorium is truly tent-like in shape and, consequently, in the median plane, inclines steeply upwards and forwards (**B**).

The falx cerebri descends from the cranial vault in the median plane into the longitudinal fissure between the cerebral hemispheres (**B**). Anteriorly, it is attached to the endocranium on the crista galli of the ethmoid; above, to the margins of the sagittal sulcus: while behind and below it is continuous along the midline with the dura of the tentorium cerebelli. The shorter free margin extends between the extremities of the attached margin above the corpus callosum.

The dural venous sinuses

These are valveless veins, containing no muscle in their walls, which are situated either between the endocranium and the dura mater, often in a bony groove, or within a dural partition. Their tributaries are of three types, veins from the brain, diploic veins from the diploë of the cranial bones, and emissary veins which connect them with extracranial veins.

The paired cavernous sinuses run from before backwards through the triangular extradural spaces already noted on either side of the hypophysial dural sac and the body of the sphenoid in **97E**.

The sinuses, which are shown within these spaces in **C**, have an unusual structure, consisting of a sponge-like mass of small, intercommunicating, endothelial-lined spaces, separated by fibrous strands which arise from both the dura and the endocranium. Because of this structure blood flow through the sinuses is slow. Furthermore, both nerves and arteries can pass through the sinuses, held in position by the fibrous septa. The largest of such structures, the internal carotid artery, is shown within the sinus in **C**.

In **D** the left cavernous sinus is shown in translucent form, viewed from the left side, after removal of the lateral part of the cranium and the dura lateral to the diaphragma sellae.

Observe that the sinus is formed just behind the medial part of the superior orbital fissure, mainly by the confluence of veins from the orbit, and ends in the angle between the apex of the petrous temporal and the dorsum sellae by dividing into superior and inferior petrosal sinuses. It is about 2.5 cm long.

Medially it is related to the body of the sphenoid, the hypophysial dural sac and the medial half of the foramen lacerum (**C**, **D**).

Its roof is formed by the diaphragma sellae and the anterior and posterior clinoid processes (**C**, **D**).

Its lateral wall consists of the sheet of dura which descends steeply from the lateral edge of the roof to reach the intracranial surface of the greater wing of the sphenoid, medial to the foramina in that bone (**C**, **D**).

It is important to visualise in **D** that if this sheet of dura is traced forwards it sweeps laterally bridging over and hiding the superior orbital fissure between the lesser and greater wings of the sphenoid. This explains how a number of nerves, which, as will be seen later, run forwards just deep to the dural lateral wall of the sinus, can continue forwards through the superior orbital fissure into the orbit.

The two cavernous sinuses are connected by narrow intercavernous sinuses which cross the midline in front of and behind the hypophysial dural sac (**D**).

The two cavernous sinuses receive tributaries from the corresponding cerebral hemispheres (see below) and are connected to veins in the infratemporal fossa by emissary veins, the largest of which traverses the foramen ovale (**D**).

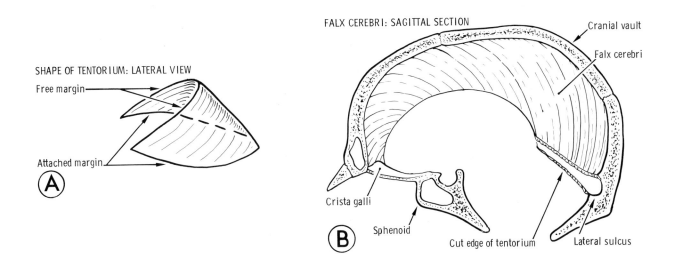

SHAPE OF TENTORIUM: LATERAL VIEW

Free margin

Attached margin

Ⓐ

FALX CEREBRI: SAGITTAL SECTION

Cranial vault

Falx cerebri

Crista galli

Sphenoid

Cut edge of tentorium

Lateral sulcus

Ⓑ

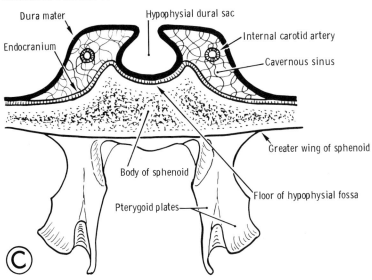

CAVERNOUS SINUSES: CORONAL SECTION

Dura mater

Hypophysial dural sac

Endocranium

Internal carotid artery

Cavernous sinus

Greater wing of sphenoid

Body of sphenoid

Floor of hypophysial fossa

Pterygoid plates

Ⓒ

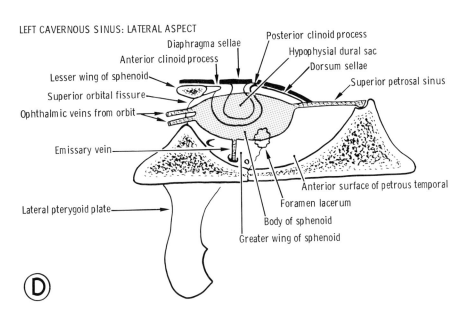

LEFT CAVERNOUS SINUS: LATERAL ASPECT

Diaphragma sellae

Anterior clinoid process

Posterior clinoid process

Hypophysial dural sac

Dorsum sellae

Lesser wing of sphenoid

Superior orbital fissure

Superior petrosal sinus

Ophthalmic veins from orbit

Emissary vein

Anterior surface of petrous temporal

Lateral pterygoid plate

Foramen lacerum

Body of sphenoid

Greater wing of sphenoid

Ⓓ

The superior sagittal sinus (**A**) begins in front of the crista galli and extends backwards, gradually expanding in size, lying in the attached margin of the falx cerebri and against the endocranium lining the sagittal sulcus (**B, C**). It ends at the internal occipital protuberance where it becomes continuous, in the majority, with the right transverse sinus (**D**) and in the minority with the left. Two or three venous lacunae (**23B**) open off the main channel on either side and extend laterally (**B, C**). Note that in infants the sinus crosses the deep aspect of the anterior and posterior fontanelles (**23C**).

The inferior sagittal sinus (**A**) is a small vessel which runs posteriorly embedded in the dura mater forming the free margin of the falx cerebri (**C**).

The straight sinus (**A**) is the continuation of the above vessel. It runs downwards and backwards in the junction between the falx cerebri and the tentorium cerebelli to the internal occipital protuberance, where it becomes continuous (**D**) with the transverse sinus which is not joined by the superior sagittal sinus (see above).

The paired transverse sinuses, and the paired sigmoid sinuses and internal jugular veins which are their continuations, are unequal in size because the superior sagittal sinus is larger than the straight sinus. Each transverse sinus runs laterally and then forwards between the dura of the attached margin of the tentorium cerebelli and the endocranium lining the transverse sulcus on the occipital bone (**D**).

The paired sigmoid sinuses are continuous with the corresponding transverse sinuses. Each turns downwards out of the attached margin of the tentorium cerebelli and runs an S-shaped course in the sigmoid sulcus to the jugular foramen (**D**). It is usually joined by a large emissary vein which passes through the mastoid foramen (**D**). The deep sigmoid sulcus is lined by endocranium and bridged over by the dura lining the posterior cranial fossa. The sinus turns downwards through the posterior part of the jugular foramen (**D**) and becomes the internal jugular vein of the neck.

The paired superior petrosal sinuses arise from the posterior ends of the corresponding cavernous sinuses. Each passes backwards and laterally along the grooved superior border of the petrous temporal in the attached margin of the tentorium cerebelli (**D**). They end by opening into the junctions of the transverse and sigmoid sinuses.

The paired inferior petrosal sinuses also arise from the posterior ends of the cavernous sinuses (**D**). They pass downwards and backwards between the endocranium and the dura of the posterior cranial fossa, overlying the junctions of the petrous temporals and the basilar parts of the sphenoid and occipital bones. They then turn downwards through the anterior parts of the jugular foramina and bend backwards just below the base of the skull to end in the internal jugular veins.

The meningeal arteries

A number of arteries, with accompanying veins, run between the endocranium and the dura mater, many of them in sharply defined grooves. Although they are called meningeal vessels the name is unfortunate because in fact they are distributed much more to the cranial bones than to the dura. One of these arteries is much larger than the others and of greater clinical significance, so it alone will be described.

The middle meningeal artery arises in the infratemporal fossa (**461A**) and enters the cranial cavity through the foramen spinosum in the floor of the lateral compartment of the middle cranial fossa (**D**). Running laterally in its groove it divides into anterior and posterior divisions which continue upwards, branching progressively, towards the vault of the skull.

SAGITTAL SINUSES & STRAIGHT SINUS

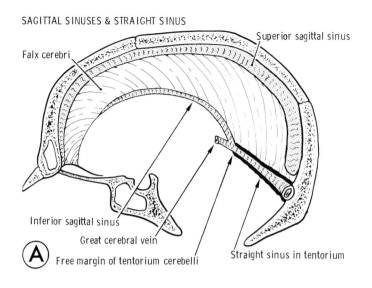

Falx cerebri

Superior sagittal sinus

Inferior sagittal sinus

Great cerebral vein

Free margin of tentorium cerebelli

Straight sinus in tentorium

(A)

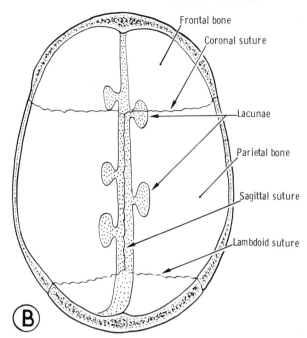

Frontal bone

Coronal suture

Lacunae

Parietal bone

Sagittal suture

Lambdoid suture

(B)

SAGITTAL SINUSES: CORONAL SECTION

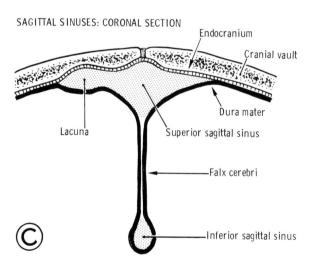

Endocranium

Cranial vault

Dura mater

Lacuna

Superior sagittal sinus

Falx cerebri

Inferior sagittal sinus

(C)

DURAL VENOUS SINUSES

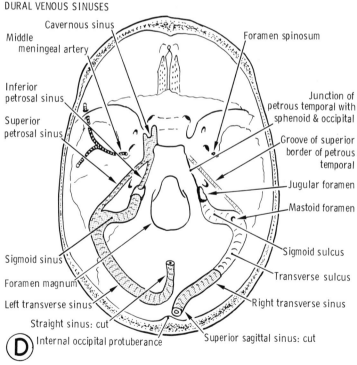

Cavernous sinus

Middle meningeal artery

Foramen spinosum

Inferior petrosal sinus

Superior petrosal sinus

Junction of petrous temporal with sphenoid & occipital

Groove of superior border of petrous temporal

Jugular foramen

Mastoid foramen

Sigmoid sulcus

Transverse sulcus

Right transverse sinus

Superior sagittal sinus: cut

Sigmoid sinus

Foramen magnum

Left transverse sinus

Straight sinus: cut

Internal occipital protuberance

(D)

101

The anterior division passes deep to the pterion (**17C**) and in some individuals the groove in which it lies deepens into a tunnel over a short distance. Above the pterion the branches of the anterior division are superficial to the motor area of the cerebral cortex (**A**). The clinical importance of the middle meningeal vessels, and particularly the anterior division, is that they may be torn by a fracture of the skull in the temporal region. The escaping blood accumulates between the dura and the bone as an extradural haemorrhage which may cause symptoms of brain compression. Because of the relationship, noted above, of the middle meningeal artery to the precentral gyrus, paralysis of the opposite side of the body is a common early feature of the condition.

The spinal dura

This is appreciably thinner than the cerebral dura with which it is continuous through the foramen magnum. It forms a loose tubular investment around the spinal cord and the elements of the cauda equina as far as the level of the second piece of the sacrum where it ends blindly (**D**).

Unlike the relationship of the cerebral dura to the cranial bones, the spinal dura is separated everywhere from the bones and ligaments forming the walls of the vertebral canal by an extradural (epidural) space of considerable dimensions. The space contains fatty areolar tissue which is pervaded by the internal vertebral venous plexus (**B**). This plexus normally receives blood from the vertebral bodies through the basivertebral veins and is drained by intervertebral veins which traverse the intervertebral foramina to join the segmental veins at all levels. Because of the absence or paucity of valves in the veins of the extradural space, it is considered by some that invasion of segmental veins by a malignant tumour may reverse their normal direction of blood flow and lead to the formation of metastases in vertebral bodies.

As each spinal nerve leaves the main spinal dural sac its two roots are enclosed within narrow tubes of dura which finally blend with the fibrous covering of the definitive nerve (epineurium) in the corresponding intervertebral foramen. These tubes are short in the upper part of the vertebral canal (**C**) but below, increase in length and obliquity with the increasing obliquity of the nerve roots until in the sacral region they are several inches long (**D**).

MIDDLE MENINGEAL ARTERY: RELATIONS TO BRAIN & SKULL

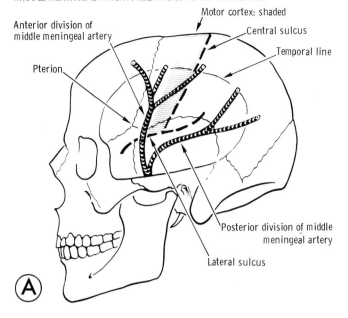

Anterior division of middle meningeal artery

Motor cortex: shaded

Central sulcus

Temporal line

Pterion

Posterior division of middle meningeal artery

Lateral sulcus

(A)

DURAL INVESTMENT OF UPPER SPINAL NERVES:
(Coronal section behind vertebral bodies)

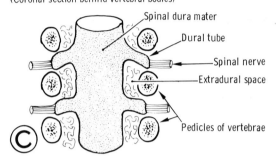

Spinal dura mater

Dural tube

Spinal nerve

Extradural space

Pedicles of vertebrae

(C)

SPINAL EXTRADURAL SPACE

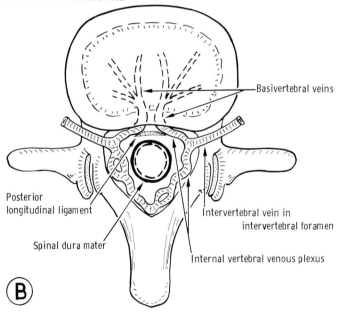

Basivertebral veins

Posterior longitudinal ligament

Spinal dura mater

Intervertebral vein in intervertebral foramen

Internal vertebral venous plexus

(B)

DURAL INVESTMENT OF LOWER SPINAL NERVES:
(Coronal section along sacral canal)

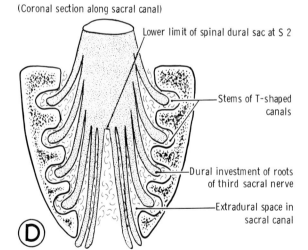

Lower limit of spinal dural sac at S 2

Stems of T-shaped canals

Dural investment of roots of third sacral nerve

Extradural space in sacral canal

(D)

The arachnoid mater

The middle of the three meningeal layers, the arachnoid is a thin translucent membrane which is separated from all parts of the dura, including its prolongations along the spinal and cranial nerves, by a very narrow subdural space. This space is lined by flat mesothelial cells and occupied by a film of fluid.

Internally, the arachnoid is separated from the pia mater by the subarachnoid space which is occupied by cerebrospinal fluid. This space varies in dimensions in different situations.

The spinal subarachnoid space is fairly wide and contains the spinal cord and the roots of the spinal nerves. The spinal cord is anchored to the spinal arachnoid by three connective tissue laminae. The posterior lamina is the subarachnoid septum which is often incomplete. On either side the paired denticulate ligaments extend laterally between the anterior and posterior roots of the spinal nerves, and are attached to the arachnoid by a series of separated pointed processes (**A**). Below the lower end of the spinal cord at the level of the second lumbar vertebra, the cerebrospinal fluid in the spinal subarachnoid space bathes the nerve roots comprising the cauda equina.

The cerebral subarachnoid space throughout most of its extent is only a few millimetres wide and is traversed by delicate strands of connective tissue (**C**). However, in some situations the arachnoid bridges over considerable irregularities on the brain surface so that the subarachnoid space is much wider and has few trabeculae. These wide parts are called the subarachnoid cisterns. Most are in and around the midline and can be observed in **B**. In addition, note that the interpeduncular and chiasmatic cisterns are continuous laterally on either side with a cistern of the lateral fossa where the arachnoid bridges the stem of the lateral sulcus.

The cerebrospinal fluid

It has been noted previously (**26**) that this watery fluid which occupies the subarachnoid space is continuously secreted by the choroid plexuses of the ventricles of the brain. It passes from the ventricular system through the median and lateral apertures in the roof of the lower part of the fourth ventricle (**45C, 45D**) into the cerebellomedullary and pontine cisterns (**B**). Although there is some interchange between the fluid in these situations and that occupying the spinal subarachnoid space, the main flow is upwards through all parts of the cerebral subarachnoid space towards the region of the cranial vault.

Although a relatively small amount of cerebrospinal fluid is lost from the subarachnoid space into lymphatic vessels associated with spinal and cranial nerves, the bulk is transferred into the superior sagittal sinus through structures called arachnoid villi. The total amount of fluid lost equals the amount formed by the choroid plexuses so that the quantity in the subarachnoid space is constant.

The arachnoid villi are small finger-like protrusions of arachnoid mater which contain finely trabeculated extensions of the subarachnoid space. These penetrate through gaps in the dura and invaginate the endothelial lining of the superior sagittal sinus mainly in its lacunae (**C**). The adjacent layers of arachnoid and venous endothelium are fenestrated (**D**). Under normal circumstances cerebrospinal fluid passes through these openings into the venous bloodstream. On the other hand if the venous pressure becomes relatively high the villi collapse, and their fenestrations close, preventing reflux of blood into the subarachnoid space. Thrombosis within the sinus naturally blocks the fenestrations in the villi and causes a progressive rise in the pressure in the subarachnoid space.

Although in youth the arachnoid villi are simple finger-like processes, as age advances they become more elaborate in form with several processes arising from a large single stem. They are then known as arachnoid granulations, and the pressure they exert against the sinus endothelium and the endocranium (**C**) often produces pit-like erosions on the inner aspects of the cranial bones at some distance from the midline (**23B**).

Lumbar and cisternal puncture are procedures in which hollow needles are passed into certain parts of the subarachnoid space, either for the assessment of its shape after the introduction of contrast media, or for the determination of the cell content, biochemical composition or pressure of the cerebrospinal fluid.

In lumbar puncture the needle is introduced in the midline posteriorly, between the spines of the third and fourth lumbar vertebrae, so that its point lies amongst the elements of the cauda equina. It will be recalled that the fourth lumbar spine is at the same level as the highest points of the iliac crests.

In the less common procedure of cisternal puncture, the needle is passed upwards and forwards in the midline between the posterior margin of the foramen magnum and the posterior arch of the atlas into the cerebellomedullary cistern (**B**).

DENTICULATE LIGAMENT IN SUBARACHNOID SPACE: ANTERIOR VIEW
(Anterior halves of spinal dura & arachnoid removed)

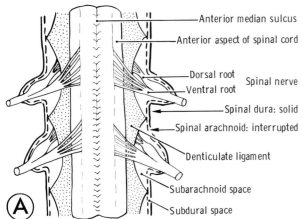

- Anterior median sulcus
- Anterior aspect of spinal cord
- Dorsal root   Spinal nerve
- Ventral root
- Spinal dura: solid
- Spinal arachnoid: interrupted
- Denticulate ligament
- Subarachnoid space
- Subdural space

(A)

SUBARACHNOID CISTERNS: MEDIAN SECTION

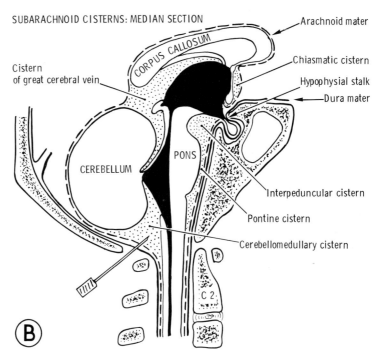

- Arachnoid mater
- Chiasmatic cistern
- Hypophysial stalk
- Dura mater
- Interpeduncular cistern
- Pontine cistern
- Cerebellomedullary cistern

Cistern of great cerebral vein

CORPUS CALLOSUM

CEREBELLUM   PONS

C 2

(B)

ARACHNOID VILLI IN VENOUS LACUNA: CORONAL SECTION

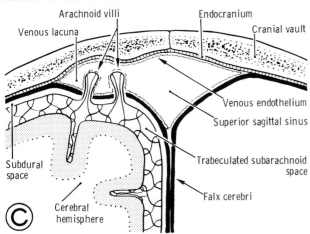

- Arachnoid villi
- Venous lacuna
- Endocranium
- Cranial vault
- Venous endothelium
- Superior sagittal sinus
- Trabeculated subarachnoid space
- Falx cerebri
- Subdural space
- Cerebral hemisphere

(C)

ARACHNOID VILLUS

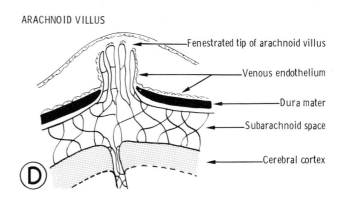

- Fenestrated tip of arachnoid villus
- Venous endothelium
- Dura mater
- Subarachnoid space
- Cerebral cortex

(D)

ARTERIES AND VEINS OF THE CENTRAL NERVOUS SYSTEM

The arterial supply to the brain

This is provided by the small branches which pass into the brain substance from larger arteries in the subarachnoid space.

The small branches within the brain may rupture causing destruction of a region of brain tissue (cerebral haemorrhage). On the other hand the larger vessels in the subarachnoid space may be obstructed by thrombosis or embolism giving rise to infarction of an area of brain tissue, or may rupture, usually at the site of a congenital aneurysm. Such a rupture causes a subarachnoid haemorrhage which produces a progressive increase in intracranial pressure. These constitute what are known colloquially as strokes and are a very common cause of illness and death.

The arteries to the brain are all ultimately derived from the paired internal carotid and vertebral arteries.

The internal carotid arteries

Each internal carotid artery ascends through the upper half of the neck and then traverses the carotid canal in the petrous part of the temporal bone (**A**), running first upwards and subsequently forwards and medially to emerge in the patent upper half of the foramen lacerum. Turning upwards and forwards, it enters the substance of the overlying cavernous sinus and passes forwards towards its anterior end (**99C**). There it turns upwards again and leaves the sinus by piercing the diaphragma sellae and the overlying arachnoid, medial to the anterior clinoid process and below the optic nerve (**B**). It will be seen later (**427B**) that in its passage through the cavernous sinus the artery is closely related to the third, fourth, fifth and sixth cranial nerves.

Turning backwards from beneath the optic nerve, the artery lies below the anterior perforated substance and lateral to the optic chiasma (**B, D**), within the interpeduncular cistern. Here it ends by dividing into anterior and middle cerebral arteries.

The vertebral arteries

Each vertebral artery ascends from the root of the neck through the foramina transversaria of all the cervical transverse processes except the seventh. Emerging from the foramen in the atlas (**C**) it bends round the lateral mass, and, passing between the groove on the posterior arch and the free margin of the posterior atlanto-occipital membrane, pierces the spinal dura and arachnoid to enter the subarachnoid space. Ascending through that part of the

space between the clivus and the medulla (**D**), in front of the several cranial nerve rootlets which emerge from that part of the brain stem (**39B**), the two vertebral arteries incline medially over the surface of the pyramids and join to form the single basilar artery at the lower border of the pons.

The basilar artery ascends in the midline through the pontine cistern (**105B**) lying between the two abducent nerves below and between the two oculomotor nerves above. It ends over the posterior perforated substance by dividing into paired posterior cerebral arteries which diverge laterally.

The branches of the vertebral and basilar arteries

These should be studied in **D** and their relationships to the third, fourth and sixth cranial nerves observed. By and large, the names of these branches indicate their distributions, but note the following additional distributions which are not shown in **D**.

1. Each anterior inferior cerebellar artery gives off a slender labyrinthine branch which accompanies the facial and vestibulocochlear nerves along the internal acoustic meatus.
2. Each posterior inferior cerebellar artery supplies branches to the choroid plexus in the roof of the fourth ventricle (**45C**) and a posterior spinal branch which descends onto the spinal cord (**111C**).

The arterial circle and the cerebral arteries

The arterial circle (of Willis) is an approximately circular anastomotic channel which links the terminations of the internal carotid and basilar arteries, and the initial parts of the anterior, middle and posterior cerebral arteries. Examine its position and parts in **D** and note the following facts.

1. The circle lies in the interpeduncular and chiasmatic cisterns and surrounds the structures forming the floor of the third ventricle.
2. The anterior communicating artery is a short single vessel joining the two anterior cerebral arteries in the chiasmatic cistern.
3. The longer posterior communicating arteries are paired vessels each of which joins the terminal part of the internal carotid artery to the corresponding posterior cerebral artery.

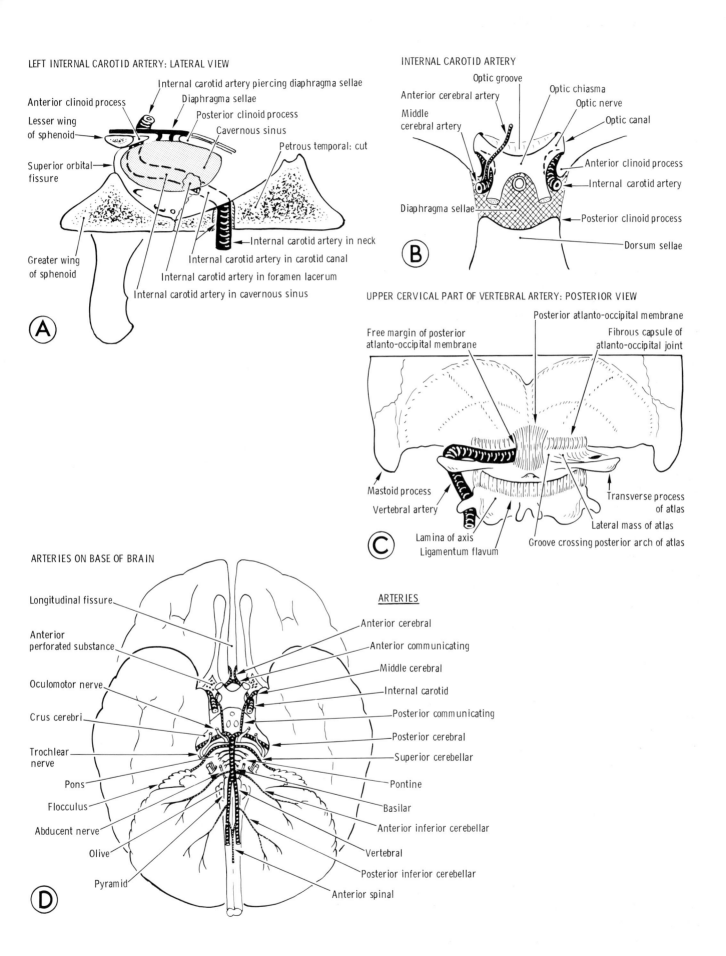

LEFT INTERNAL CAROTID ARTERY: LATERAL VIEW

Internal carotid artery piercing diaphragma sellae
Anterior clinoid process
Diaphragma sellae
Lesser wing of sphenoid
Posterior clinoid process
Cavernous sinus
Petrous temporal: cut
Superior orbital fissure
Greater wing of sphenoid
Internal carotid artery in neck
Internal carotid artery in carotid canal
Internal carotid artery in foramen lacerum
Internal carotid artery in cavernous sinus

A

INTERNAL CAROTID ARTERY

Optic groove
Anterior cerebral artery
Optic chiasma
Optic nerve
Middle cerebral artery
Optic canal
Anterior clinoid process
Internal carotid artery
Diaphragma sellae
Posterior clinoid process
Dorsum sellae

B

UPPER CERVICAL PART OF VERTEBRAL ARTERY: POSTERIOR VIEW

Posterior atlanto-occipital membrane
Free margin of posterior atlanto-occipital membrane
Fibrous capsule of atlanto-occipital joint
Mastoid process
Vertebral artery
Transverse process of atlas
Lateral mass of atlas
Groove crossing posterior arch of atlas
Lamina of axis
Ligamentum flavum

C

ARTERIES ON BASE OF BRAIN

Longitudinal fissure
Anterior perforated substance
Oculomotor nerve
Crus cerebri
Trochlear nerve
Pons
Flocculus
Abducent nerve
Olive
Pyramid

ARTERIES

Anterior cerebral
Anterior communicating
Middle cerebral
Internal carotid
Posterior communicating
Posterior cerebral
Superior cerebellar
Pontine
Basilar
Anterior inferior cerebellar
Vertebral
Posterior inferior cerebellar
Anterior spinal

D

Because of the large calibre of the main cerebral arteries, the anastomoses provided by the arterial circle is not usually sufficient to provide an efficient collateral circulation if one of the internal carotid arteries or the basilar artery is occluded. It seems that the physiological purpose of the circle is to be related rather to the equalisation of pressures within the normal cerebral arteries.

The anterior cerebral artery is the smaller of the terminal branches of the internal carotid. It passes forwards and medially, above the optic nerve to the lowest part of the longitudinal fissure, where it is linked to the corresponding vessel of the opposite side by the single, short anterior communicating artery (**107B, 107D**). Thereafter, it runs on the medial surface of the cerebral hemisphere a short distance from the free surfaces of the lamina terminalis and the corpus callosum as far as the splenium (**A**). Observe the area of cerebral cortex shown as white in **A** and **B** which the branches of the anterior cerebral artery supply, and note that this area includes those parts of the main somatomotor and somatosensory cortices which are associated with the perineum and lower limb (**69**).

The middle cerebral artery is the other terminal branch of the internal carotid (**107D**). It lies initially below the anterior perforated substance (**C**) and subsequently runs in the depth of the stem of the lateral sulcus (**C**) to the surface of the insula. Branches emerge onto the superolateral surface of the hemisphere through the lateral sulcus to supply the cortical region which is crosshatched in **A** and **B**. Note that this region includes the greater parts of the main somatomotor and somatosensory areas and the acoustic area of the cortex (**69**).

The posterior cerebral arteries are the terminal branches of the single basilar artery (**107D**). After being connected to the corresponding internal carotid, each winds round the cerebral peduncle above the superior cerebellar artery and separated from it by the oculomotor and trochlear nerves. It reaches the medial surface of the temporal lobe near the uncus and runs backwards in the general line of the calcarine and parieto-occipital sulci (**A**). Finally its branches turn round the occipital pole to reach the superolateral surface of the hemisphere (**B**). Its surface branches spread over an area (stippled) which consists of the medial and inferior aspects of the temporal lobe except near its pole (**A**) and over all surfaces of the occipital lobe (**B**). Note that this region includes the visual and olfactory cortical areas.

Branches of the arterial circle and cerebral arteries

These branches fall into three categories, cortical, central and choroidal.

The cortical branches to the whole cerebrum arise from the surface branches of the three cerebral arteries in the respective areas of distribution discussed above. After ramifying in the pia mater they penetrate the cortex perpendicularly as end arteries. Although their main distribution is to the cortex some extend beyond the surface grey matter into the adjacent white matter.

The central branches arise in the groups indicated in (**D**) from the arterial circle or the proximal parts of the cerebral arteries.

1. The anterior group supply the optic chiasma, the lamina terminalis and the anterior part of the corpus striatum.
2. Each anterolateral or striate group arises from the corresponding middle cerebral artery and penetrates the anterior perforated substance (**C**). The medial striate vessels curve upwards and then medially through the globus pallidus and the internal capsule into the thalamus, while the lateral striate follow a similarly curved course through the putamen and internal capsule to the head and body of the caudate nucleus.
3. Each posterolateral group arises from the posterior cerebral after it has wound round the midbrain. The vessels supply the colliculi, the geniculate bodies, the pineal body and the pulvinar of the thalamus.
4. The posterior group penetrate the posterior perforated substance and give branches to the midbrain and the posterior part of the floor of the third ventricle.

Choroidal branches supply the choroid plexuses of the forebrain. The anterior choroidal arises from the internal carotid, just before its division, and supplies the choroid plexus of the inferior horn of the lateral ventricle (not shown in **A**). The posterior choroidal is a branch of the posterior cerebral which passes forwards into the tela choroidea and supplies the plexuses of the central part of the lateral ventricle and the third ventricle (**A**).

FOREBRAIN & MIDBRAIN: MEDIAN SECTION

(Cortical distribution of cerebral arteries:
Anterior - white: Posterior - stippled: Middle - hatched)

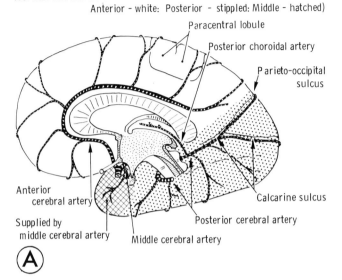

Paracentral lobule

Posterior choroidal artery

Parieto-occipital sulcus

Anterior cerebral artery

Supplied by middle cerebral artery

Middle cerebral artery

Posterior cerebral artery

Calcarine sulcus

(A)

CEREBRAL HEMISPHERE: LATERAL ASPECT

(Cortical distribution of cerebral arteries as indicated in A)

Branches of anterior cerebral artery

Parieto-occipital sulcus

Central sulcus

Branches of middle cerebral artery

Lateral sulcus

Branches of posterior cerebral artery

(B)

MIDDLE CEREBRAL & STRIATE ARTERIES: OBLIQUE SECTION

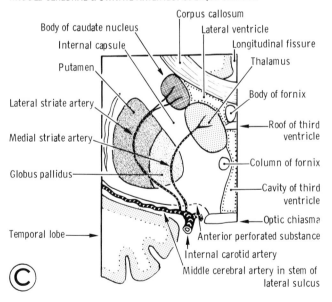

Body of caudate nucleus

Corpus callosum

Lateral ventricle

Internal capsule

Longitudinal fissure

Putamen

Thalamus

Lateral striate artery

Body of fornix

Medial striate artery

Roof of third ventricle

Globus pallidus

Column of fornix

Cavity of third ventricle

Temporal lobe

Optic chiasma

Anterior perforated substance

Internal carotid artery

Middle cerebral artery in stem of lateral sulcus

(C)

ORIGINS OF GROUPS OF CENTRAL ARTERIAL BRANCHES

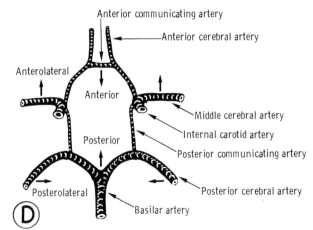

Anterior communicating artery

Anterior cerebral artery

Anterolateral

Anterior

Middle cerebral artery

Internal carotid artery

Posterior

Posterior communicating artery

Posterolateral

Posterior cerebral artery

Basilar artery

(D)

The venous drainage of the brain

The veins of the brain are thin-walled valveless vessels, running mainly in the subarachnoid space, which drain into the dural venous sinuses and thus eventually into the internal jugular veins of the neck. To open into the dural sinuses, the veins must pierce both the arachnoid and dura and cross the narrow subdural space (**A**). In the latter situation they may be torn by injuries which cause a momentary shift of one part of the brain surface away from the rigidly fixed dura. Thus a subdural haemorrhage is often purely venous in contrast to a subarachnoid haemorrhage which is usually arterial.

The cerebral veins

The superficial cerebral venous plexuses cover the surfaces of the cerebral hemispheres and receive tributaries largely from the cortex. From the upper and anterior parts of each plexus, veins pass upwards and forwards to open into the main channel, but not the lacunae, of the superior sagittal sinus (**A**). From the lower part veins pass downwards into the cavernous, superior petrosal and transverse sinuses.

Paired internal cerebral veins form within the tela choroidea of the third and fourth ventricles (**B**) by the junction of choroidal veins and deep veins from the interiors of the hemispheres. The two vessels run backwards and, between the splenium of the corpus callosum and the pineal body, unite in the midline to form the great cerebral vein (**B**). This vessel continues backwards in the cistern named after it (**105B**) and, piercing the anterior margin of the tentorium cerebelli, joins the beginning of the straight sinus (**101A**).

A basal vein is formed on each side over the anterior perforated substance by the union of the deep middle cerebral vein, which runs downwards from the insular cortex in the depths of the stem of the lateral sulcus, and the striate veins which issue from the region of the internal capsule and the corpus striatum. It winds round the midbrain and joins the great cerebral vein (**B**).

The cerebellar and brain stem veins

Those from the superior vermis of the cerebellum and from the midbrain usually drain into the basal veins or the great cerebral vein.

From the rest of the region the veins open into those dural venous sinuses which lie in the walls of the posterior cranial fossa, that is, the straight, transverse, sigmoid and petrosal sinuses (**101D**).

The arteries and veins of the spinal cord

The upper part of the spinal cord receives a single anterior spinal artery which arises by two stems from the terminal parts of the vertebral arteries on the anterior surface of the medulla (**107D**), and two posterior spinal arteries each of which springs from the corresponding posterior inferior cerebellar artery (**107D**) and soon divides into two branches. These descending vessels lie in the pia covering the cord, and their relationships to the median fissure and the dorsal roots of the spinal nerves should be observed in **C**.

Although these arteries are small, they are joined as they pass downwards by other vessels, so that they maintain their original calibre and are able to extend as far as the lower end of the spinal cord. The augmenting vessels are derived from the spinal branches of intersegmental arteries which enter the vertebral canal through the intervertebral foramina or the pevlic sacral foramina. Some twigs from these spinal branches ramify in the extradural space. Others piece the spinal dura and arachnoid with the spinal nerves and run with the ventral and dorsal nerve roots to the spinal cord to join the anterior and posterior spinal arteries respectively (**C**).

Six longitudinal veins run along the surface of the length of the cord in the positions indicated in **C**. They are drained by small vessels which accompany the spinal nerve roots and open into the intervertebral veins (**103B**).

ENTRANCE OF CEREBRAL VEIN INTO DURAL VENOUS SINUS

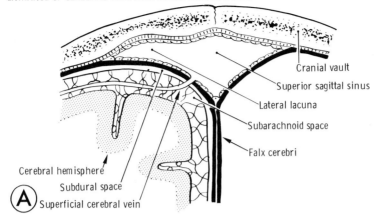

Cranial vault
Superior sagittal sinus
Lateral lacuna
Subarachnoid space
Falx cerebri
Cerebral hemisphere
Subdural space
(A) Superficial cerebral vein

MEDIAN SECTION OF FOREBRAIN & MIDBRAIN: CEREBRAL VEINS

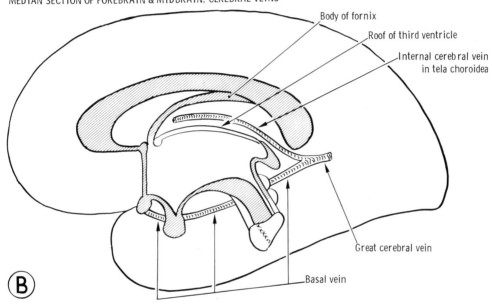

Body of fornix
Roof of third ventricle
Internal cerebral vein
in tela choroidea
Great cerebral vein
Basal vein
(B)

TRANSVERSE SECTION OF SPINAL CORD:
BLOOD SUPPLY OF CORD

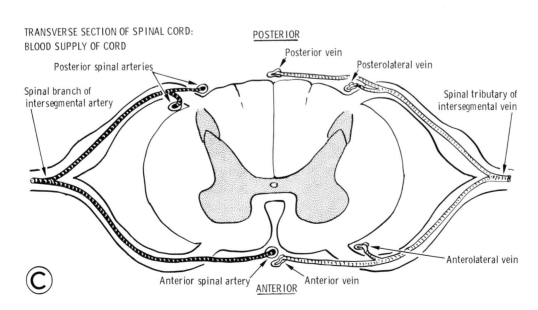

POSTERIOR
Posterior vein
Posterolateral vein
Posterior spinal arteries
Spinal branch of
intersegmental artery
Spinal tributary of
intersegmental vein
Anterolateral vein
Anterior spinal artery
Anterior vein
(C)
ANTERIOR

111

THE HYPOPHYSIS CEREBRI

This important structure is considered at this late stage because a knowledge of its blood vessels and of its relations to the dura mater and dural venous sinuses is necessary to its understanding.

It has been seen previously that the part of the hypothalamus which forms the floor of the third ventricle between the mamillary bodies and the optic chiasma is a prominent region of grey matter called the tuber cinereum (**A**). From the summit of this prominence the slender hypophysial stalk extends downwards and then expands into the more or less spherical body of the hypophysis (**B**).

In the adult, the body consists from before backwards of a large pars anterior, a narrow cleft or row of vesicles, a very narrow pars intermedia and a pars posterior (**B**). The stalk consists of two parts (**B**). The infundibulum, which contains a tapering extension of the lumen of the third ventricle, is continuous above with the tuber cinereum and below with the pars posterior. The pars tuberalis clothes the anterior and lateral aspects of the infundibulum. Although it is continuous below with the pars anterior, it has a different structure and its function is unclear.

In an alternative terminology the body and stalk of the hypophysis together are divided into two parts on embryological grounds.

1. The adenohypophysis (stippled in **B**) consists of the pars anterior, the pars intermedia and the pars tuberalis.
2. The neurohypophysis (clear in **B**) comprises the pars posterior and the infundibulum.

Relations

The hypophysial stalk crosses the interpeduncular subarachnoid cistern (**105B**) from the tuber cinereum to the central part of the dural diaphragma sellae (**C, D**). Here that layer of dura and the overlying arachnoid fuse to form a common fibrous sac which is flask-like in form and descends into the hypophysial fossa on the superior aspect of the body of the sphenoid. The body of the gland is enclosed within this fibrous hypophysial sac, no subarachnoid space intervening.

Note the relationships of the hypophysis to the following structures.

1. The cavernous (**D**) and intercavernous venous sinuses (**C**).
2. The internal carotid arteries (**D**). An aneurysm of the artery where it lies in the cavernous sinus may cause pressure on the hypophysis.
3. The optic chiasma (**C**). The effects of pressure on the chiasma by an enlarged hypophysis have been discussed previously (**84**).
4. The sphenoidal sinuses (**C**) are air-filled spaces within the sphenoid which open forwards into the nasal cavity and provide one surgical approach to the hypophysis.

Blood vessels

The hypophysis and its stalk have a peculiar vascular pattern (**E**) with functions additional to those of nourishment and the transport of hypophysial hormones into the general circulation.

The inferior hypophysial arteries arise on either side from the internal carotids as they lie within the cavernous sinuses. Their branches penetrate the hypophysial dural sac and terminate in a sinusoidal capillary bed in the pars posterior.

The superior hypophysial arteries arise on both sides from the internal carotid arteries immediately above the diaphragma sellae and reach the junction of the tuber cinereum and the hypophysial stalk. Some branches descend through the pars tuberalis and end in sinusoidal capillaries in the pars anterior. They constitute the main arterial supply to the adenohypophysis. Other branches enter the infundibulum either directly or through the pars tuberalis and in that part end in discrete clusters of capillaries. These capillaries are drained by venules which leave the infundibulum and pass downwards through the pars tuberalis to open into the sinusoids of the pars anterior. This second vascular pathway from the superior hypophysial arteries to the pars anterior thus traverses successively two groups of capillaries or sinusoids and is consequently known as the hypophysial portal system.

The hypophysial veins which carry the hormones produced by the hypophysis into the general circulation are short vessels which open through the surrounding fibrous sac into the cavernous and intercavernous sinuses.

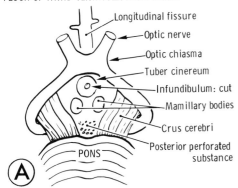

FLOOR OF THIRD VENTRICLE: FROM BELOW

- Longitudinal fissure
- Optic nerve
- Optic chiasma
- Tuber cinereum
- Infundibulum: cut
- Mamillary bodies
- Crus cerebri
- Posterior perforated substance

PONS

Ⓐ

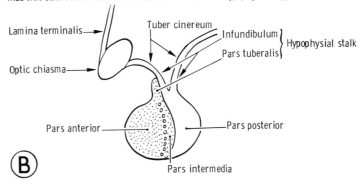

MEDIAN SECTION OF HYPOPHYSIS CEREBRI (Adenohypophysis stippled)

- Lamina terminalis
- Optic chiasma
- Tuber cinereum
- Infundibulum ⎫ Hypophysial stalk
- Pars tuberalis ⎭
- Pars anterior
- Pars posterior
- Pars intermedia

Ⓑ

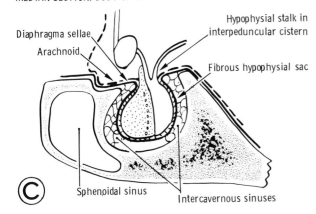

MEDIAN SECTION: BODY OF SPHENOID & HYPOPHYSIS

- Diaphragma sellae
- Arachnoid
- Hypophysial stalk in interpeduncular cistern
- Fibrous hypophysial sac
- Sphenoidal sinus
- Intercavernous sinuses

Ⓒ

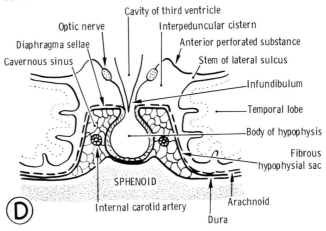

CORONAL SECTION: HYPOPHYSIS CEREBRI

- Optic nerve
- Cavity of third ventricle
- Diaphragma sellae
- Interpeduncular cistern
- Cavernous sinus
- Anterior perforated substance
- Stem of lateral sulcus
- Infundibulum
- Temporal lobe
- Body of hypophysis
- Fibrous hypophysial sac
- SPHENOID
- Internal carotid artery
- Arachnoid
- Dura

Ⓓ

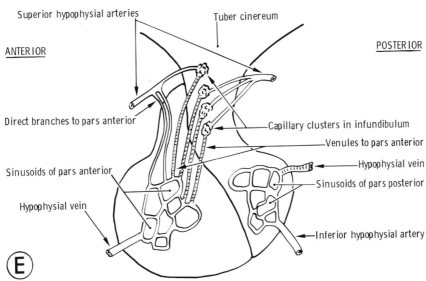

DIAGRAMMATIC REPRESENTATION OF HYPOPHYSIAL BLOOD VESSELS

- Superior hypophysial arteries
- Tuber cinereum
- ANTERIOR
- POSTERIOR
- Direct branches to pars anterior
- Capillary clusters in infundibulum
- Venules to pars anterior
- Hypophysial vein
- Sinusoids of pars anterior
- Sinusoids of pars posterior
- Hypophysial vein
- Inferior hypophysial artery

Ⓔ

Nervous connections

No nerve fibres are present in the adenohypophysis although, as will be seen below, the activity of that part is controlled indirectly by neurons.

In contrast, the axons of neurons whose cell bodies are situated in various parts of the hypothalamus pervade both parts of the neurohypophysis constituting the hypothalamo-hypophysial tract (**A**).

All these neurons exhibit the phenomenon of neurosecretion, in which a number of different hormones are elaborated by the endoplasmic reticulum and transported along the axons to be released at the axon terminals. The neurons fall into two groups (**A**).

1. The axons of one group terminate close to the sinusoids of the pars posterior. Here they liberate two hormones (the antidiurectic hormone and oxytocin) which pass through the sinusoid walls into the general circulation.

2. The axons of the other group terminate in close relationship to the capillary clusters in the infundibulum. Here they liberate hormones which enter the capillaries and pass through the venules of the hypophysial portal system to the sinusoids in the adenohypophysis. These are known as releasing hormones, or perhaps better as hormone-regulating factors, as, passing through the sinusoidal walls, they exercise control over the elaboration and release of the several hormones produced by the cells of the pars anterior.

THE AUTONOMIC NERVOUS SYSTEM

It has been noted already (**26**) that in this text the autonomic system is treated as a purely motor system which, with other factors, exercises a degree of involuntary control over the secretory activities of exocrine glands and the contraction of smooth and cardiac muscle. In other descriptions visceral sensory neurons are included in the same system. In this text such neurons will be considered separately in another section.

The autonomic system as defined above consists of sympathetic and parasympathetic parts which differ in their sites of origin in the central nervous system, their distributions and their functions. Both parts, as has been noted (**33D**), consist of nervous pathways in which two multipolar neurons are linked in series by a synapse. The proximal or preganglionic neurons have their cell bodies in the grey matter of the spinal cord or brain stem, and their axons are medullated. The cell bodies of the distal or postganglionic neurons lie either in compact groups called autonomic ganglia or in more widely dispersed collections called autonomic plexuses. The axons of these neurons are unmyelinated.

It is convenient to consider the general features of these autonomic ganglia and plexuses here.

Parasympathetic ganglia

These are essentially sites of synapse between preganglionic and postganglionic parasympathetic neurons, but many are also traversed by other functional types of neurons without synapse. The latter may be postganglionic sympathetic, sensory or branchial motor (**B**).

They are small, compact structures which lie near to, but not on the course of, certain cranial nerves or their branches in the regions of head and neck.

Sympathetic ganglia

These are also small compact structures which are sites of synapse between preganglionic and postganglionic sympathetic neurons. Most are also traversed by preganglionic sympathetic and visceral sensory neurons without relay, but they are never associated in any way with parasympathetic neurons.

In contrast to the individual nature of the parasympathetic ganglia described above, adjacent sympathetic ganglia are joined by narrow cords of nerve fibres to form the long paired sympathetic trunks (**C**). These extend in a paravertebral position from the base of the skull to the coccyx where they end by fusing in the small, single ganglion impar.

The number of ganglia on the pelvic, lumbar and thoracic parts of each trunk may correspond to the number of spinal nerves in those regions. But not infrequently the number in one of these regions is reduced by one or even two so that one or two of the remaining ganglia are associated with more than one spinal nerve. This phenomenon is most pronounced in the cervical region where the number of ganglia is reduced to three (**C**). The elongated superior cervical ganglion is associated with the first four cervical nerves, the small middle ganglion with the fifth and sixth cervical nerves, and the inferior ganglion with the seventh and eighth cervical nerves. Commonly the latter is fused to the first thoracic ganglion forming what is called a cervicothoracic ganglion.

HYPOTHALAMOHYPOPHYSIAL TRACT

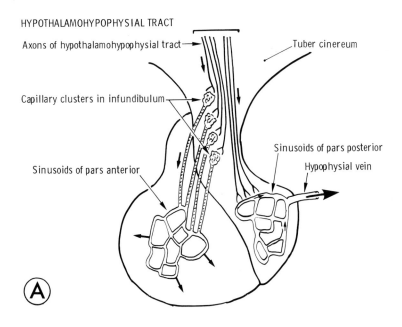

Axons of hypothalamohypophysial tract →
Tuber cinereum
Capillary clusters in infundibulum →
Sinusoids of pars posterior
Hypophysial vein
Sinusoids of pars anterior

A

EXAMPLE (DIAGRAMMATIC) OF PARASYMPATHETIC GANGLION

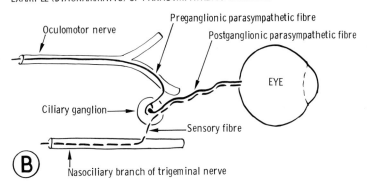

Oculomotor nerve
Preganglionic parasympathetic fibre
Postganglionic parasympathetic fibre
EYE
Ciliary ganglion →
Sensory fibre
B
Nasociliary branch of trigeminal nerve

SYMPATHETIC TRUNK: UPPER PART

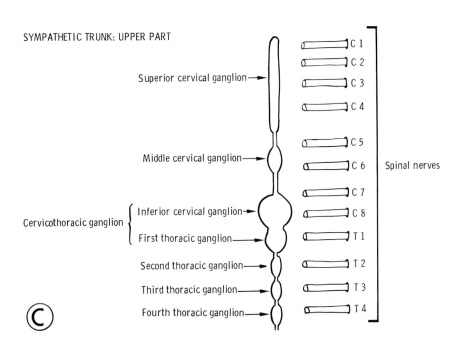

Superior cervical ganglion →
C 1
C 2
C 3
C 4
C 5
Middle cervical ganglion →
C 6
Spinal nerves
C 7
Cervicothoracic ganglion { Inferior cervical ganglion →
C 8
First thoracic ganglion →
T 1
Second thoracic ganglion →
T 2
Third thoracic ganglion →
T 3
C
Fourth thoracic ganglion →
T 4

The autonomic plexuses

Autonomic plexuses contain in varying proportions the cell bodies and axons of both sympathetic and parasympathetic neurons.

A number of central plexuses are situated near the midline in the thorax and along the posterior wall of the abdomen. The positions of these are indicated in **A**. Although their names are given in that figure for convenience, it is not suggested that they should be learnt at this time.

From these central plexuses many slender branch plexuses extend to the thoracic and abdominal viscera, either along the walls of the corresponding visceral arteries or along independent courses.

Terminal plexuses are present in the walls of hollow viscera and in the substance of solid viscera.

The general features of the parasympathetic system

The cell bodies of all preganglionic parasympathetic neurons are situated either in the nuclei which comprise the visceral motor grey columns in the brain stem (**49A**) or in the intermediate grey matter in the second, third and often the fourth sacral segments of the spinal cord (**37F**). The outflow from the central nervous system is consequently described as craniosacral.

1. In three of the cranial parasympathetic pathways the preganglionic axons emerge in the oculomotor, facial and glossopharyngeal nerves. After leaving those nerves they relay in parasympathetic ganglia and thereafter the postganglionic neurons innervate much of the smooth muscle of the eye, the lacrimal and salivary glands and the mucosal glands of the nose, pharynx and mouth (**49A, 51B, 53A**). Their distribution is thus restricted to the regions of the head and neck.
2. In a fourth cranial parasympathetic pathway the preganglionic axons emerge in the vagus nerves. In contrast to those in the three pathways described above, these axons do not end in an individual parasympathetic ganglion. On the contrary, they leave the vagus either in the neck or the thorax and pass into the system of autonomic plexuses in the thorax and the upper abdomen, reaching as far as the superior mesenteric and its associated branch plexuses (**A**). Some relay in central plexuses and others in branch plexuses, but most synapse with short postganglionic neurons in the terminal plexuses in viscera. The pathway provides parasympathetic innervation to the thoracic viscera and to many abdominal viscera including the gastrointestinal tract as far as about the midpoint of the large intestine.
3. The preganglionic parasympathetic axons which

constitute the sacral outflow emerge through the ventral roots into the second, third and fourth sacral spinal nerves, and pass thereafter into the ventral rami. They leave the ventral rami as distinct branches called the pelvic splanchnic nerves. These join the system of autonomic plexuses in the lower abdomen, spreading to the inferior and superior hypogastric plexuses and the inferior mesenteric plexus (**A**) and through the associated branch plexuses. As in the case of the vagal fibres, some axons relay in the central plexuses and others in branch plexuses, but most synapse with short postganglionic parasympathetic neurons in the terminal plexuses in viscera. This pathway provides parasympathetic innervation to the pelvic viscera, the distal half or so of the large intestine and the erectile tissues of the genital organs.

The general features of the sympathetic system

Inflow into the sympathetic trunk

The cell bodies of all preganglionic sympathetic neurons lie in the intermediolateral nucleus (**37D**) which extends continuously along the lateral grey column of the spinal cord from the first thoracic to the second lumbar segment. The axons emerge into the corresponding spinal nerves through their ventral roots (**B**). The sympathetic outflow from the central into the peripheral nervous systems is thus described as being thoracolumbar, in contrast to the craniosacral parasympathetic outflow described above. All the preganglionic sympathetic axons subsequently leave the spinal nerves in which they have emerged, in branches which arise a short distance along their ventral rami, and pass to the corresponding ganglia of the sympathetic trunk (**B**). As the preganglionic axons are medullated these branches appear white and are called white rami communicantes. Thus white rami communicantes are associated with all thoracic and upper lumbar spinal nerves, but not with the higher and lower nerves of the spinal series into which no preganglionic axons have emerged from the spinal cord (**C, D**). Put in another way the cervical, lower lumbar and sacral ganglia on the sympathetic trunk are 'isolated' in the sense that they have no direct preganglionic inflow from the spinal cord.

Many of the preganglionic axons traversing the white rami communicantes do not progress within the sympathetic trunk beyond the ganglion they first reach. However others, having reached the trunk, turn either upwards to reach one of the cervical ganglia (**C**) or downwards to reach one of the lower lumbar or sacral ganglia (**D**). Thus, despite the restriction of sympathetic outflow to the thoracolumbar segments of the spinal cord, all ganglia on the sympathetic trunk receive preganglionic sympathetic axons either directly or indirectly.

POSITIONS OF CENTRAL, BRANCH & TERMINAL AUTONOMIC PLEXUSES

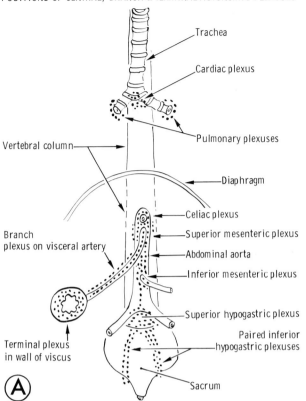

Trachea

Cardiac plexus

Pulmonary plexuses

Vertebral column

Diaphragm

Celiac plexus

Superior mesenteric plexus

Abdominal aorta

Inferior mesenteric plexus

Branch plexus on visceral artery

Superior hypogastric plexus

Paired inferior hypogastric plexuses

Terminal plexus in wall of viscus

Sacrum

(A)

SYMPATHETIC OUTFLOW FROM THORACOLUMBAR SPINAL CORD

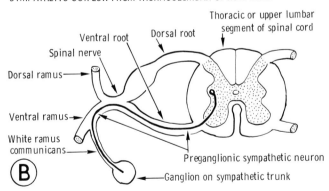

Ventral root

Dorsal root

Thoracic or upper lumbar segment of spinal cord

Spinal nerve

Dorsal ramus

Ventral ramus

White ramus communicans

Preganglionic sympathetic neuron

Ganglion on sympathetic trunk

(B)

UPPER PART OF SYMPATHETIC TRUNK: PREGANGLIONIC FIBRES

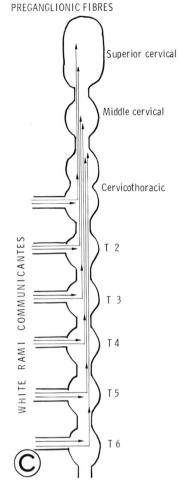

Superior cervical

Middle cervical

Cervicothoracic

T 2

T 3

T 4

T 5

T 6

WHITE RAMI COMMUNICANTES

(C)

LOWER PART OF SYMPATHETIC TRUNK: PREGANGLIONIC FIBRES

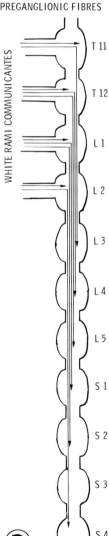

T 11

T 12

L 1

L 2

L 3

L 4

L 5

S 1

S 2

S 3

S 4

WHITE RAMI COMMUNICANTES

(D)

Branches of the sympathetic trunk

Once preganglionic sympathetic axons reach their definitive ganglia on the sympathetic trunk, the pathways of which they are part may continue in a number of different ways.

1. After relay within the ganglia, some postganglionic axons pass in vascular branches onto the walls of adjacent somatic arteries, where they form periarterial plexuses. It should be noted particularly that such somatic periarterial plexuses differ from the thoracic and abdominal autonomic plexuses described above, in that postganglionic sympathetic axons are their only autonomic component.

   The plexuses control the activities of the smooth muscle in the arterial walls, but some may also provide routes by which postganglionic sympathetic axons can be distributed to other distant structures. For example, a major part of the pathway followed by postganglionic sympathetic neurons to the eye is through the periarterial plexus on the wall of the internal carotid artery which is derived from the superior cervical ganglion as shown diagrammatically in **A**.

2. Other postganglionic axons pass in lateral branches of the trunk ganglia to the ventral rami of the corresponding spinal nerves. Because these branches consist of unmyelinated axons, they have a grey appearance and are called grey rami communicantes. Every spinal nerve receives a grey ramus in contrast to the limited distribution of white rami noted above (**B**). A trunk ganglion which corresponds to one spinal nerve sends one grey ramus to that nerve, whereas trunk ganglia which correspond to more than one spinal nerve have a corresponding number of grey rami e.g. the superior cervical ganglion has four grey rami which pass to the first four cervical nerves.

The postganglionic axons are then distributed through the branches of both rami of the spinal nerves. Through cutaneous branches they innervate the sweat glands, the smooth muscles associated with hair follicles and the smooth muscle in the walls of small skin arteries, while through muscular branches they innervate the smooth muscle in the walls of vessels within the muscles. In addition fine branches arise from nerve trunks at intervals which join and reinforce the periarterial plexuses on neighbouring large arteries (**C**), except for their most proximal parts, where as seen above the plexuses are formed by direct arterial branches from the sympathetic trunk.

3. The medial branches of the ganglia of the sympathetic trunk are concerned in the innervation of thoracic and abdominal viscera and their vessels. They pass medially and usually downwards from all the trunk ganglia to join central autonomic plexuses in either the thorax or the abdomen.

   In the pathways to the thoracic viscera the synapses between preganglionic and postganglionic neurons are predominantly situated in the cervical and upper thoracic trunk ganglia, and the medial branches of these ganglia therefore carry postganglionic sympathetic axons which pass without further interruption through thoracic central, branch and terminal plexuses. On the other hand in the pathways to abdominal viscera there are, in general, no synapses within the trunk ganglia. Preganglionic axons pass directly from the lower thoracic, lumbar and sacral ganglia through their medial branches and relay in the abdominal central autonomic plexuses. Postganglionic axons then continue through the branch and terminal plexuses. This peculiar difference in the constitutions of thoracic and abdominal central autonomic plexuses is summarised diagrammatically in **D**.

EXAMPLE OF VASCULAR BRANCH OF SYMPATHETIC TRUNK

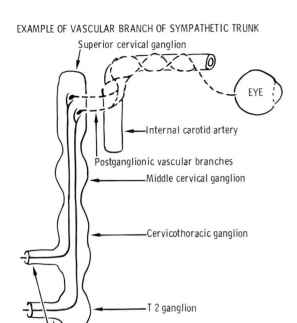

Superior cervical ganglion

EYE

Internal carotid artery

Postganglionic vascular branches

Middle cervical ganglion

Cervicothoracic ganglion

T 2 ganglion

(A)

White rami communicantes

INNERVATION OF SOMATIC ARTERY

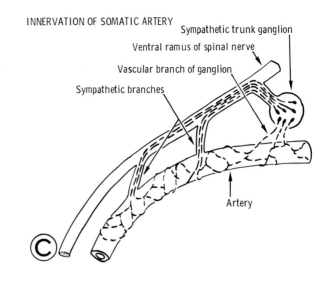

Sympathetic trunk ganglion

Ventral ramus of spinal nerve

Vascular branch of ganglion

Sympathetic branches

Artery

(C)

RAMI COMMUNICANTES OF SYMPATHETIC GANGLIA

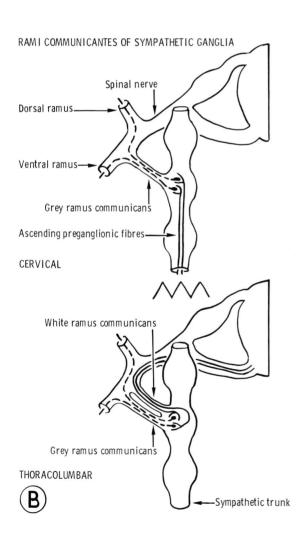

Spinal nerve

Dorsal ramus

Ventral ramus

Grey ramus communicans

Ascending preganglionic fibres

CERVICAL

White ramus communicans

Grey ramus communicans

THORACOLUMBAR

(B)

Sympathetic trunk

MEDIAL BRANCHES TO THORACIC & ABDOMINAL AUTONOMIC PLEXUSES

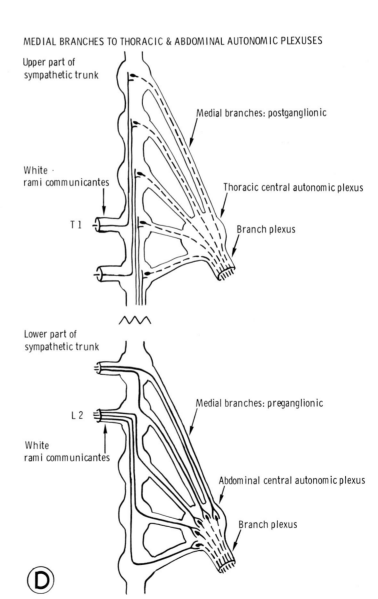

Upper part of sympathetic trunk

Medial branches: postganglionic

White rami communicantes

Thoracic central autonomic plexus

T 1

Branch plexus

Lower part of sympathetic trunk

Medial branches: preganglionic

L 2

White rami communicantes

Abdominal central autonomic plexus

Branch plexus

(D)

119

THE VISCERAL SENSORY SYSTEM

It has been noted in the previous pages that the pathways which mediate the motor innervation of viscera and blood vessels consist of two multipolar neurons in series, and that the preganglionic and postganglionic neurons synapse in autonomic ganglia or plexuses. In contrast, the pathways which transmit sensory information from viscera and from blood vessels are formed by single pseudo-unipolar neurons whose cell bodies lie in sensory ganglia on the posterior roots of spinal nerves and on certain cranial nerves.

It is because of these differences that in this text the visceral sensory system is not regarded as part of the autonomic system, even though in many situations, as will be seen, the fibres of the two systems are intimately intermingled.

Of the impulses which reach the brain stem and spinal cord through visceral sensory pathways, some initiate reflex activity in autonomic neurons, while others reach levels of consciousness along tracts which are not yet certainly identified.

The visceral sensory neurons which transmit information concerning blood pressure (baroreceptors) and the chemical composition of the blood (chemoreceptors) are components of the glossopharyngeal and vagus nerves. Their cell bodies are in the sensory ganglia which lie on the upper parts of those nerves, and their central processes enter the brain stem where they are involved in the reflex control of the circulation and respiration.

Visceral sensations which are consciously appreciated are of two general kinds.

Visceral pain may be due to an inflammatory lesion such as a duodenal ulcer, or to excessive contraction of plain muscle in the wall of a hollow viscus in an attempt to overcome obstruction of its lumen, or to vascular inadequacy as in angina pectoris.

The peripheral processes of most visceral sensory neurons transmitting pain impulses from viscera run successively through branch and central autonomic plexuses (**A**) and reach the sympathetic trunks by way of their medial branches (**A**). Within the trunks these peripheral processes may ascend or descend to reach the spinal level of sympathetic outflow to the viscus concerned. They then leave the sympathetic trunks in the corresponding white rami communicantes and reach their cell bodies in the sensory ganglia on the corresponding spinal nerves (**A**). The central processes of the same neurons enter the spinal cord.

Visceral pain is usually experienced in or about the midline, irrespective of the position of the viscus concerned, and it cannot be localised by the patients with any precision. However an inflammatory process, initially confined to a viscus, may subsequently spread to the deeper layers of the adjacent body wall. Pain is then experienced through the appropriate sensory spinal nerves and can be accurately localised by the patient. Thus pain from an inflamed vermiform appendix is experienced at first around the umbilicus, but after some time 'shifts' to the right side.

Visceral distension may excite sensations of different qualities depending on the hollow viscus concerned, e.g. stomach, rectum, urinary bladder. The peripheral processes of visceral sensory neurons concerned with these kinds of sensation, like those concerned with visceral pain, at first pass through branch and central autonomic plexuses (**B, C**). However, subsequently, instead of following predominantly sympathetic routes, they continue along one of two predominantly parasympathetic routes.

1. Some pass successively through the pelvic splanchnic nerves and the ventral rami and posterior roots of the second, third and fourth sacral spinal nerves. Their cell bodies are in the sensory ganglia on those spinal nerves and their central processes pass into the corresponding segments of the spinal cord (**B**).
2. Others join the vagus nerves. Their cell bodies are in the vagal ganglia on the upper part of the nerve and their central processes enter the brain stem (**C**).

EXAMPLE OF VISCERAL SENSORY NEURONS: SENSATION OF PAIN

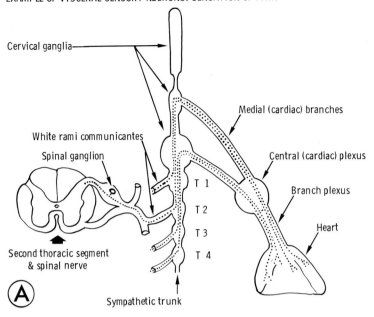

Cervical ganglia

White rami communicantes

Spinal ganglion

Medial (cardiac) branches

Central (cardiac) plexus

Branch plexus

Heart

T 1

T 2

T 3

T 4

Second thoracic segment
& spinal nerve

Sympathetic trunk

(A)

EXAMPLE OF VISCERAL SENSORY NEURON: SENSATION OF DISTENSION

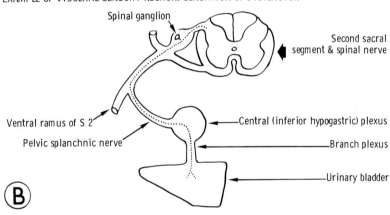

Spinal ganglion

Second sacral
segment & spinal nerve

Ventral ramus of S 2

Pelvic splanchnic nerve

Central (inferior hypogastric) plexus

Branch plexus

Urinary bladder

(B)

EXAMPLE OF VISCERAL SENSORY NEURONS: SENSATION OF DISTENSION

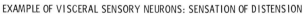
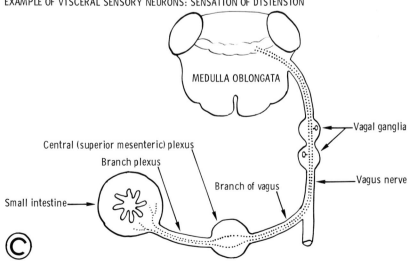

MEDULLA OBLONGATA

Central (superior mesenteric) plexus

Branch plexus

Branch of vagus

Vagal ganglia

Vagus nerve

Small intestine

(C)

CHAPTER 3

The thorax

INTRODUCTION

The thorax is the upper compartment of the trunk. Below, it is separated from the abdomen by a muscular partition called the diaphragm; above, it is continuous with the tissues of the neck (**A**).

The chest wall is formed anteriorly by the flat sternum (**B**), posteriorly by the thoracic part of the vertebral column (**A**) and laterally by the ribs and costal cartilages separated by the intercostal muscles and membranes (**B**). In the coronal plane (**C**) the thorax is a truncated cone and, owing to the upward convexity of the diaphragm, the vertical diameter is appreciably less centrally than it is on either side. In a horizontal plane (**D**) the transverse diameter is greater than the anteroposterior, and the thoracic cavity is reniform owing to the forward projection of the thoracic vertebral bodies.

The thoracic inlet (**B**) is the term applied to the space surrounded by the first thoracic vertebra, the first ribs and costal cartilages and the upper border of the manubrium sterni through which the thoracic cavity becomes continuous with the tissues of the neck. In adults it is steeply inclined downwards and forwards, (**A**) but this obliquity is much less marked in infants.

The infrasternal angle (**B**) is formed by the divergent inferior margins of the thoracic cage consisting of the costal cartilages 7–12. Its size varies in individuals of different build.

The thoracic cavity is divided into two parts by a broad septum, the mediastinum, which extends between the vertebral column, sternum, and diaphragm, and is continuous above with the tissues of the neck (**C, D**). The mediastinum contains the heart, its associated great vessels and a number of viscera.

The cavities on either side of the mediastinum are occupied by the lungs, which invaginate the serous pleural sacs (**C, D**). The lungs are thus covered by a layer of visceral pleura, while the walls of the cavities in which they lie are lined by parietal pleura. Through the site of invagination of the pleural sacs, the lungs are in structural continuity with the mediastinum through the roots of the lungs.

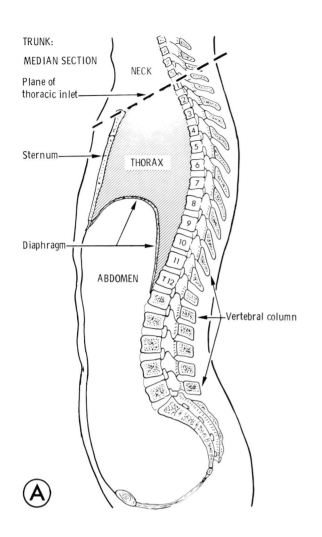

TRUNK:
MEDIAN SECTION

NECK

Plane of
thoracic inlet

Sternum

THORAX

Diaphragm

ABDOMEN

Vertebral column

Ⓐ

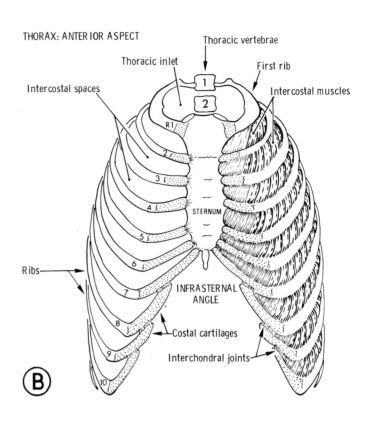

THORAX: ANTERIOR ASPECT

Thoracic inlet

Thoracic vertebrae

First rib

Intercostal spaces

Intercostal muscles

Ribs

STERNUM

INFRASTERNAL
ANGLE

Costal cartilages

Interchondral joints

Ⓑ

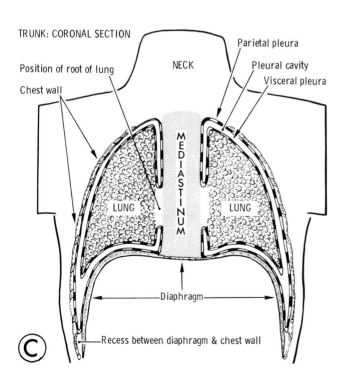

TRUNK: CORONAL SECTION

Parietal pleura

Position of root of lung

NECK

Pleural cavity

Chest wall

Visceral pleura

MEDIASTINUM

LUNG

LUNG

Diaphragm

Recess between diaphragm & chest wall

Ⓒ

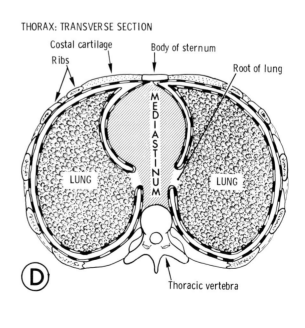

THORAX: TRANSVERSE SECTION

Costal cartilage

Body of sternum

Ribs

Root of lung

MEDIASTINUM

LUNG

LUNG

Ⓓ

Thoracic vertebra

THE THORACIC WALL

The thoracic wall gives some measure of protection to the viscera which it surrounds and is very closely associated with the process of respiration.

The bones and joints

The central part of the posterior wall of the thorax is formed by the twelve thoracic vertebrae which have been considered already (**3A, 7F**).

The sternum

This lies in the central part of the anterior thoracic wall (**A, B, C**). It consists of three parts, the manubrium, the body and the xiphoid process, which are joined by the manubriosternal and xiphisternal joints. These are both symphyses (secondary cartilaginous joints), the adjacent bone edges being coated by cartilage while the paired cartilage plates are joined by a thin zone of fibrous tissue (**3E**).

The manubrium is shown in outline **B**. Its inferior margin is appreciably narrower than the superior. Note the jugular notch (suprasternal notch), the cartilage-covered clavicular notches, with which the medial ends of the clavicles articulate, and the rough lateral angles which, in life, are structurally continuous with the costal cartilages of the first ribs.

The body is broader at its upper border than its lower, and broadest at the junction of its upper three-quarters and its lower quarter (**B**).

The xiphoid process (**B**) varies in size but is always considerably smaller than the other two parts. In a few individuals it is perforate or bifid. It is cartilaginous in youth but becomes more or less completely ossified in most adults.

The sternal angle is the slight angulation, open backwards, between the manubrium and body at the manubriosternal joint (**C**). Above and below the joint the anterior surface of the bone is slightly raised so that the angle can be readily palpated through the skin as a thick ridge. This feature is an important landmark on the thoracic wall.

The level of the sternum during quiet respiration in adults varies little. The manubrium is situated in front of the third and fourth thoracic vertebral bodies (**B**), and the body in front of the fifth to the ninth vertebrae. In infants the sternum lies at a higher level, the jugular notch being level with the first thoracic vertebra. This relationship has an important influence of the effects of rib movements on inspiration at this age.

The ribs and costal cartilages

The walls of the thorax between the vertebrae and sternum contain two sets of twelve ribs, each of which is continuous anteriorly with a cartilaginous rod, of similar cross sectional area, known as a costal cartilage (**D**). Each rib articulates posteriorly with the thoracic vertebral column. The costal cartilages on ribs 1–7 articulate directly with the lateral margin of the sternum (**A**), and the corresponding ribs are called vertebrosternal. The cartilages of ribs 8–10 articulate with the cartilages immediately above them (**A**). These ribs are classed as vertebrochondral. The cartilages of ribs 11 and 12 end freely in the body wall and these ribs are described as vertebral.

Rib 1 and ribs 10, 11, and 12 have peculiar features, but the characteristics of the other members of the series (the typical ribs) are similar.

Examine a dried specimen of one of the typical ribs in conjunction with the diagrams in (**D**). The rib consists of head, neck, tubercle and shaft. The head is at the posterior end and the anterior end of the shaft is in continuity with its costal cartilage. Note particularly the following features.

1. The head carries upper and lower articular facets, set at an angle to one another and separated by a nonarticular strip of bone.
2. The tubercle consists of two parts, a medial part which carries a small articular facet and a lateral which is nonarticular.
3. The shaft has inner and outer surfaces, a rounded upper margin and a sharp lower margin.
4. The costal groove extends along the lower part of the inner surface of the shaft.
5. At the angle, a short distance lateral to the tubercle, the curvature of the shaft is more acute than elsewhere along its length.

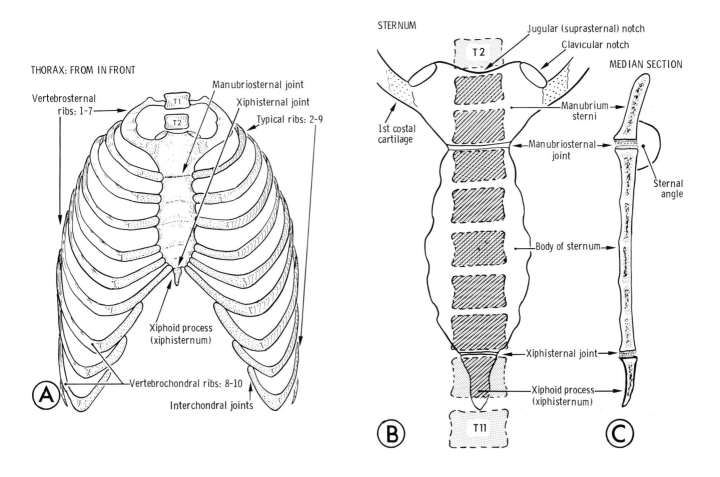

THORAX: FROM IN FRONT

Vertebrosternal ribs: 1-7

Manubriosternal joint

Xiphisternal joint

Typical ribs: 2-9

Xiphoid process (xiphisternum)

Vertebrochondral ribs: 8-10

Interchondral joints

A

STERNUM

Jugular (suprasternal) notch

Clavicular notch

MEDIAN SECTION

1st costal cartilage

Manubrium sterni

Manubriosternal joint

Sternal angle

Body of sternum

Xiphisternal joint

Xiphoid process (xiphisternum)

B

C

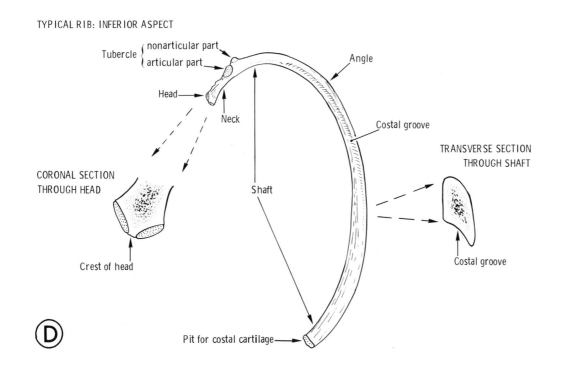

TYPICAL RIB: INFERIOR ASPECT

Tubercle { nonarticular part
          { articular part

Angle

Head

Neck

Costal groove

CORONAL SECTION THROUGH HEAD

TRANSVERSE SECTION THROUGH SHAFT

Shaft

Crest of head

Costal groove

Pit for costal cartilage

D

The costal joints

1. The first costal cartilage is directly continuous with the lateral angle of the manubrium (**127B**). The first sternocostal joint is thus a synchondrosis (primary carilaginous joint) between rib and sternum, and it is notable that this is the only joint of this type which persists into adult life. The extremities of cartilages 2–7 are separated from the lateral margin of the sternum by small synovial sternocostal joints (**127A**). Note that cartilage 2 articulates with both the manubrium and body of the sternum and consequently with the manubriosternal joint (**127A**). This relationship of the second costal cartilage to the readily palpable sternal angle is important, because in life the first rib is usually obscured by the clavicle (**381F**). It is consequently convenient when counting the ribs on the anterior chest wall to start from the second. Cartilages 8, 9 and 10 articulate by synovial interchondral joints with the cartilages immediately above them (**127A**). From above down the three joints lie progressively further from the midline. Cartilages 11 and 12 end freely without articulation.
2. The heads of all the ribs articulate by costovertebral synovial joints with the lateral aspects of thoracic vertebral bodies. The typical ribs (2–9) articulate with the adjacent borders of two vertebral bodies, that corresponding in number to the rib and that immediately above it (**A**). The atypical ribs (1, 10, 11 and 12) articulate only with the one numerically-corresponding vertebral body.
3. The tubercles of all ribs except 11 and 12 articulate with the numerically-corresponding transverse process at synovial costotransverse joints (**A**). The facets on the transverse processes 1–7 are concave forwards (**B**). At joints 8, 9 and 10 the facets are plane and nearly horizontally disposed (**C**).

The movements of the ribs

All the rib shafts incline downwards as well as forwards as they pass round the chest wall (**A**) while all the costal cartilages except those of ribs 1, 2, 11 and 12 incline upwards and medially (**A, 127A**). From the point of view of rib movements it is particularly important to note the following features of vertebrosternal ribs.

1. The anterior end of each costal cartilage lies at an appreciably lower level than the head of the corresponding rib (**A**).
2. The lateral part of each rib lies at a lower level than a plane traversing its head and the anterior end of its costal cartilage (**A**).

The movements of the ribs reflect their orientation and the character of their joints.

1. In the case of the vertebrosternal ribs, upward movement around an axis through the costovertebral and costotransverse joints carries the anterior ends of the costal cartilages, and the sternum to which they are attached, upwards and forwards (**E**). This movement increases the anteroposterior diameter of the thorax. It is important to note that this kind of displacement of the sternum and the vertebrosternal ribs does not require that an upward force should be applied to all seven of the vertebrosternal ribs or their costal cartilages. An upward force applied even to one rib or its cartilage, or indeed to the sternum itself, will produce the same collective displacement.
2. Because, as has been noted above, the lateral part of each vertebrosternal rib shaft lies at a lower level than a plane traversing its head and the anterior end of its costal cartilage, elevation of the rib around an axis through its costotransverse and sternocostal joints (**F**) moves the rib shaft outwards as well as upwards and increases the transverse diameter of the thorax (bucket-handle movement).
3. Because of the near horizontal orientation of their costotransverse facets (**C**), the vertebrochondral ribs tend to move round vertical axes which pass through the costovertebral joints, so that their costal cartilages move laterally on the cartilages immediately above them at the interchondral joints (**D**). This movement increases the transverse diameter of the thorax and also, be it noted, the transverse diameter of the upper abdomen. When the three vertebrochondral ribs move simultaneously in this way the size of the infrasternal angle is increased. Because of the steep upward inclination of the cartilages of the lower vertebrosternal and vertebrochondral ribs, lateral movement of one vertebrochondral cartilage tends to cause upward displacement of the cartilage immediately above it. Upward displacement of the seventh cartilage in this way is in fact the same movement as that discussed in 1 above and has the same effect on thoracic capacity (**G**).

TYPICAL RIB: LATERAL VIEW

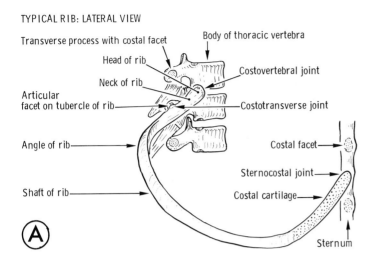

Transverse process with costal facet

Head of rib

Neck of rib

Articular facet on tubercle of rib

Angle of rib

Shaft of rib

Body of thoracic vertebra

Costovertebral joint

Costotransverse joint

Costal facet

Sternocostal joint

Costal cartilage

Sternum

(A)

COSTOTRANSVERSE JOINT OF VERTEBROSTERNAL RIB: TRANSVERSE SECTION

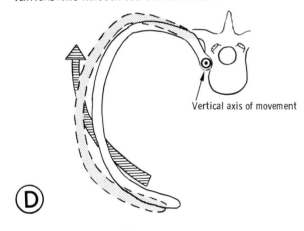

(B) Transverse process — Rib

COSTOTRANSVERSE JOINT OF VERTEBROCHONDRAL RIB: TRANSVERSE SECTION

Rib

(C) Transverse process

SUPERIOR VIEW OF VERTEBROCHONDRAL RIB: MOVEMENT AROUND VERTICAL AXIS THROUGH COSTOVERTEBRAL JOINT

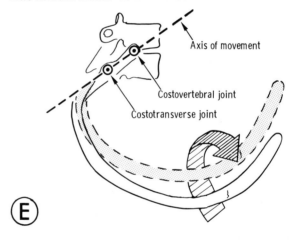

Vertical axis of movement

(D)

LATERAL VIEW OF VERTEBROSTERNAL RIB: UPWARD MOVEMENT AROUND AXIS THROUGH COSTOTRANSVERSE & COSTOVERTEBRAL JOINTS

Axis of movement

Costovertebral joint

Costotransverse joint

(E)

ANTERIOR VIEW OF VERTEBROSTERNAL RIB: UPWARD MOVEMENT AROUND AXIS THROUGH COSTOTRANSVERSE & COSTOSTERNAL JOINTS

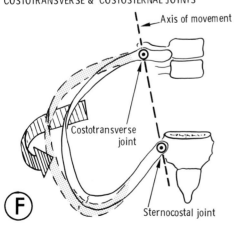

Axis of movement

Costotransverse joint

Sternocostal joint

(F)

SEVENTH & EIGHTH COSTAL CARTILAGES

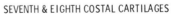
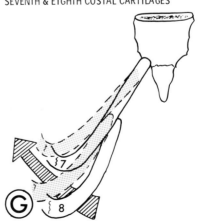

7

8

(G)

The muscles

The diaphragm

The diaphragm is a thin dome-shaped muscle which is concave downwards (**A**). Its origin encircles the deep aspect of the body wall, lying at the level of the xiphisternum in front and the upper lumbar vertebrae behind. From this origin the muscle fibres run upwards and centrally and are inserted into an area of dense connective tissue within the muscle called the central tendon. This tendon is of trefoil shape, one process extending forwards and two backwards (**C**). The sternal fibres are two short muscular slips which spring from the back of the xiphoid process (**C**). The costal fibres, which are much longer, arise by six slips from the deep aspects of the costal cartilages 7–12 (**C**). The origin of the lumbar fibres is from the twelfth rib, the upper lumbar vertebrae and the fascia between them (**B**): the details of this part of the origin will be considered in relation to the abdomen from where it can be studied more profitably (**201B**). The upper part or dome of the diaphragm is in the form of two cupolae (**B**) separated by the slightly lower central tendon. In expiration the uppermost part of the diaphragm is at the level of the fourth costal cartilages and the intervertebral disc between the eighth and ninth thoracic vertebrae.

Because of its domed shape, the peripheral part of the diaphragm is separated from the thoracic wall by a deep narrow gutter known as the costodiaphragmatic recess (**B, C**).

The diaphragm contains three major apertures (**B, C**).

1. The vena caval opening is a short distance to the right of the midline in the central tendon. Because it is in the tendon it is not constricted when the muscle contracts.
2. The oesophageal opening is in the posterior muscular part of the diaphragm, a little to the left of the midline, and at the level of the tenth thoracic vertebra.
3. The aortic opening is behind, rather than in, the diaphragm. It lies centrally in the lumbar part of the muscle in front of the first and second lumbar vertebrae.

The intercostal muscles

Three layers of tissue, each of which consists partly of muscle and partly of membrane, occupy the intercostal spaces between each adjacent pair of ribs and costal cartilages (**125B, 133A, 133B**).

1. The outer layer consists of the external intercostal muscle in the lateral and posterior parts of the space and the external intercostal membrane in the anterior part. The muscle fibres incline forwards round the chest wall as they descend between the adjacent rib margins.
2. The middle layer consists of the internal intercostal muscle anteriorly and laterally and the internal intercostal membrane posteriorly. The muscle fibres in this layer incline backwards round the chest wall as they descend. Note that they arise from the floor of the costal groove rather than the inferior margin of the rib.
3. The inner layer is composed of anterior, lateral and posterior groups of muscle fibres, many of which extend across more than one intercostal space. The three groups may be described collectively as the innermost intercostal muscle.

The postvertebral muscles

These comprise the thoracic part of the mass of muscles which are called collectively the erector spinae (**133B**). This muscle complex extends from the sacrum and pelvis below to the skull above (**133C**). In the thoracic region it occupies the gutter between the vertebral spines and the transverse processes and ribs, extending as far laterally as the angles of the ribs (**133D**). It is covered posteriorly by the thoracolumbar fascia which, in this region, consists of a single layer continuous below with the posterior lamina of the lumbar part of the same fascia (**133D**). The muscle is innervated by the dorsal rami of the thoracic nerves. It extends the thoracic vertebral column, a movement which increases the vertical diameter of the thoracic cavity.

Additional muscles

The bones of the thoracic skeleton give attachment to many muscles whose primary functions are concerned with other regions, but which in exceptional circumstances play a part in the process of respiration. They can be divided into three groups.

1. Muscles which extend downwards from the cervical vertebrae and skull to the upper ribs and sternum (**391A, 401B**).
2. Those which pass upwards from the ribs and sternum to the bones of the shoulder girdle and humerus (**493, 501D**).
3. The muscles of the anterior and lateral parts of the abdominal wall, which are attached to the lower ribs (**207, 209**).

It would be inappropriate to describe these muscles at this stage but their involvement in respiration in some circumstances is discussed below.

DIAPHRAGM AFTER REMOVAL OF LATERAL BODY WALL

CORONAL SECTION OF THORAX:
POSTERIOR HALF OF DIAPHRAGM

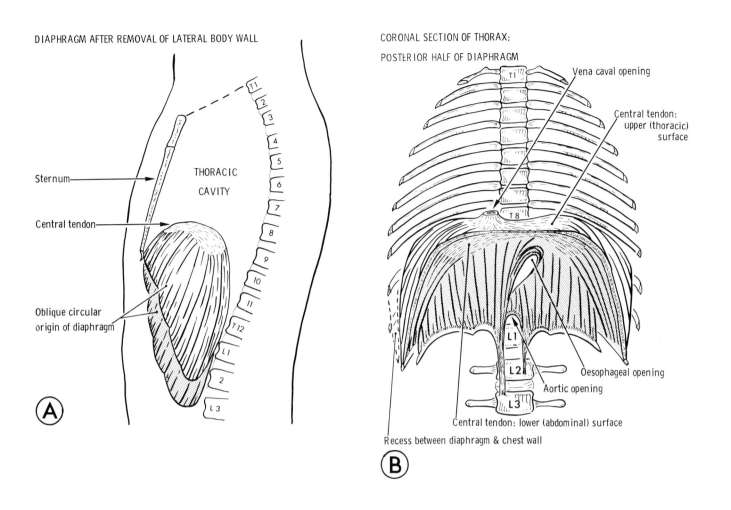

Sternum

Central tendon

Oblique circular
origin of diaphragm

THORACIC
CAVITY

(A)

Vena caval opening

Central tendon:
upper (thoracic)
surface

Oesophageal opening

Aortic opening

Central tendon: lower (abdominal) surface

Recess between diaphragm & chest wall

(B)

UPPER SURFACE OF DIAPHRAGM

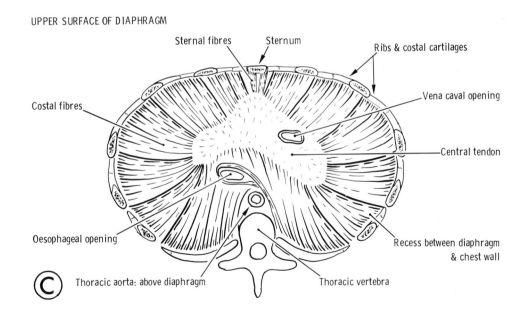

Sternal fibres   Sternum   Ribs & costal cartilages

Costal fibres

Vena caval opening

Central tendon

Oesophageal opening

Recess between diaphragm
& chest wall

(C)   Thoracic aorta: above diaphragm   Thoracic vertebra

131

The mechanics of respiration

Each cycle of respiration consists of two phases. In the inspiratory phase the volume of the thoracic cavity is increased by the activity of several muscles, so that a subatmospheric pressure is created in the pleural cavities. As a result the lungs expand to fill the vacuum and air is sucked into them. In quiet respiration about 500 ml of air is inspired in each cycle. About a third of this volume occupies the non-respiratory parts of the respiratory tract, while the rest reaches the alveoli, the thin-walled sacs where gaseous interchange occurs between the air and the pulmonary capillaries.

The expiratory phase, except in certain special circumstances, such as coughing, sneezing and blowing, is a passive process dependent on the elastic recoil of the lungs.

It is important to realise at the outset that the intercostal muscles do not contribute to the rib movements involved in inspiration. Nevertheless they are important because, throughout that process, their contraction prevents the subatmospheric pressure in the thorax sucking the intercostal tissues inwards.

In minimal inspiration in a normal subject, often called quiet inspiration, the thoracic capacity is increased solely by contraction of the diaphragm. The effect of this contraction is to increase the vertical, transverse and anteroposterior diameters.

1. The dome of the diaphragm descends about 1.5 cm and the vertical thoracic diameter is correspondingly increased.
2. The descent of the diaphragm necessarily displaces abdominal viscera. The additional abdominal capacity required by the displaced viscera is partly obtained by relaxation of the anterior abdominal muscles, which incidentally relieves the lower ribs of the downward pull of these muscles. Usually, however, the greater part of the additional capacity is produced by the displaced viscera pushing the lower ribs laterally (**129D**), a movement which increases the transverse diameters of both the upper part of the abdomen and the lower part of the thorax (**128**).
3. The lateral displacement of the vertebrochondral ribs described in the previous paragraph forces the seventh costal cartilage, and the sternum to which it is attached, upwards and forwards and thus increases the anteroposterior thoracic diameter (**129G**).

In deeper inspiration, the diaphragm is assisted by other muscles.

1. After the diaphragmatic effects described above, downward movement of the dome of the diaphragm is arrested when no further reserve abdominal

capacity is available. Thereafter further contraction of the diaphragm, now acting from the fixed central tendon, pulls costal cartilages 7–12 and the xiphsternum, and therefore the rest of the sternum, upwards and forwards increasing still more the anteroposterior thoracic diameter (**129E**).
2. The anteroposterior diameter is also increased by upward pull of certain cervical muscles (scalene muscles) on the first and second ribs.
3. The erector spinae muscles extend the concave thoracic vertebral column and thus increase the vertical diameter of the thorax.

Forced inspiration occurs during very violent exertion or when pulmonary efficiency is reduced by respiratory or cardiac diseases. In those circumstances the diaphragm, erector spinae and scalene muscles act in the ways described above, as strongly as possible. In addition, however, if the shoulder girdle can be fixed by the subject holding on to a stationary object, the muscles which pass from the vertebrosternal ribs to the scapula and humerus, particularly the pectoralis minor (**493D**), lift the lateral parts of those ribs around the axes passing through the costotransverse (**129F**) and costosternal joints, and thus increase the transverse diameter of the upper thorax.

Expiration, as has been noted, is usually a passive process depending on the relaxation of all the inspiratory muscles and the contraction of the abundant elastic tissue in the lungs.

However, on many occasions, expiration is an active process in which air is actively forced out of the lungs. The main forces in such active expiration comes from the contraction of the muscles of the anterior and lateral abdominal walls. All these muscles, but particularly the internal oblique and transversus abdominis muscles (**207C**, **207E**) raise the intra-abdominal pressure, forcing the diaphragm upwards and reducing the vertical thoracic diameter. Furthermore, all these muscles, but particularly rectus abdominis and external oblique (**205E**, **209A**, **209B**), pull the ribs from the fifth to the twelfth downwards, rotating these ribs around both their axes (**129E**, **129F**) and reducing both the anteroposterior and transverse thoracic diameters.

Forced respiration is often associated with temporary closure, followed by sudden opening, of part of the upper respiratory tract. Thus, in coughing the lumen of the larynx is closed and then suddenly opened when intrathoracic pressure is maximal, so that air rushes upwards cleaning the air passages of irritating material. In sneezing the mouth and the communication between the nose and pharynx (**463A**) are closed and then the latter is opened so that air is forced rapidly through the nose. And in blowing, the aperture of the mouth is partially closed so that the velocity of the expired air is increased.

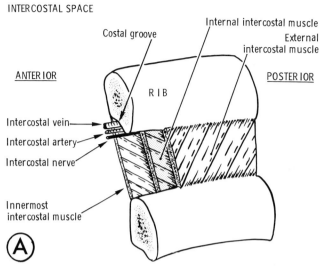

INTERCOSTAL SPACE

Costal groove

Internal intercostal muscle

External intercostal muscle

ANTERIOR

POSTERIOR

RIB

Intercostal vein

Intercostal artery

Intercostal nerve

Innermost intercostal muscle

(A)

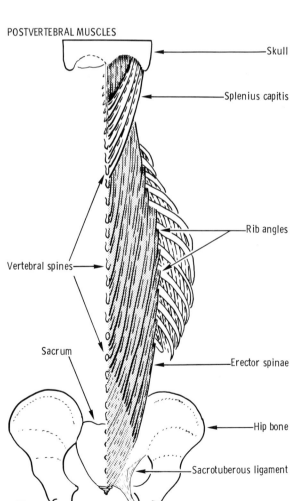

POSTVERTEBRAL MUSCLES

Skull

Splenius capitis

Rib angles

Vertebral spines

Erector spinae

Sacrum

Hip bone

Sacrotuberous ligament

(C)

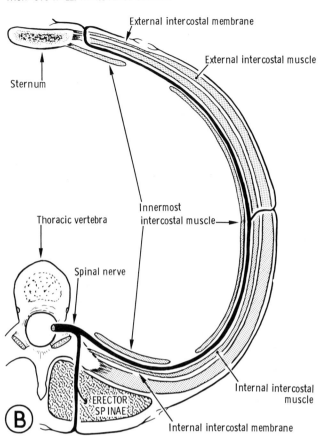

THORACIC WALL: TRANSVERSE SECTION

External intercostal membrane

External intercostal muscle

Sternum

Innermost intercostal muscle

Thoracic vertebra

Spinal nerve

Internal intercostal muscle

ERECTOR SPINAE

Internal intercostal membrane

(B)

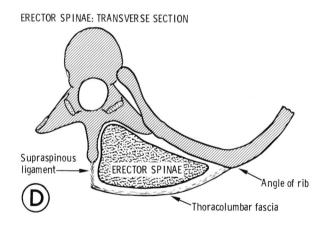

ERECTOR SPINAE: TRANSVERSE SECTION

Supraspinous ligament

ERECTOR SPINAE

Angle of rib

Thoracolumbar fascia

(D)

The nerves of the thoracic wall

Each thoracic nerve emerges through the intervertebral foramen below the numerically corresponding vertebra and immediately divides into a dorsal and a larger ventral ramus (**133B**).

The dorsal rami of the thoracic nerves

All the dorsal rami have similar courses. They pass backwards between two transverse processes and through the erector spinae muscle which they supply. They then traverse, but do not supply, the overlying muscles of the shoulder girdle (trapezius and latissimus dorsi, **493C**, **501C**) and end as cutaneous branches (**133B**). These incline downwards and laterally, the downward inclination increasing along the series, and supply corresponding strips of skin (**A**). The strip supplied by the twelfth thoracic dorsal ramus ends as low as the hip bone.

The ventral rami of the thoracic nerves

The ventral rami pass laterally into the posterior ends of the corresponding intercostal spaces, except that of the twelfth thoracic nerve which is placed below the twelfth rib.

1. The ventral rami of T3–6 are similar and are regarded as the typical members of the series. They pass round the corresponding intercostal spaces lying in the upper part of the neurovascular plane between the innermost and middle layers of intercostal muscles (**B, 133B**), and are consequently known as intercostal nerves. Note how the nerves (and accompanying vessels) are contained in the costal grooves and are thus protected from external trauma. Each nerve supplies the intercostal muscles in its own space and the subjacent strip of costal pleura. Furthermore, through a large lateral cutaneous branch and a small anterior cutaneous branch, each supplies an intercostal strip of skin which reaches the midline anteriorly and stretches backwards into continuity with the strip innervated by the corresponding dorsal ramus (**C**). It should be noted that there is considerable overlap in the nerve supply of successive dermatomes. Each is supplied by its own nerve and by those above and below it, so that division of one intercostal nerve does not usually result in any appreciable area of anaesthesia.
2. The ventral ramus of T1 is atypical, in that, in the proximal part of the first intercostal space, it gives off an ascending branch which passes upwards and

laterally across the neck of the first rib (**D**). This branch joins the ventral ramus of C8, on the upper surface of the shaft of the rib, to form the lower trunk of the brachial plexus. This plexus is distributed to the upper limb and is considered with that region (**511A**).

The remainder of the ventral ramus becomes the first intercostal nerve. It runs round the uppermost part of the first intercostal space in the neurovascular plane between the middle and innermost layers of intercostal muscles, supplying these muscles and the costal pleura deep to them. It differs from a typical intercostal nerve in being devoid of cutaneous branches. The skin over the anterior part of the first intercostal space is innervated by fibres which descend from the C4 spinal segment in the supraclavicular nerves (**C**) while the lateral part of the same space is not covered by skin as it faces into the axilla (armpit).

3. The ventral ramus of T2 (the second intercostal nerve) is atypical only in respect of its lateral cutaneous branch. As the lateral aspect of the second intercostal space faces into the armpit and is not directly covered by skin, this branch crosses that region and supplies skin on the upper part of the medial side of the arm (**C**). It is consequently called the intercostobrachial nerve, and the second thoracic dermatome lies partly on the thoracic wall and partly on the arm (**C**). Note the break in the orderly sequence of cutaneous innervation on the anterior thoracic wall at the level of the second rib. Above that level the skin is innervated by C4, below by T2. The 'missing' nerves are those which innervate the tissues of the upper limb.
4. The ventral rami of T7–11, otherwise called the intercostal nerves of those numbers, are initially similar to the typical intercostal nerves. However their intercostal spaces fail by progressively greater distances to reach the sternum and end in structural continuity with the tissues of the abdominal wall. Consequently each member of this group passes from the anterior end of its intercostal space, between adjacent digitations of the diaphragm, and the rest of its course lies in the abdominal wall (**215D**). Its lateral cutaneous branch arises while it is still in its intercostal space but its anterior cutaneous branch arises in the anterior part of the abdominal wall. The dermatomes which these branches supply lie partly on the thoracic and partly on the abdominal wall (**C**).
5. The ventral ramus of T12 is the subcostal nerve. It lies below the twelfth rib and passes behind the lumbar origin of the diaphragm into the abdominal wall, where it will be considered further (**205C**).

THORACIC DORSAL RAMI: CUTANEOUS DISTRIBUTION

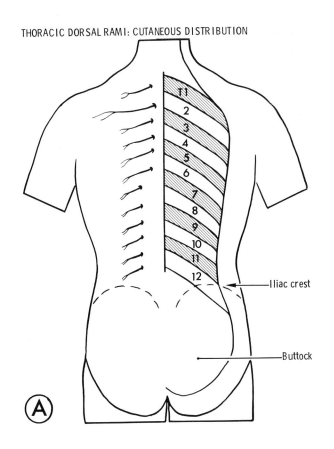

T1
2
3
4
5
6
7
8
9
10
11
12

Iliac crest

Buttock

A

THORACIC VENTRAL RAMI: DISTRIBUTION OF ANTERIOR & LATERAL CUTANEOUS BRANCHES

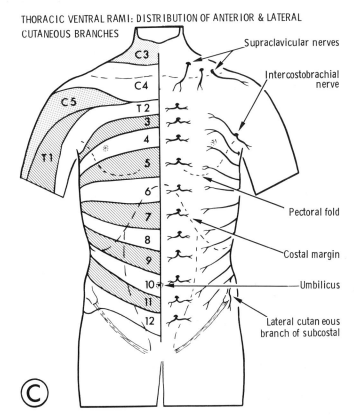

C3
C4
C5
T2
3
4
5
6
7
8
9
10
11
12
T1

Supraclavicular nerves

Intercostobrachial nerve

Pectoral fold

Costal margin

Umbilicus

Lateral cutaneous branch of subcostal

C

INTERCOSTAL SPACE IN SECTION

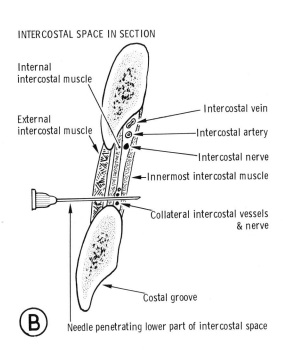

Internal intercostal muscle

External intercostal muscle

Intercostal vein

Intercostal artery

Intercostal nerve

Innermost intercostal muscle

Collateral intercostal vessels & nerve

Costal groove

Needle penetrating lower part of intercostal space

B

VENTRAL RAMUS OF FIRST THORACIC NERVE

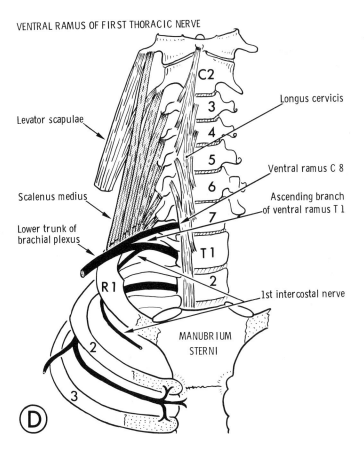

Levator scapulae

Scalenus medius

Lower trunk of brachial plexus

C2
3
4
5
6
7
T1
2
R1
2
3

Longus cervicis

Ventral ramus C 8

Ascending branch of ventral ramus T 1

1st intercostal nerve

MANUBRIUM STERNI

D

The thoracic part of the sympathetic trunk

The thoracic part of the sympathetic trunk consists of 12 ganglia connected by narrow intervening strands. Traced from above downwards the trunk gradually inclines in a medial direction. The first ganglion lies in front of and a little above the neck of the first rib. The majority of the ganglia are situated in front of the heads of the numerically corresponding ribs while the lower two or three ganglia are placed on the lateral aspects of the corresponding vertebral bodies (**A**). Below, the thoracic part of the trunk is continuous with the lumbar part behind the lumbar origin of the diaphragm (**291B**). Above, it is continued as the cervical part of the trunk to the base of the skull. The cervical trunk, which, as will be described below, gives branches to the thoracic viscera as well as to the regions of the head and the neck, carries only three ganglia, which are called superior, middle and inferior (**A**). The inferior cervical and first thoracic ganglia are often fused forming the cervicothoracic (stellate) ganglion.

Each thoracic sympathetic ganglion is joined to the ventral ramus of the corresponding thoracic nerve by a white ramus communicans which is about 1 cm long and runs from the ganglion laterally and backwards (**B, C**). These white rami carry nearly all the preganglionic sympathetic fibres which arise from the central nervous system. Many therefore spread upwards and downwards in the sympathetic trunk, so that collectively they constitute the entire preganglionic inflow to the cervical and thoracic ganglia and part of the inflow to the lumbar and sacral ganglia.

Many of the preganglionic fibres which reach the thoracic sympathetic trunk through the white rami end immediately by synapsing with postganglionic cells in the corresponding ganglia (**C**). The nonmyelinated axons of these cells pass to the ventral ramus of the corresponding thoracic nerve in a grey ramus communicans which runs parallel to but a little medial to the white ramus (**B, C**). These fibres are distributed through both the ventral and dorsal rami of the thoracic nerves to the thoracic and abdominal parietes, except for the skin over the highest and lowest parts which are not innervated by the thoracic nerves.

All the ganglia on the sympathetic trunk give off medial (visceral) branches. Some of those arising from the cervical ganglia and those arising from the upper five thoracic ganglia pass to central autonomic plexuses within the thorax (**B, D**) and are concerned in the innervation of thoracic viscera (**184**).

The larger medial branches which arise from the lower thoracic sympathetic ganglia contribute to the autonomic innervation of abdominal viscera (**B**). They run downwards, anterior and medial to the sympathetic trunk on the lateral aspects of the thoracic vertebral bodies. Medial branches from the ganglia T5–9 join to form the greater splanchnic nerve, branches from ganglia T10 and 11 join to form the lesser splanchnic nerve, while the medial branch of the lowest thoracic ganglion constitutes the least splanchnic nerve. The three splanchnic nerves pass into the abdomen, through or behind the lumbar fibres of the diaphragm. They reach the abdominal central autonomic plexuses.

The arteries and veins of the chest wall

A number of arteries arise from the axillary artery which lies in the armpit (axilla), and pass downwards to be distributed to the superficial muscles and superficial fascia of the chest wall. They are accompanied by veins which drain upwards into the axillary vein.

These vessels are closely associated topographically and functionally with the upper limb and will be considered with that region (**509A**).

Intercostal arteries and veins run longitudinally in each intercostal space. Each space contains a posterior intercostal artery running forwards and a smaller and shorter anterior intercostal artery running backwards. The two vessels anastomose in the region of the costochondral junction.

Note the position of these arteries in relation to the costal groove of the rib above and to the tissue layers in the intercostal space (**135B**). Observe that they are accompanied by anterior and posterior intercostal veins and by the numerically corresponding intercostal nerve, in the same neurovascular plane.

It is often recommended that in aspiration of the pleural cavity the intercostal vessels and nerves should be avoided by inserting the aspirating needle through the lower part of an intercostal space. However, this part of the space usually contains collateral branches of the main vessels and nerve so that the procedure does not have great advantage.

SYMPATHETIC TRUNK: CERVICAL & THORACIC PARTS: FROM IN FRONT

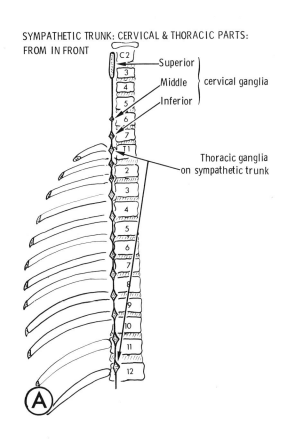

C2

Superior
Middle } cervical ganglia
Inferior

Thoracic ganglia on sympathetic trunk

A

SYMPATHETIC TRUNK: CERVICAL & THORACIC PARTS: FROM THE SIDE

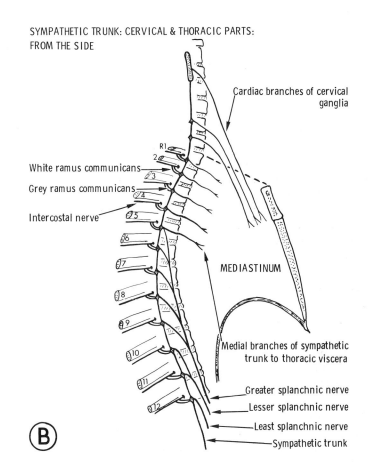

Cardiac branches of cervical ganglia

R1

White ramus communicans

Grey ramus communicans

Intercostal nerve

MEDIASTINUM

Medial branches of sympathetic trunk to thoracic viscera

Greater splanchnic nerve
Lesser splanchnic nerve
Least splanchnic nerve
Sympathetic trunk

B

SYMPATHETIC TRUNK: CONNECTIONS IN HORIZONTAL SECTION

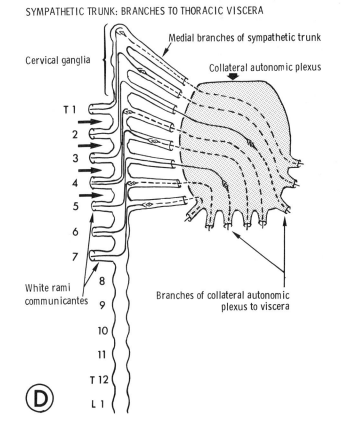

Spinal (dorsal root) ganglion

Dorsal root

Lateral grey horn: with cells of preganglionic fibres

Dorsal ramus

Ventral root

Ventral ramus

Ganglion on sympathetic trunk: with cells of postganglionic fibres

White ramus communicans

Grey ramus communicans

C

—————◇ Sympathetic preganglionic fibres
- - - - - ◇ Sympathetic postganglionic fibres

SYMPATHETIC TRUNK: BRANCHES TO THORACIC VISCERA

Cervical ganglia

Medial branches of sympathetic trunk

Collateral autonomic plexus

T 1
2
3
4
5
6
7

White rami communicantes

8
9
10
11
T 12
L 1

Branches of collateral autonomic plexus to viscera

D

137

The posterior intercostal arteries arise either from the descending thoracic aorta (**143B**) or the subclavian arteries, while the corresponding veins drain into the veins of the azygos system or the brachiocephalic veins. These connections lie in the mediastinum and the root of the neck, and will be considered when the major vessels are described in those regions.

The subcostal artery is in series with the posterior intercostal arteries. It arises from the descending thoracic aorta and follows the subcostal nerve below the twelfth rib and behind the lumbar origin of the diaphragm into the abdominal wall. It is accompanied by the subcostal vein (**143B**).

The internal thoracic artery arises in the root of the neck from the subclavian artery which will be described later. From its origin it runs vertically downwards on the anterior thoracic wall a centimetre or so from the sternum (**A**), passing deep to the costal cartilages and superficial to the innermost intercostal muscles (**B**). Behind the sixth intercostal space it divides into two branches. The superior epigastric artery passes between the costal and sternal fibres of the diaphragm into the anterior abdominal wall. The musculophrenic artery runs downwards and laterally in the costodiaphragmatic recess, deep to the anterior ends of the lower intercostal spaces (**A**).

The internal thoracic and musculophrenic arteries give off all the anterior intercostal arteries which pass laterally in the intercostal neurovascular plane to anastomose with the posterior intercostal arteries (**A**). The internal thoracic artery also supplies perforating branches which pierce the overlying intercostal and pectoral muscles to reach the superficial fascia of the anterior thoracic wall close to the sternum (**A, B**). In the female these contribute to the blood supply of the mammary gland and become considerably enlarged during a period of lactation.

The internal thoracic artery and its branches are accompanied by veins which end in the brachiocephalic veins, which will be considered later (**141D**).

The parietal pleura

The thorax contains two serous pleural sacs which are separated centrally by the mediastinum (**125C, 125D**). The free surfaces of the pleural membranes are covered by a single layer of flattened cells which lie upon a layer of fibro-elastic tissue.

The sacs are invaginated from the medial sides by the lungs, so that each lung is covered by visceral pleura while the walls of the cavity in which it lies are lined by parietal pleura (**125C**). On either side, at the site of invagination, a number of structures pass between the mediastinum and the lung, and are surrounded by a short pleural tube through which the visceral and parietal pleurae are continuous (**125C, 125D**).

Normally the space between the visceral and parietal pleurae is only a potential space occupied by a lubricating capillary film of fluid. However, in diagrams it is usually convenient to show an appreciable separation between the two layers.

The partietal pleura on each side may be divided into distinct regions which line different parts of the cavity containing the lung.

The diaphragmatic pleura covers the upper surface of the diaphragm lateral to the mediastinum (**C**). Peripherally, it dips down into the ever narrowing recess between the diaphragm and the lower ribs before being reflected upwards as the costal pleura. The resulting narrow lower part of the pleural sac is the costodiaphragmatic recess. It is important to learn the surface markings of the costodiaphragmatic line of reflection on the anterior, lateral and posterior aspects of the body as illustrated in **D, E**. Medially the diaphragmatic pleura becomes continuous with the mediastinal pleura at about a right angle (**C**)

The costal pleura lines the ribs, costal cartilages and intercostal muscles, much of the sternum and the lateral aspects of the thoracic vertebral bodies and intervertebral discs. Posteriorly, it becomes continuous with the mediastinal pleura at an obtuse angle where the latter turns forwards from the anterolateral aspect of the vertebrae (**C**). Anteriorly, the continuity with the mediastinal pleura is much more acute, forming a costomediastinal pleural recess (**C**). It is convenient to postpone consideration of the positions of the costomediastinal lines of reflection till later (**161B**).

The mediastinal pleura covers the lateral aspects of the mediastinum, but again it is convenient to postpone consideration of its exact disposition until the mediastinal structures themselves have been described (**159B, 159C**).

The cervical pleura forms the upper limit of the pleural cavity and is smoothly continuous with the mediastinal and costal pleurae. It rises as a dome through the thoracic inlet as high as the neck of the first rib which lies 3–4 cm above the level of the first costal cartilage (**F, 141A**). The cervical pleurae thus lie outside the anatomical limits of the thorax in the root of the neck.

The nerve supply of the parietal pleura consists of sensory fibres in spinal nerves, so that pain is experienced when stimuli adequate for other somatic tissues are applied to the membrane. The costal pleura and the peripheral part of the diaphragmatic pleura are innervated by the intercostal nerves. The cervical, the mediastinal and the central diaphragmatic regions of the pleura are innervated by the phrenic nerve. Although this nerve will not be considered till later, it may be noted now that, since it arises mainly from the C4 spinal segment, irritation of the pleural regions it supplies frequently gives rise to referred pain in the lower part of the neck and the shoulder, where the skin is innervated from the same spinal segment through the supraclavicular nerves (**135C**).

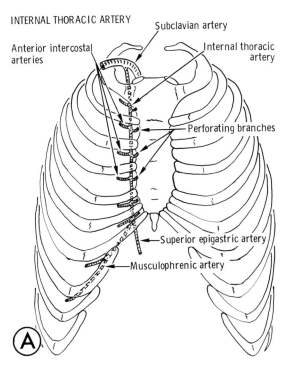

INTERNAL THORACIC ARTERY

Subclavian artery

Anterior intercostal arteries

Internal thoracic artery

Perforating branches

Superior epigastric artery

Musculophrenic artery

(A)

INTERNAL THORACIC ARTERY:
HORIZONTAL SECTION

Perforating branch

External intercostal membrane

Internal intercostal muscle

STERNUM

(B) Internal thoracic artery
& venae comitantes

Innermost intercostal muscle

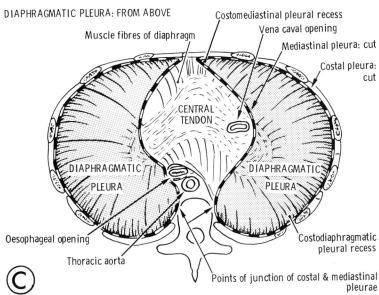

DIAPHRAGMATIC PLEURA: FROM ABOVE

Muscle fibres of diaphragm

Costomediastinal pleural recess

Vena caval opening

Mediastinal pleura: cut

Costal pleura: cut

CENTRAL TENDON

DIAPHRAGMATIC PLEURA

DIAPHRAGMATIC PLEURA

Oesophageal opening

Thoracic aorta

Costodiaphragmatic pleural recess

Points of junction of costal & mediastinal pleurae

(C)

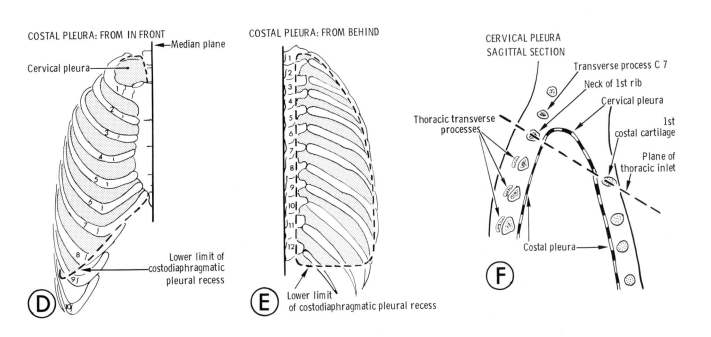

COSTAL PLEURA: FROM IN FRONT

Median plane

Cervical pleura

Lower limit of costodiaphragmatic pleural recess

(D)

COSTAL PLEURA: FROM BEHIND

Lower limit of costodiaphragmatic pleural recess

(E)

CERVICAL PLEURA
SAGITTAL SECTION

Transverse process C 7

Neck of 1st rib

Cervical pleura

1st costal cartilage

Thoracic transverse processes

Plane of thoracic inlet

Costal pleura

(F)

THE MEDIASTINUM AND ITS CONTENTS

It has been observed already that the mediastinum is the central region in the thorax which lies between the mediastinal parts of the parietal pleurae (**125C**). Its posterior limit is the anterior aspect of the thoracic vertebral column (**C**). Its anterior limit is very narrow in its upper part, where the right and left costomediastinal pleural recesses are closely approximated: lower down it is wider, where the left costomediastinal recess diverges from the midline (**161B, 161C**). Its lower boundary is the convex upper surface of the diaphragm including the greater part of its central tendon (**139C**). Above it is continuous through the thoracic inlet with the tissues in the root of the neck.

It is customary to divide the mediastinum into superior and inferior parts by a transverse plane which passes through the manubriosternal joint and the lower part of the fourth thoracic vertebral body (**A**). The inferior mediastinum may be further subdivided into anterior, middle and posterior parts, but this partition is not of great value and will be ignored in this text.

A group of structures, collectively known as the root of the lung, passes between the lateral aspect of the inferior mediastinum and the hilus of the lung on either side at the level of the fifth, sixth and seventh thoracic vertebral bodies (**A**). These structures are enclosed within pleural tubes which connect the mediastinal pleurae with the visceral pleurae on the lungs, and are pear-shaped in sagittal section (**A**). The structures of the root are congregated in the broad upper part of the tube. The narrow lower part which is often called the pulmonary ligament (**A**) is usually occupied by areolar tissue. It is important to note, however, that occasionally it contains an accessory bronchial artery which may be troublesome in operations on the lung.

The azygos vein

The azygos vein (**B**) is formed on the right side of the anterior aspect of the twelfth thoracic vertebral body by the union of the right subcostal vein and the right ascending lumbar vein which emerges from the upper part of the right psoas major muscle (**B**). (This is a muscle of the posterior abdominal wall which will be considered in another chapter.)

The vessel passes directly up the right side of the anterior aspect of the vertebral column, covered on its lateral side by the most posterior part of the mediastinal pleura (**B, C**). In front of the fourth thoracic vertebral body it turns forwards towards its junction with the superior vena cava in the anterior part of the mediastinum (**157B**).

It receives all the right posterior intercostal veins except the first. The second, third, and fourth are received through a common trunk called the right superior intercostal vein (**B**) and the others individually. These tributaries leave their respective intercostal spaces, pass behind the sympathetic trunk and incline forwards across the lateral aspects of the vertebral bodies (**B, C**). The azygos vein is also joined by visceral tributaries from the right extrapulmonary bronchi and from the oesophagus (**147A**).

The hemiazygos veins

A similar venous channel lies along the left side of the anterior aspect of the thoracic vertebral bodies (**C**), but usually consists of two separate parts (**B**). The lower is called the hemiazygos vein and the upper the accessory hemiazygos. The former is formed in the same way as the azygos and ascends as far as the eighth thoracic vertebra, where it turns sharply to the right and, passing across the vertebral body, ends in the azygos vein. The accessory hemiazygos descends from the fourth to the eighth thoracic vertebra where it ends in the same way.

The two veins receive all the left posterior intercostal veins below the third (compare with azygos), and visceral tributaries from the left extrapulmonary bronchus and from the oesophagus.

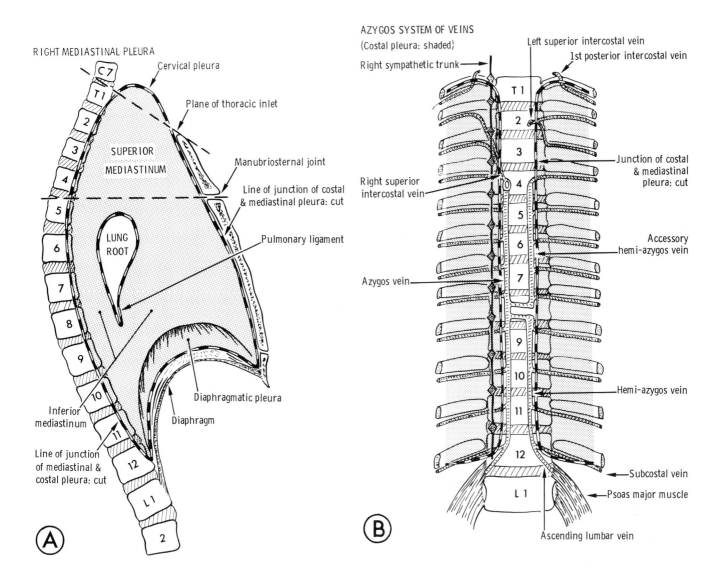

RIGHT MEDIASTINAL PLEURA

- C7
- T1
- 2
- 3
- 4
- 5
- 6
- 7
- 8
- 9
- 10
- 11
- 12
- L1
- 2

Cervical pleura

Plane of thoracic inlet

SUPERIOR MEDIASTINUM

Manubriosternal joint

Line of junction of costal & mediastinal pleura: cut

Pulmonary ligament

LUNG ROOT

Inferior mediastinum

Diaphragmatic pleura

Diaphragm

Line of junction of mediastinal & costal pleura: cut

Ⓐ

AZYGOS SYSTEM OF VEINS
(Costal pleura: shaded)

Right sympathetic trunk

Left superior intercostal vein

1st posterior intercostal vein

T1
- 2
- 3
- 4
- 5
- 6
- 7
- 9
- 10
- 11
- 12
- L1

Right superior intercostal vein

Azygos vein

Junction of costal & mediastinal pleura: cut

Accessory hemi-azygos vein

Hemi-azygos vein

Subcostal vein

Psoas major muscle

Ascending lumbar vein

Ⓑ

AZYGOS & HEMI-AZYGOS VEINS: TRANSVERSE SECTION

Hemi-azygos vein

Azygos vein

Junction of costal & mediastinal pleura

Sympathetic trunk

Right posterior intercostal vein

Ⓒ

THE BRACHIOCEPHALIC VEINS

Internal jugular vein

Subclavian vein

R1

T1

T2

Right brachiocephalic vein

Superior vena cava

Left brachiocephalic vein

Manubrium sterni

Ⓓ

The brachiocephalic veins are illustrated in **141D** as they lie in the anterior part of the root of the neck and the superior mediastinum. They will be considered in detail later but they are shown here because they receive the following tributaries.

1. Each first posterior intercostal vein turns upwards in front of the neck of the first rib and thereafter curves forwards and downwards over the cervical pleura (**141B**).
2. The left second and third posterior intercostal veins join to form the left superior intercostal which runs forwards across the left side of the mediastinum to join the left brachiocephalic vein (**153E**).
3. The internal thoracic veins which receive all the anterior intercostal veins.

The descending thoracic aorta

The great artery which carries oxygenated blood from the heart to the tissues of the body is the aorta. Observe its general course in the thorax (**A**) and note the names applied to its three parts. The heart and ascending aorta lie anteriorly, and the descending aorta posteriorly, in the inferior mediastinum: the arch of the aorta is situated in the superior mediastinum and passes backwards as well as to the left.

The descending aorta, which can be considered here, is continuous with the arch of the aorta on the left side of the lower border of the fourth thoracic vertebral body, that is at the level of the plane demarcating superior and inferior mediastina (**A**). It passes downwards along the vertebral column, gradually inclining medially until it passes through the aortic opening of the diaphragm into the abdomen (**B**). It lies in front of and largely hides the two hemiazygos veins (cf. **B** with **141B**). Its left surface is covered throughout by the left mediastinal pleura (**B, C**).

The vessel gives off the subcostal arteries and all the posterior intercostal arteries of both sides except the first and second (**B**). The asymmetrical position of the descending aorta accounts for differences in the initial parts of the left and right branches (**B, C**). The right posterior intercostal arteries arise from the right posterior aspect of the aorta, and cross the anterior aspects of the vertebral bodies before passing behind the azygos vein (**B, C**). Passing out of the mediastinum the arteries turn backwards, across the lateral aspects of the vertebral bodies and behind the sympathetic trunk and its medial branches, into their intercostal spaces (**C**). The arteries of the left side arise from the posterior aspect of the aorta and pass directly backwards, usually on the lateral side of the hemiazygos veins (**C**).

Visceral branches are also supplied and will be considered later.

The thoracic duct

This begins in front of the twelfth thoracic vertebral body as a continuation of a fusiform sac called the cisterna chyli (**B**). This cisterna chyli lies in front of the first and second lumbar vertebrae, in the aortic opening of the diaphragm, on the right side of the aorta. It receives the lymph from the lower limbs and the greater part of the abdominal cavity. The lymph from the small intestine is milky in appearance because fat is absorbed from that part of the gut into lymphatic vessels as minute particles called chylomicra. The lymph in the cisterna chyli and thoracic duct consequently has a similar milky appearance.

The duct ascends in a sagittal plane as far as the fifth thoracic vertebra. Note in (**B**) the structures which lie behind and on either side of it in this part of its course.

In front of the fifth thoracic vertebral body the duct moves to the left anterior aspect of the vertebral column and it remains in that position as it ascends through the superior mediastinum and the thoracic inlet into the root of the neck (**B**). As will be seen later it then diverges sharply to the left and joins the venous system in the angle between the internal jugular and subclavian veins (**395B**).

The tributaries of the thoracic duct are considered later (**189**).

AORTA

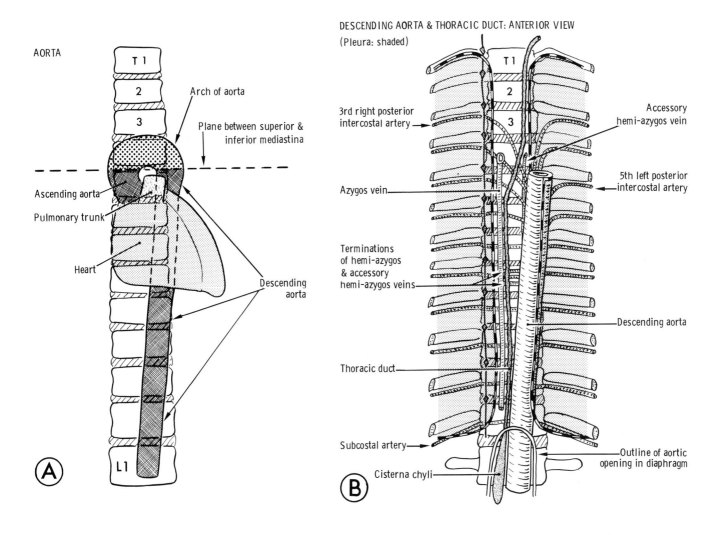

T 1
2
3

Arch of aorta

Plane between superior & inferior mediastina

Ascending aorta
Pulmonary trunk
Heart

Descending aorta

L1

(A)

T 1
2
3

3rd right posterior intercostal artery

Accessory hemi-azygos vein

Azygos vein

5th left posterior intercostal artery

Terminations of hemi-azygos & accessory hemi-azygos veins

Descending aorta

Thoracic duct

Subcostal artery

Cisterna chyli

Outline of aortic opening in diaphragm

(B)

DESCENDING AORTA:
TRANSVERSE SECTION

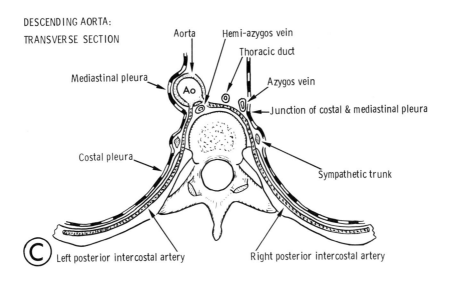

Aorta
Hemi-azygos vein
Thoracic duct
Mediastinal pleura
Ao
Azygos vein
Junction of costal & mediastinal pleura
Costal pleura
Sympathetic trunk
Left posterior intercostal artery
Right posterior intercostal artery

(C)

143

The oesophagus

This muscular tube connects the pharynx to the stomach. It begins in the midline of the neck in front of the sixth cervical vertebral body (**391**) and it is important to note, in connection with the passage of instruments along the upper part of the digestive tract, that this origin is some 15 cm from the incisor teeth in adults.

The oesophagus passes downwards through the lower part of the neck and the mediastinum and enters the abdomen through the oesophageal opening in the diaphragm (**131B**, **131C**). It will be recalled that this opening lies in the lumbar fibres of that muscle 2 cm or so to the left of the median plane and at the same level as the tenth thoracic vertebral body. The abdominal part of the oesophagus is only a little more than 1 cm long. Although the total length of the oesophagus varies in individuals of different builds, on average it is about 25 cm.

The lumen of the oesophagus is comparatively narrow where it passes through the diaphragm. Radiological examination of the viscus while a contrast medium is being swallowed (a barium swallow) indicates that it is also constricted at two other levels where, as will be seen later, it is closely related to the arch of the aorta (**157A**) and the left principal bronchus (**147B**).

Observe the following features of the course of the viscus (**A**, **B**).

1. Between the sixth cervical and fifth thoracic vertebrae it follows the sagittal curvatures of the vertebral column (**B**) and diverges a little to the left before returning to the median plane (**A**).
2. Between T1 and T4 the thoracic duct is situated along its left side (**A**).
3. At the levels of T4, 5 and 6 it passes anterior to the thoracic duct and the third, fourth, fifth, and sixth right posterior intercostal arteries. The azygos vein is to its right and the accessory hemiazygos vein and the descending aorta to its left (**A**).
4. Below the sixth thoracic vertebra the oesophagus inclines forwards and to the left (**B**) so that it loses contact with the vertebral column and passes across the anterior aspect of the descending aorta (**A**, **B**, **C**). The azygos vein and the thoracic duct are on its right side.
5. Below the eighth thoracic vertebra the oesophagus lies behind the posterior part of the diaphragm (**C**).

The muscular wall of the oesophagus consists of inner circular and outer longitudinal layers. The longitudinal fibres arise from the posterior surface of the cricoid cartilage (**D**) which can be felt in the lower part of the neck immediately below the thyroid cartilage (Adam's apple). As they descend they expand round the sides of the oesophagus to its posterior aspect and subsequently provide a uniform longitudinal coat around the oesophageal wall. As a result of this arrangement a triangular area on the uppermost part of the posterior oesophageal wall is devoid of longitudinal fibres. The character of the muscle fibres in both layers changes along the length of the viscus. In the upper third or so they are striated while in the lower third they are nonstriated. Between these two regions fibres of both types are present but the proportion of nonstriated fibres increases progressively from above down.

The arterial supply of the oesophagus is derived from three sources.

1. The cervical and upper thoracic regions are supplied by descending branches of the inferior thyroid artery (**393A**).
2. The supply to the greater parts of the thoracic oesophagus is through branches of the descending aorta. These are short and fairly wide and are consequently rather difficult to secure and tie off at operation.
3. The abdominal and the very lowest thoracic regions of the viscus are supplied by ascending branches from the left gastric artery which is one of the main vessels of the stomach (**251B**).

The venous drainage of the same three regions is into the brachiocephalic veins through their inferior thyroid tributaries (**485A**), into the azygos and hemiazygos veins and into the abdominal portal system through the left gastric veins (**253C**). It will be seen later that the anastomosis which occurs between the tributaries of the azygos veins and the left gastric veins in the lower part of the oesophagus is of great clinical importance.

The nerve supply of all parts of the oesophagus is derived mainly from the vagus nerves and will be discussed later in this chapter.

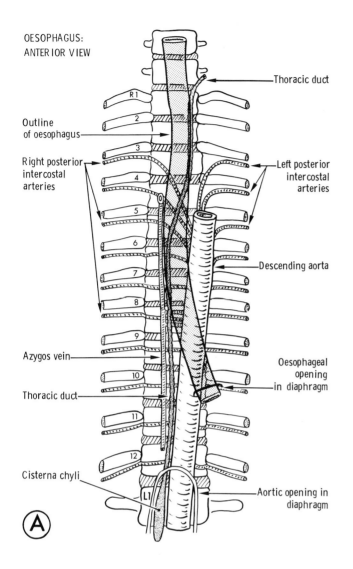

OESOPHAGUS:
ANTERIOR VIEW

Thoracic duct

Outline
of oesophagus

R1
2
3

Right posterior
intercostal
arteries

4

Left posterior
intercostal
arteries

5

6

7

Descending aorta

8

9

Azygos vein

10

Oesophageal
opening
in diaphragm

Thoracic duct

11

12

Cisterna chyli

L1

Aortic opening in
diaphragm

A

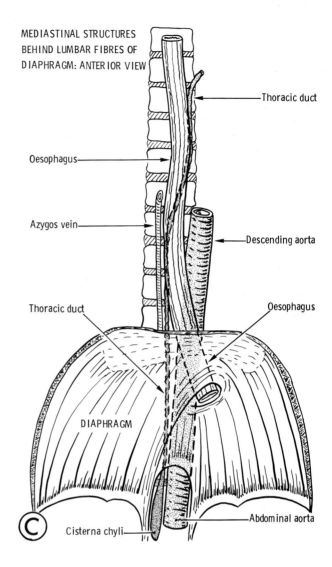

MEDIASTINAL STRUCTURES
BEHIND LUMBAR FIBRES OF
DIAPHRAGM: ANTERIOR VIEW

Thoracic duct

Oesophagus

Azygos vein

Descending aorta

Thoracic duct

Oesophagus

DIAPHRAGM

Abdominal aorta

C

Cisterna chyli

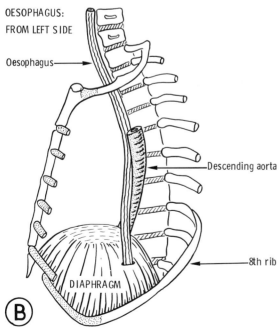

OESOPHAGUS:
FROM LEFT SIDE

Oesophagus

Descending aorta

DIAPHRAGM

8th rib

B

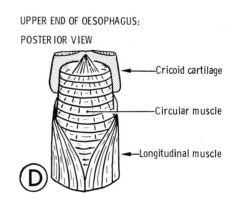

UPPER END OF OESOPHAGUS:
POSTERIOR VIEW

Cricoid cartilage

Circular muscle

Longitudinal muscle

D

145

The trachea and principal bronchi

The trachea, which is in continuity with the larynx, begins in the midline immediately in front of the commencement of the oesophagus at the level of the sixth cervical vertebral body (**A**, **B**). From there it passes downwards and backwards through the root of the neck and the superior mediastinum, with a continual slight inclination to the right (**A**) so that it lies anterior and to the right of the oesophagus. It bifurcates into two principal bronchi in the uppermost part of the inferior mediastinum, at the level of the upper border of the fifth thoracic vertebral body, just in front of the right edge of the oesophagus (**A**).

The principal bronchi pass laterally and downwards through the roots of the lungs towards the lungs at their hila. The two bronchi differ in a number of ways (**A**).

1. The tracheal bifurcation is to the right of the median plane, while, because of the position of the heart, the hilus of the left lung lies farther from the midline than that of the right lung. Consequently the left bronchus is comparatively long (5 cm) and more nearly horizontal than vertical, whereas the right bronchus is shorter (2.5 cm) and more nearly vertical than horizontal.
2. Because the capacity of the right lung is greater than that of the left (**179C**, **179D**), the right bronchus is wider than the left.
3. Because of the differences in their orientation and calibre, an aspirated foreign body is more likely to pass into the right bronchus than the left.
4. The first branch of the right principal bronchus (right upper lobe bronchus) arises in the root of the lung, while the primary division of the left principal bronchus is situated just within the substance of the left lung.
5. The right bronchus passes in front of the azygos vein. The left crosses anterior to the oesophagus and the descending aorta, producing some degree of constriction of the oesophageal lumen (**A**).

The structures of the trachea and extrapulmonary bronchi are similar (**C**). The anterior two-thirds or so of their walls contain transverse C-shaped bars of hyaline cartilage, while between and behind these cartilages the wall is formed by an extensible membrane consisting of collagenous, elastic and plain muscle fibres. The last of the eighteen or so tracheal cartilages also forms the first cartilages of the two bronchi by virtue of a process (the carina) which passes downwards and backwards between them (**A**).

This structure of the air passages is functionally important because it ensures both longitudinal extensibility and the permanent maintenance of a patent lumen.

The blood supply of the upper part of the trachea is derived from descending branches of the inferior thyroid arteries which lie in the neck (**393A**). The lower part of the trachea and the principal bronchi are supplied by the two bronchial arteries which arise either directly from the descending aorta or from the posterior intercostal branches of that vessel.

The veins of the upper trachea drain into the inferior thyroid veins. The rest of the extrapulmonary air passages are drained by superficial bronchial veins into the azygos and hemiazygos veins. The deep bronchial veins are considered with the lungs (**182**).

The heart and great vessels

The heart is a muscular pump which provides by far the greater part of the force required for the circulation of the blood. It is very roughly conical in form. The base is directed backwards and the apex forwards, downwards and to the left (**F**). Thus the long axis of the heart extends from behind forwards, downwards and to the left at about 45° to coronal and sagittal planes.

The organ consists of right and left channels. Each (**D**) consists of two chambers, a thin-walled atrium behind, which receives blood through veins, and a comparatively thick-walled ventricle in front, which delivers blood into a large artery arising from its upper posterior part. The muscular wall of each ventricle is separated from the walls of the corresponding atrium and artery by fibrous rings (**E**, **D**). Each atrium gives off a small blind conical diverticulum from its upper anterior part, known as the auricle (**F**).

The two channels are joined side to side so that to a large extent they share a common septum which is approximately aligned with the cardiac axis (**E**). The posterior part of the septum separates the two atria and is called the interatrial septum, while the anterior part intervenes mainly between the two ventricles and is called the interventricular septum (**E**).

On the external surface of the heart there is little evidence of the boundary between the two atria (**E**). In contrast the boundary between the ventricles is marked by anterior (**F**) and inferior interventricular grooves which overlie the margins of the interventricular septum, and the two atria and their auricles are demarcated from the ventricles by a continuous groove called the coronary sulcus (**E**, **F**).

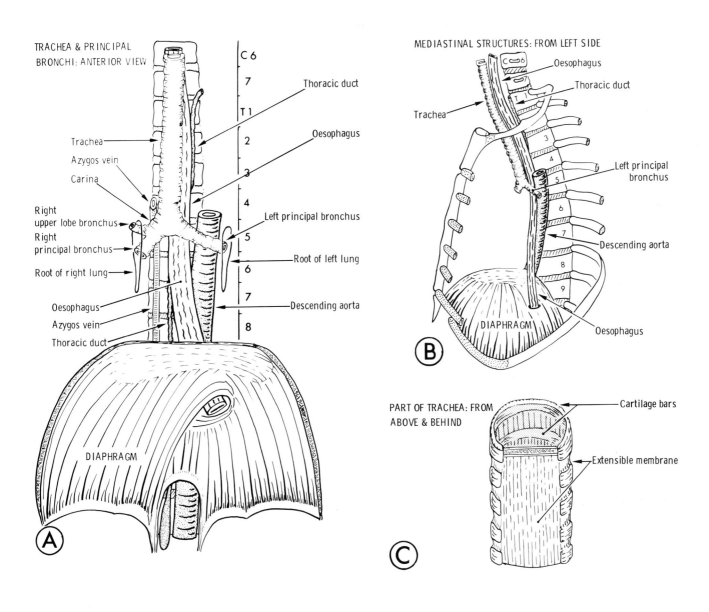

TRACHEA & PRINCIPAL
BRONCHI: ANTERIOR VIEW

C 6
7
T 1
2
3
4
5
6
7
8

Trachea
Azygos vein
Carina
Right
upper lobe bronchus
Right
principal bronchus
Root of right lung
Oesophagus
Azygos vein
Thoracic duct
DIAPHRAGM

Thoracic duct
Oesophagus
Left principal bronchus
Root of left lung
Descending aorta

Ⓐ

MEDIASTINAL STRUCTURES: FROM LEFT SIDE

C 6
1
3
4
5
6
7
8
9

Oesophagus
Thoracic duct
Trachea
Left principal
bronchus
Descending aorta
DIAPHRAGM
Oesophagus

Ⓑ

PART OF TRACHEA: FROM
ABOVE & BEHIND

Cartilage bars
Extensible membrane

Ⓒ

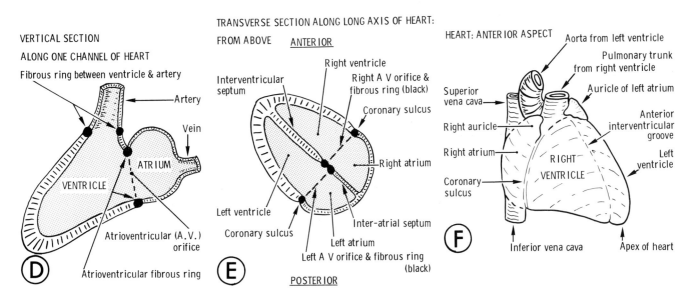

VERTICAL SECTION
ALONG ONE CHANNEL OF HEART

Fibrous ring between ventricle & artery
Artery
Vein
ATRIUM
VENTRICLE
Atrioventricular (A.V.)
orifice
Atrioventricular fibrous ring

Ⓓ

TRANSVERSE SECTION ALONG LONG AXIS OF HEART:
FROM ABOVE   ANTERIOR

Interventricular
septum
Right ventricle
Right A V orifice &
fibrous ring (black)
Coronary sulcus
Right atrium
Left ventricle
Coronary sulcus
Inter-atrial septum
Left atrium
Left A V orifice & fibrous ring
(black)

Ⓔ

POSTERIOR

HEART: ANTERIOR ASPECT

Aorta from left ventricle
Pulmonary trunk
from right ventricle
Auricle of left atrium
Anterior
interventricular
groove
Left
ventricle
Superior
vena cava
Right auricle
Right atrium
Coronary
sulcus
RIGHT
VENTRICLE
Inferior vena cava
Apex of heart

Ⓕ

In the circulation of the blood (**A**), the right atrium receives deoxygenated blood from the systemic circulation through three veins, the superior vena cava carrying blood from the upper part of the body, the inferior vena cava draining the abdomen and lower limbs, and the coronary sinus from the heart itself. This blood is then passed successively through the right atrioventricular orifice, the right ventricle, and the pulmonary orifice and carried by the pulmonary trunk and two pulmonary arteries to the pulmonary circulation.

Here the blood takes up oxygen from, and gives up carbon dioxide to, the air within the alveoli of the lungs, and returns to the left atrium through two pulmonary veins on each side. After passing successively through the left atrioventricular orifice, the left ventricle and aortic orifice, it is carried into the systemic circulation once again through the aorta.

The heart is invaginated into a serous sac, the serous pericardium, so that its outer surface is intimately covered by the visceral pericardium which is separated by only a potential space from the encapsulating parietal pericardium. The parietal pericardium is in turn closely surrounded by a fibrous sac, the fibrous pericardium. Having noted the presence of these two pericardial sacs, it is an advantage to ignore them while the form, position and relations of the heart and great vessels are considered. Thereafter they will be described in detail.

The external form of the heart

In an obliquely-placed conical organ such as the heart the surfaces and borders are not exactly demarcated and may be regarded more in the nature of aspects. It is usual to recognise in this way a base and an apex, right and upper borders, and anterior (sternocostal), inferior (diaphragmatic) and left surfaces (**B, C**).

Examine these several aspects of the heart. Observe the chambers which contribute to them, and the positions of the interventricular grooves and the coronary sulcus.

The position of the heart

The heart lies in the inferior mediastinum some distance in front of the sixth, seventh, and eighth thoracic vertebrae (**D**). The left atrial part of the base is separated from the vertebrae by the terminations of the pulmonary veins (**C**) and by the oesophagus and the descending aorta (**D**). The right atrial part of this aspect, which does not reach as high a level as the left atrium, is separated from the vertebrae by the lower right pulmonary vein (**C**) and the azygos vein and thoracic duct (**D**).

The inferior surface of the heart is related to the central tendon, and a small part of the muscular substance of the left cupola, of the diaphragm.

The right border and left surface are related, through the mediastinal pleurae, with the pleural cavities and the medial surfaces of the lungs (**F**).

The relations of the anterior (sternocostal) surface to the thoracic cage are indicated in **G**. It should be noted, however, that parts of the anterior surface are separated from these relations by the pleural cavities, the lungs and the thymus, as will be described later. Observe that in the adult the apex of the heart normally lies deep to the fifth intercostal space some 8 cm from the midline where its pulsations can usually be palpated.

The pulmonary veins

Two pulmonary veins, superior and inferior, leave the hilus of each lung anterior to and below the principal bronchus and pass initially through the corresponding lung root (**E**). They open through the upper part of the posterior wall of the left atrium.

The right veins pass in front of the azygos vein and the thoracic duct, the upper one lying behind the superior vena cava and the lower behind the right atrium (**C, E**). The left veins pass between the left edges of the left atrium and the descending aorta (**C, E**).

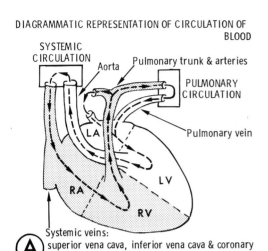

DIAGRAMMATIC REPRESENTATION OF CIRCULATION OF
BLOOD

SYSTEMIC
CIRCULATION

Aorta

Pulmonary trunk & arteries

PULMONARY
CIRCULATION

Pulmonary vein

LA

LV

RA

RV

Systemic veins:
superior vena cava, inferior vena cava & coronary
sinus

(A)

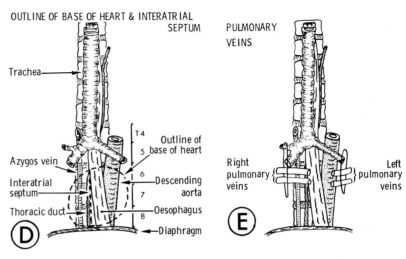

OUTLINE OF BASE OF HEART & INTERATRIAL
SEPTUM

Trachea

Azygos vein

Interatrial
septum

Thoracic duct

T 4
5
Outline of
base of heart
6
Descending
aorta
7
Oesophagus
8
Diaphragm

(D)

PULMONARY
VEINS

Right
pulmonary
veins

Left
pulmonary
veins

(E)

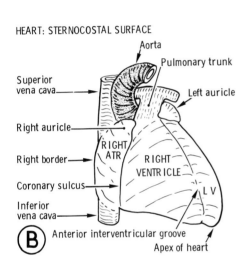

HEART: STERNOCOSTAL SURFACE

Aorta

Pulmonary trunk

Superior
vena cava

Left auricle

Right auricle

Right border

RIGHT
ATR

RIGHT
VENTRICLE

LV

Coronary sulcus

Inferior
vena cava

Anterior interventricular groove

Apex of heart

(B)

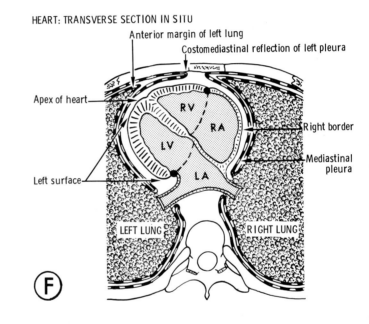

HEART: TRANSVERSE SECTION IN SITU

Anterior margin of left lung

Costomediastinal reflection of left pleura

Apex of heart

RV

RA

Right border

LV

Left surface

LA

Mediastinal
pleura

LEFT LUNG

RIGHT LUNG

(F)

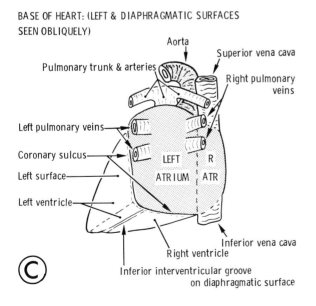

BASE OF HEART: (LEFT & DIAPHRAGMATIC SURFACES
SEEN OBLIQUELY)

Aorta

Superior vena cava

Pulmonary trunk & arteries

Right pulmonary
veins

Left pulmonary veins

Coronary sulcus

LEFT
ATRIUM

R
ATR

Left surface

Left ventricle

Inferior vena cava

Right ventricle

Inferior interventricular groove
on diaphragmatic surface

(C)

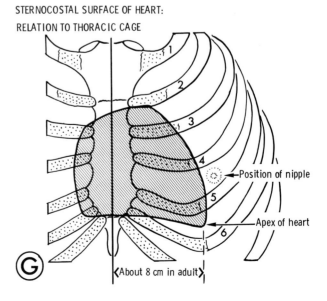

STERNOCOSTAL SURFACE OF HEART:
RELATION TO THORACIC CAGE

1

2

3

4

Position of nipple

5

Apex of heart

6

‹About 8 cm in adult›

(G)

The pulmonary trunk

This large vessel, having a diameter of about 3 cm, leaves the upper part of the right ventricle (the infundibulum) (**A, B**) and follows a spiral course, inclining first upwards, backwards and to the left, and then upwards and backwards. Below, it is situated in front of the lower part of the ascending aorta (see below) while above it lies in front of the uppermost part of the left atrium (**A, B**). Its projection on the anterior chest wall is shown in **D** but it will be noted later that it is separated from the sternum and costal cartilages by other structures.

Immediately above the pulmonary orifice, the trunk exhibits three slight dilatations which lie above the three cusps of the pulmonary valve and are called the posterior, left anterior and right anterior pulmonary sinuses.

Just below and to the left of the bifurcation of the trachea, and some distance in front of the oesophagus, the pulmonary trunk divides into right and left pulmonary arteries (**A, B**).

The pulmonary arteries

These arteries pass laterally from the bifurcation of the pulmonary trunk, above the level of the pulmonary veins, and traverse the roots of the lungs (**A**). The right artery passes in front of the right principal bronchus, below the origin of the right upper lobe bronchus, which is consequently sometimes described as the eparterial bronchus. The left artery crosses the left principal bronchus, which separates it from the descending aorta (**A, C**), above the origin of the left upper lobe bronchus, which may therefore be described as hyparterial.

The ascending aorta

The ascending aorta, which has about the same calibre as the pulmonary trunk but a considerably thicker wall, begins at the aortic orifice of the left ventricle. The orifice lies behind the infundibulum of the right ventricle and is situated below, behind and a little to the right of the pulmonary orifice (**B**). The vessel passes upwards, in a gentle curve which is convex forwards and to the right (**B, C**), and becomes continuous with the aortic arch behind the second right costal cartilage at the level of the sternal angle (**D**).

Immediately above the aortic orifice the lumen of the aorta exhibits three dilatations. These are the anterior and the left and right posterior aortic sinuses. The orifices of the right and left coronary arteries lie in the upper parts of the anterior and left posterior sinuses respectively.

Observe the following relations of the ascending aorta.

1. The infundibulum of the right ventricle on the left, and the right auricle on the right, cover and obscure its lowest part (**C**).

2. The pulmonary trunk winds spirally upwards and backwards across its left side (**C**).
3. Posteriorly, it is related to the upper part of the left atrium, the right pulmonary artery and the left edge of the superior vena cava (**B, C**).
4. Its projection on the anterior thoracic wall is shown in **D**, but it will be noted later that it is separated from the chest wall by other structures.

The arch of the aorta

This part of the aorta lies in the lower half of the superior mediastinum. It follows a complexly curved course, which is convex upwards, forwards and to the left, between the ascending aorta and the descending aorta (**143A**), both of which have been considered already.

Its early part curves upwards and to the left across the anterior aspect of the trachea a short distance above the tracheal bifurcation (**C**). It then bends downwards and backwards with an inclination to the left across the left sides of the trachea, the oesophagus and the thoracic duct, to the left side of the lower border of the fourth thoracic vertebral body (**E**). Below it lies the bifurcation of the pulmonary trunk, the origins of the two pulmonary arteries and the left bronchus (**C**).

From the upper aspect of the aortic arch three large vessels arise which constitute the blood supply to the upper limbs (the subclavian arteries) and the region of the head and neck (the common carotid arteries). The right subclavian and right common carotid arteries arise by a common stem called the brachiocephalic trunk, whereas the left common carotid and left subclavian arteries arise directly from the arch (**C**).

Observe the projections of the aortic arch and the mediastinal parts of its branches on the anterior thoracic wall in **D**. Note that the aortic arch is behind the lower half of the manubrium sterni and the branches behind the upper half.

The brachiocephalic trunk arises from the highest part of the aortic arch in front of the trachea (**C**). It curls upwards, backwards and to the right, to the right aspect of the trachea behind the highest part of the clavicular notch of the manubrium sterni, and there divides into its terminal branches (**D**).

PULMONARY TRUNK & ARTERIES

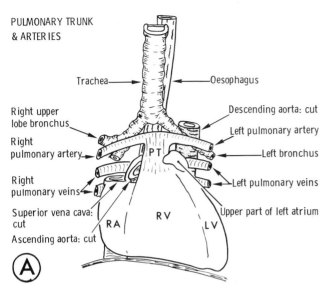

Trachea

Oesophagus

Right upper lobe bronchus

Descending aorta: cut

Right pulmonary artery

Left pulmonary artery

Left bronchus

Right pulmonary veins

Left pulmonary veins

Superior vena cava: cut

Upper part of left atrium

Ascending aorta: cut

PT

RA   RV   LV

(A)

SAGITTAL SECTION OF HEART & GREAT VESSELS: FROM LEFT

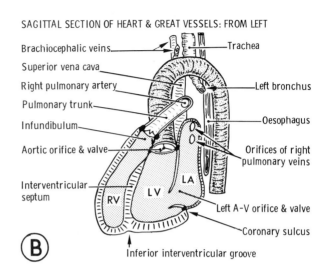

Brachiocephalic veins

Trachea

Superior vena cava

Right pulmonary artery

Left bronchus

Pulmonary trunk

Oesophagus

Infundibulum

Aortic orifice & valve

Orifices of right pulmonary veins

Interventricular septum

RV   LV   LA

Left A-V orifice & valve

Coronary sulcus

(B)

Inferior interventricular groove

ASCENDING AORTA & AORTIC ARCH

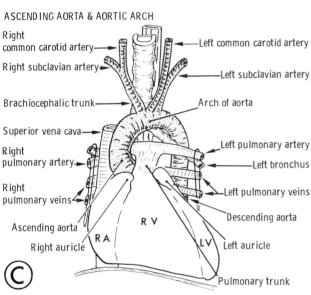

Right common carotid artery

Left common carotid artery

Right subclavian artery

Left subclavian artery

Brachiocephalic trunk

Arch of aorta

Superior vena cava

Left pulmonary artery

Right pulmonary artery

Left bronchus

Right pulmonary veins

Left pulmonary veins

Descending aorta

Ascending aorta

RA   RV   LV

Right auricle

Left auricle

Pulmonary trunk

(C)

PROJECTION OF GREAT VESSELS ON ANTERIOR THORACIC WALL

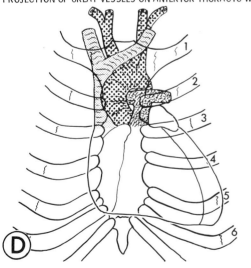

1
2
3
4
5
6

(D)

MEDIASTINUM: FROM LEFT SIDE
(Interrupted line surrounds structures forming root of left lung)

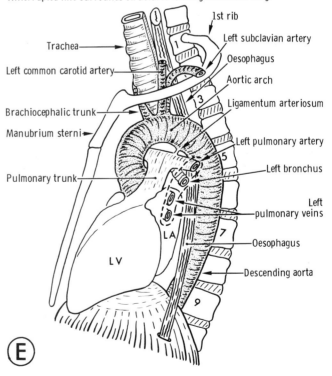

1st rib

Trachea

Left subclavian artery

Oesophagus

Left common carotid artery

Aortic arch

Brachiocephalic trunk

Ligamentum arteriosum

Manubrium sterni

Left pulmonary artery

Left bronchus

Pulmonary trunk

Left pulmonary veins

LA

Oesophagus

LV

Descending aorta

3
5
7
9

(E)

The right subclavian artery curves laterally with an upward convexity across the anterior aspect of the cervical pleura and across the upper surface of the shaft of the first rib immediately behind the insertion of a cervical muscle named scalenus anterior (**A**). It gives off two branches which are concerned with the supply of the thoracic wall. The internal thoracic artery (**139A**) passes downwards on to the deep aspect of the anterior thoracic wall (**A**). The costocervical trunk arises from the posterior aspect of the subclavian artery and runs backwards over the cervical pleura to divide at the neck of the first rib. The superior intercostal branch turns downwards into the thorax between the chest wall and the cervical pleura (**B**) and supplies the first two posterior intercostal arteries (**C**). The deep cervical branch continues backwards into the muscles at the back of the neck (**A, B**).

The right common carotid artery passes upwards and a little laterally into the right side of the neck (**A**).

The left common carotid artery is considerably smaller than the brachiocephalic. It arises a little to the left of the midline and passes upwards, backwards and to the left from the left anterior to the left side of the trachea (**A**). The left subclavian artery runs parallel to and behind it. Reaching the level of the upper part of the clavicular notch of the manubrium, it becomes symmetrical with the right common carotid artery.

The left subclavian artery arises behind and a little to the left of the left common carotid (**A**), this relationship reflecting the strong backward inclination of the second part of the aortic arch. It ascends through the superior mediastinum behind the left common carotid artery, on the left side of the trachea and in front of the thoracic duct and the left edge of the oesophagus. Behind the upper limit of the clavicular notch of the manubrium it turns laterally and becomes symmetrical as regards position and branches with the corresponding artery of the right side.

The thyroidea ima artery is an inconstant narrow vessel which, when present, runs upwards to the thyroid gland in the lower part of the neck. It has a variable origin from the aortic arch or from any of its three branches described above.

The ligamentum arteriosum can be conveniently mentioned here although it is not a branch of the aortic arch. In the adult, it is a thick short fibrous cord, which is attached below to the upper aspect of the termination of the pulmonary trunk or the beginning of the left pulmonary artery, and above to the undersurface of the arch of the aorta a short distance beyond the origin of the left subclavian artery (**E**). It is the fibrosed remnant of the ductus arteriosus which is a large and important vessel in foetal life but becomes obliterated at or soon after birth (**175D**).

The brachiocephalic veins

The brachiocephalic veins are each formed by the junction of the corresponding internal jugular and subclavian veins (**D**). The internal jugular descends from the head and neck on the lateral side of the common carotid artery and medial to scalenus anterior (**D**); the subclavian vein passes medially, below and in front of the subclavian artery, separated from it by scalenus anterior (**D**).

The veins are formed at symmetrical points in the thoracic inlet, but then follow dissimilar courses. The right vein is short (2.5 cm) and almost vertical. It descends along the anterolateral aspect of the brachiocephalic artery. The left vein is comparatively long (6 cm) and nearly horizontal, and passes from left to right across the anterior aspects of the three branches of the aortic arch. The two veins join behind the lower border of the first right costal cartilage to form the superior vena cava (**D**).

Observe the projection of the brachiocephalic veins on the anterior thoracic wall (**151D**), and notice particularly the normal adult relationship of the left brachiocephalic vein to the upper half of the manubrium sterni. In the early years of life this vein often lies at a rather higher level and may project above the jugular notch of the manubrium. This is of surgical importance when it is necessary to make an artificial opening into the trachea between the thyroid gland and the manubrium (**486**).

The tributaries of the brachiocephalic veins are not identical. Both veins receive the corresponding internal thoracic veins, the first posterior intercostal veins, which turn forwards over the cervical pleura (**C**), and vertebral veins from the neck (**395B**). A network of veins descends from the thyroid gland into the superior mediastinum. Most of these vessels join the left brachiocephalic vein but a few join the right brachiocephalic. The second and third left posterior intercostal veins join to form the left superior intercostal vein. This vessel runs forwards beneath the mediastinal pleura across the left side of the arch of the aorta to join the left brachiocephalic vein (**E**). Its importance lies in the fact that it passes close to the ligamentum arteriosum (or the ductus arteriosus) and constitutes a landmark for the latter structure when it has to be ligated in infancy.

ROOT OF NECK

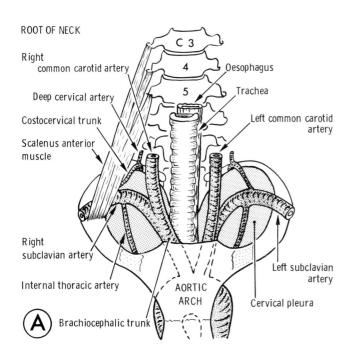

- Right common carotid artery
- C 3
- 4
- 5
- Oesophagus
- Trachea
- Deep cervical artery
- Costocervical trunk
- Scalenus anterior muscle
- Left common carotid artery
- Right subclavian artery
- Internal thoracic artery
- AORTIC ARCH
- Left subclavian artery
- Cervical pleura
- Brachiocephalic trunk
- (A)

SAGITTAL SECTION THROUGH THORACIC INLET

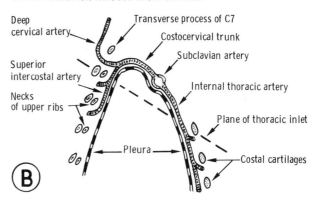

- Deep cervical artery
- Transverse process of C7
- Costocervical trunk
- Subclavian artery
- Superior intercostal artery
- Necks of upper ribs
- Internal thoracic artery
- Plane of thoracic inlet
- Pleura
- Costal cartilages
- (B)

POSTERIOR CHEST WALL: UPPER PART

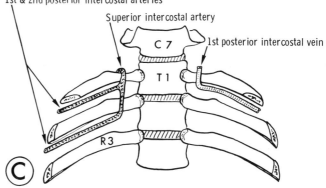

- 1st & 2nd posterior intercostal arteries
- Superior intercostal artery
- C 7
- 1st posterior intercostal vein
- T 1
- R 3
- (C)

ROOT OF NECK AFTER REMOVAL OF STERNUM

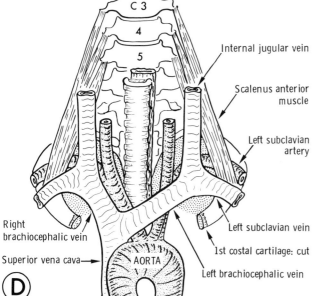

- C 3
- 4
- 5
- Internal jugular vein
- Scalenus anterior muscle
- Left subclavian artery
- Right brachiocephalic vein
- Superior vena cava
- AORTA
- Left subclavian vein
- 1st costal cartilage: cut
- Left brachiocephalic vein
- (D)

SUPERIOR MEDIASTINUM & ROOT OF NECK FROM LEFT

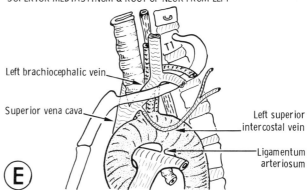

- Left brachiocephalic vein
- T 1
- Superior vena cava
- Left superior intercostal vein
- Ligamentum arteriosum
- (E)

153

The superior vena cava

This large vessel is formed by the union of the two brachiocephalic veins behind the lower border of the first right costal cartilage (**153D**), and descends vertically to open into the upper part of the right atrium, behind the third right sternocostal joint (**A, 151D**). Because of the effect of gravity in the upright position, neither it nor the brachiocephalic veins are equipped with valves.

In its upper part, the vessel lies against the groove between the ascending aorta and the aortic arch in front and the trachea behind (**A**). Its lower part is posterolateral to the ascending aorta and in front of the structures in the root of the right lung, particularly the right pulmonary artery and upper right pulmonary vein (**A**).

The azygos vein was considered earlier in this chapter as far as the point at which it lay on the right anterior aspect of the fourth thoracic body (**141B**). It can now be observed that from that point the vessel curves forwards to join the middle part of the superior vena cava (**A**). This arch of the azygos vein crosses the right side of the lowest part of the trachea and lies above the uppermost structures in the root of the right lung.

The thoracic part of the inferior vena cava

The inferior vena cava carries nearly all the venous blood from the body below the diaphragm. It enters the thorax through the vena caval opening in the right part of the central tendon of that muscle, at the level of the eighth thoracic vertebral body in quiet respiration (**131B, 131C**). Almost immediately thereafter it opens into the lowest part of the right atrium on the diaphragmatic surface of the heart. In its short thoracic course it lies in front of the azygos vein (**A**).

The pericardium

The serous pericardium is one of the serous membranes of the body and similar in structure to the pleura and the peritoneum. It is invaginated from its upper posterior aspect by the heart and the adjacent parts of the great vessels associated with it. The heart and vessels are thus covered by a visceral pericardial layer which can move freely with negligible friction on a parietal pericardial layer which lines the immediately surrounding structures. The visceral pericardium may be regarded as a broad mesentery or mesocardium. But as its posterosuperior part contains an aperture (**B**) this part consists of an arterial tube above and a venous tube behind.

The arterial pericardial tube contains two arteries, namely the ascending aorta and the pulmonary trunk, and is very approximately cylindrical (**C**). The venous tube is deeply grooved on its inferior aspect so that it is ∩-shaped in coronal section (**C**). Observe that its short left limb encloses the terminal parts of the two left pulmonary veins. The longer right limb encloses the lower half of the superior vena cava, the terminal parts of the two right pulmonary veins and the inferior vena cava (**C**).

The recess of the pericardial cavity which invaginates the venous tube from below (**C, D**) is called the oblique sinus. It lies between the visceral pericardium covering the posterior wall of the left atrium between the pulmonary veins, and the parietal pericardium covering the anterior aspects of the oesophagus and the ascending aorta (**149D**).

In postnatal life the deficiency in the mesocardium is in the form of a channel, known as the transverse sinus, which passes from side to side between the arterial and venous tubes (**D, E**). It extends from the interval between the ascending aorta and the superior vena cava on the right to that between the pulmonary trunk and the left atrium on the left. One finger can be passed through it (large arrow in **C**).

MEDIASTINUM: FROM RIGHT SIDE

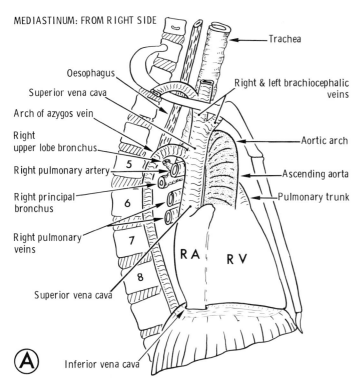

- Oesophagus
- Superior vena cava
- Arch of azygos vein
- Right upper lobe bronchus
- Right pulmonary artery — 5
- Right principal bronchus — 6
- Right pulmonary veins — 7
- 8
- Superior vena cava

RA   RV

- Trachea
- Right & left brachiocephalic veins
- Aortic arch
- Ascending aorta
- Pulmonary trunk

(A)

- Inferior vena cava

DIAGRAMMATIC REPRESENTATION OF INVAGINATION OF SEROUS PERICARDIUM BY HEART & GREAT VESSELS

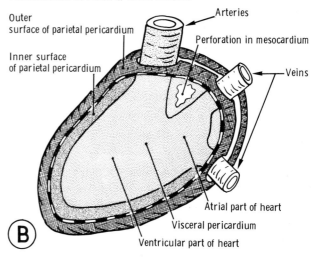

- Outer surface of parietal pericardium
- Inner surface of parietal pericardium
- Arteries
- Perforation in mesocardium
- Veins
- Atrial part of heart
- Visceral pericardium
- Ventricular part of heart

(B)

HEART WITH VISCERAL PERICARDIUM: FROM BEHIND

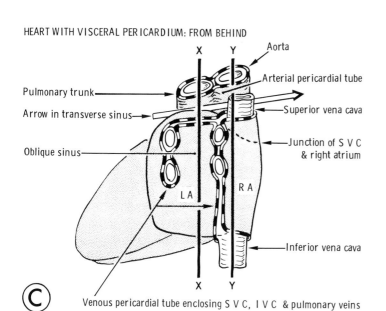

X   Y

- Pulmonary trunk
- Arrow in transverse sinus
- Oblique sinus
- Aorta
- Arterial pericardial tube
- Superior vena cava
- Junction of S V C & right atrium

LA   RA

- Inferior vena cava

X   Y

(C)

- Venous pericardial tube enclosing S V C, I V C & pulmonary veins

SAGITTAL SECTION ALONG PLANE X-X IN C

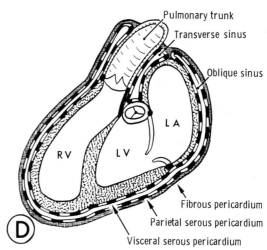

- Pulmonary trunk
- Transverse sinus
- Oblique sinus

RV   LV   LA

- Fibrous pericardium
- Parietal serous pericardium
- Visceral serous pericardium

(D)

SAGITTAL SECTION ALONG PLANE Y-Y IN C

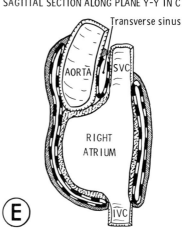

- Transverse sinus

AORTA   SVC

RIGHT ATRIUM

IVC

(E)

The fibrous pericardium is a fibrous sac, adherent to the parietal layer of the serous pericardium (**A, B**). Its base is firmly attached to the central tendon of the diaphragm and is perforated by the inferior vena cava (**B**). Above, its limit is less exact, the fibrous layer disappearing as a definite structure by blending with the adventitial coats of the superior vena cava, the ascending aorta, the right and left pulmonary arteries and the four pulmonary veins, beyond the limits of the serous pericardium.

The roots of the lungs

It has been noted previously that on either side a number of structures leave the inferior mediastinum and pass laterally, within a pear-shaped pleural tube, to the hilus of the corresponding lung. The structures which comprise this root of the lung are the principal bronchus, the pulmonary artery and veins and the bronchial arteries and veins. Observe their relationship to one another on the left and right sides (**A, B**). Note also that the root of the left lung (**A**) lies in front of the descending aorta, below the aortic arch and behind the fibrous pericardium covering the pulmonary trunk, whereas the root of the right lung (**B**) is in front of the azygos vein, below the arch of that vein and behind the fibrous pericardium covering the superior vena cava.

The phrenic nerves

Although the paired phrenic nerves contain an appreciable component of afferent fibres which will be considered later, their principal function is to supply efferent fibres to all the muscle of the diaphragm. Despite their distribution to this muscle, the nerves arise in the middle region of the neck from the ventral rami of C3, 4 and 5, particularly from C4. Because of this high origin the nerves have a cervical course, which will be described in the appropriate chapter (**393A**), and then descend along the whole length of the lateral aspects of the mediastinum. They lie immediately deep to the mediastinal pleura and each passes in front of the root of the corresponding lung. Both nerves enter the thorax by inclining downwards and medially across the internal thoracic artery (**C**) above the first costal cartilage and in front of the cervical pleura. Thereafter, because of the asymmetry of the main mediastinal structures, their relations differ. Observe in **B** the successive relations of the right phrenic to the right brachiocephalic vein, the upper half of the superior vena cava and the right side of the fibrous pericardium. In **A** note that the left nerve descends between the left common carotid and subclavian arteries, behind the left brachiocephalic vein, crosses the left aspect of the aortic arch and finally descends on the left side of the fibrous pericardium.

Reaching the diaphragm, each nerve pierces the muscle and radiates branches across its inferior surface to the muscle fibres of the corresponding cupola.

The afferent fibres in the nerves are of two kinds. First, proprioceptive fibres pass centrally from the diaphragm. Secondly, there are fibres which, in disease processes, may convey the sensation of pain from the parietal layer of any of three serous membranes, namely the cervical and mediastinal pleurae and all but the most peripheral parts of the diaphragmatic pleura, the parietal serous pericardium and some regions of peritoneum in the upper part of the abdominal cavity. Such sensory impulses from the serous membranes may give rise to referred pain in the skin area innervated by C4, that is the skin over the lower part of the neck and the point of the shoulder.

Each nerve is accompanied in the inferior mediastinum by the long slender pericardiacophrenic branch of the internal thoracic artery.

The vagus nerves

These are the tenth in the series of cranial nerves. They arise from the medulla oblongata, traverse the base of the skull and pass downwards, as one of the components of the main neurovascular bundle of the neck, to the thoracic inlet. Their fibres, though not the original nerves themselves, continue through the whole length of the thorax and end in the upper part of the abdominal cavity.

The nerves contain three types of fibres.

1. Preganglionic parasympathetic which arise from cells in the medial part of the dorsal vagal nucleus (**53A**).
2. Branchial efferent motor fibres, that is fibres which innervate striated muscle developed from the mesoderm of branchial arches. They arise from cells in the nucleus ambiguus (**53A, 53B**).
3. Visceral afferent fibres which transmit a number of different types of impulses. Their cells of origin are situated in two sensory ganglia which lie on the proximal part of each vagus nerve. The central processes of these cells end in the lateral part of the dorsal vagal nucleus.

In the neck the two vagus nerves follow symmetrical courses, and reach the root of the neck lying posterolateral to the corresponding common carotid arteries (**C**). They give off a number of cervical branches. Some of these are concerned wholly with cervical structures and will not be considered at this time. Others are concerned wholly or in part with thoracic structures and these will be described below. In the upper part of the thorax the courses of the two nerves are dissimilar.

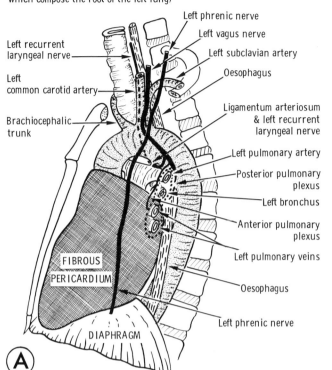

LEFT ASPECT OF MEDIASTINUM (The dotted line surrounds the structures which compose the root of the left lung)

Left recurrent laryngeal nerve

Left common carotid artery

Brachiocephalic trunk

Left phrenic nerve

Left vagus nerve

Left subclavian artery

Oesophagus

Ligamentum arteriosum & left recurrent laryngeal nerve

Left pulmonary artery

Posterior pulmonary plexus

Left bronchus

Anterior pulmonary plexus

Left pulmonary veins

Oesophagus

Left phrenic nerve

FIBROUS PERICARDIUM

DIAPHRAGM

A

RIGHT ASPECT OF MEDIASTINUM (The dotted line surrounds the structures which compose the root of the right lung)

Right phrenic nerve

Right subclavian artery

Right subclavian vein

Oesophagus

Right vagus nerve

Right upper lobe bronchus

Right pulmonary artery

Right principal bronchus

Right pulmonary veins

Azygos vein

Inferior vena cava

Right vagus nerve

Right recurrent laryngeal nerve

Right common carotid artery

Brachiocephalic trunk

Left common carotid artery

Left brachiocephalic vein

Aortic arch

Superior vena cava

FIBROUS PERICARDIUM

DIAPHRAGM

B

Right phrenic nerve

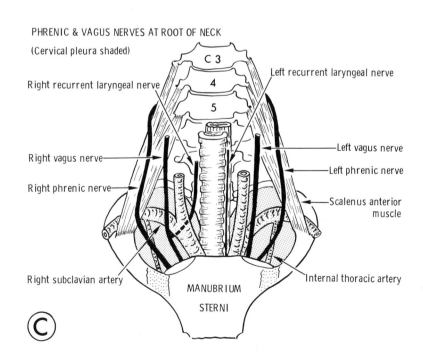

PHRENIC & VAGUS NERVES AT ROOT OF NECK
(Cervical pleura shaded)

C 3

4

5

Right recurrent laryngeal nerve

Right vagus nerve

Right phrenic nerve

Right subclavian artery

Left recurrent laryngeal nerve

Left vagus nerve

Left phrenic nerve

Scalenus anterior muscle

Internal thoracic artery

MANUBRIUM STERNI

C

The right vagus enters the thorax by passing in front of the right subclavian artery (**157B**, **157C**), medial to the phrenic nerve. It is important to note that, at this point, the vagus gives off the right recurrent laryngeal nerve because although, as its name indicates, that branch is primarily distributed to the larynx, it is also involved to some extent in the innervation of mediastinal viscera. The recurrent laryngeal nerve hooks backwards and upwards round the subclavian artery, and ascends in the neck in the groove between the right aspects of the trachea and the oesophagus (**157C**).

Having given off this branch, the vagus nerve itself inclines downwards and backwards, across the right side of the trachea (**157B**) in the superior mediastinum, until it reaches the posterior aspect of the root of the right lung. Observe (**C**) this part of its course and its relationships to the right brachiocephalic vein, the upper half of the superior vena cava and the arch of the azygos vein.

Reaching the root of the lung, the vagus divides abruptly into a large number of fine branches which run into the posterior pulmonary plexus and, to a lesser extent, the anterior pulmonary plexus (**C, 157A**).

The left vagus enters the thorax between the left subclavian and left common carotid arteries (**157A, 157C**). It passes behind the left brachiocephalic vein and is crossed from behind forwards by the phrenic nerve (**B**). The nerve then inclines downwards and backwards across the left side of the aortic arch to reach a point posterior to the ligamentum arteriosum (**B, 399B**).

Here the nerve gives off the left recurrent laryngeal nerve which hooks beneath the aortic arch, behind the ligamentum arteriosum, to reach the groove between the trachea and the oesophagus in which it ascends into the neck (**157A**). Notice in particular the different level of origin of the left and right recurrent laryngeal nerves (**157A, 157B, 399B**).

From the aortic arch the vagus nerve sends fine branches into the left posterior pulmonary plexus, and to a lesser extent into the left anterior pulmonary plexus, on the posterior and anterior aspects of the root of the left lung (**B, 157A**).

In the lower part of the thorax, fibres derived from both vagus nerves leave the posterior pulmonary plexuses and pass downwards into the oesophageal plexus on the wall of the lower part of the thoracic oesophagus (**187A**). Just above the diaphragm, some of these vagal fibres become aggregated into two distinct nerves called the anterior and posterior vagal trunks, which pass into the abdominal cavity on the respective aspects of the abdominal oesophagus. The course and distribution of these nerves are considered later (**295A**).

The thymus

The thymus is an essential component of the lymphoid system. It is pinkish grey and consists of closely packed lobules in which lymphocytes occupy the interstices within a network of branched epithelial reticular cells. Developmentally, the organ consists of right and left lobes but in most individuals, although it still shows evidence of its bilateral origin, the two halves are fused to a considerable extent (**A**).

The thymus enlarges from birth to puberty. Thereafter, there is a progressive reduction in size as both lymphocytes and reticular cells are gradually replaced by fat and fibrous tissue. By this process of involution, the organ in later adult life (and therefore in nearly all dissecting room cadavers) is reduced to a fibrous strand which is difficult to identify with certainty by naked-eye examination.

In the young, the viscus lies in the anterior part of the mediastinum from the level of the fourth costal cartilages to about the upper border of the manubrium sterni, but in some individuals it continues upwards for a variable distance into the neck towards the thyroid gland. Observe in **A** its close relationship to the upper half of the fibrous pericardium, the arch of the aorta and its branches, the left brachiocephalic vein and the trachea.

The main arterial supply in the thorax is derived from the internal thoracic arteries which lie to its lateral sides. In the neck it receives descending twigs from the inferior thyroid arteries (**393A**). The venous return is into the corresponding veins and into the left brachiocephalic vein.

The mediastinal pleurae

In general the mediastinal pleura extends forwards across the lateral aspects of the mediastinal structures from the anterolateral aspects of the thoracic vertebral column (**B, C**).

On each side it is continuous by means of a short pleural tube with the visceral pleura on the medial surface of the corresponding lung. The tubes arise immediately behind the fibrous pericardium, at the level of T5, 6 and 7 and are pear-shaped in sagittal section (**B, C**). The broad upper part of each tube contains the structures which comprise the root of the lung. The narrow lower part, called the pulmonary ligament, usually contains only areolar tissue but in a few individuals it contains a bronchial artery which may be troublesome in the operation of removal of the lung (pneumonectomy).

THYMUS: ANTERIOR VIEW
(Interrupted lines indicate outlines of sternum & costal cartilages)

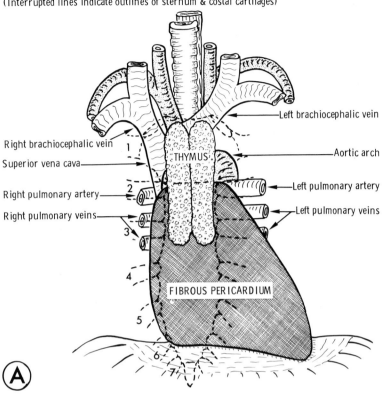

Right brachiocephalic vein

Superior vena cava

Right pulmonary artery

Right pulmonary veins

Left brachiocephalic vein

Aortic arch

THYMUS

Left pulmonary artery

Left pulmonary veins

FIBROUS PERICARDIUM

(A)

LEFT MEDIASTINAL PLEURA

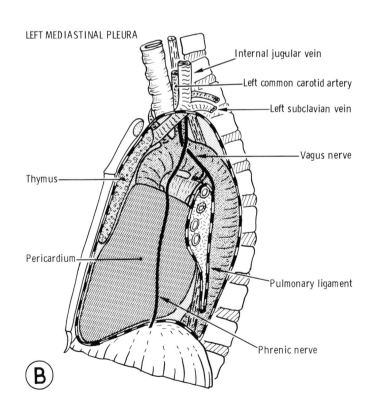

Internal jugular vein

Left common carotid artery

Left subclavian vein

Vagus nerve

Thymus

Pericardium

Pulmonary ligament

Phrenic nerve

(B)

RIGHT MEDIASTINAL PLEURA

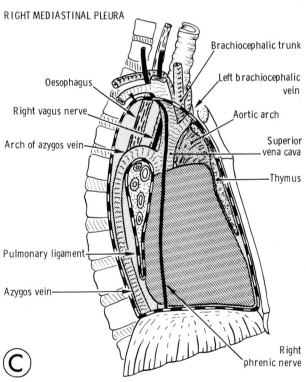

Oesophagus

Right vagus nerve

Arch of azygos vein

Brachiocephalic trunk

Left brachiocephalic vein

Aortic arch

Superior vena cava

Thymus

Pulmonary ligament

Azygos vein

Right phrenic nerve

(C)

The mediastinal pleurae are closely moulded over the mediastinal structures but in certain regions they are insinuated towards the midline forming a series of pleural recesses (**138**).

1. On the left side of the inferior mediastinum, after bulging to the left over the descending aorta, the pleura frequently dips medially between the aorta and the oesophagus forming a left retro-oesophageal recess (**A**).

2. On the right side of the inferior mediastinum, in some individuals, the pleura dips medially, both in front of and behind the azygos vein, so that the vessel lies in the free margin of a short mesentery and is separated from the oesophagus by a right retro-oesophageal recess (**A**). When deep retro-oesophageal recesses are present on both sides they almost meet each other across the posterior aspect of the middle part of the oesophagus.

3. Anteriorly, each layer of mediastinal pleura is insinuated medially, between the anterior aspect of the mediastinum and the chest wall, forming the right and left costomediastinal pleural recesses (**A, B, C**). Behind the manubrium sterni, both recesses reach an oblique line which runs from the lateral angle of that bone to the centre of the manubriosternal joint (**B**). Below that level, the right recess extends to the midline as far as the xiphisternal joint, whereas, although the left recess also reaches the midline as far as the level of the fourth costal cartilage, it then diverges to the left and descends deep to the left margin of the body of the sternum as far as the sixth costal cartilage (**B**).

Note the mediastinal structures, particularly the upper part of the thymus and the lower part of the pericardium, which are situated between the two costomediastinal pleural recesses and are consequently in direct relationship to the sternum (**C**).

THE STRUCTURE OF THE HEART

As has been seen, the outer surface of the heart is intimately covered by the visceral layer of the serous pericardium. That layer, together with a variable amount of fat which lies deep to it, constitute the epicardium.

The greater part of the thickness of the walls of the heart chambers is formed by cardiac muscle fibres which constitute the myocardium. However, the myocardium of the ventricles is discontinuous with that of the atria and with the muscle in the walls of the aorta and pulmonary trunk. The separation is effected by a continuous zone of fibrous tissue which surrounds and connects the orifices between the atria and ventricles, and between the ventricles and the great arteries, and is known as the fibrous skeleton of the heart. In contrast, there is no such abrupt fibrous discontinuity between the walls of the atria and the walls of the veins which enter those chambers.

The interior of all the heart chambers is lined by smooth endothelium which is continuous with that of the arteries and veins. In the heart it is known as the endocardium.

The fibrous skeleton of the heart

The right and left atrioventricular (AV) orifices, by which the atria communicate with the ventricles, are equipped with endocardial valves which determine the direction of blood flow between the chambers. The valves are attached to thick fibrous rings interposed between the atrial and ventricular musculature. The rings lie approximately in vertical planes both of which are at right angles to the cardiac axis (**D, E**). The right ring is a little larger and extends a little lower than the left and its plane is somewhat farther forwards in reference to the cardiac axis. The adjacent parts of the two rings are joined by a broad zone of fibrous tissue which is interposed between the interatrial and interventricular septa (**D, E**). The outer margin of the rings, and their connecting fibrous zone, form the floor of the coronary sulcus which demarcates ventricles from atria on the outer surface of the heart.

The orifices, through which the left and right ventricles open into the aorta and pulmonary trunk respectively, are also equipped with valves attached to fibrous rings. The aortic ring lies above and in front of the AV rings and faces upwards and somewhat forwards and to the right (**E**). Its posterior margin is continuous with the fibrous zone which has been seen to join the two AV rings. The pulmonary ring lies anterior to, and at an appreciably higher level than, the aortic ring in a plane which faces upwards and somewhat backwards and to the left (**E**). It is connected to the aortic ring by a narrow strip of fibrous tissue called, for reasons which will be evident later, the tendon of the infundibulum.

The four orifices can thus be regarded as apertures in a bent plate of fibrous tissue of which the lower part is approximately vertical and the upper part approximately horizontal (**F**).

MEDIASTINUM: HORIZONTAL SECTION AT LEVEL OF T 5

Costomediastinal pleural recesses

Fibrous pericardium

Pulmonary trunk & arteries

Ascending aorta

SVC

Root of lung

Root of lung

Left retro-oesophageal recess

Oesophagus

Right retro-oesophageal recess

Descending aorta

T 5

Azygos vein

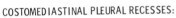

(A)

COSTOMEDIASTINAL PLEURAL RECESSES:
RELATION TO STERNUM & COSTAL CARTILAGES

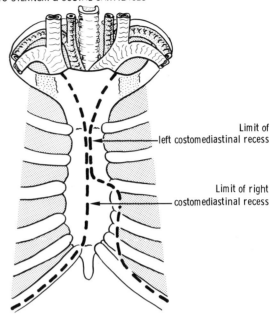

Limit of left costomediastinal recess

Limit of right costomediastinal recess

(B)

COSTOMEDIASTINAL PLEURAL RECESSES:
RELATION TO MEDIASTINAL STRUCTURES

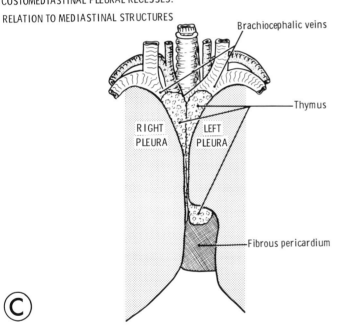

Brachiocephalic veins

Thymus

RIGHT PLEURA

LEFT PLEURA

Fibrous pericardium

(C)

VENTRICULAR PART OF HEART: VIEWED FROM BEHIND
AFTER REMOVAL OF ATRIA & GREAT VESSELS

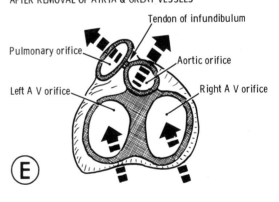

Tendon of infundibulum

Pulmonary orifice

Aortic orifice

Left A V orifice

Right A V orifice

(E)

TRANSVERSE SECTION OF HEART: FIBROUS ZONES IN BLACK

Right atrioventricular ring

Fibrous zone connecting A V rings

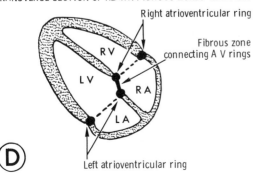

RV

LV

RA

LA

Left atrioventricular ring

(D)

FIBROUS SKELETON OF HEART: DIAGRAMMATIC CONCEPT

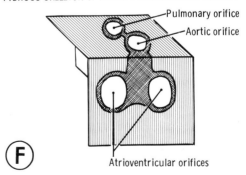

Pulmonary orifice

Aortic orifice

Atrioventricular orifices

(F)

161

General features of the heart valves

The two atrioventricular (AV) valves each consist of a number of endocardial folds, known as cusps, which protrude into the cardiac lumen from the corresponding AV fibrous ring. They permit blood flow from atria to ventricles and prevent flow in the opposite direction. The atrial aspect of each cusp is smooth and featureless. On the other hand the cusp margin and, in most cusps, the ventricular surface also give attachment to fine tendons, the chordae tendineae, which arise from the apices of papillary muscles. The latter are conical masses of cardiac muscle which are continuous at their bases with the muscular walls of the ventricles (**A, B**).

When the atrial pressure exceeds that of the ventricle, the cusps separate so that the AV orifice becomes patent (**A**). When the ventricular pressure is the greater, the marginal parts of the atrial surfaces of the cusps come into apposition, closing the orifice, and are held in that position by contraction of the papillary muscles and the resultant tension in the chordae tendineae (**B**).

The aortic and pulmonary valves each consist of three cup-shaped endocardial cusps which are markedly concave towards the lumen of the corresponding artery (**A**). Each cusp is strengthened by fibrous tissue between the endocardial layers, which thickens the centre of the free margin forming the nodule and radiates from that region to the attached margin (**C**). Crescentic areas abutting on the free margin on either side of the nodule contain little fibrous tissue. They are consequently more translucent than the rest of the cusp and are called lunules.

Immediately above each cusp, as has been noted already, (**150**) the corresponding artery exhibits a dilatation or sinus.

When the ventricular pressure exceeds the arterial, the cusps are pushed upwards into the sinuses and the orifice becomes patent, allowing passage of blood from ventricle to artery (**B**). When the pressure difference is in the opposite direction the orifice is closed by the cusps coming into apposition (**A**). Displacement of the cusps beyond this position into the ventricles is pevented by the rigidity conferred by their cup-shaped form.

Observe the number, position and names of the cusps of each of the four heart valves (**D**). Note that the terms anterior and inferior, which are applied to two of the cusps of the tricuspid valve, refer to their relationships to the anterior (sternocostal) and inferior (diaphragmatic) surfaces of the heart and not to their relationship to each other.

The cardiac cycle

Each cardiac cycle involves successive periods of contraction (systole) and relaxation (diastole) of the cardiac muscle. Normally the two atria operate simultaneously, and the two ventricles also operate in phase, but a little later than the atria.

During ventricular systole the rising pressures in those chambers first close the AV valves. Soon afterwards the interventricular pressures reach sufficient levels to open the aortic and pulmonary valves, and the ventricles empty their blood into the arteries, the pulse expanding the elastic arterial walls (**B**). Meanwhile the atria are in diastole and are passively filling with blood flowing into them from the veins.

As the ventricles pass into diastole, their internal pressures fall sharply, and the elastic recoil of the arterial walls forces blood back towards the ventricles and closes the aortic and pulmonary valves (**A**). As ventricular diastole continues the atria are also still in diastole. But blood from the full atria opens the AV valves, and passes through the patent AV orifices into the ventricles. When the greater part of the atrial contents has passed passively into the ventricles in this way, the transfer is completed and the ventricles are fully filled by a short atrial systole. Atrial systole is followed after a short interval (**170**) by ventricular systole and the cycle is repeated.

When the heart is examined by means of a stethoscope (auscultation) two heart sounds are heard in each cardiac cycle. Traditionally the softer first sound is expressed verbally as 'lubb' and the more highly pitched and staccato second sound as 'dup'. In large measure the first sound reflects the closure of the AV valves at the beginning of ventricular systole while the second sound is caused by the closure of the aortic and pulmonary valves by arterial rebound at the end of ventricular systole.

HEART VALVES IN VENTRICULAR DIASTOLE:
ARROWS INDICATE PRESSURE GRADIENTS

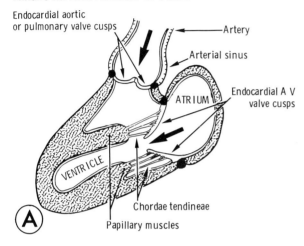

Endocardial aortic
or pulmonary valve cusps

Artery

Arterial sinus

Endocardial A V
valve cusps

ATRIUM

VENTRICLE

Chordae tendineae

Papillary muscles

A

HEART VALVES IN VENTRICULAR SYSTOLE:
ARROWS INDICATE PRESSURE GRADIENTS

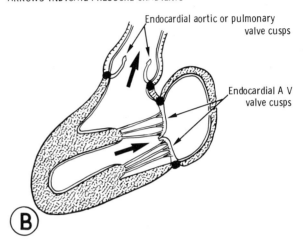

Endocardial aortic or pulmonary
valve cusps

Endocardial A V
valve cusps

B

VALVE OF GREAT ARTERY

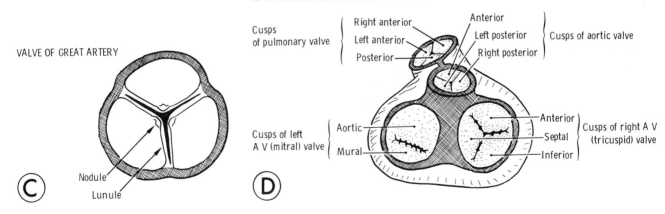

Nodule

Lunule

C

HEART VALVES FROM BEHIND: ATRIA & GREAT ARTERIES REMOVED

Cusps
of pulmonary valve
{
Right anterior
Left anterior
Posterior
}

Anterior
Left posterior
Right posterior
}
Cusps of aortic valve

Cusps of left
A V (mitral) valve
{
Aortic
Mural
}

Anterior
Septal
Inferior
}
Cusps of right A V
(tricuspid) valve

D

The interior of the heart chambers

The left atrium

The left atrium is smaller, shorter from before backwards, and situated at a higher level than the right atrium (**A, C**). From its upper left corner a small ear-like diverticulum, the auricle, curls forwards round the left side of the pulmonary trunk (**149B**). In the auricle the muscle bundles raise the endocardium into interlacing ridges, but in the main chamber the inner aspects of the walls are smooth. Posterior, left anterior and right anterior or septal walls can be recognised (**A**). In the upper part of the posterior wall are the four valveless orifices of the pulmonary veins, two coming from each lung (**C, D, 149C**). The lower part of the left anterior wall is occupied by the left AV orifice (**D**), while the upper part extends upwards behind the pulmonary trunk and aorta. The septal wall is flat. In some specimens, it exhibits a faint curved ridge, concave upwards, surrounding a shallow semilunar depression. These features are to be correlated with corresponding features which will be noted on the septal wall of the right atrium.

The left ventricle

The left ventricle extends from the left AV orifice, forwards, downwards, and to the left to the apex of the heart (**A, D**). Because the peripheral resistance offered by the systemic circulation is considerably greater than that of the pulmonary circulation, its wall is some three times as thick as that of the right ventricle (**A, B**). The thickness of the interventricular septum corresponds to that of the other left ventricular walls. It bulges markedly towards the right and consequently the lumen of the left ventricle is approximately circular in cross section (**B**). The cavity is roughly conical, with the left AV orifice occupying its base and the aortic orifice lying in the most posterior parts of its anterosuperior wall (**D**). The inner aspect of the greater part of the rest of the wall exhibits a complex of interlacing, endocardium-covered muscular bundles called the trabeculae carneae. Some of these are simple ridges on the ventricular wall, others are attached to the wall at either end but free between, while still others, called papillary muscles, are conical and have a basal attachment to the ventricular wall and a free apex from which chordae tendineae pass to the left AV valve cusps. Only the papillary muscles are shown in (**D**). In the left ventricle there are two of these papillary muscles, an anterior on the sternocostal wall and an inferior on the diaphragmatic wall (**D**).

The left atrioventricular (mitral) valve

The left atrioventricular or mitral valve consists of cusps of unequal size which are usually continuous peripherally (**D, 163D**). The longer aortic cusp, which is about 17 mm long, is attached to the AV fibrous ring above and to the right, close to the attachment of the left posterior cusp of the aortic valve. The smaller mural cusp is about 11 mm long and arises from the lower and left parts of the AV ring (**D, 163D**). Chordae tendineae from each papillary muscle in the left ventricle are attached to both cusps. The tendinous attachments to the mural cusp are placed on both its margin and its ventricular surface. In contrast, because blood has to flow over the ventricular surface of the aortic cusp as it passes from the ventricle to the aorta, the tendinous attachments to this cusp are restricted to its margin alone (**D**). In the normal heart the mitral valve will admit the tips of two fingers.

The aortic valve

The aortic valve consists of right posterior, left posterior, and anterior cusps (**D, 163D**). The aortic sinuses lie immediately above them in corresponding positions. In conformity with the high pressure which they withstand during aortic reflux, the aortic cusps are thicker and stronger than those of the pulmonary valve.

The right atrium

The right atrium lies to the right and in front of the left atrium and at a lower level (**A, C**). It has septal and left anterior walls, while the rest of the wall forms a continuous curve round the anterior, right and posterior aspects of the chamber (**A**). From its upper part, above the right AV orifice, an auricle, similar in form to that of the left atrium, curls forwards and to the left round the root of the aorta (**149B**).

The inner surface of the right wall of the atrium is marked by a ridge called the crista terminalis (**167B**). This ends, above, in the interval between the superior vena caval orifice and the auricle, and below, to the right and a little in front of the inferior vena cava. Behind this ridge the endocardium is smooth, but in front of it the lining membrane is raised into parallel ridges by muscle bundles called the musculi pectinati, which run forwards towards the right and upper aspects of the right AV orifice and into the auricle. These two morphologically different parts of the chamber reflect its development from two originally distinct chambers of the embryonic heart. The smooth region develops from the sinus venosus. It is often described in the adult as the sinus venarum and the ridged part which develops from the embryonic atrium as the right atrium proper.

TRANSVERSE SECTION ALONG CARDIAC AXIS

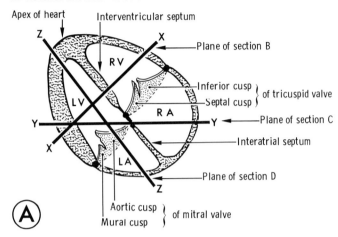

Apex of heart
Interventricular septum
Z
X
RV
Plane of section B
Inferior cusp } of tricuspid valve
Septal cusp
LV
RA
Plane of section C
Y
Y
Interatrial septum
X
LA
Plane of section D
Z
Aortic cusp } of mitral valve
Mural cusp

(A)

VERTICAL SECTION ALONG PLANE X-X SHOWN IN A

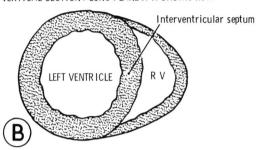

Interventricular septum
LEFT VENTRICLE
RV

(B)

CORONAL SECTION ALONG PLANE Y-Y SHOWN IN A:
SEEN FROM IN FRONT

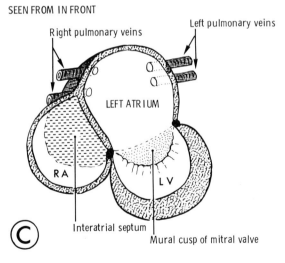

Right pulmonary veins
Left pulmonary veins
LEFT ATRIUM
RA
LV
(C)
Interatrial septum
Mural cusp of mitral valve

VERTICAL SECTION ALONG PLANE Z-Z SHOWN IN A:
SEEN FROM RIGHT

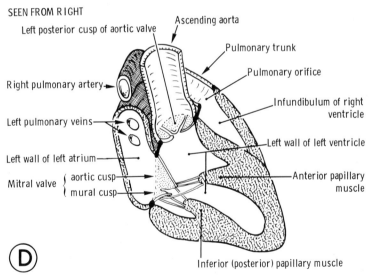

Left posterior cusp of aortic valve
Ascending aorta
Pulmonary trunk
Right pulmonary artery
Pulmonary orifice
Infundibulum of right ventricle
Left pulmonary veins
Left wall of left atrium
Left wall of left ventricle
Mitral valve { aortic cusp
mural cusp
Anterior papillary muscle
(D)
Inferior (posterior) papillary muscle

165

All but the uppermost part of the left anterior wall of the atrium is occupied by the right AV orifice and valve (see below).

The septal wall (**C**) is smooth. In its lower part an oval depression, the fossa ovalis, is bounded above, in front and behind by a prominent margin, the limbus fossae ovalis. The faint markings on the left aspect of the interatrial septum which correspond to these features have been noted above. The floor of the fossa is thin and in some individuals there is a valvular slit-like opening between its upper margin and the left aspect of the upper part of the limbus (**D**).

Because after birth the pressure in the left atrium is normally somewhat higher than in the right, such a valve-like opening does not allow passage of blood between the two atria unless some other cardiac or vascular abnormality causes a rise in pressure in the right atrium.

Three large veins open into the sinus venarum portion of the atrium. The opening of the superior vena cava is in the upper posterior part and has no valve (**B, C**). The inferior vena cava opens into the posterior part of the floor of the chamber, some distance behind the AV orifice (**B, C**). From the anterior margin of the opening a single crescentic endocardial cusp extends upwards as the valve of the inferior vena cava. The left end of the cusp (**C**) is attached to the anterior limb of the limbus fossae ovalis while the right end (**B**) runs into the lower extremity of the crista terminalis. After birth the valve is functionless and is indeed often fenestrated. The coronary sinus carries most of the venous blood from the heart, though several small additional veins do open into the atrium independently (**175B**). Its opening (**C**) lies in the angle between the septal wall, the right anterior wall and the floor of the atrium, and therefore between the limbus fossae ovalis and the valve of the inferior vena cava behind and the right AV orifice in front. It is associated with a single valve cusp arising from its lower margin which is probably non-functional.

The right ventricle

The right ventricle, in comparison to the left, has a thinner wall, its lumen is crescentic in cross section (**165B**) and it is shorter, so that its anterior end does not reach the apex of the heart (**A**).

In longitudinal section it is distinctly U-shaped in form (**C**). The lower or inflow limb extends back to the right AV orifice, and its upper or outflow limb, which is known as the infundibulum because of its somewhat conical form, leads upwards and backwards to the pulmonary orifice. The two parts are separated by a thick and prominent zone of muscle, the supraventricular crest, which is interposed between the right AV and pulmonary orifices to the right of the aortic orifice (**C**).

The infundibulum differs in its development from the rest of the ventricle and can be regarded as a conical muscular pouch passing upwards from the main ventricular cavity. It rises above the level of the left ventricle and aortic valve, so that its upper part lies in front and to the left of the initial part of the ascending aorta, and the interventricular septum does not contribute to its wall (**E**).

The walls of the main part of the chamber exhibit trabeculae carneae similar to those already noted in the left ventricle. There are two papillary muscles, an anterior on the sternocostal wall and an inferior on the diaphragmatic wall (**B**). One thick muscular band is attached to the septal wall and extends freely across the cavity to the base of the anterior papillary muscle (**A**). It is now called the septomarginal trabecula but its previous name, which is sometimes still used, was the moderator band. In contrast to the main part of the ventricle the walls of the infundibulum are smooth.

The right atrioventricular (tricuspid) valve

The right atrioventricular or tricuspid valve consists of three endocardial cusps, the peripheral parts of which tend to be continuous. The cusps arise from the upper right, lower right and medial parts of the fibrous ring surrounding the orifice and are called anterior, inferior and septal respectively (**163D**). Their atrial surfaces are smooth but their free margins and ventricular aspects give attachment to chordae tendineae (**B**). Each cusp is usually associated with tendons from both of the papillary muscles of the right ventricle.

The pulmonary valve

The pulmonary valve has three cusps, right anterior, left anterior and posterior. Above each cusp the wall of the pulmonary trunk presents a dilatation or sinus (**C, E, 163D**).

The interventricular septum

The septum lies mainly between the left ventricle and the main part of the right ventricle. It is muscular, apart from the small region described below. As has been noted already, its width is similar to that of the wall of the left ventricle and it bulges towards the right making the cavities of the left and right ventricles circular and crescentic respectively in cross section (**165B**).

TRANSVERSE SECTION ALONG CARDIAC AXIS

Septomarginal trabecula

Anterior papillary muscle of right ventricle

Plane of section E

X

Y —————— Y

LV

RA

LA

X

Plane of sections B & C

(A)

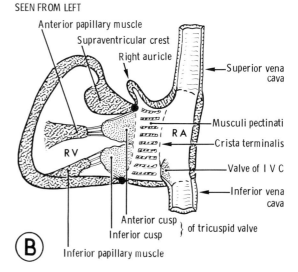

VERTICAL SECTION ALONG PLANE X-X SHOWN IN A: SEEN FROM LEFT

Anterior papillary muscle

Supraventricular crest

Right auricle

Superior vena cava

Musculi pectinati

Crista terminalis

Valve of I V C

Inferior vena cava

RV

RA

Anterior cusp
Inferior cusp } of tricuspid valve

Inferior papillary muscle

(B)

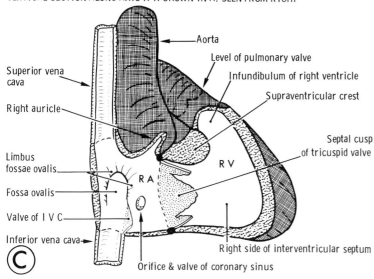

VERTICAL SECTION ALONG AXIS X-X SHOWN IN A: SEEN FROM RIGHT

Aorta

Level of pulmonary valve

Infundibulum of right ventricle

Supraventricular crest

Superior vena cava

Right auricle

Limbus fossae ovalis

Fossa ovalis

Valve of I V C

Inferior vena cava

Septal cusp of tricuspid valve

RA

RV

Right side of interventricular septum

Orifice & valve of coronary sinus

(C)

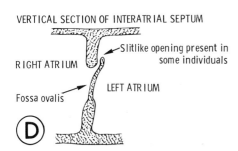

VERTICAL SECTION OF INTERATRIAL SEPTUM

RIGHT ATRIUM

Slitlike opening present in some individuals

LEFT ATRIUM

Fossa ovalis

(D)

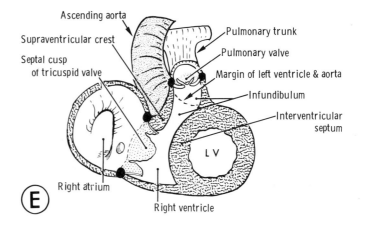

CORONAL SECTION OF HEART ALONG PLANE Y-Y SHOWN IN A: SEEN FROM IN FRONT

Ascending aorta

Pulmonary trunk

Supraventricular crest

Pulmonary valve

Septal cusp of tricuspid valve

Margin of left ventricle & aorta

Infundibulum

Interventricular septum

LV

Right atrium

Right ventricle

(E)

One small oval region, known as the membranous part of the septum, is thin and translucent and consists solely of fibrous tissue between two layers of endocardium (**A**). Seen from the left ventricle this part lies in the angle between the aortic and mitral orifices (**B**). Seen from the right side of the heart (**C**) it lies just below the supraventricular crest and, because the right AV ring lies a little anterior to the left (**A**), it is crossed about its centre by the attached margin of the septal cusp of the tricuspid valve (**A, C**). Consequently, the anterior half of the membranous part of the septum is truly interventricular, whereas the posterior half is situated in the anterior part of the septal wall of the right atrium and separates that cavity from the left ventricle (**A**). Indeed, it is sometimes called the atrioventricular part of the septum. Occasionally the membranous part of the septum is congenitally deficient. Because of the pressure differences, blood is then shunted from the high pressure left ventricle into the low pressure right heart chambers and so into the pulmonary circulation. The rest of the muscular interventricular septum is separated from the muscular interatrial septum by that part of the fibrous skeleton of the heart which joins the fibrous rings of the right and left AV orifices (**161F**).

The conducting system of the heart

This system consists of a number of zones and tracts of specialised cardiac muscle fibres. It initiates the contractions of the atrial muscle fibres (atrial systole) and, because part of the system passes through the fibrous skeleton which separates the ordinary muscle fibres of the atria and ventricles, it allows the spread of impulses from the contracting atrial muscle to the ventricular muscle, where they produce ventricular systole.

The sinuatrial (SA) node lies in the right wall of the sinus venarum part of the right atrium (**D**). It is about 10 mm long and extends downwards and to the right from the anterior aspect of the superior vena caval orifice along the posterior margin of the upper part of the crista terminalis. Because of the fundamental importance of the node to the function of the heart this region is avoided in heart surgery. The node consists of a network of fibres which have many of the histological features of ordinary cardiac muscle fibres but are much narrower. At the periphery of the node these nodal fibres become directly continuous with adjacent ordinary atrial muscle fibres. Numerous nerve cells lie around the node and many non-myelinated nerve fibres penetrate into its substance though they lack specialised endings in association with the nodal fibres.

The fibres of the sinuatrial node are characterised by the property of spontaneous alternate contraction and re-laxation. The frequency of the cycle can be slowed by vagal stimulation and increased by sympathetic stimulation. With each depolarisation of the nodal fibres, electrical activity spreads through the atrial muscle fibres which are continuous with them, to all the atrial muscle. The atria consequently normally beat with the rhythm dictated by the SA node. And because, as will be seen below, the atria in turn impose their rhythm on the ventricles, the SA node is often known as the cardiac pacemaker.

The atrioventricular (AV) node lies in the muscular wall of the anterior part of the interatrial septum, between the orifice of the coronary sinus below and the membranous part of the interventricular septum above (**B, C**). Its structure is similar to that of the SA node, though its fibres are somewhat larger, and like the SA node, it is surrounded by nerve cells. The nodal fibres form an intricate meshwork, and are continuous in one direction with the atrial muscle fibres and in the other with the conducting tissue of the atrioventricular (AV) bundle.

The atrioventricular (AV) bundle (**B, C**), often alternatively known as the bundle of His, is composed of fibres similar to those of the AV node but orientated parallel to one another. It extends upwards and forwards from the AV node, through the fibrous tissue between the two AV rings (**161D**), to the lower margin of the membranous part of the interventricular septum. In the anterior part of this membranous area it divides into right and left bundle branches, which exhibit the same structure as the main bundle and straddle the adjacent margin of the muscular part of the septum.

The left bundle branch (**B**) usually takes the form of a broad band or a number of parallel fasciculi, and runs downwards and forwards along the left aspect of the muscular interventricular septum, beneath the endo-cardium, to reach the bases of the two papillary muscles.

The right bundle branch (**C**) is more compact and rounded. It runs subendocardially along the right side of the interventricular septum and thereafter along the septomarginal trabecula (**167A**) to the base of the anterior papillary muscle.

The Purkinje fibres form plexuses of conducting tissue which arise from the terminations of the bundle branches in both ventricles, and ramify into all parts of the ventricular myocardium, to end by becoming continuous with the ventricular muscle fibres. The fibres consist of Purkinje cells orientated parallel to one another. These cells are much larger than cardiac muscle cells and contain comparatively few myofibrils.

The continuous conducting tissue of the AV bundle, the two bundle branches and the Purkinje fibres are separated and insulated, except at their terminations, from the adjacent cardiac muscle by a thin fibrous sheath.

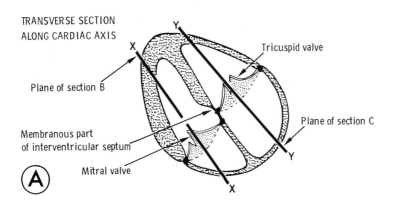

TRANSVERSE SECTION
ALONG CARDIAC AXIS

Tricuspid valve

Plane of section B

Plane of section C

Membranous part
of interventricular septum

Mitral valve

(A)

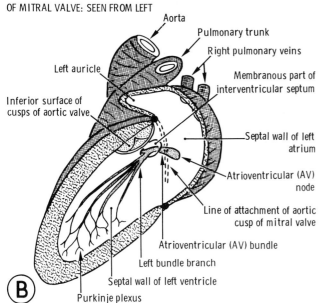

VERTICAL SECTION ALONG PLANE X-X SHOWN IN A AFTER REMOVAL
OF MITRAL VALVE: SEEN FROM LEFT

Aorta

Pulmonary trunk

Right pulmonary veins

Left auricle

Membranous part of
interventricular septum

Inferior surface of
cusps of aortic valve

Septal wall of left
atrium

Atrioventricular (AV)
node

Line of attachment of aortic
cusp of mitral valve

Atrioventricular (AV) bundle

Left bundle branch

Septal wall of left ventricle

Purkinje plexus

(B)

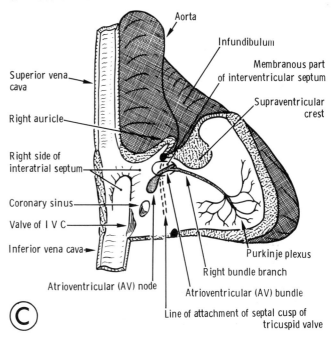

VERTICAL SECTION ALONG PLANE Y-Y SHOWN IN A AFTER REMOVAL
OF TRICUSPID VALVE: SEEN FROM RIGHT

Aorta

Infundibulum

Membranous part
of interventricular septum

Superior vena
cava

Supraventricular
crest

Right auricle

Right side of
interatrial septum

Coronary sinus

Valve of I V C

Inferior vena cava

Purkinje plexus

Right bundle branch

Atrioventricular (AV) node

Atrioventricular (AV) bundle

Line of attachment of septal cusp of
tricuspid valve

(C)

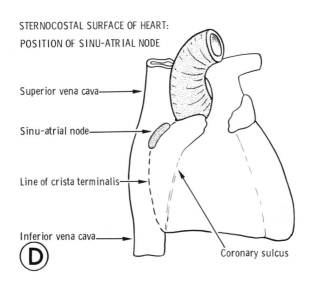

STERNOCOSTAL SURFACE OF HEART:
POSITION OF SINU-ATRIAL NODE

Superior vena cava

Sinu-atrial node

Line of crista terminalis

Inferior vena cava

Coronary sulcus

(D)

169

The function of the AV conducting tissue is to transmit electrical impulses from the atrial muscle with which it is continuous at its atrial end, to the ventricular muscle with which it is continuous anteriorly, thereby producing ventricular contraction. It will be evident that, because the impulses for ventricular contraction are derived in this way from atrial contraction, and atrial contraction is initiated by the rhythmic activity of the fibres of the SA node, both atria and ventricles beat at the same frequency, which is dictated by the SA node. But because atrial and ventricular muscle are separated by the cardiac fibrous skeleton, there is a delay between atrial and ventricular contractions of some 0.2 s, which is equal to the transmission time through the AV conducting tissue. This interval is functionally important because it provides sufficient time for atrial systole to complete the filling of the relaxed ventricles before ventricular systole ensues (**162**).

Electrocardiography

The electrical changes occurring in the myocardium during each cardiac cycle are conducted through the body fluids to the body surface, and can be recorded through strategically placed surface electrodes. Such a recording is known as an electrocardiogram and normally consists of a regular repetition of a number of waves and peaks (**A**). The P wave represents atrial systole, the QRS complex the slightly asynchronous contractions of different parts of the ventricles, while the T wave is caused by repolarisation of the ventricular muscle. The duration of the P–R interval is a measure of the time taken for the impulse to pass over the atria and along the AV conducting tissue. The interval between the end of the S wave and the beginning of the T wave corresponds closely to the period of maximal ejection during ventricular systole.

Heart block

Heart block is a group of conditions in which changes in the cardiac cycle result from defective conduction, or failure of conduction, in some part of the conducting system of the heart.

Although the abnormality may occasionally occur in the SA node, it is more usually associated with the AV conducting tissue.

Surface marking of the heart and great vessels

The projections on the anterior chest wall of the heart and its valvular orifices, and those of the great vessels, should be studied in **B**. Percussion of the chest wall indicates an area of dullness produced by the presence of the heart and vessels, but, because of the considerable overlap by the anterior margins of the lungs (**149F**), the correspondence between the area of dullness and the surface projection is not usually very close. The size and position of the heart and great vessels are better assessed by radiological techniques (**176**).

It should also be noted that, although it is helpful to know the relative positions of the cardiac valves as shown by their surface projections (**B**), in auscultation, using a stethoscope, the heart sounds produced by closure of the valves (**162**) are not heard most clearly in these positions. The sounds tends to be conducted distal to each valve in relation to the blood flow, and thus tend to be best heard where the chamber or vessel distal to the valve is closest to the chest wall. The regions of maximum intensity for each valve sound are shown by asterisks in **B**.

Valvular defects

The heart valves may exhibit congenital deformities or be affected by disease processes during life. In these circumstances a valve may be unable to open to its normal extent (stenosis) so that there is obstruction to the onward flow of blood. Alternatively, it may be unable to close efficiently so that blood leaks back into a chamber after it has been ejected by contraction of that chamber (incompetence). In each case, strain is placed primarily on the chamber proximal to the abnormal valve, for example the left atrium in the case of mitral stenosis or incompetence and the right ventricle in cases of abnormalities of the pulmonary valve.

The abnormal blood flow through a stenosed or incompetent valve produces a sound, known as a murmur, which can be heard during auscultation, and the nature and situation of the defect may be diagnosed by noting the position of maximum intensity of the murmur and its relation in time to the two normal sounds of the cardiac cycle. Thus in aortic stenosis the murmur is heard maximally over the second right sternocostal joint (aortic valve area) and occurs between the two normal heart sounds, that is during ventricular systole.

The arterial supply to the heart

The heart receives its blood supply through the right and left coronary arteries, of which the left is usually the larger. These arteries are branches of the ascending aorta arising from the upper parts of, or even slightly above, the anterior and left posterior aortic sinuses. The positions of their origins precludes their occlusion by the cusps of the aortic valve during ventricular systole. The main branches of the arteries run on the outer surface of the heart immediately deep to the visceral pericardium. The fine terminal branches of the two arteries anastomose in the myocardium to a considerable extent. In general, it appears that if occlusion occurs gradually in one of the smaller arterial branches, this anastomosis may be sufficient to maintain an

ELECTROCARDIOGRAM: BIPOLAR LIMB LEADS

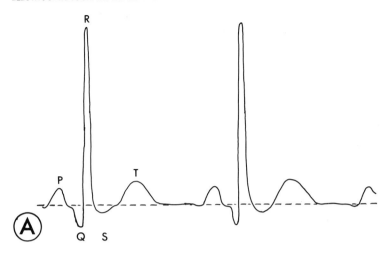

PROJECTION OF HEART, HEART VALVES & GREAT VESSELS ON THE ANTERIOR CHEST WALL
(T, tricuspid: M, mitral: A, aortic: P, pulmonary)

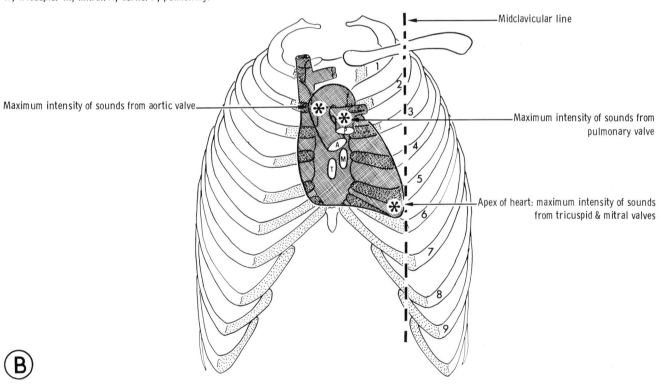

adequate blood supply to the affected area of myocardium. But if the obstruction occurs suddenly, or affects a major branch, the anastomosis is usually insufficient to support the infarcted tissue and the tissue dies.

The left coronary artery

This vessel arises from the left posterior aortic sinus, passes to the left between the pulmonary trunk and the left atrium and curls forwards to appear between the trunk and the left auricle, where it divides into two branches.

The anterior interventricular branch passes forwards and downwards along the anterior interventricular groove on the sternocostal surface of the heart (**A**). Usually it then turns onto the diaphragmatic surface, just to the right of the apex, and runs back for a variable distance along the inferior (posterior) interventricular groove (**B**). It gives branches to both ventricles and the interventricular septum.

The circumflex branch is smaller and passes downwards along the left part of the coronary sulcus (**A**, **B**) and usually ends before the junction of that sulcus with the inferior interventricular groove (see below). It supplies branches to the left atrium and ventricle.

The right coronary artery

Whereas the left coronary artery is only about 3 cm long before it divides into two terminal branches, the individual part of the right coronary is much longer (**A**). Running forwards from its origin from the anterior aortic sinus, it enters the coronary sulcus behind the tip of the right auricle and thereafter continues along the right part of the sulcus to the inferior margin of the sternocostal surface of the heart, supplying branches to the right atrium and ventricle. The vessel then turns to the left into the inferior part of the coronary sulcus (**B**) and ends by anastomosing with the circumflex branch of the left coronary. In its course it gives off two major branches.

The marginal branch runs forwards along the inferior margin of the sternocostal surface, supplying the right ventricle (**A**).

The inferior (posterior) interventricular branch arises at the junction of the coronary sulcus and the inferior interventricular groove (**B**). A variable distance along the groove it ends by anastomosing with the anterior interventricular branch of the left coronary.

The blood supply of the conducting tissue

The SA node may be supplied from the right or left coronary arteries or from both (**A**). The branch from the right coronary arises close to its origin and passes backwards between the aorta and the right auricle to the roof of the right atrium at its junction with the superior vena cava. That from the left coronary usually arises from the early part of its circumflex branch. It passes behind the pulmonary trunk and aorta to reach the right atrium.

The artery to the AV node usually arises from the right coronary artery while that vessel lies in the inferior part of the coronary sulcus close to the origin of its inferior interventricular branch. It runs upwards in the interatrial septum.

Variations of the coronary artery pattern

As with arterial supplies elsewhere in the body, the coronary arterial pattern is fairly constant amongst the population. However, variations are by no means rare and the most important, from a clinical point of view, relate to the origin of the inferior interventricular artery. Most commonly, as indicated in the above description, this vessel is a branch of the right coronary artery (**A**, **B**). This arrangement is described as right coronary artery dominance. In some individuals it is a direct continuation of the circumflex branch of the left coronary, and the right coronary terminates in the coronary sulcus before it reaches the inferior interventricular groove (**C**). This is called left coronary artery dominance. In still others, the right coronary and circumflex arteries join to form the inferior interventricular artery at the posterior end of the inferior interventricular groove (**D**). This is balanced dominance.

The venous drainage of the heart

The greater part of the heart is drained through a large vein, the coronary sinus, whose opening into the right atrium has been studied already (**167C**).

CORONARY ARTERIES: RIGHT CORONARY ARTERY DOMINANCE

(Auricles turned aside & section of pulmonary trunk removed)

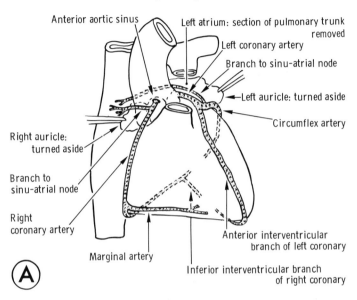

Anterior aortic sinus

Left atrium: section of pulmonary trunk removed

Left coronary artery

Branch to sinu-atrial node

Left auricle: turned aside

Circumflex artery

Right auricle: turned aside

Branch to sinu-atrial node

Right coronary artery

Marginal artery

Anterior interventricular branch of left coronary

Inferior interventricular branch of right coronary

CORONARY ARTERIES: AS IN (A) FROM BEHIND & BELOW

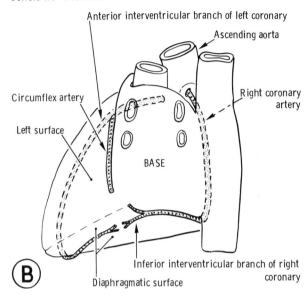

Anterior interventricular branch of left coronary

Ascending aorta

Circumflex artery

Left surface

Right coronary artery

BASE

Inferior interventricular branch of right coronary

Diaphragmatic surface

CORONARY ARTERIES: LEFT CORONARY ARTERY DOMINANCE (Compare with A)

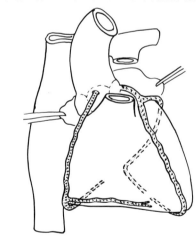

CORONARY ARTERIES: BALANCED DOMINANCE (Compare with A)

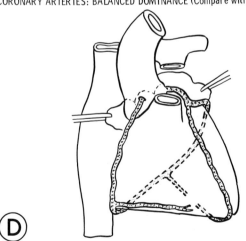

The sinus begins as a continuation of the great cardiac vein, which runs upwards alongside the anterior interventricular branch of the left coronary artery in the anterior interventricular groove (**B**). Turning to the left it descends in the left part of the coronary sulcus to its junction with the inferior interventricular groove (**A**) and thereafter runs upwards for a short distance in the interatrial septum to open into the right atrium (**167C**). It receives a number of large veins from the left aspect of the left ventricle (**A**) and is joined near its termination by the middle and small cardiac veins (**A**). The former runs backwards in the inferior interventricular groove while the latter, having received tributaries from the right ventricle and the marginal vein (**B**), runs to the left in the inferior part of the coronary sulcus (**A**).

The most important of the veins which do not join the coronary sinus are several small vessels which run backwards across the sternocostal surface of the right ventricle and open directly into the right atrium (**B**).

The foetal circulation

In the foetus very little blood passes through the pulmonary vessels and the foetal blood is oxygenated in the placenta and not in the lungs. Consequently, the circulation as a whole differs in a number of ways from that which occurs after birth.

Observe the following features of the prenatal heart and vessels.

1. Note the system of large veins associated with the liver (**C**). The inferior vena cava, carrying deoxygenated blood from the abdomen and lower limbs, passes upwards across the posterior surface of the liver and receives hepatic veins draining the system of sinusoids within that viscus. The portal vein, carrying deoxygenated blood from the gastro-intestinal tract, divides on the inferior surface of the liver into right and left branches. The blood in the right branch passes through liver sinusoids and hepatic veins to the inferior vena cava. Some of that in the left branch follows a similar route, but the rest passes directly to the inferior vena cava through a wide bypass channel on the posterior surface of the liver called the ductus venosus. The single, large umbilical vein, present throughout the later stages of prenatal development, passes from the placenta to the umbilicus in the umbilical cord. Thereafter it passes upwards in the abdominal cavity to the inferior surface of the liver, where it joins the left branch of the portal vein opposite the attachment of the ductus venosus.

2. Before birth the interatrial septum contains an oblique opening, the foramen ovale (**C**). It lies between the floor of the fossa ovalis (the septum primum) and the left side of the limbus fossae ovalis (the septum secundum) and is consequently valvular,

allowing the passage of blood from right to left but not in the opposite direction.

3. Note in **D** the wide short vessel called the ductus arteriosus which, in prenatal life, joins the bifurcation of the pulmonary trunk to the arch of the aorta immediately beyond the origin of the left subclavian artery.

4. Observe the two umbilical arteries which arise from the internal iliac arteries (**C**). They pass upwards in the abdominal cavity to the umbilicus and traverse the umbilical cord to the placenta.

In the foetus the blood circulates along the following route.

1. Deoxygenated blood is carried from the foetus to the placenta through the umbilical arteries (**D**) and oxygenated blood is returned through the umbilical vein.

2. Most of the oxygenated blood is shunted to the inferior vena cava through the ductus venosus (**C**) while the rest passes to the vena cava through liver sinusoids.

3. Blood arriving at the right atrium through the inferior vena cava is thus a mix of oxygenated blood from the umbilical vein and deoxygenated blood from the lower part of the inferior vena cava and the portal vein.

4. This blood is directed by the valve of the inferior vena cava across the right atrium towards the foramen ovale. Because little blood is returning to the left atrium from the lungs, its pressure is low and blood consequently passes through the foramen ovale into the left atrium (**C**). Thereafter, it traverses the left AV orifice, the left ventricle and the ascending aorta to reach the aortic arch.

5. This blood is the most highly oxygenated in the foetus and although a small part of it continues into the descending aorta the greater part is distributed to the heart, through the coronary arteries, and to the head, neck and upper limbs through the branches of the aortic arch (**C**).

6. Deoxygenated blood is returned to the right atrium from these tissues via the superior vena cava and the coronary sinus (**D**) and traverses the right AV orifice, the right ventricle and the pulmonary trunk (**D**).

7. As little blood passes to the lungs before birth, most of this stream passes through the ductus arteriosus into the aortic arch where it joins with some oxygenated blood (see 5) and passes into the descending aorta for distribution to the thoracic walls, the abdomen and lower limbs. Thus the upper part of the body, including the heart, receives more highly oxygenated blood than does the lower part.

8. The circuit is completed by some of this blood passing from the regions noted in (7) into the inferior and superior venae cavae and the portal vein, while the rest returns to the placenta for reoxygenation through the umbilical arteries.

CARDIAC VEINS: FROM BEHIND & BELOW

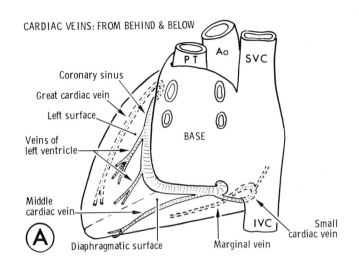

Coronary sinus
Great cardiac vein
Left surface
Veins of left ventricle
Middle cardiac vein
Diaphragmatic surface
Marginal vein
Small cardiac vein
PT
Ao
SVC
BASE
IVC

A

CARDIAC VEINS: STERNOCOSTAL ASPECT (Auricles turned aside)

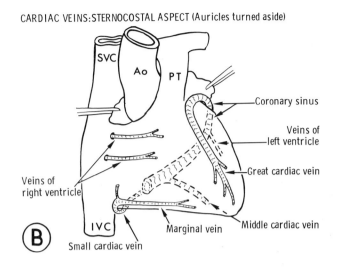

SVC
Ao
PT
Coronary sinus
Veins of left ventricle
Great cardiac vein
Middle cardiac vein
Marginal vein
Small cardiac vein
IVC
Veins of right ventricle

B

THE FOETAL CIRCULATION: I

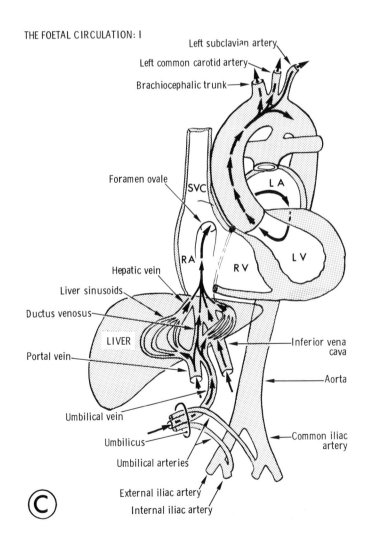

Left subclavian artery
Left common carotid artery
Brachiocephalic trunk
Foramen ovale
Hepatic vein
Liver sinusoids
Ductus venosus
Portal vein
Umbilical vein
Umbilicus
Umbilical arteries
External iliac artery
Internal iliac artery
SVC
LA
RA
RV
LV
LIVER
Inferior vena cava
Aorta
Common iliac artery

C

THE FOETAL CIRCULATION: II

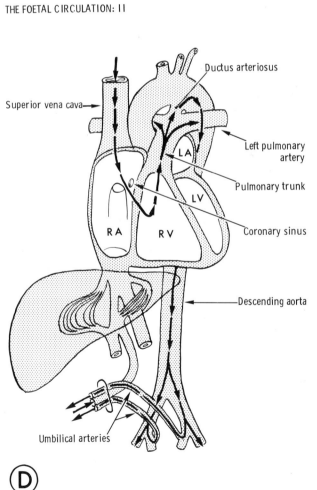

Superior vena cava
Ductus arteriosus
Left pulmonary artery
Pulmonary trunk
Coronary sinus
Descending aorta
Umbilical arteries
LA
RA
RV
LV

D

175

9. Note that, since both ventricles are pumping blood into the systemic circulation, they develop similar pressures and their walls are consequently of similar thickness. The disparity between the thickness of the ventricular walls, characteristic of the adult heart, does not begin to develop until the circulation changes at birth.

Changes in the circulation at birth

Immediately after birth, two events occur which bring about profound changes in the pattern of the circulation. These are the commencement of respiration and the ligation of the umbilical cord.

With the commencement of respiration, the vessels of the pulmonary circulation open up, so that all the blood from the right ventricle and pulmonary trunk passes to the lungs through the pulmonary arteries and returns to the left atrium through the pulmonary veins. As a result the pressure in the left atrium rises.

Ligation of the umbilical cord results in closure of the umbilical arteries, the umbilical vein, and the ductus venosus, so that the volume of blood reaching the right atrium through the inferior vena cava is reduced and the right atrial pressure falls to that in the left atrium.

As a result of the equalisation of pressures in the two atria, the valvular foramen ovale closes, first by apposition and later by fusion of the septum primum and septum secundum. Thereafter, all right atrial blood passes into the right ventricle and the pulmonary circulation.

With the establishment of the pulmonary circulation the ductus arteriosus closes. A little blood continues to pass through it for some time after birth, but in the direction from the aortic arch to the pulmonary trunk, and this flow may give rise to loud murmurs over the left chest. Complete occlusion of the ductus takes several weeks. As a result of the closure of the ductus, the blood leaving the left ventricle is no longer restricted to the ascending aorta and the aortic arch and their branches, but passes through the descending aorta to the rest of the systemic circulation.

The vessels which are closed at or soon after birth become converted into solid fibrous cords which persist throughout life. The umbilical arteries become known as the medial umbilical ligaments (**275E**), the umbilical vein as the ligamentum teres (**227A**), the ductus venosus as the ligamentum venosum (**227B**), and the ductus arteriosus as the ligamentum arteriosum (**151E**).

Two defects which may occur in the process of change from the foetal to the postnatal circulation should be noted.

A patent forament ovale may persist owing to failure of fusion of the septum primum and septum secundum. Some degree of this condition exists in over 10% of adults, and is of no significance except when some other cardiac or vascular abnormality causes the right atrial pressure to exceed that of the left.

A patent ductus arteriosus may persist. It allows diversion of aortic arch blood at higher pressure into the pulmonary circulation. This results in excessive blood flow through the lungs, left atrium and left ventricle and also increased pressure in the pulmonary artery if the pulmonary circulation fails to adapt to the increased blood flow.

Techniques of cardiac investigation

The assessment of the shape and size of the heart by percussion, the study of heart sounds and murmurs by auscultation and the investigation of electric changes in the heart by electrocardiography have all been mentioned briefly in the preceding pages.

Radiographic examination of the heart and great vessels is another common investigative procedure. Study the features of the heart which are evident in a postero-anterior view (**A**).

There are now a number of more sophisticated radiological techniques in use. For example cardiac catheterisation involves the introduction of a long narrow flexible tube into a peripheral artery or vein and its passage into one of the chambers of the heart or even into the coronary arteries.

Angiocardiography involves the injection of a contrast medium through such a cardiac catheter so that features of the heart chambers of the great vessels may be clearly visualised on subsequent radiography. Thus in **B** and **C** contrast medium has been injected through a catheter passed via a femoral vein into the right atrium. In **B** the medium is seen flowing through the right chambers of the heart and the pulmonary arteries. After flowing through the pulmonary capillaries the medium returns through the pulmonary veins into the left chambers of the heart and the aorta (**C**).

POSTERO-ANTERIOR RADIOGRAPH OF CHEST

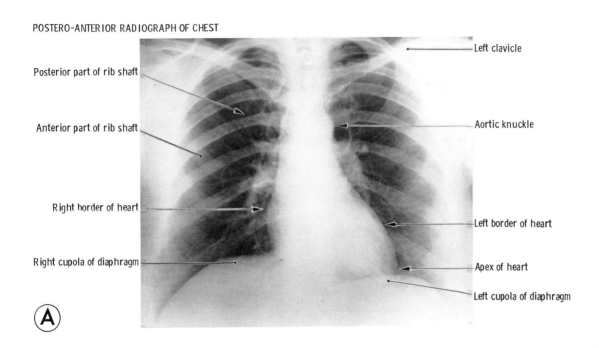

Left clavicle

Posterior part of rib shaft

Anterior part of rib shaft

Aortic knuckle

Right border of heart

Left border of heart

Right cupola of diaphragm

Apex of heart

Left cupola of diaphragm

A

ANGIOCARDIOGRAPHY

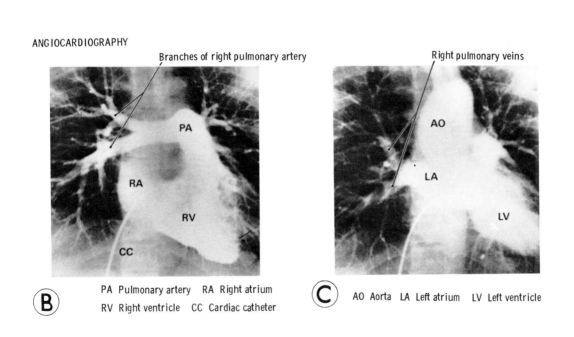

Branches of right pulmonary artery

PA

RA

RV

CC

B

PA Pulmonary artery   RA Right atrium
RV Right ventricle   CC Cardiac catheter

Right pulmonary veins

AO

LA

LV

C   AO Aorta   LA Left atrium   LV Left ventricle

177

THE LUNGS

Each lung invaginates the corresponding pleural sac from its medial side, so that it is entirely covered by visceral pleura except over a pear-shaped area, the hilus (**C, D**). Around the hilus the visceral pleura becomes continuous with the mediastinal part of the parietal pleura, the short connecting tube constituting the root of the lung in its broad upper part and the pulmonary ligament in its narrower lower part. The root of the lung, as has been noted previously (**157A, 157B**), contains respiratory passages, the pulmonary and bronchial vessels, and the anterior and posterior pulmonary nerve plexuses. It will be observed later that they also contain many lymphatics.

The opposed surfaces of the visceral and parietal pleura are smooth and glistening, and are normally separated by only a capillary film of fluid, which facilitates movement of the lung on the parietal pleura and the structures it covers. However, the lung contains a large amount of elastic tissue. Contraction of this tissue is normally responsible for the expulsion of air from the lungs during quiet expiration, but if the pleural sac becomes open to the exterior, either by injury to the lung surface or injury to the thoracic wall, the elastic tissue contracts to its full extent. As a result, the lung retracts towards its root and the pleural sac becomes a widely patent air-filled cavity (pneumothorax).

Because the heart projects a good deal farther to the left than the right, the right lung is larger than the left (**A**), this difference in capacity being reflected in the different diameter of the primary bronchi (**147A**).

Each lung is roughly conical. Note the names applied to its surfaces and borders (**A, B, C, D**) and observe particularly the following features regarding its position.

1. The narrow rounded apex (**E, F**) fits snugly beneath the cervical pleura, so that it reaches the level of the neck of the first rib which is 3–4 cm above that of the first costal cartilage.
2. The greater part of the medial surface is apposed to the mediastinal pleura and its related mediastinal viscera and vessels, in front, behind and above the lung root and the pulmonary ligament (**157A, 157B**). In front of the root and ligament the surface exhibits a concave cardiac impression, where it is related to the pericardium. The impression is deeper on the left lung than on the right (**A, C, D**).
3. The posterior part of the medial surface is related to the costal pleura where it covers the lateral aspect of the vertebral bodies and discs (**A**).
4. The blunt rounded posterior border lies in the groove between the vertebrae and the heads and necks of the ribs (**A**).
5. The inferior margin of the lung is thin and sharp where it separates the costal surface of the lung from the base (**C, D**). In quiet respiration it does not extend to the lower limit of the costodiaphragmatic pleural recess (**B**). Anteriorly, it underlies the sixth costal cartilage (**E**). Laterally (mid-axillary line), it is about a hand's breadth above the limit of the pleural recess, deep to the eighth rib (**E, F**). Posteriorly, it lies at the level of the tenth thoracic spine (**F**). Because of the relationship of lung and pleural cavity in this region, aspiration of fluid which may form in the pleural cavity is usually performed through the ninth intercostal space in the mid-axillary line (**B**).
6. The anterior border is thin and sharp (**A, C, D**) except in its upper part (**C, D**) where it and the covering pleura are crossed, on the right, by the brachiocephalic vein and subclavian artery. On the right the border extends, along its whole length, into the depths of the costomediastinal pleural recess (**A**). On the left side it bears the same relationship to the pleura as far down as the level of the fourth costal cartilage, but below that level it presents a deep cardiac notch and falls some 3 cm short of the pleural limit (**E**).

By comparing **161C** and **E** it can be appreciated that the only part of the pericardium which is not covered anteriorly by either the sternum or the lungs is that small region which is separated by the costomediastinal pleural recess from the anterior ends of the left fourth and fifth intercostal spaces. Consequently, aspiration of fluid from the pericardial cavity is accomplished by the introduction of a hollow needle through one of these spaces about 1 cm from the sternal margin.

The lobes of the lungs

The lungs are divided into lobes by deep fissures, which extend from the peripheral surface nearly to the hilus and are lined throughout by visceral pleura. Each lobe receives one branch of the corresponding primary bronchus (lobar or secondary bronchi).

The right lung is divided into three lobes, superior, middle and inferior, by two fissures described as oblique and horizontal. The oblique fissure cuts the posterior border of the lung some 6 cm below the apex, at a point which is about 2 cm from the median plane and at a level between the spines of the third and fourth thoracic vertebra (**F**). Below, it cuts the inferior border a little short of its anterior end, deep to the sixth right costochondral junction (**E**). The horizontal fissure may be traced on the surface of the lung from the anterior margin at the level of the fourth costal cartilage to the oblique fissure in the mid-axillary line (**E**). The inferior lobe thus occupies the posterior and lower parts of the lung, while the superior lobe comprises

LUNGS: T.S. AT LEVEL OF T 6

Costomediastinal pleural recess

Anterior border
of left lung

Cardiac impressions

MEDIASTINUM

T 6

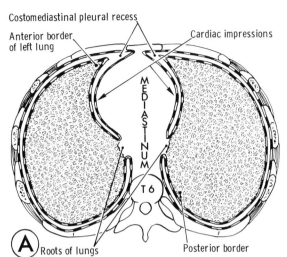

Roots of lungs

Posterior border

LUNGS: CORONAL SECTION
IN MIDAXILLARY PLANE

Apices of lungs

Roots of lungs

Pulmonary ligaments

Diaphragm

Aspiration
of pleural cavity

MEDIASTINUM

Inferior margins

Costodiaphragmatic
pleural recess

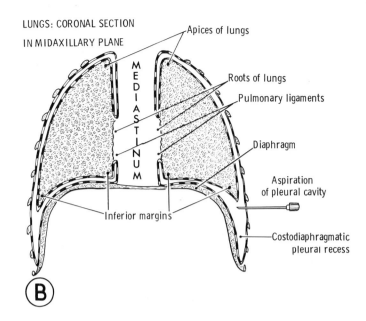

RIGHT LUNG: FROM MEDIAL SIDE

Apex of lung

Brachiocephalic vessels

Hilus of lung

UPPER LOBE

ROOT OF LUNG
Right upper lobe bronchus

Right pulmonary artery

Right principal bronchus

Right pulmonary veins

Horizontal
fissure

Anterior margin

MIDDLE
LOBE

Oblique fissure

LOWER
LOBE

Cut edge of pleura

Posterior margin

Inferior
margin

BASE

Pulmonary ligament

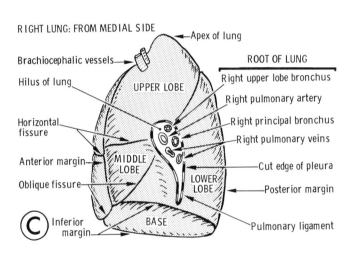

LEFT LUNG: FROM MEDIAL SIDE

Apex of lung

Cut edge of pleura

Hilus of lung

UPPER LOBE

Left subclavian artery
& left brachiocephalic vein

ROOT OF LUNG

Left pulmonary artery

Left principal bronchus

Left pulmonary veins

Anterior margin

Cardiac notch

Posterior
margin

LOWER
LOBE

LINGULA

Oblique
fissure

BASE

Inferior margin

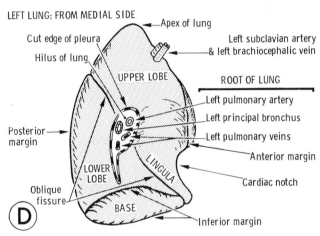

LUNG & PLEURA IN THORACIC CAGE:
ANTERIOR VIEW

Apex of lung: cervical pleura

Horizontal fissure of
lung

Anterior margin of lung:
costomediastinal pleural recess

Cardiac notch: anterior
border of left lung

Costomediastinal
pleural recess

Oblique fissure

Costodiaphragmatic
pleural recess

Oblique fissure

Inferior margin of lung

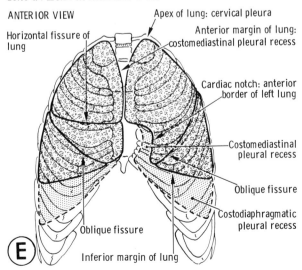

LUNG & PLEURA IN THORACIC CAGE:
POSTERIOR VIEW

Apex of lung

Oblique fissure

Posterior border of lung

Inferior margin of lung

Costodiaphragmatic
pleural recess

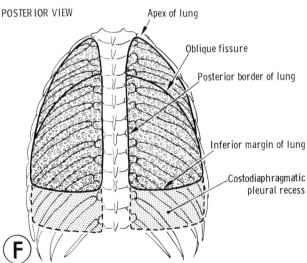

the upper anterior part, and the wedge-shaped middle lobe the lower anterior part.

The left lung is divided into superior and inferior lobes by a single oblique fissure, the position of which is similar to that of the oblique fissure of the right lung (**179E, 179F**). The part of the left superior lobe which corresponds to the right middle lobe, but is not demarcated by a fissure, is known as the lingula.

The bronchopulmonary segments

Within each lobe the lobar bronchi divide into smaller branches of similar structure, each of which supplies a specific region of the lobe demarcated from adjacent regions by fibrous septa. These regions, which are roughly pyramidal with their bases at the lung surface, are known as bronchopulmonary segments, and the branches of the bronchi which supply them are called segmental or tertiary bronchi.

The segments are named according to their positions within the lobes. In **A** the segments are shown as they appear on the medial and lateral aspects of the lungs. Each is numbered, and in the table below, the names corresponding to these numbers are shown.

Note that the positions of the segments are very similar in the two lungs, except that the middle lobe of the right lung consists of lateral and medial segments, whereas the corresponding lingula of the left lung consists of superior lingular and inferior lingular segments, and the medial basal segment present in the right lung is absent in the left probably because of the depth of the cardiac impression on that side.

	RIGHT LUNG		LEFT LUNG	
Lobes	Bronchopulmonary segments	*Lobes*	Bronchopulmonary segments	
Superior	2 Apical 3 Posterior 4 Anterior	*Superior*	3 Apical 4 Posterior 5 Anterior 7 Sup. lingular 8 Inf. lingular	
Middle	6 Lateral 7 Medial			
Inferior	9 Superior 10 Posterior basal 11 Lateral basal 12 Anterior basal 13 Medial basal	*Inferior*	10 Superior 11 Posterior basal 12 Lateral basal 13 Anterior basal	

The lobar and segmental bronchi

Each principal bronchus divides into lobar bronchi, which are each associated with a single lung lobe, and the lobar bronchi in turn divide into segmental bronchi, which are associated with individual bronchopulmonary segments. The intrapulmonary bronchi differ from the extrapul-

monary in that the cartilages in their walls are complete rings rather than horseshoe-shaped bars.

The bronchial trees of the right and left lungs are shown diagrammatically from the lateral and anterior aspects in **B**. The names of the bronchi corresponding to the numbers in (**B**) and their directions, in the upright posture, are tabulated below.

Right lung

Superior lobar (1) superolateral
    Apical segmental (2) superolateral
    Posterior segmental (3) posterolateral
    Anterior segmental (4) antero-inferior
Middle lobar (5) anterolateral
    Lateral segmental (6) anterolateral
    Medial segmental (7) anteromedial
Inferior lobar (8) postero-inferior
    Superior segmental (9) posterosuperior
    Post. basal segmental (10) postero-inferior
    Lat. basal segmental (11) inferolateral
    Ant. basal segmental (12) antero-inferior
    Med. basal segmental (13) inferomedial

Left lung

Superior lobar (1) lateral
    Superior division (2) superolateral
      Apical segmental (3) superolateral
      Posterior segmental (4) posterolateral
      Anterior segmental (5) antero-inferior
    Inferior (lingular) division (6) anterior
      Superior segmental (7) anterior
      Inferior segmental (8) antero-inferior
Inferior lobar (9) inferolateral
    Superior segmental (10) posterosuperior
    Post. basal segmental (11) postero-inferior
    Lat. basal segmental (12) inferolateral
    Ant. basal segmental (13) antero-inferior

The bronchial tree can be demonstrated radiologically after injection of a contrast medium through a fine catheter introduced through the mouth or nose and fed downwards through the larynx and trachea. The contrast medium does not, of course, fill the air passages: it merely coats their walls as far as the smaller branches of the segmental bronchi. Nevertheless, this is sufficient to give a clear picture of the bronchial pattern throughout most of the lung. A lateral bronchogram of the right lung and an anteroposterior bronchogram of both lungs, labelled in the same manner as in **B**, are shown in **C** and **D**.

Notice that the bronchial patterns in the right and left lungs differ in some respects.

1. There is no middle lobar bronchus on the left side, its place being taken by the inferior (lingular) division of the superior lobar bronchus.

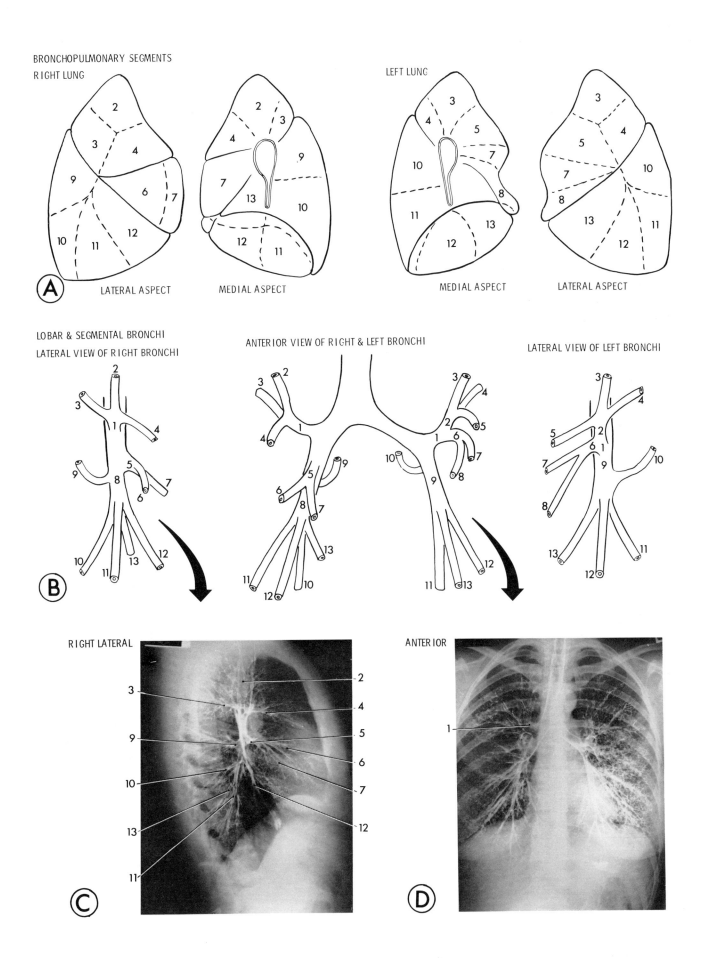

BRONCHOPULMONARY SEGMENTS
RIGHT LUNG

LATERAL ASPECT   MEDIAL ASPECT

LEFT LUNG

MEDIAL ASPECT   LATERAL ASPECT

A

LOBAR & SEGMENTAL BRONCHI
LATERAL VIEW OF RIGHT BRONCHI

ANTERIOR VIEW OF RIGHT & LEFT BRONCHI

LATERAL VIEW OF LEFT BRONCHI

B

RIGHT LATERAL

ANTERIOR

C

D

2. The directions of the two segmental bronchi arising from the right middle lobar bronchus differ from those of the two segmental bronchi arising from the comparable inferior division of the left superior lobar bronchus.
3. A medial basal segmental bronchus is present in the right lung but is usually absent in the left lung.

A knowledge of the pattern of the bronchial tree and in particular the directions of the lobar and segmental bronchi is of clinical importance for two reasons.

1. The interior of the proximal parts of the air passages can be examined in the living person after the introduction of a flexible fibre optic telescope, known as a bronchoscope, through the mouth, larynx and trachea. By suitable manipulation of the instrument, the lumina of the primary bronchi and the orifices of the segmental bronchi can be visualised and the presence of any disease process in their lining membrane determined. It is of interest to note that when the left primary bronchus is examined the pulsations of the descending aorta which lies immediately behind it are usually clearly visible.
2. Exudate from one diseased bronchopulmonary segment can be drained into the upper air passages—from which they can be removed by coughing—by placing the patient in a position in which the proximal end of the relevant segmental bronchus is inclined sharply downwards (postural drainage). As one example, the position adopted in drainage of the posterior basal segments is illustrated in **A**. The inclination of the left posterior basal segmental bronchus with the patient in this position is shown in **B**.

The lung lobules

The segmental bronchi divide repeatedly into progressively smaller branches. Eventually, the cartilage rings disappear from their walls, which become purely fibromuscular in structure. These passages are called bronchioles and they continue to branch until the terminal bronchioles are reduced to a lumen of about 0.5 mm in diameter. The terminal bronchioles then open into regions of tortuous thin-walled air passages, which are in communication with thin-walled spaces or alveoli. These regions are pyramidal in form and are demarcated from similar adjacent regions by delicate planes of connective tissue. They form the units of respiratory substance of the lung and are known as lobules. The bases of many of the lung lobules reach the lung surface, and the connective tissue planes which separate them, especially if they contain deposited carbon particles, outline polygonal areas over the lung surface.

The blood vessels in the lung

The pulmonary arteries enter the lungs through the hila anterior to the bronchi (**151A**). Each divides repeatedly in a synchronous fashion with the bronchi and bronchioles which they follow closely. Eventually, their terminal branches enter the lung lobules and open into the extensive capillary plexus in the alveolar walls. It is in this situation that gaseous interchange between the alveolar air and the blood occurs.

The pulmonary veins originate from the interalveolar plexus, but for the greater part of their course they run towards the hila, independently of the air passage and pulmonary arteries, in the septa which separate the bronchopulmonary segments. Thus, whereas a single branch of a pulmonary artery supplies each bronchopulmonary segment, the tributaries of the pulmonary veins tend to be associated with two or more segments. Towards the hila, the number of veins is reduced to two in each lung and these pass into the lung roots, below and anterior to the bronchi and pulmonary arteries (**157A, 157B**).

The bronchial vessels are concerned with the blood supply and venous drainage of the air passages below the bifurcation of the trachea. The arteries arise from the thoracic aorta or from posterior intercostal arteries. The veins consist of a deep set, which drain the intrapulmonary air passages, and a superficial set, which drain the extrapulmonary bronchi and the hilar lymph nodes (**189C**). Both sets end in the azygos and accessory hemiazygos veins.

It is important to note that the bronchial vessels anastomose to an appreciable extent with those of the pulmonary circulation, so that some of the blood carried to the lungs in the bronchial arteries returns through the pulmonary veins.

Radiographic examination of the lungs

In an ordinary postero-anterior radiograph of the lungs (**C**), the air which they contain renders them radiolucent and much of the lung fields consequently appear dark. This dark background is crossed by branching light tracts which radiate from the regions of the hila. The great majority of these tracts represent pulmonary blood vessels, their opacity being due to the blood they contain. The distribution of these vessel shadows depends on posture. In the erect posture about twice as many vessels are visible in the lower parts of the lungs as in the upper, but this difference disappears if the patient is supine.

It is very important to avoid the mistake of interpreting these vascular shadows as representing the bronchial tree. Because the air passages contain air they have the same translucency as the general lung substance and are equally dark in radiographs. A bronchus is only visible if it is seen end on. Then the wall appears as a light ring around the dark air-containing lumen. In contrast, a blood vessel viewed end on is seen as a uniformly white circle

POSTURAL DRAINAGE OF POSTERIOR BASAL
BRONCHOPULMONARY SEGMENT

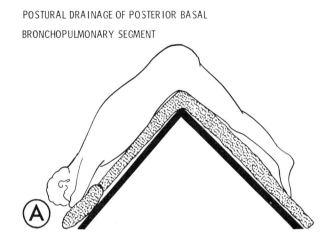

LEFT BRONCHIAL TREE FROM LATERAL SIDE WITH
PATIENT IN POSITION SHOWN

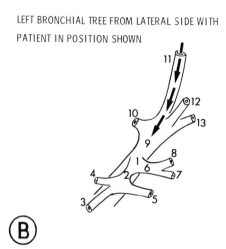

POSTERO-ANTERIOR RADIOGRAPH OF CHEST

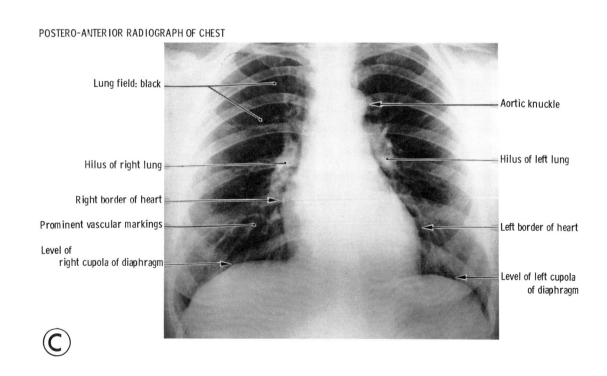

Lung field: black

Aortic knuckle

Hilus of right lung

Hilus of left lung

Right border of heart

Prominent vascular markings

Left border of heart

Level of
right cupola of diaphragm

Level of left cupola
of diaphragm

THE NERVE SUPPLY OF THE THORACIC VISCERA

The thoracic viscera are innervated by branches of the vagus nerve (**57**) and by medial branches of the cervical and upper four or five thoracic ganglia of the sympathetic trunk (**137D**).

The heart

The heart is innervated through the cardiac plexus. Although this structure is often described as consisting of superficial and deep parts, the distinction between them is seldom clear. The whole plexus is situated in the interval in front of and below the tracheal bifurcation, above the proximal part of the right pulmonary artery, below the aortic arch and to the right of the ligamentum arteriosum (**A**).

The cardiac plexus distributes branches to the great arteries and veins of the thorax and becomes continuous below with right and left coronary plexuses. These run on the walls of the corresponding arteries and send branches to the sinuatrial and atrioventricular nodes. Several functionally distinct types of neurons are involved in these plexuses.

1. Preganglionic sympathetic fibres arise from cells in the lateral grey column of the upper four thoracic segments of the spinal cord, and traverse the corresponding white rami communicantes to the sympathetic trunk, in which they spread to reach the three cervical ganglia and the upper four thoracic ganglia (**B**). From these ganglia the sympathetic pathway continues through cardiac medial branches to the cardiac plexus, and thereafter to the heart and great vessels. The preganglionic-postganglionic synapses on this pathway may be situated in the ganglia of the trunk, or in the cardiac nerves, or in the cardiac plexus. The effects of sympathetic stimulation are:
    a) constriction of the great vessels
    b) dilatation of the coronary arteries
    c) acceleration of the spontaneous rhythm of the SA node and increase of the conduction velocity through the AV conducting tissue. Thus the heart rate is increased and the P–R interval in electrocardiograms is shortened.
    d) increase in the force of contraction of atrial and ventricular myocardium.
2. Visceral afferent neurons conveying the sensation of pain have their cells of origin in the spinal (posterior root) ganglia of the upper thoracic spinal nerves (**C**). The peripheral processes of these cells follow the sympathetic pathway described above, with the exception of the cardiac branch of the superior cervical ganglia, to the myocardium and visceral pericardium and to the walls of the great vessels. The central processes enter the spinal cord where impulses may spread to other sensory nerves in the same segments. Thus pain caused by a lesion in the heart or great vessels may be referred to the medial side of the arm, which has a cutaneous innervation from T1 and 2, and to the anterior chest wall, where the skin is innervated by the upper intercostal nerves.

3. Preganglionic parasympathetic fibres arise in the brain stem and run uninterrupted courses through the cardiac branches of the vagus nerves which arise in the neck and through the cardiac branches of the recurrent laryngeal branches of the vagi (**D**). They relay with postganglionic neurons in the cardiac plexus, or in the coronary plexuses, or in the substance of the heart, and these fibres end on the coronary arteries, or in the atrial myocardium, particularly in association with the SA and AV nodes. The effects of parasympathetic stimulation are:
    a) deceleration of the spontaneous rhythm of the SA node and decrease in the conduction velocity of the AV conducting tissue, so that the heart rate is decreased and the P–R interval lengthened.
    b) depression of the contractility of atrial myocardium, though there appears to be no effect on the ventricular muscle.
    c) vasoconstriction of the coronary arteries.
4. The visceral afferent neurons which transmit information concerning distension of the great vessels and heart chambers have their cells in the two sensory ganglia which lie on the vagus nerve just below the base of the skull (**D**). Their central processes enter the brain stem. Their peripheral processes follow the parasympathetic pathways described above to the cardiac plexus and thereafter to a number of mechanoreceptor (baroreceptor) areas. These are situated in the walls of the coronary arteries, the aortic arch, the pulmonary trunk, the proximal parts of the pulmonary arteries, in the walls of the right and left atria close to the orifices of the venae cavae and the pulmonary veins and in the walls of the ventricles.

Sensory information transmitted along these pathways causes reflex stimulation of the parasympathetic supply to the heart, and consequently slowing of the heart rate and a fall in systemic blood pressure.

POSITION OF CARDIAC PLEXUS

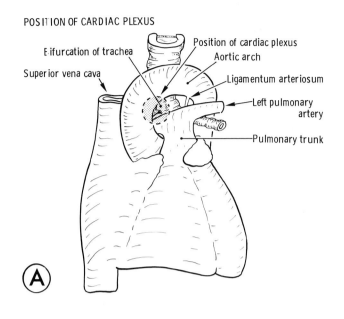

Bifurcation of trachea
Position of cardiac plexus
Aortic arch
Superior vena cava
Ligamentum arteriosum
Left pulmonary artery
Pulmonary trunk

(A)

SYMPATHETIC PATHWAYS TO HEART & GREAT VESSELS

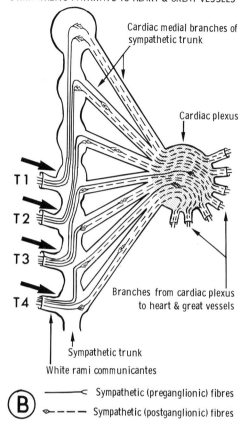

Cardiac medial branches of sympathetic trunk
Cardiac plexus
T1
T2
T3
T4
Branches from cardiac plexus to heart & great vessels
Sympathetic trunk
White rami communicantes

(B)
———< Sympathetic (preganglionic) fibres
- - -⟨ Sympathetic (postganglionic) fibres

VISCERAL AFFERENT (PAIN) PATHWAYS FROM HEART & GREAT VESSELS

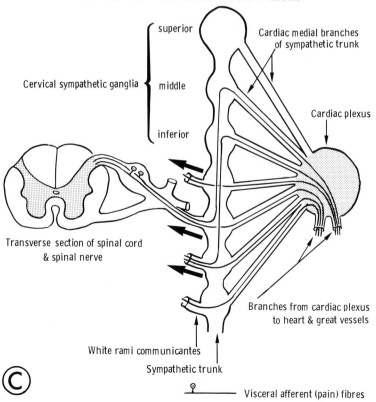

superior
middle
inferior
Cervical sympathetic ganglia
Cardiac medial branches of sympathetic trunk
Cardiac plexus
Transverse section of spinal cord & spinal nerve
Branches from cardiac plexus to heart & great vessels
White rami communicantes
Sympathetic trunk

(C)
⟜ Visceral afferent (pain) fibres

PARASYMPATHETIC PATHWAYS TO & FROM HEART & GREAT VESSELS

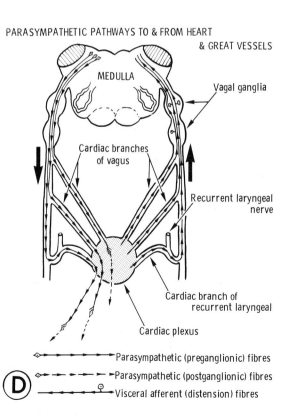

MEDULLA
Vagal ganglia
Cardiac branches of vagus
Recurrent laryngeal nerve
Cardiac branch of recurrent laryngeal
Cardiac plexus

(D)
Parasympathetic (preganglionic) fibres
Parasympathetic (postganglionic) fibres
Visceral afferent (distension) fibres

The oesophagus

The superior mediastinal and cervical parts of the oesophagus are innervated from the right vagus nerve and both right and left recurrent laryngeal nerves (**A**) and from the medial branches of the upper thoracic ganglia (**B**). The inferior mediastinal part receives its nerve supply through the diffuse oesophageal plexus on its wall (**A**). This plexus is formed by fine branches which pass through the posterior pulmonary plexuses from the vagus nerves (**A**) and additional branches from the upper thoracic sympathetic ganglia and the greater splanchnic nerves (**B**).

Four functional types of fibres are involved.

1. Branchial efferent fibres pass through the vagus and recurrent laryngeal nerves from the nucleus ambiguus and supply the striated muscle in the uppermost part of the oesophagus.
2. Preganglionic parasympathetic fibres originate in the dorsal vagal nucleus and traverse the vagus nerves and the posterior pulmonary plexuses to reach the oesophageal plexus. Most relay in the wall of the oesophagus, and the resulting postganglionic fibres are motor to the plain muscle of the viscus. Others pass through the oesophageal plexus without relay and continue into the abdomen in the anterior and posterior vagal trunks (**158**).
3. The postganglionic sympathetic fibres reaching the oesophagus through the medial branches of the sympathetic trunk appear to be solely vasomotor to the arteries in its wall.
4. Visceral afferent fibres of pain reach the sympathetic trunk through its medial branches and thereafter pass by the white rami communicantes to their cell bodies in the posterior root ganglia of the corresponding spinal nerves.

The lungs

A nerve supply enters the lungs from a diffuse autonomic nerve plexus which surrounds the lung root and is usually somewhat arbitrarily divided into smaller anterior and larger posterior pulmonary plexuses. Both parts receive fibres through the vagus nerves and the medial branches of the upper thoracic sympathetic ganglia, and send fine plexuses into the lung along the walls of the blood vessels and air passages as far as the visceral pleura. Nerve cells are distributed throughout these plexuses.

A number of functionally distinct nerve fibres are involved.

1. Postganglionic sympathetic fibres originate in the upper thoracic sympathetic ganglia. They are inhibitory to the bronchial musculature and glands, and vasoconstrictor to the blood vessels.
2. Preganglionic parasympathetic vagal fibres originate in the dorsal vagal nucleus in the brain stem, and synapse with the cells already noted in the pulmonary plexus and along the intrapulmonary air passages. The postganglionic fibres arising from these cells are motor to the bronchial muscle and glands.
3. All the sensory fibres from the lungs pass along the vagus nerves and are the peripheral processes of cells in the jugular and nodose ganglia on the upper part of that nerve (**A**). The central processes pass into the brain stem. Some of the sensory fibres transmit information concerning the degree of distension of the lung from stretch receptors associated with the air passages and the visceral pleura. Others respond to irritation of the air passages and are involved in the cough reflex. Additional sensory nerve endings are situated in the walls of the pulmonary blood vessels and transmit information conerned with the reflex control of blood pressure and heart rate.

VAGAL PATHWAYS TO OESOPHAGUS

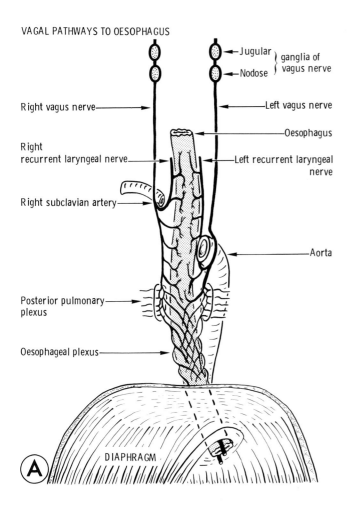

Jugular — ⎫ ganglia of
Nodose — ⎬ vagus nerve

Right vagus nerve

Left vagus nerve

Oesophagus

Right recurrent laryngeal nerve

Left recurrent laryngeal nerve

Right subclavian artery

Aorta

Posterior pulmonary plexus

Oesophageal plexus

DIAPHRAGM

A

POSTGANGLIONIC SYMPATHETIC PATHWAYS TO OESOPHAGUS

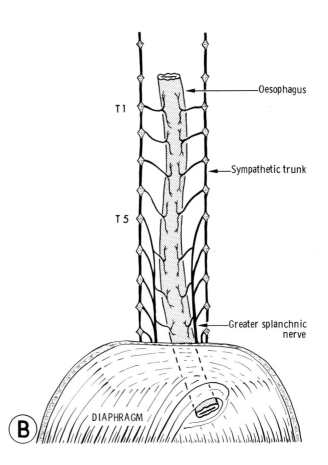

Oesophagus

T 1

T 5

Sympathetic trunk

Greater splanchnic nerve

DIAPHRAGM

B

187

THE LYMPHATICS OF THE THORAX

The superficial tissues

The skin of the thorax, and the superficial fascia, with the mammary gland which it contains in the female, are drained by lymphatics which are very closely, though not entirely, associated with those of the upper limb. They will be considered in the chapter on that region (**513A, 515D**).

The deep tissues

The deeper structures of the thoracic walls and the thoracic viscera are drained into three major lymph trunks, namely the single thoracic duct and the paired right and left bronchomediastinal trunks.

The thoracic duct

The thoracic duct has already been considered. Its origin and its course within the thorax (**143B, 145B**) should now be revised. As will be seen in greater detail later (**395B**) the vessel ends symmetrically in the root of the neck. It sweeps laterally from the left margin of the oesophagus behind the left common carotid artery and internal jugular vein (**A**) and, turning downwards, opens into the angle between the left internal jugular and subclavian veins.

It receives the lymph from the greater part of the abdomen and the lower limbs through the cisterna chyli. In the thorax it receives tributaries from the following groups of lymph nodes.

Posterior intercostal nodes which lie at the posterior end of each intercostal space (**B**). These receive lymph from the posterior three-quarters or so of the spaces and the associated parietal pleura. It should be noted that in some individuals the efferents from the nodes in the upper six spaces on the right side drain into the right broncho-mediastinal trunk (**A, C**) instead of the thoracic duct.

Posterior mediastinal nodes which lie in the posterior part of the inferior mediastinum around the oesophagus and the descending aorta (**B**). They drain the greater part of the oesophagus and the posterior part of the mediastinum.

Diaphragmatic nodes which lie on the upper surfaces of the diaphragm around the terminal parts of the phrenic nerves (**B**). Their efferents pass to the thoracic duct via the posterior mediastinal nodes but also into the broncho-mediastinal trunks via the parasternal nodes (see below).

The diaphragmatic nodes on the right side are the more important group because, besides receiving lymph from the diaphragm and the diaphragmatic pleura, they are joined by vessels which drain the upper and posterior parts of the liver and follow the terminal part of the inferior vena cava (**304**).

The bronchomediastinal trunks

The bronchomediastinal lymph trunks form as distinct vessels in the lower part of the superior mediastinum and end by opening individually into the proximal parts of the corresponding brachiocephalic veins (**A, C**). The tributaries of the bronchomediastinal trunks are derived from three groups of lymph nodes.

The parasternal nodes (**D**) form two symmetrical chains on the deep aspect of the chest wall along the courses of the internal thoracic vessels. Each chain drains the anterior ends of the upper six intercostal spaces, and also receives important tributaries from the superficial tissues of the chest wall including the mammary gland (**515D**) and from the diaphragmatic nodes (see above).

The brachiocephalic nodes (**A**) lie around the left brachiocephalic vein and the major branches of the aortic arch. They receive descending tributaries from the thyroid gland in the neck and vessels from the thymus and the pericardium.

The tracheobronchial nodes constitute a large and important group which drain the lungs, the principal bronchi and the trachea (**C**).

In the lungs, lymphatic vessels lie both peripherally beneath the visceral pleura and deeply along the courses of the bronchioles and bronchi. There are no vessels in the walls of the alveoli.

The lymph vessels converge on the hila of the lungs, some of them passing through small pulmonary nodes in the lung substance. Thereafter they traverse the several subgroups of the tracheobronchial group shown in **C**.

Many of the tracheobronchial nodes are very large and in city dwellers they are dark or even black in colour. The colour is due to the presence of carbon particles carried to them through the lymphatic vessels by phagocytes from the lungs.

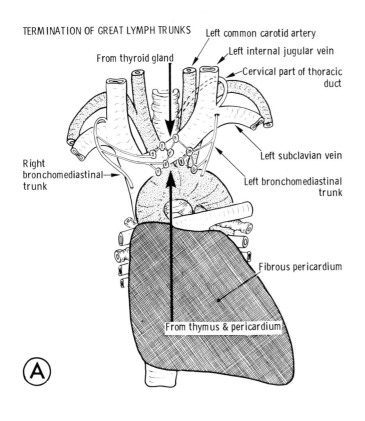

TERMINATION OF GREAT LYMPH TRUNKS

From thyroid gland

Left common carotid artery

Left internal jugular vein

Cervical part of thoracic duct

Right bronchomediastinal trunk

Left subclavian vein

Left bronchomediastinal trunk

From thymus & pericardium

Fibrous pericardium

A

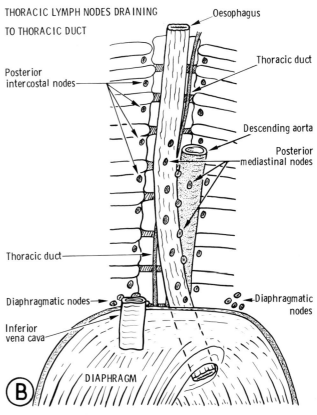

THORACIC LYMPH NODES DRAINING TO THORACIC DUCT

Oesophagus

Posterior intercostal nodes

Thoracic duct

Descending aorta

Posterior mediastinal nodes

Thoracic duct

Diaphragmatic nodes

Diaphragmatic nodes

Inferior vena cava

DIAPHRAGM

B

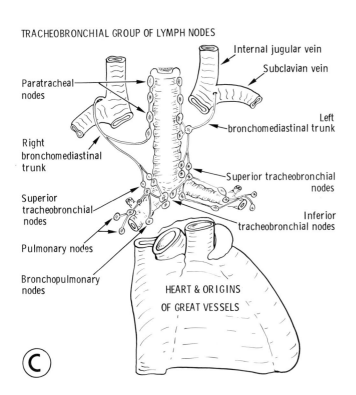

TRACHEOBRONCHIAL GROUP OF LYMPH NODES

Internal jugular vein

Subclavian vein

Paratracheal nodes

Left bronchomediastinal trunk

Right bronchomediastinal trunk

Superior tracheobronchial nodes

Superior tracheobronchial nodes

Inferior tracheobronchial nodes

Pulmonary nodes

Bronchopulmonary nodes

HEART & ORIGINS OF GREAT VESSELS

C

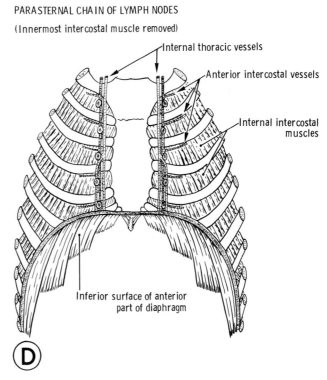

PARASTERNAL CHAIN OF LYMPH NODES
(Innermost intercostal muscle removed)

Internal thoracic vessels

Anterior intercostal vessels

Internal intercostal muscles

Inferior surface of anterior part of diaphragm

D

CHAPTER 4

The abdomen
and perineum

INTRODUCTION

The abdominal cavity lies within the lower part of the trunk. Above, it is separated from the thoracic cavity by a dome-like muscular partition, the diaphragm. Below it is demarcated from the perineum by another muscular partition called the pelvic diaphragm (**A**). The perineum is a region of connective tissue, between the pelvic diaphragm above and the skin between the thighs below. It is traversed by the terminal parts of the gastro-intestinal and urogenital systems.

BONES AND JOINTS OF THE ABDOMINAL WALLS

The vertebral column

The lumbar, sacral and coccygeal parts of the vertebral column form the central part of the posterior abdominal wall. They have been considered already (**3A**) but they should now be revised, particular attention being paid to the following features.

1. The anterior convexity of the lumbar vertebral column.
2. The orientation of the lumbar articular facets, and the consequent restriction of rotatory movements between lumbar vertebrae (**9A**).
3. The boundaries of the lumbar and lumbosacral intervertebral foramina.
4. The lumbosacral angle, the lumbosacral intervertebral disc and the sacral promontory (**9D, 9E**).
5. The cartilage-covered auricular facet which lies on the upper half of the lateral aspect of the sacrum (**9G**).

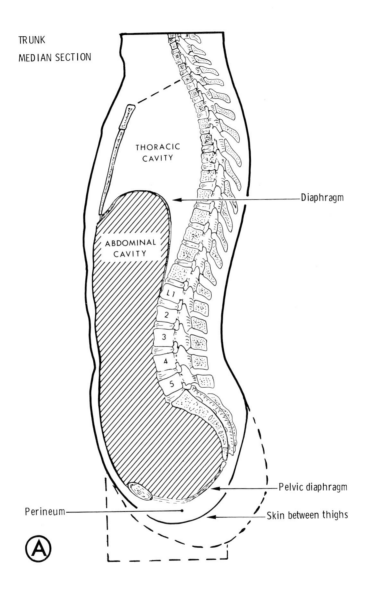

TRUNK

MEDIAN SECTION

THORACIC CAVITY

ABDOMINAL CAVITY

Diaphragm

L 1

2

3

4

5

Pelvic diaphragm

Perineum

Skin between thighs

Ⓐ

193

The costal margin

The lower six ribs and their costal cartilages, which form the costal margin, give attachment to part of the diaphragm and to the muscles of the anterior abdominal wall.

Revise the form of the costal margin (**125B**), noting particularly the following features.

1. The costochondral junctions lie progressively farther from the median plane from above downwards.
2. The seventh costal cartilage articulates with the lateral aspect of the xiphisternal joint.
3. The eighth, ninth and tenth costal cartilages turn upwards and medially to articulate with the costal cartilages immediately above them, by synovial interchondral joints.
4. The costal cartilages of the eleventh and twelfth ribs end freely without articulating with other skeletal elements.

The bony pelvis

The bony pelvis is a complex bony ring which makes large contributions to the walls of the lower part of the abdominal cavity and the perineum. It is formed by the sacrum and coccyx behind, and the two hip bones (**A**). In front, the hip bones articulate with each other in the median plane at the pubic symphysis (**E**). Behind, each articulates with the auricular facet on the sacrum at the sacroiliac joint (**A, D**).

The bony pelvis has three functions.

1. It forms a bony ring which surrounds and protects the lower abdominal viscera.
2. It provides attachments for numerous muscles, most of which act on the hip and knee joints.
3. It transmits the force of body weight from the lumbar vertebral column to the bones of the lower limbs.

The hip bone

The hip bone is grossly irregular in shape. Seen from the lateral side (**B**) its major features are the cup-shaped acetabulum, which is the proximal articular surface of the hip joint, and below that, a large aperture named the obturator foramen. In life the greater part of this foramen is occupied by a thick lamina of tough connective tissue called the obturator membrane. Only the upper anterior corner of the foramen remains patent as the obturator canal.

The cartilaginous precursor of the hip bone is ossified from three primary centres which remain separated throughout the growth period by a triradiate zone of cartilage centred on the acetabulum (**C**). The bone formed from the upper centre is called the ilium, that formed from the anterior centre is the pubis, while that derived from the posterior centre is the ischium. After the three zones of bone fuse at puberty, by ossification of the triradiate cartilage, the regions of the consolidated hip bone retain their original names.

Note that the pubis consists of a body, anteriorly, and superior and inferior rami which diverge, laterally and backwards, above and below the obturator foramen (**C**). In contrast the ischium consists of a body, lying behind the obturator foramen, and one ramus passing forwards below it (**C**). The single ischial ramus is continuous with the inferior pubic ramus below the obturator foramen, the two together constituting the conjoint or ischiopubic ramus.

By study of (**D**) and examination of a dried bone learn the names and positions of the many features associated with the medial aspect of the hip bone.

The pubic symphysis

This symphysis (secondary cartilaginous joint) lies in the median plane between the pubic parts of the two hip bones. The medial surface of the body of each pubis is coated by a thin layer of hyaline cartilage (**E**), and the two plates of cartilage are joined by a zone of fibrocartilage. The joint allows no appreciable movement, but, by virtue of the elasticity of its tissues, it resists the tensile stresses which are created in the region by the transfer of body weight from the lumbar vertebral column to the femoral heads.

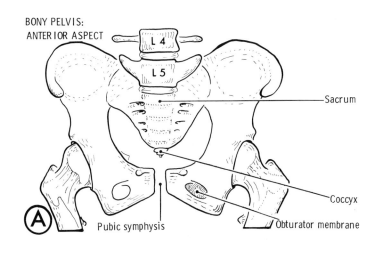

BONY PELVIS: ANTERIOR ASPECT

L 4
L 5

Sacrum

Coccyx

Pubic symphysis

Obturator membrane

A

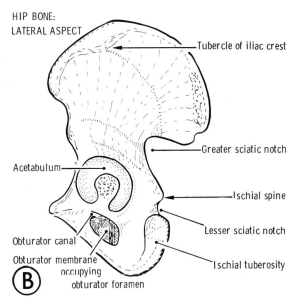

HIP BONE: LATERAL ASPECT

Tubercle of iliac crest

Greater sciatic notch

Acetabulum

Ischial spine

Lesser sciatic notch

Obturator canal

Ischial tuberosity

Obturator membrane occupying obturator foramen

B

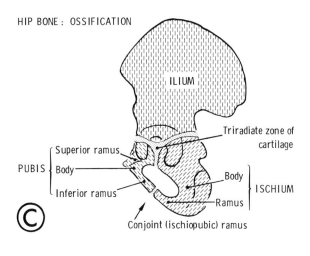

HIP BONE: OSSIFICATION

ILIUM

Triradiate zone of cartilage

PUBIS
Superior ramus
Body
Inferior ramus

Body
ISCHIUM
Ramus

Conjoint (ischiopubic) ramus

C

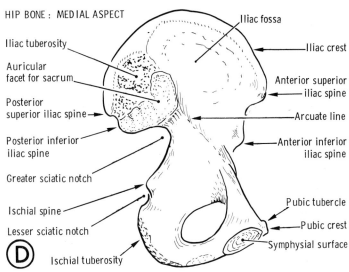

HIP BONE: MEDIAL ASPECT

Iliac fossa

Iliac tuberosity

Auricular facet for sacrum

Iliac crest

Posterior superior iliac spine

Anterior superior iliac spine

Arcuate line

Posterior inferior iliac spine

Anterior inferior iliac spine

Greater sciatic notch

Ischial spine

Pubic tubercle

Lesser sciatic notch

Pubic crest

Ischial tuberosity

Symphysial surface

D

PUBIC SYMPHYSIS: CORONAL SECTION

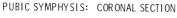

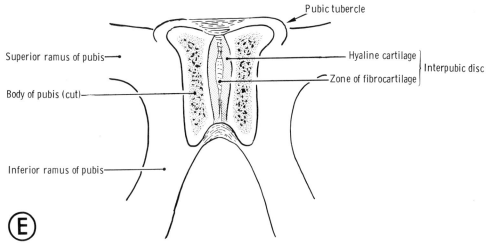

Pubic tubercle

Superior ramus of pubis

Hyaline cartilage

Interpubic disc

Zone of fibrocartilage

Body of pubis (cut)

Inferior ramus of pubis

E

The sacro-iliac joint

On either side of the median plane the large synovial sacro-iliac joint separates the sacrum from the iliac part of the hip bone. The positions and outlines of the cartilaginous auricular articular surfaces of the joint have been noted already (**195D, 9G**). These surfaces are irregular in contour, small eminences on one fitting into reciprocal recesses on the other. In conformity with this interlocking relationship, little movement occurs at the joint and it is to be regarded, like the pubic symphysis, as a shock absorber. The joint cavity is enclosed by a fibrous capsule. However, on some aspects this capsule is thin and weak and the stability of the joint, and the restriction of its mobility, are dependent on several very large accessory ligaments. These are so placed that they resist the tendency of the force of body weight, acting along the lumbar vertebral column (**A**) to rotate the sacrum so that its upper part moves downwards and its lower part upwards and backwards.

The interosseous sacro-iliac ligament is short but of massive thickness (**B**). It lies above and behind the joint and bridges the narrow cleft between the tuberosity of the ilium (**195D**) and the dorsolateral aspect of the sacrum. It prevents downward displacement of the upper part of the sacrum (**A**).

The sacrotuberous ligament (**C**) has a broad upper attachment to the posterior iliac spines and the dorsal aspects of the sacrum and coccyx. Its fibres converge as they pass downwards and are attached, below, to the medial margin of the ischial tuberosity. It prevents rotation of the lower part of the sacrum upwards (**A**).

The sacrospinous ligament (**C**) is comparatively thin and consequently of less mechanical significance, though it does play some part in stabilising the sacrum in the same manner as the sacrotuberous ligament.

The obturator membrane and the ligaments of both the pubic symphysis and the sacro-iliac joints are so closely associated with the bony pelvis in contributing to the formation of the body wall, that the name osteoligamentous pelvis is often used as an inclusive term (**C**).

Orientation of the osteoligamentous pelvis

In standing, the osteoligamentous pelvis is orientated so that the anterior superior iliac spines and the anterior aspect of the pubic symphysis lie in the same coronal plane (**D**). In sitting, on the other hand, the pelvis is rotated somewhat backwards, so that one coronal plane traverses the anterior superior iliac spines and the central parts of the acetabula (**E**).

The relationship of the osteoligamentous pelvis to the compartments of the trunk

Around the inner aspect of the osteoligamentous pelvis there is a circular ridge called the brim of the pelvis. It is composed on both sides by several features in continuity (**C, F**) namely, the sacral promontory, the upper surface of the lateral parts of the sacrum (**9E**), the arcuate line of the ilium, the pecten pubis (pectineal line), the pubic crest and the upper border of the pubic symphysis. In the erect posture the plane of the pelvic brim extends upwards and backwards at an angle of about 60° to the horizontal (**J**).

The part of the osteoligamentous pelvis which lies above the brim is named the false pelvis, while the cylindrical part which lies behind and below the brim is the true pelvis (greater and lesser segments of the pelvis). The true pelvis is itself divided into upper and lower regions by the pelvic diaphragm already noted (**192**) which stretches across its lumen (**G**).

It has been noted already that the abdominal cavity extends from the diaphragm above to the pelvic diaphragm below. It can now be appreciated that the abdominal cavity consists of two compartments in broad continuity through the pelvic brim. The larger upper compartment is the abdominal cavity proper, and the false pelvis contributes to its walls. The smaller lower compartment lying within the true pelvis is the pelvic cavity. Below the level of the pelvic diaphragm the true pelvis surrounds the perineum (**G**).

It is evident that the terminology in this region tends to be confusing. It is most important that the different meanings of the terms bony pelvis, osteoligamentous pelvis, false pelvis, true pelvis and pelvic cavity should be clearly understood.

The female bony pelvis

During the process of birth, the child must pass through the cavity of the osteoligamentous pelvis to reach the exterior. Consequently obstetricians use the terms pelvic inlet and pelvic outlet.

The inlet is the communication between the false pelvis and the true pelvis and is surrounded by the pelvic brim (**J**). The outlet is the lower margin of the true pelvis and its associated ligaments, and it is thus also the lower limit of the side walls of the perineum. It is formed by the pubic symphysis and the coccyx, and on either side by the paired ischiopubic rami, ischial tuberosities, and sacrotuberous ligaments (**H**). In the erect posture the plane of the outlet is inclined upwards and backwards at 15° to the horizontal (**J**).

DISPLACEMENT TENDENCY

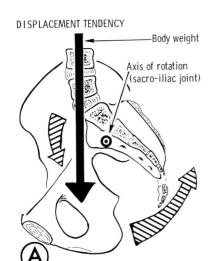

- Body weight
- Axis of rotation (sacro-iliac joint)

(A)

SACRO-ILIAC JOINT IN SECTION

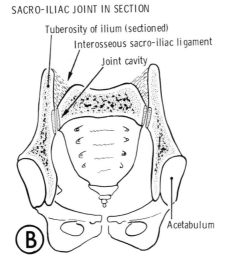

- Tuberosity of ilium (sectioned)
- Interosseous sacro-iliac ligament
- Joint cavity
- Acetabulum

(B)

OSTEOLIGAMENTOUS PELVIS: LIGAMENTS

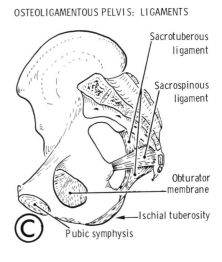

- Sacrotuberous ligament
- Sacrospinous ligament
- Obturator membrane
- Ischial tuberosity
- Pubic symphysis

(C)

STANDING

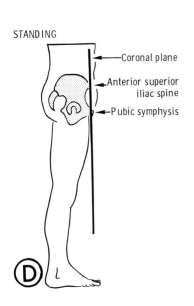

- Coronal plane
- Anterior superior iliac spine
- Pubic symphysis

(D)

SITTING

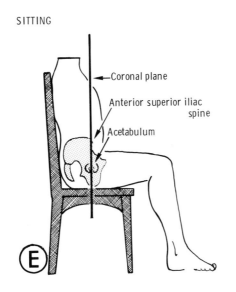

- Coronal plane
- Anterior superior iliac spine
- Acetabulum

(E)

PELVIC BRIM

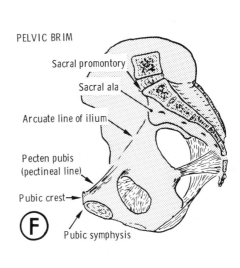

- Sacral promontory
- Sacral ala
- Arcuate line of ilium
- Pecten pubis (pectineal line)
- Pubic crest
- Pubic symphysis

(F)

PELVIS: CORONAL SECTION

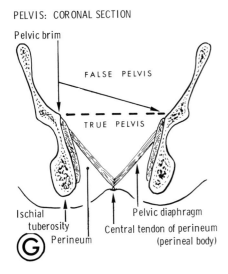

- Pelvic brim
- FALSE PELVIS
- TRUE PELVIS
- Ischial tuberosity
- Perineum
- Pelvic diaphragm
- Central tendon of perineum (perineal body)

(G)

PELVIC OUTLET FEMALE

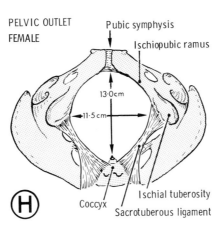

- Pubic symphysis
- Ischiopubic ramus
- 13.0 cm
- 11.5 cm
- Coccyx
- Ischial tuberosity
- Sacrotuberous ligament

(H)

OSTEOLIGAMENTOUS PELVIS: ORIENTATION

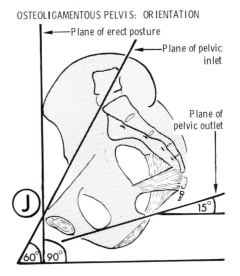

- Plane of erect posture
- Plane of pelvic inlet
- Plane of pelvic outlet
- 15°
- 60°
- 90°

(J)

In the female the superior pubic rami are widely divergent and the sacral promontory projects less in front of the lateral parts of the sacrum (A) than it does in the male. The pelvic inlet is consequently wide and circular whereas in the male it is comparatively narrow and heart shaped (A). The female pelvic outlet is also comparatively wide, the pubic arch, formed by the diverging inferior pubic rami, being greater than 90° and the ischial tuberosities being curved laterally (everted) (A).

The average measurements (diameters) of the inlet and outlet of the female pelvis are shown in A, 197H.

Sex differences are more obvious in the pelvis than in other parts of the skeleton. They are therefore frequently used in forensic practice to determine the sex of human remains.

THE ABDOMINAL CAVITY PROPER

The posterior wall

The posterior wall of the abdominal cavity proper extends from the twelfth ribs to the brim of the pelvis. Centrally it contains the lumbar vertebral column, and below and laterally the false pelvis (C).

The erector spinae muscle

Along the posterior aspect of the body numerous small postvertebral muscles, which collectively extend from the sacrum to the skull, are closely associated in one bulky longitudinal mass. It is usually convenient to consider this as a single functional unit named the erector spinae muscle. This arises from the dorsal surfaces of the sacrum and sacrotuberous ligament (B). After passing upwards in the gutter bounded by the spinous processes, laminae and transverse processes of the lumbar vertebrae (D), it continues upwards onto the posterior aspects of the thoracic cage and the cervical vertebral column (133C). Functionally, the erector spinae is the extensor muscle of the vertebral column. It is innervated by the dorsal rami of all the spinal nerves.

The quadratus lumborum

This muscle lies lateral to the vertebral column. Observe its attachments to the twelfth rib, the iliac crest and the lumbar transverse processes (C, D).

It is a lateral flexor of the vertebral column. It has also been claimed that during inspiration, the muscles of both sides, acting together, prevent elevation of the twelfth ribs, and thus stabilise the origin of those fibres of the diaphragm which arise from these ribs.

The thoracolumbar fascia

This zone of dense connective tissue extends from the iliac crest to the twelfth rib, lateral to quadratus lumborum (C).

Medially it divides into anterior, middle and posterior laminae (D). Note the relationship of these laminae to the quadratus lumborum and erector spinae muscles. Most of the anterior lamina is thin and translucent but its upper part forms a thick fascial band passing across the upper part of quadratus lumborum. This is the lateral arcuate ligament (C).

The iliopsoas muscle

The iliopsoas muscle is inserted by a single large tendon into the femur (331B) but in the abdomen it consists of two separate muscular heads named iliacus and psoas major. Observe (C) the origins of psoas major from the intervertebral discs and transverse processes between T12 and L5, and from the series of fibrous arches which are slung across the concave lateral aspects of the upper four lumbar vertebral bodies (E).

In a transverse section through one of these four vertebral bodies, it is evident how psoas major bulges laterally in front of quadratus lumborum, and how a psoas canal passes from beneath each fibrous arch, backwards between psoas major and a lumbar vertebral body to the region of an intervertebral foramen (D).

From this extensive origin psoas major extends downwards and somewhat laterally, just above the pelvic brim into the anterior aspect of the thigh (E).

The iliacus arises from the iliac fossa of the hip bone (195D). Its fibres converge on the lateral border of psoas major and pass with it into the thigh (E).

The iliopsoas is a flexor of the hip joint (331B) and a lateral flexor of the lumbar vertebral column. In addition, however, the psoas parts of the two iliopsoas muscles flex the lumbar vertebral column when that movement is made against the force of gravity as in rising from the supine position.

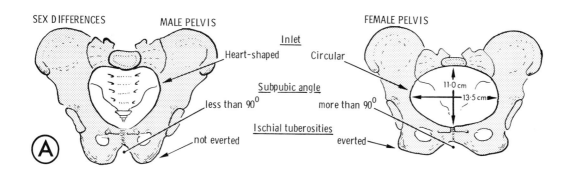

SEX DIFFERENCES   MALE PELVIS

FEMALE PELVIS

Inlet
Heart-shaped   Circular

11·0 cm
13·5 cm

Subpubic angle
less than 90°   more than 90°

Ischial tuberosities
not everted   everted

(A)

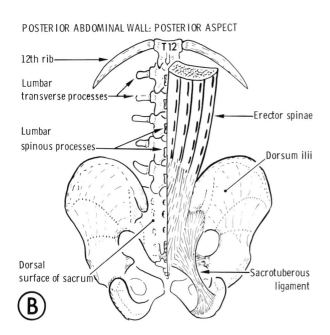

POSTERIOR ABDOMINAL WALL: POSTERIOR ASPECT

T 12

12th rib

Lumbar transverse processes

Erector spinae

Lumbar spinous processes

Dorsum ilii

Dorsal surface of sacrum

Sacrotuberous ligament

(B)

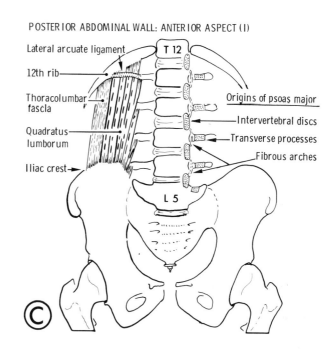

POSTERIOR ABDOMINAL WALL: ANTERIOR ASPECT (I)

Lateral arcuate ligament   T 12

12th rib

Thoracolumbar fascia

Origins of psoas major

Intervertebral discs

Quadratus lumborum

Transverse processes

Fibrous arches

Iliac crest

L 5

(C)

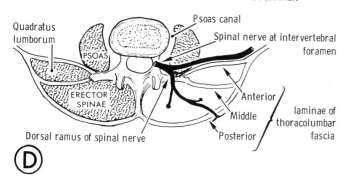

POSTERIOR ABDOMINAL WALL: T. S. AT INTERVERTEBRAL FORAMEN

Quadratus lumborum

Psoas canal

PSOAS

Spinal nerve at intervertebral foramen

ERECTOR SPINAE

Anterior

Middle

laminae of thoracolumbar fascia

Dorsal ramus of spinal nerve

Posterior

(D)

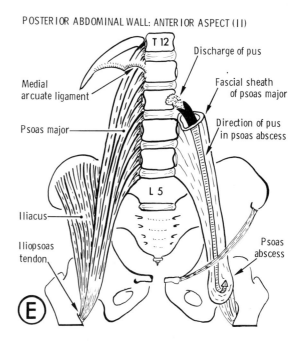

POSTERIOR ABDOMINAL WALL: ANTERIOR ASPECT (II)

T 12   Discharge of pus

Medial arcuate ligament

Fascial sheath of psoas major

Psoas major

Direction of pus in psoas abscess

L 5

Iliacus

Iliopsoas tendon

Psoas abscess

(E)

199

The iliopsoas fascia

A thin fascial layer covers the anterior aspect of the iliacus and psoas major heads of iliopsoas in both abdomen and thigh. Above, a thickened band of the same fascia crosses the upper part of psoas major. This is the medial arcuate ligament which is continuous laterally with the lateral arcuate ligament (**199E**).

Because the iliopsoas fascia covers both the abdominal and femoral parts of iliopsoas, pus originating from a disease process in the lumbar vertebrae, and accumulating under the fascia, tends to track downwards until it eventually forms a swelling in the upper part of the thigh (psoas abscess).

The latissimus dorsi

This large thin sheet of muscle fibres is inserted into the humerus and is functionally associated with the upper limb. Its tendinous origin arises from the lower six thoracic spines, the posterior lamina of the thoracolumbar fascia and the posterior part of the iliac crest (**A**). Note how its lateral border passes upwards over the undivided region of the thoracolumbar fascia.

The diaphragm

The muscular diaphragm forms the roof of the abdominal cavity. Many of its features, including its nerve supply, have been considered already in relation to the thorax (**131**), but it is helpful to reconsider the muscle at this stage. In general it is dome-shaped, but the central part of the dome is at a slightly lower level than the more lateral parts, which are called the cupolae (**B, C**). The thin sheet of muscle fibres has an oblique circular origin from the deep aspect of the body wall, the anterior part of the circle being considerably higher than the posterior (**C**). From this origin the muscle fibres incline upwards and centrally to end in a fibrous zone of trefoil shape (**131C**). Although this is situated at the highest part of the diaphragm, and consequently much nearer the anterior than the posterior part of its origin, it is nevertheless called the central tendon. The anterior (sternal) fibres of the muscle arise from the xiphoid process of the sternum, and the lateral (costal) fibres from the lower six costal cartilages. The posterior (lumbar) fibres originate from the lateral and medial arcuate ligaments (**B**), and from the upper lumbar vertebral bodies by two separate thick bundles, the right and left crura (**B**). Although they are separate below, the two crura unite at the level of the twelfth thoracic vertebral body, their union being coated by tendinous fibres which constitute the median arcuate ligament (**B**).

In many individuals the costal and lumbar fibres of the diaphragm are separated, on one or both sides, by a triangular fibrous zone devoid of muscular fibres and named the vertebrocostal trigone (**B**).

The level of the diaphragm varies considerably in different circumstances. In expiration, when the body is in the supine position, the projection of the uppermost part of the diaphragm on to the anterior chest wall lies at the level of the xiphisternal joint, and extends laterally on either side to cross the fifth rib at the lateral line. Posteriorly, this level corresponds to the eighth thoracic vertebral body (**C**). In inspiration the diaphragm descends to a lower level (**132**). It can be seen from **C** that the upper part of the abdominal cavity is covered and protected by the rib cage.

Besides varying throughout the respiratory cycle, the level of the diaphragm also varies significantly with posture. It descends slightly in the erect posture, owing to the gravitational pull of the abdominal viscera, and to a greater degree in the sitting position because the anterior abdominal muscles are then relaxed. Lying on one side results in the lower diaphragmatic cupola rising to a high level and the upper cupola descending to a lower level.

Communications between the thorax and abdomen

There are three such openings in the diaphragm.

The aortic opening lies behind, rather than within, the diaphragm. Observe its almost vertical disposition and its boundaries (**B**). Its upper margin lies at the level of the lower border of the twelfth thoracic vertebral body. The opening transmits the continuity between the thoracic and abdominal aortae (**203C**), and the cisterna chyli (**303A**).

The oesophageal opening is situated in the lumbar muscle fibres of the diaphragm, slightly to the left of the median plane and at the level of the tenth thoracic vertebral body (**B**). Because it is placed in the muscular substance of the diaphragm, the oesophageal opening is constricted during each inspiration. Later in this chapter it will be noted that this opening is traversed not only by the oesophagus but by the important arteries and veins associated with that viscus (**251B, 253C**), and by the anterior and posterior vagal trunks (**295A**).

The vena caval opening is placed in the central tendon of the diaphragm about 2 cm or so to the right of the median plane and opposite the eighth thoracic vertebral body in the supine position (**B**). Because of its relationship to the central tendon the lumen of the inferior vena cava is not affected by respiration. The opening also transmits some of the terminal branches of the right phrenic nerve (**157B**), and lymphatic vessels from the liver (**305A**).

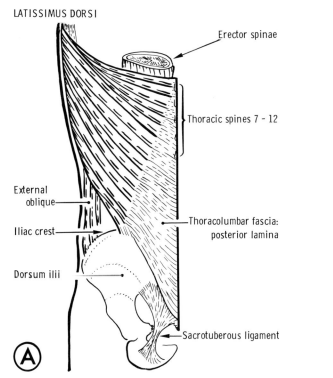

LATISSIMUS DORSI

Erector spinae

Thoracic spines 7 - 12

External oblique

Iliac crest

Dorsum ilii

Thoracolumbar fascia: posterior lamina

Sacrotuberous ligament

(A)

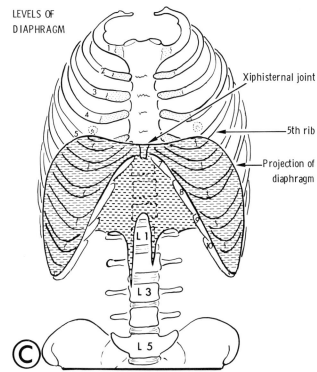

LEVELS OF DIAPHRAGM

Xiphisternal joint

5th rib

Projection of diaphragm

L 1

L 3

L 5

(C)

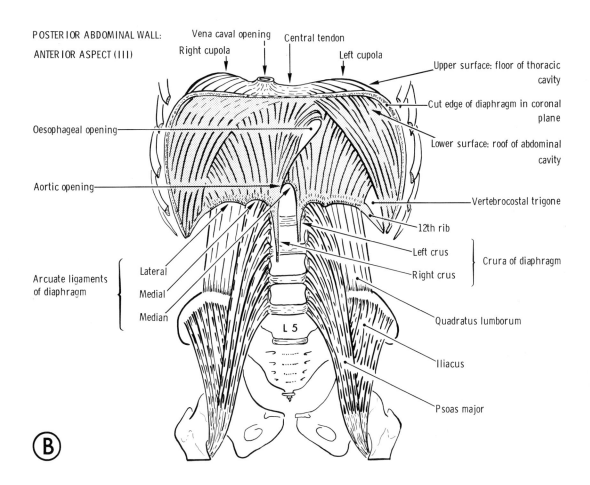

POSTERIOR ABDOMINAL WALL:
ANTERIOR ASPECT (III)

Vena caval opening

Right cupola

Central tendon

Left cupola

Upper surface: floor of thoracic cavity

Cut edge of diaphragm in coronal plane

Oesophageal opening

Lower surface: roof of abdominal cavity

Aortic opening

Vertebrocostal trigone

12th rib

Left crus

Right crus

Crura of diaphragm

Arcuate ligaments of diaphragm

Lateral

Medial

Median

L 5

Quadratus lumborum

Iliacus

Psoas major

(B)

The fascial envelope and extraperitoneal tissue of the abdomen

The muscular and bony walls of the abdominal cavity are lined by three concentric tissue layers (**A**). The outermost is the fascial envelope. The innermost is a serous membrane called the peritoneum. Although it is shown in **A** as a single sac it should be noted that it has, in fact, a very complex disposition, which will be considered in detail later. Between the fascial envelope and the peritoneum is a layer of fatty areolar tissue, named the extraperitoneal tissue. It varies in thickness in different situations and in different individuals, reaching several centimetres in those who are obese.

Although the fascial layer forms a complete and continuous envelope, it varies in character, and in name, in different situations. In some places it consists of fascia lining the deep aspects of an abdominal muscle, in others of a thick zone of dense connective tissue such as the undivided part of the thoracolumbar fascia. And thirdly, where the abdominal wall is bony, the fascial envelope is formed by periosteum.

The part of the fascial envelope associated with the anterior and lateral aspects of the abdominal cavity proper lines the deep aspect of an extensive flat muscle called the transversus abdominis. This part is consequently named the transversalis fascia (**A**).

The abdominal arterial stem

Observe the vessels which form the main arterial stem in the extraperitoneal tissue on the posterior wall of the abdominal cavity (**C**). Note particularly the following features.

1. The continuity of the abdominal aorta and the descending thoracic aorta at the aortic opening behind the diaphragm.
2. The position of the aorta just to the left of the median plane.
3. The bifurcation of the abdominal aorta in front of the fourth lumbar vertebral body.
4. The bifurcation of each common iliac artery in front of the sacroiliac joint at the level of the lumbosacral intervertebral disc.
5. The passage of the internal iliac artery along the pelvic cavity.
6. The course of the external iliac artery along the medial border of iliopsoas at the brim of the pelvis, and its continuation into the lower limb as the femoral artery.

These major vessels supply visceral and parietal branches to the abdominal and pelvic cavities. The more important of the abdominal parietal branches are considered below.

The paired phrenic arteries diverge from the uppermost part of the aorta onto the under surface of the diaphragm (**C**).

Four lumbar arteries arise from each side of the aorta, and are in series with the posterior intercostal arteries in the thorax. Each passes deep to one of the fibrous arches of psoas major and runs backwards through a psoas canal towards the corresponding intervertebral foramen (**B, C**). The arteries there divide into branches which pass both laterally and backwards to supply the tissues of the posterior abdominal wall. All the lumbar arteries give off fine, but important, spinal branches which traverse the lumbar intervertebral foramina and contribute to the blood supply of the lowest part of the spinal cord and the nerve roots of the cauda equina (**B**).

The inferior epigastric artery arises from the external iliac immediately above the mid-inguinal point (midway between the anterior superior iliac spine and the public symphysis). It passes upwards and medially along the anterior abdominal wall lying in the extraperitoneal tissue, and, therefore, deep to the transversalis fascia. About halfway between the umbilicus and the pubic symphysis the vessel pierces this fascial layer and comes into relationship with the deep aspect of the rectus abdominis muscle (**221C**). Its subsequent course will be considered later.

The inferior vena cava and its tributaries

The external and internal iliac veins join to form the common iliac veins (**D**). These in turn unite in front of the fifth lumbar vertebral body, to the right of the median plane to form the inferior vena cava (**D**). Because of the eccentric origin of the inferior vena cava the left common iliac vein is longer than the right. Observe the relationships of these veins to the corresponding arteries (**D**).

The inferior vena cava originates at a lower level than the termination of the aorta. It ascends in front of the lumbar vertebral column, immediately to the right of the aorta. Thereafter it inclines gradually to the right, lying on the right crus of the diaphragm, to reach the vena caval opening in the central tendon of that muscle.

Veins corresponding to the phrenic and lumbar arteries join the inferior vena cava. Parietal veins from the wall of the pelvic cavity join the internal iliac veins. The inferior epigastric veins pass into the external iliac veins.

The inferior vena cava and the internal iliac veins also receive visceral tributaries which will be considered later.

The nerves of the posterior abdominal wall

These are the twelfth thoracic nerve and the upper four lumbar nerves. The fifth lumbar nerve is more conveniently considered in relationship to the pelvic cavity.

LINING OF ABDOMINAL WALLS

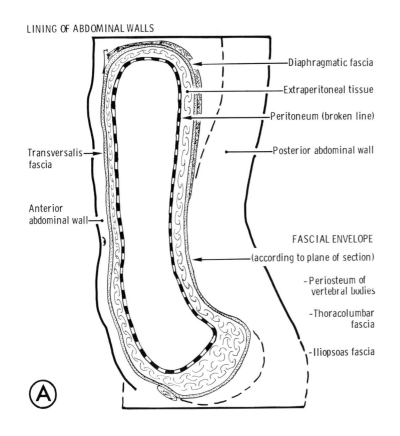

- Diaphragmatic fascia
- Extraperitoneal tissue
- Peritoneum (broken line)
- Posterior abdominal wall

Transversalis fascia

Anterior abdominal wall

FASCIAL ENVELOPE
(according to plane of section)
- Periosteum of vertebral bodies
- Thoracolumbar fascia
- Iliopsoas fascia

Ⓐ

POSTERIOR ABDOMINAL WALL
T.S. AT INTERVERTEBRAL FORAMEN

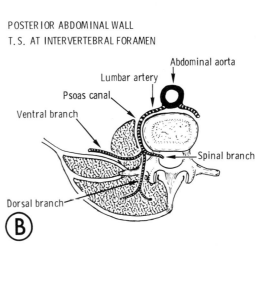

Abdominal aorta

Lumbar artery

Psoas canal

Ventral branch

Spinal branch

Dorsal branch

Ⓑ

ABDOMINAL ARTERIAL STEM

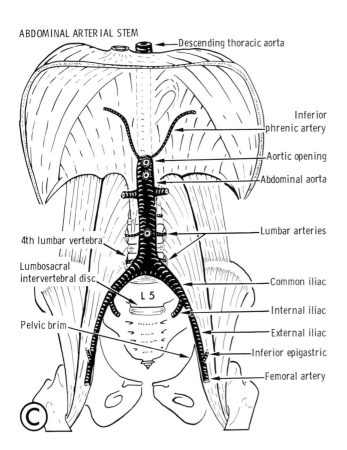

- Descending thoracic aorta

Inferior phrenic artery

Aortic opening

Abdominal aorta

Lumbar arteries

4th lumbar vertebra

Lumbosacral intervertebral disc

L 5

Pelvic brim

Common iliac

Internal iliac

External iliac

Inferior epigastric

Femoral artery

Ⓒ

INFERIOR VENA CAVA

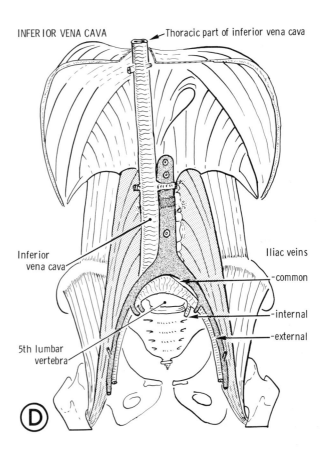

Thoracic part of inferior vena cava

Inferior vena cava

Iliac veins
- common
- internal
- external

5th lumbar vertebra

Ⓓ

Each nerve leaves the vertebral canal through the intervertebral foramen, which lies below the vertebra of corresponding number, and immediately divides into a dorsal and a ventral ramus (**A**).

The dorsal rami turn backwards and give branches to the erector spinae muscle (**A**) and to successive strips of skin on the posterior aspect of the trunk and the upper part of the buttock (**B**).

The ventral rami innervate the quadratus lumborum and iliopsoas muscles. That of T12 is known as the subcostal nerve. It appears from behind the lateral arcuate ligament, crosses quadratus lumborum below the twelfth rib and passes into the substance of the thoracolumbar fascia (**C**). The ventral rami L1–4 form the roots of the lumbar nerve plexus.

The lumbar plexus

The roots of the plexus run laterally into the psoas major muscle (**A**), the plexus itself lies in the substance of the muscle, and the plexus branches emerge from one or other surface of the muscle. Study the structure of the plexus and the names and root origins of its branches (**C**).

The iliohypogastric nerve (L1) emerges from the lateral aspect of psoas, runs downwards and laterally across quadratus lumborum and enters the substance of the thoracolumbar fascia.

The ilio-inguinal nerve (L1) accompanies the iliohypogastric at a slightly lower level and crosses the iliac crest on to iliacus.

The lateral cutaneous nerve of the thigh (L2, 3) emerges from the lateral border of psoas and extends downwards and laterally across iliacus to a position immediately below the anterior superior iliac spine, from where it enters the thigh.

The femoral nerve (L2, 3, 4) is considerably larger than the other branches. It passes downwards into the thigh in the groove between psoas and iliacus (**C, 207B, 331C**).

The genitofemoral nerve (L1, 2) runs steeply downwards and emerges through the anterior aspect of psoas major (**C**). It soon divides into femoral and genital branches, which will be considered later (**213A, 335E**).

The obturator nerve (L2, 3, 4) and the descending branch of the ventral ramus of L4 emerge from the medial aspect of the psoas muscle and turn downwards over the brim of the pelvis into the pelvic cavity. They will be considered with that region (**269A, 269B**).

It is important that the tissue planes in which two of these nerves lie should be appreciated, because it will be found that these relationships clarify the anatomy of certain regions which will be considered later (**258**). The femoral nerve lies outside the fascial envelope of the abdomen, between fascia and muscle. On the other hand, the genitofemoral nerve quickly pierces the iliopsoas fascia and its branches descend inside the fascial envelope, that is, in the extraperitoneal tissue.

Anterior and lateral abdominal walls

The muscles of these regions lie immediately superficial to the fascial envelope of the abdomen (**D**). On either side of the median plane there is a longitudinal strap-like muscle, the rectus abdominis, and three concentric sheet-like muscles, named from without inwards, the external and internal oblique and transversus abdominis muscles. In general, each of the sheet-like muscles consists of muscular fibres laterally, which give way to aponeuroses medially. The three pairs of aponeuroses are inserted, in large measure, by interlacing in the median plane, forming a dense zone of connective tissue. This extends from the xiphoid process of the sternum to the pubic symphysis and from its white appearance is called the linea alba (**D, E**).

The rectus abdominis muscle

Each rectus abdominis muscle arises from the front of the body of the pubis and passes upwards alongside the linea alba, increasing progressively in width. Above, it crosses superficial to the costal margin onto the lower part of the thoracic cage. The lateral fibres are inserted into the fifth costal cartilage, the middle into the sixth, and the medial into the seventh (**E**).

Three transverse zones of fibrous tissue known as tendinous intersections cross the muscle (**E**). Relate their levels to the xiphoid process and the umbilicus. Note that they extend to the anterior surface of the muscle, but not to its posterior surface, which is purely muscular.

The lowest part of the rectus abdominis is covered anteriorly by a small triangular muscle, the pyramidalis (**E**).

The inguinal ligament

The fibres of the aponeurosis of external oblique (the most superficial of the three sheet-like abdominal muscles) run downwards and medially (see below). The inferior part of this aponeurosis passes across the interval between the anterior superior iliac spine and the pubic tubercle (**E, 207A, 207B**). Traditionally, but not entirely appropriately, this part of the aponeurosis is called the inguinal ligament. The ligament curls backwards and then upwards, so that it has a grooved upper surface and a free posterior margin, but no definite anterior margin.

The lacunar part of the ligament is formed by the backward deflection of its posterior fibres into the pectineal line. It is triangular, with a sharp sickle-shaped lateral margin, and lies approximately in the horizontal plane (**207A, 207B**).

SPINAL NERVE IN OBLIQUE TRANSVERSE SECTION

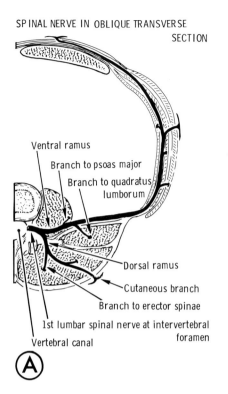

Ventral ramus
Branch to psoas major
Branch to quadratus lumborum
Dorsal ramus
Cutaneous branch
Branch to erector spinae
1st lumbar spinal nerve at intervertebral foramen
Vertebral canal

(A)

DORSAL RAMI: CUTANEOUS DISTRIBUTION

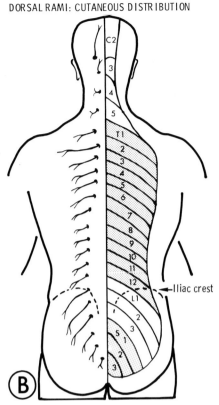

C2
3
4
5
T1
2
3
4
5
6
7
8
9
10
11
12
L1
2
3
4
5
S1
2
3
Iliac crest

(B)

ABDOMINAL WALLS

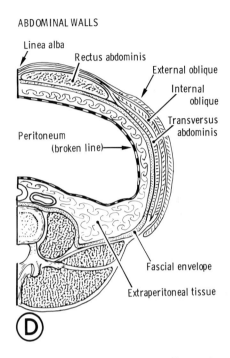

Linea alba
Rectus abdominis
External oblique
Internal oblique
Transversus abdominis
Peritoneum (broken line)
Fascial envelope
Extraperitoneal tissue

(D)

LUMBAR PLEXUS

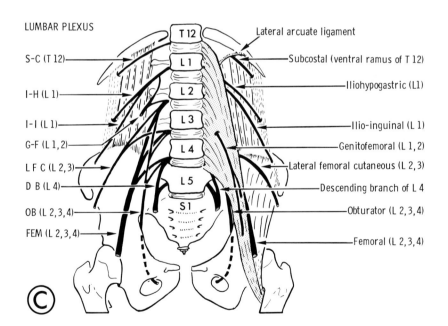

S-C (T 12)
I-H (L 1)
I-I (L 1)
G-F (L 1, 2)
L F C (L 2, 3)
D B (L 4)
OB (L 2, 3, 4)
FEM (L 2, 3, 4)

T 12
L 1
L 2
L 3
L 4
L 5
S 1

Lateral arcuate ligament
Subcostal (ventral ramus of T 12)
Iliohypogastric (L1)
Ilio-inguinal (L 1)
Genitofemoral (L 1, 2)
Lateral femoral cutaneous (L 2, 3)
Descending branch of L 4
Obturator (L 2, 3, 4)
Femoral (L 2, 3, 4)

(C)

RECTUS ABDOMINIS

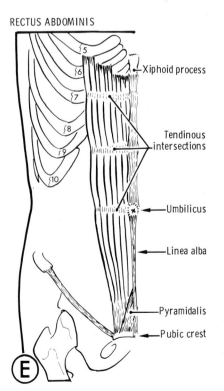

5
6
7
8
9
10
Xiphoid process
Tendinous intersections
Umbilicus
Linea alba
Pyramidalis
Pubic crest

(E)

The transversus abdominis muscle

This is the deepest of the three flat muscles. Trace the origin of the fibres of this muscle along the C-shaped line formed by the lower six costal cartilages, the lateral edge of the thoracolumbar fascia, the anterior two-thirds of the iliac crest and the lateral half of the grooved upper surface of the inguinal ligament (**C, D**). In general the muscle fibres are horizontally disposed. Note the position of the musculo-aponeurotic junction, particularly its relation to the rectus abdominis muscle (**C**). Most of the aponeurosis is inserted into the linea alba. From the xiphoid process to half way between the umbilicus and the pubic symphysis the aponeurosis passes behind the rectus muscle (**C**) and has a sharp lower margin called the arcuate line. Between the arcuate line and the pubic symphysis the aponeurosis passes in front of both rectus abdominis and pyramidalis (**C**), so that the rectus muscle lies directly on the transversalis fascia. The lowest part of the aponeurosis, which is continuous with that described above, has a distinct lower margin and curves downwards and medially into the pubic crest and the pectineal line. It constitutes the deeper fibres of the conjoint tendon (**C, D**).

The internal oblique muscle

This is the middle of the three flat muscles.

Follow the line of origin of its muscle fibres from the lateral two-thirds of the upper surface of the inguinal ligament (compare to the transversus abdominis), the anterior two-thirds of the iliac crest, and the lateral edge of the thoracolumbar fascia (**E, F**). The general direction of the muscle fibres is upwards and forwards round the abdominal wall (**E, F**). The uppermost are inserted into the lower three ribs (**E**). The rest of the muscle becomes aponeurotic along a line which is convex medially (**F**).

As far down as the arcuate line (see above) this aponeurosis splits into anterior and posterior laminae which pass across the corresponding aspects of rectus abdominis to the linea alba (**E, 209C**). Above, both laminae are attached to the thoracic cage. At the arcuate line the posterior lamina ceases abruptly (**E**), and from that level to the pubic symphysis the aponeurosis passes undivided across the anterior aspect of rectus and pyramidalis (**209C**). The lowest part of the aponeurosis (derived from the muscle fibres coming from the inguinal ligament) arches downwards and medially, and fuses with the corresponding part of the aponeurosis of transversus to form the conjoint tendon. This is inserted into the pubic crest and the pectineal line at right angles to the lacunar part of the inguinal ligament (**E**).

The external oblique muscle

This, the most superficial of the flat abdominal muscles,

has an origin which differs markedly from those described above. It arises by eight digitations, which spring from the outer surface of the lower eight ribs, in a straight line between the costochondral junctions of the fifth and twelfth ribs (**209A, 209B**).

The posterior muscle fibres descend almost vertically to reach the anterior half of the iliac crest (**209B**). They form a free posterior margin which overlies the thoracolumbar fascia (**201A**). The other muscle fibres reach a musculo-aponeurotic junction along an angled line which descends vertically from the ninth costal cartilage and then turns laterally along the line joining the umbilicus and anterior superior iliac spine (**209A, 209B**). The fibres of the aponeurosis run downwards and medially, superficial to rectus abdominis and the aponeuroses of internal oblique and transversus abdominis, to the linea alba and the pubic crest and tubercle (**209A, 209C**). The lower margin of the aponeurosis is the inguinal ligament.

The lower medial part of the external oblique aponeurosis presents a triangular opening called the superficial inguinal ring. Its base is the pubic crest and its long axis is in line with the fibres of the aponeurosis (**209C**).

The rectus sheath

The rectus abdominis muscle is enclosed within a sheath formed by parts of the other layers of the anterior abdominal wall. As the majority of abdominal surgical incisions are made through the sheath, a clear understanding of its anatomy is very important.

The structure of the sheath is conveniently considered in three parts.

1. The uppermost part of the muscle overlies the fifth, sixth, seventh and eighth costal cartilages, and the anterior intercostal membranes and interchondral joints which lie between them (**C**). Here the muscle is covered by the anterior lamina of the aponeurosis of internal oblique and the undivided aponeurosis of external oblique, which are intimately fused. The superficial surface of this composite layer gives origin to the lowest fibres of the pectoralis major muscle (**501D**).

2. Between the costal margin and halfway between the umbilicus and the pubic symphysis (the level of the arcuate line), the anterior wall of the sheath consists of the aponeurosis of external oblique closely united to the anterior lamina of that of internal oblique, while the posterior wall is formed by the posterior lamina of the aponeurosis of internal oblique and the aponeurosis of transversus abdominis (**209C**). For some distance below the costal margin, the uppermost muscle fibres of transversus abdominis almost reach the linea alba and consequently lie in the posterior wall of the sheath (**C**). Below, both components of the posterior wall end at the free

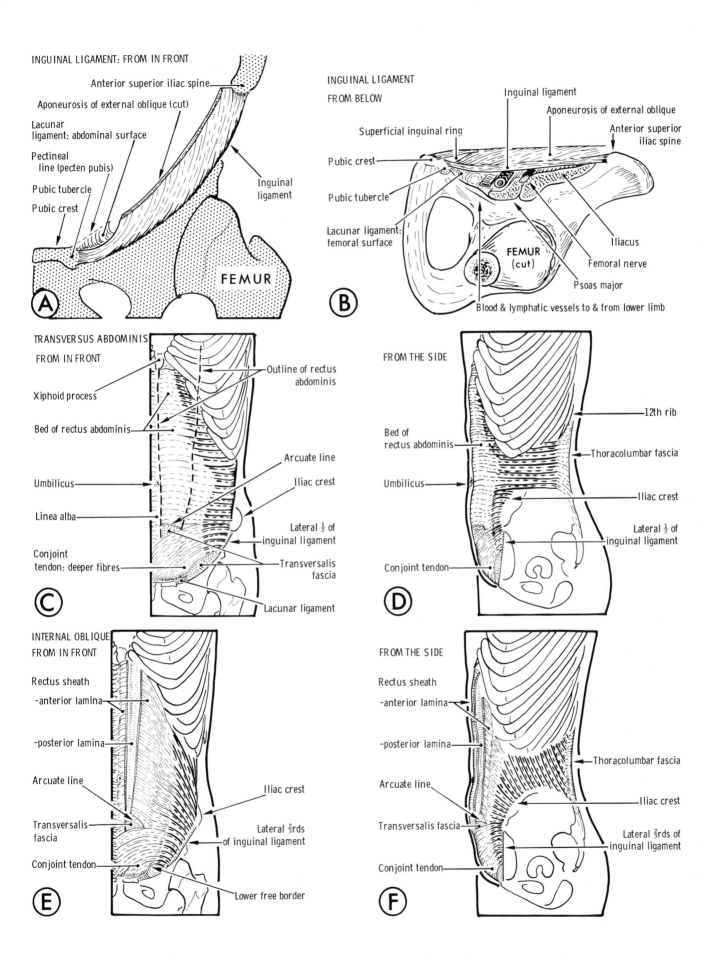

INGUINAL LIGAMENT: FROM IN FRONT

- Anterior superior iliac spine
- Aponeurosis of external oblique (cut)
- Lacunar ligament: abdominal surface
- Pectineal line (pecten pubis)
- Pubic tubercle
- Pubic crest
- Inguinal ligament
- FEMUR

(A)

INGUINAL LIGAMENT FROM BELOW

- Superficial inguinal ring
- Inguinal ligament
- Aponeurosis of external oblique
- Anterior superior iliac spine
- Pubic crest
- Pubic tubercle
- Lacunar ligament: femoral surface
- Iliacus
- Femoral nerve
- FEMUR (cut)
- Psoas major
- Blood & lymphatic vessels to & from lower limb

(B)

TRANSVERSUS ABDOMINIS FROM IN FRONT

- Xiphoid process
- Outline of rectus abdominis
- Bed of rectus abdominis
- Umbilicus
- Linea alba
- Conjoint tendon: deeper fibres
- Arcuate line
- Iliac crest
- Lateral ½ of inguinal ligament
- Transversalis fascia
- Lacunar ligament

(C)

FROM THE SIDE

- Bed of rectus abdominis
- Umbilicus
- Conjoint tendon
- 12th rib
- Thoracolumbar fascia
- Iliac crest
- Lateral ½ of inguinal ligament

(D)

INTERNAL OBLIQUE FROM IN FRONT

- Rectus sheath
  - -anterior lamina
  - -posterior lamina
- Arcuate line
- Transversalis fascia
- Conjoint tendon
- Iliac crest
- Lateral ⅔rds of inguinal ligament
- Lower free border

(E)

FROM THE SIDE

- Rectus sheath
  - -anterior lamina
  - -posterior lamina
- Arcuate line
- Transversalis fascia
- Conjoint tendon
- Thoracolumbar fascia
- Iliac crest
- Lateral ⅔rds of inguinal ligament

(F)

border of the arcuate line. It is very important to note that, whereas the anterior wall of this part of the sheath is firmly fused to the three tendinous intersections in the rectus abdominis (**205E**), the posterior wall is not so connected, as the intersections do not reach the posterior aspect of the muscle.

3. Between the arcuate line and the pubic symphysis, the aponeuroses of all three flat muscles of the abdominal wall are undivided, and all pass in front of rectus abdominis and pyramidalis to the linea alba (**C**). The lowest part of the aponeurosis of external oblique contains the superficial inguinal ring (**A, C, E**), while the lowest parts of the aponeurosis of internal oblique and transversus abdominis constitute the conjoint tendon (**C, 207E**). This lowest part of rectus abdominis lies directly on the transversalis fascia (**C**) so that there is no real lateral limit to the sheath.

Besides the rectus abdominis, this sheath contains the superior and inferior epigastric vessels and the terminal parts of the nerves of the anterior abdominal wall. All of these will be considered later (**215D, 217A**).

The actions of the anterior abdominal muscles

The rectus abdominis is a strong flexor of the lumbar vertebral column, acting against gravity when the body is supine, but only when flexion is resisted by some external force when the body is upright.

Because they follow the curvature of the abdominal wall, all the anterior abdominal muscles raise the intra-abdominal pressure, provided the diaphragm is fixed by its contraction. They thus come into play while respiration is temporarily arrested in defaecation, vomiting, and childbirth.

If the diaphragm is not fixed, contraction of the abdominal muscles drives it upwards, and at the same time pulls the lower ribs downwards, thus producing forced expiration as in coughing or sneezing.

The fascia and skin of the abdominal wall and external genitalia

The muscles and aponeuroses of the abdominal wall are covered by superficial fascia and skin. Over the lower part of the abdomen the fascia consists of two layers, a superficial fatty areolar layer, which varies greatly in thickness in different individuals, and a deep fibro-elastic, membranous layer, which acts rather as a corset around the region against which the abdominal viscera exert pressure in the upright posture (**D**).

As they pass downwards from the central part of the abdominal wall, both the skin and the superficial fascia pass backwards into the perineum. In the male they cover the scrotum and in the female the mons pubis and the major labia.

The scrotum is a cutaneous pouch which contains the testes. The skin is lined by a continuation of the membranous layer of the superficial fascia, which here contains bundles of involuntary muscle fibres constituting the dartos muscle (**E**). And this musculo-fascial layer passes as a median septum from the scrotal skin to the penis dividing the scrotum into two halves. The dartos muscle reacts principally to temperature. In cold conditions it contracts, and wrinkles and thickens the overlying skin, whereas in warm conditions it relaxes and the overlying skin becomes thin and smooth. This is a mechanism which tends to maintain the testes at their optimal functional temperature.

In thin muscular individuals the abdominal skin shows a number of rounded ridges and grooves which reflect the form of the underlying rectus abdominis (**215C**).

1. The linea semilunaris is a ridge which overlies the lateral border of the muscle and consequently runs downwards from the ninth costal cartilage.
2. Three transverse sulci mark the positions of the tendinous intersections between the more prominent intervening parts of the muscles.
3. On the upper half of the abdominal wall, a broad shallow groove overlies the linea alba between the two recti.

The umbilicus

The umbilicus is a deeply depressed wrinkled scar which is situated about halfway down the midline of the anterior abdominal wall. It is formed by the separation of the stump of the umbilical cord some time after birth. At birth this stump still contains the two umbilical arteries and the single umbilical vein which connected the foetal and placental circulations (**211A**). Some newborn infants are affected by abnormalities of the blood and blood forming tissues, which necessitate an exchange transfusion. The umbilical vessels are cannulated and the baby's own abnormal blood is drawn off through the umbilical arteries and replaced, through the umbilical vein, by healthy blood from a donor.

Umbilical herniae are of two types.

1. During early development, the primitive peritoneal cavity extends as a sac into the proximal part of the umbilical cord, and contains the apical part of the midgut loop (**211B**). Normally this sac becomes obliterated and the gut returns to the peritoneal cavity proper by the end of the third month of development. In a few individuals obliteration does not occur and the sac persists as a hernial sac at the time of birth. Most of these congenital umbilical herniae close spontaneously by the end of the first year, but a few require operative treatment.

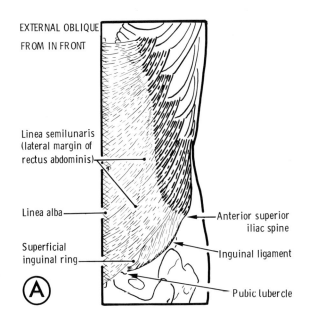

EXERNAL OBLIQUE
FROM IN FRONT

Linea semilunaris
(lateral margin of
rectus abdominis)

Linea alba

Superficial
inguinal ring

Anterior superior
iliac spine

Inguinal ligament

Pubic tubercle

(A)

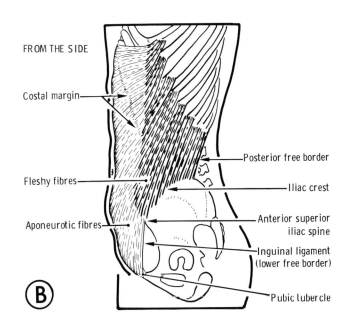

FROM THE SIDE

Costal margin

Fleshy fibres

Aponeurotic fibres

Posterior free border

Iliac crest

Anterior superior
iliac spine

Inguinal ligament
(lower free border)

Pubic tubercle

(B)

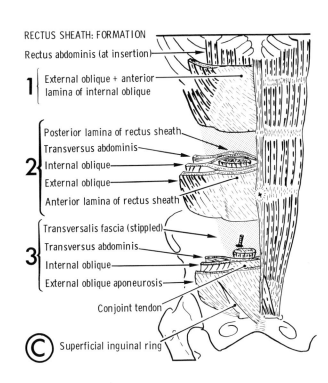

RECTUS SHEATH: FORMATION

Rectus abdominis (at insertion)

1 { External oblique + anterior
lamina of internal oblique

2 {
Posterior lamina of rectus sheath
Transversus abdominis
Internal oblique
External oblique
Anterior lamina of rectus sheath

3 {
Transversalis fascia (stippled)
Transversus abdominis
Internal oblique
External oblique aponeurosis

Conjoint tendon

(C) Superficial inguinal ring

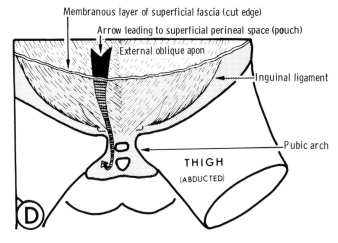

SUPERFICIAL FASCIA: MEMBRANOUS LAYER

Membranous layer of superficial fascia (cut edge)

Arrow leading to superficial perineal space (pouch)

External oblique apon

Inguinal ligament

Pubic arch

THIGH
(ABDUCTED)

(D)

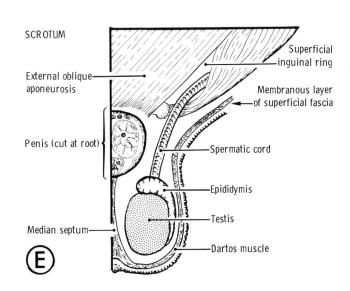

SCROTUM

External oblique
aponeurosis

Penis (cut at root)

Median septum

Superficial
inguinal ring

Membranous layer
of superficial fascia

Spermatic cord

Epididymis

Testis

Dartos muscle

(E)

2. An acquired umbilical hernia appears in middle-aged or elderly adults who are usually obese. The umbilicus weakens and a bulge of extraperitoneal fat and a peritoneal sac protrudes.

The inguinal region

In this region, the transversalis fascia passes up the anterior abdominal wall from the free posterior margin of the inguinal ligament. The inferior epigastric artery and its associated venae comitantes pass upwards and medially from the midinguinal point deep to this layer of fascia (**C**).

In males a tubular diverticulum arises from the transversalis fascia about a centimetre above the mid-inguinal point, just lateral to the inferior epigastric artery and deep to the lowest fibres of the internal oblique muscle (**C**). The diverticulum is the internal spermatic fascia, and its ring-like line of continuity with the transversalis fascia is the deep inguinal ring. The ring is usually oval with its long axis vertical. The tube passes medially and downwards, traverses the superficial inguinal ring in the aponeurosis of external oblique (**213A, 213B**), and descends into one half of the scrotum.

Throughout some of its course it is surrounded by two concentric tissue layers. The inner of these is the cremasteric fascia, which is derived from the internal oblique muscle and consists of both fascia and muscle fibres. The latter are striated but not under voluntary control. They raise the testis in response to cold or fear. The outermost layer is the external spermatic fascia which arises from the margins of the superficial inguinal ring.

This three-layered tubular structure contains the testis at its blind lower end. The rest of it contains a number of structures which connect the testis with the abdominal extraperitoneal tissue through the deep inguinal ring and constitute the spermatic cord.

In females, similar though narrower fascial tubes pass into the major labium. They contain a fibromuscular cord, the round ligament of the uterus.

The oblique track of the spermatic cord or its homologue in the female between the deep and superficial inguinal rings is the inguinal canal (see below).

The testis and epididymis

The testis is the male gonad and lies at the lower end of the spermatic cord within one half of the scrotum. The left usually lies somewhat lower than the right. It is broadly almond-shaped with upper and lower poles and anterior and posterior borders (**D**). Its tough fibrous coat is the tunica albuginea (**D, E**). Numerous septa pass from the deep aspect of the tunica and divide the testis into compartments or lobules which contain the seminiferous tubules (**D**). Posteriorly, these tubules join a plexus, called the rete testis, which is embedded in a mass of fibrous tissue called the mediastinum (**D**). Above, this plexus drains into the epididymis by twelve or so efferent ductules (**D**). These are intensely coiled and bound to one another by delicate fibres, so that they appear to form a single body lying over the upper pole of the testis. This is the head of the epididymis (**D**). Traced downwards, the efferent ductules coalesce to form the single, narrow, thin-walled canal of the epididymis. This is also intricately coiled and bound together to form the body of the epididymis which lies along the posterolateral margin of the testis (**D, E**). Its exact position is important in the differentiation of epididymal and testicular lesions. Near the lower pole of the testis the epididymis turns backwards as the tail (**D**), and thereafter the canal of the epididymis straightens out, and acquires a thick muscular wall as it turns upwards to become the ductus deferens. This ascends behind the epididymis into the spermatic cord (**D**).

The testis and epididymis invaginate a serous cavity, the tunica vaginalis, from behind. The tunica is derived from the peritoneum and consists of parietal and visceral parts. Observe the aspects of the testis and epididymis, which are covered by the visceral layer (**D, E**), and in particular the serous recess which intervenes between the testis and the body of the epididymis from the lateral side (**E**).

The spermatic cord

The spermatic cord consists of a number of structures which pass between the abdominal cavity and the testis, through the deep inguinal ring and the concentric internal spermatic, cremasteric and external spermatic fasciae.

UMBILICAL VESSELS

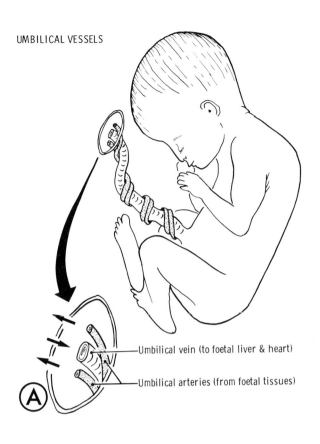

Umbilical vein (to foetal liver & heart)

Umbilical arteries (from foetal tissues)

PHYSIOLOGICAL HERNIATION
OF GUT INTO UMBILICAL CORD
IN EARLY DEVELOPMENT

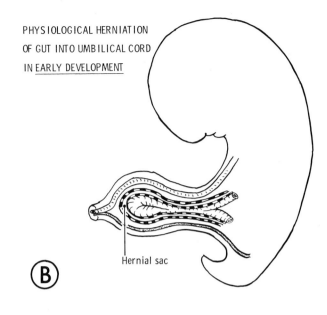

Hernial sac

INGUINAL REGION

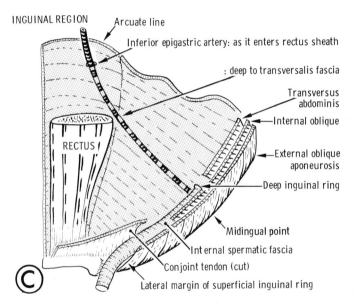

Arcuate line

Inferior epigastric artery: as it enters rectus sheath

: deep to transversalis fascia

Transversus abdominis

Internal oblique

External oblique aponeurosis

Deep inguinal ring

RECTUS

Midingual point

Internal spermatic fascia

Conjoint tendon (cut)

Lateral margin of superficial inguinal ring

TESTIS & EPIDIDYMIS: VERTICAL SECTION

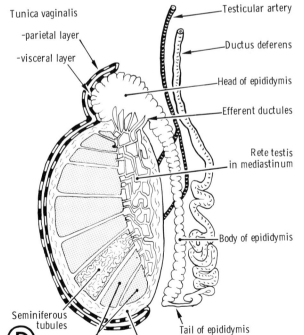

Tunica vaginalis

-parietal layer

-visceral layer

Testicular artery

Ductus deferens

Head of epididymis

Efferent ductules

Rete testis in mediastinum

Body of epididymis

Seminiferous tubules

Lobules (empty)

Tunica albuginea

Tail of epididymis

TESTIS & EPIDIDYMIS
TRANSVERSE SECTION

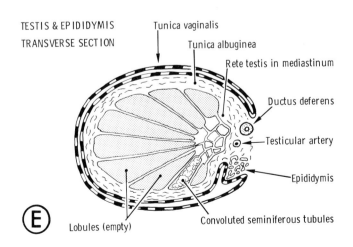

Tunica vaginalis

Tunica albuginea

Rete testis in mediastinum

Ductus deferens

Testicular artery

Epididymis

Lobules (empty)

Convoluted seminiferous tubules

211

The main structures within the cord are the following.

1. *The ductus deferens* (see above) has a thick muscular wall around a narrow lumen, and is consequently easily palpable through the scrotal skin as a firm cord-like structure (**A**).
2. *The testicular artery* is one of the bilateral branches of the abdominal aorta and arises high up that vessel in front of the disc between L1 and L2 (**231C, 259A**). After passing down the posterior abdominal wall and through the deep inguinal ring it travels down the spermatic cord (**A**) to the testis and epididymis.
3. *The pampiniform plexus of veins* returns the venous blood from the testis and epididymis, and forms the main bulk of the spermatic cord (**A**). Passing through the deep inguinal ring, the plexus is reduced to one or two veins which ascend along the posterior abdominal wall (**259A**). The testicular veins drain asymmetrically. The right vein joins the inferior vena cava while the left passes into the left renal vein (**237A**).
4. The genital branch of the genitofemoral nerve has already been observed on the posterior abdominal wall (**205C**). In the cord it innervates the cremaster muscle fibres.
5. Lymphatic vessels which drain the testis and epididymis traverse the spermatic cord and pass through the deep inguinal ring into the abdominal cavity.

The inguinal canal

The inguinal canal, which is of clinical importance as a frequent site of herniae (see below), is the track along which the spermatic cord, or its homologue in the female, passes obliquely through the abdominal wall from the deep inguinal ring in the transversalis fascia to the superficial inguinal ring in the external oblique aponeurosis. In adults the canal is about 4 cm long. In children it is shorter and less oblique, while in infants the two rings are almost superimposed.

1. The floor, on which the spermatic cord rests, consists of the medial half of the grooved upper surface of the inguinal ligament and the lacunar ligament.
2. The posterior wall is deficient laterally at the deep inguinal ring; in the central part of the canal it is formed by the transversalis fascia and the inferior epigastric artery; medially it consists of the conjoint tendon lying in front of the transversalis fascia (**B**).
3. The anterior wall is formed at its lateral end by the lowest fibres of internal oblique and the aponeurosis of external oblique: its middle part consists of the aponeurosis of external oblique alone; medially it is deficient at the superficial inguinal ring (**B**).
4. The fibres of internal oblique and transversus abdominis arch above the spermatic cord, from the

plane of the anterior wall of the canal to that of its posterior wall, forming what can be regarded as a roof (**B**).

Because of the presence of the two inguinal rings the canal is potentially weak in response to intra-abdominal pressure. However, this weakness is mitigated by the apposition of each ring to the strongest part of the apposing wall of the canal (**B**). The deep inguinal ring faces the double layered lateral end of the anterior wall of the canal formed by internal oblique and the aponeurosis of external oblique, while the superficial ring is backed by the two layers of the conjoint tendon and the transversalis fascia (**B**).

Inguinal herniae

The most common type of hernia observed in clinical practice are those associated with the inguinal region. They are of two distinct types.

Oblique (indirect) inguinal herniae usually occur in young people and more often in males than in females. The peritoneum of the anterior abdominal wall protrudes as a sac through the deep inguinal ring and thus comes to lie within the concentric fascial coverings of the spermatic cord or its female homologue, and usually in front of the normal contents of the cord (**C**). The sac varies in length in different cases. It may be restricted to the inguinal canal, or may traverse the superficial inguinal ring and pass into the scrotum or the major labium. It is an important diagnostic feature at operation that, because the sac traverses the deep inguinal ring, its neck is usually narrow and always lies lateral to the inferior epigastric artery (**C**).

Most, indeed perhaps all, oblique inguinal herniae are due to a congenital defect. During development the deep inguinal ring and the inguinal canal are traversed in both sexes by a tubular process of peritoneum, the processus vaginalis, before either the testis or the ovary has migrated from the posterior abdominal wall to its definitive position (**D**). In the male the testis 'slides' along the processus into the scrotum during the seventh month of intrauterine life (**E**).

Thereafter the processus becomes obliterated except for its terminal part, which persists throughout life as the tunica vaginalis (see above) (**F**). In females the ovary never becomes associated with the processus vaginalis, as it migrates into the pelvic cavity, and the whole processus vaginalis is normally obliterated.

Obliteration of the processus vaginalis may fail to a greater or lesser degree, leaving a persistent peritoneal sac into which abdominal viscera may be forced by a sudden rise in intra-abdominal pressure (**G**). Frequently, although a sac is present from birth, an adequate rise in pressure, and the consequent development of an evident hernia, does not occur until early adult life.

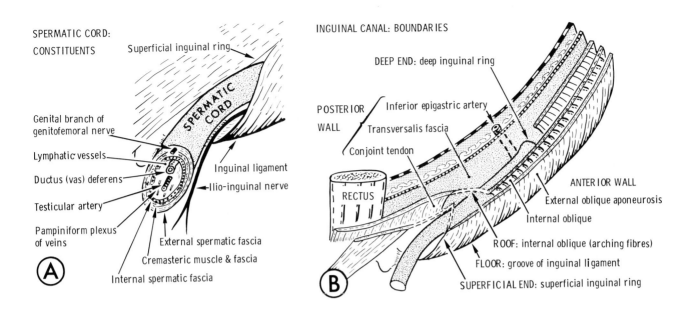

SPERMATIC CORD: CONSTITUENTS

Superficial inguinal ring

SPERMATIC CORD

Genital branch of genitofemoral nerve
Lymphatic vessels
Ductus (vas) deferens
Testicular artery
Pampiniform plexus of veins

Inguinal ligament
Ilio-inguinal nerve

External spermatic fascia
Cremasteric muscle & fascia
Internal spermatic fascia

Ⓐ

INGUINAL CANAL: BOUNDARIES

DEEP END: deep inguinal ring

POSTERIOR WALL
Inferior epigastric artery
Transversalis fascia
Conjoint tendon

RECTUS

ANTERIOR WALL
External oblique aponeurosis
Internal oblique

ROOF: internal oblique (arching fibres)
FLOOR: groove of inguinal ligament
SUPERFICIAL END: superficial inguinal ring

Ⓑ

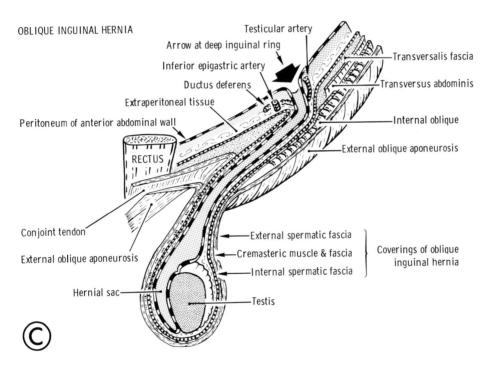

OBLIQUE INGUINAL HERNIA

Testicular artery
Arrow at deep inguinal ring
Inferior epigastric artery
Ductus deferens
Extraperitoneal tissue
Peritoneum of anterior abdominal wall

Transversalis fascia
Transversus abdominis
Internal oblique
External oblique aponeurosis

RECTUS

Conjoint tendon
External oblique aponeurosis

Hernial sac

External spermatic fascia
Cremasteric muscle & fascia
Internal spermatic fascia
} Coverings of oblique inguinal hernia

Testis

Ⓒ

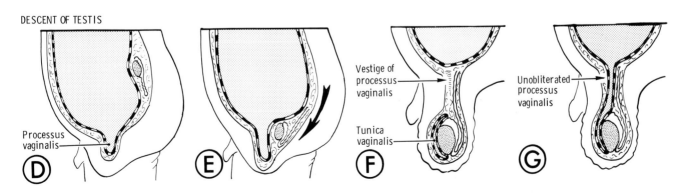

DESCENT OF TESTIS

Processus vaginalis

Ⓓ

Ⓔ

Vestige of processus vaginalis
Tunica vaginalis

Ⓕ

Unobliterated processus vaginalis

Ⓖ

If obliteration fails completely the hernial contents descend into the tunica vaginalis in the scrotum or into the major labium. On the other hand obliteration may occur in the middle part of the processus but fail in its upper part: the hernia is then confined to the inguinal canal. These are sometimes called 'complete' or 'incomplete' oblique inguinal hernia depending upon the degree of failure of obliteration.

Sometimes the normal obliteration of the processus vaginalis fails only over a short segment above the middle of the spermatic cord. The persistent segment may fill with fluid at any age, producing a tense cyst known as a hydrocele of the cord.

Direct inguinal herniae usually occur in the elderly, and are due to the association of a chronic rise of intra-abdominal pressure and senile degeneration of the fibrous structures in the posterior wall of the inguinal canal. In this case the hernial sac is a wide bulge of peritoneum through the posterior wall of the canal, between the lateral margin of the rectus abdominis and the inferior epigastric vessels (**A**). Thus, in contrast to an oblique inguinal hernia, the neck of a direct hernia is wide and lies medial to the inferior epigastric vessels.

According to its exact position a direct hernia pushes either the transversalis fascia alone, or both this fascia and the attenuated conjoint tendon, into the medial part of the inguinal canal behind the spermatic cord or its female homologue. As it enlarges it may bulge a short distance through the superficial inguinal ring on the medial side of the cord, both structures being covered by external spermatic fascia.

The nerves of the anterior and lateral abdominal walls

Both the nerves and the deep vessels of these parts of the abdominal wall run the greater parts of their courses round the body wall in a neurovascular plane between transversus abdominis and internal oblique (**B**).

The seventh, eighth, ninth, tenth and eleventh intercostal nerves enter this plane by passing from the corresponding intercostal spaces, deep to the costal cartilages and between the adjacent costal digitations of origin of transversus abdominis. The subcostal and the iliohypogastric nerves have already been observed entering the substance of the thoracolumbar fascia (**205C**). Thereafter, they enter the abdominal neurovascular plane between the two muscles which arise from that fascia. The ilio-inguinal nerve passes from iliacus (**205C**) back across the iliac crest on to the deep surface of transversus abdominis, which it pierces to enter the neurovascular plane. The nerves pass forwards round the abdominal wall with different obliquities and end by supplying successive areas of skin over the rectus abdominis.

1. The seventh and eighth intercostal nerves emerge from their intercostal spaces behind the upper part of rectus abdominis and consequently enter the neurovascular plane in the uppermost part of the posterior wall of the rectus sheath (**D**). They are directed upwards and medially and pierce in succession the posterior lamina of the aponeurosis of internal oblique (**D**), rectus abdominis and the anterior rectus sheath wall, before emerging as anterior cutaneous branches (**C**).

2. The ninth, tenth, and eleventh intercostals and the subcostal nerve reach the neurovascular plane at increasing distances lateral to rectus abdominis, and run in the plane to the lateral border of the rectus sheath, the ninth following a horizontal course while the others incline downwards. The subcostal nerve reaches the rectus sheath just above the level of the arcuate line. Note the manner in which these nerves then traverse rectus abdominis and its sheath to become cutaneous (**E**). The tenth intercostal usually supplies the skin around the umbilicus (**C**).

3. The iliohypogastric nerve leaves the neurovascular plane by piercing the muscle fibres of internal oblique well lateral to the rectus sheath, about 2 cm medial to the anterior superior iliac spine (**C**). After continuing downwards and medially between the internal and external oblique aponeuroses (**F**), it becomes cutaneous a short distance above the superficial inguinal ring (**C**).

4. The ilio-inguinal nerve passes through internal oblique a little below and lateral to the iliohypogastric and travels medially and downwards along the inguinal canal, lying below or anterior to, and separate from, the spermatic cord or the round ligament of the uterus (**213A**). Knowledge of its position is important in any operation on the inguinal canal. The nerve emerges through the superficial inguinal ring and supplies cutaneous branches to the area of skin shown in **C**.

Lateral branches of large size arise from all the nerves of the anterior abdominal wall, except the ilio-inguinal, and pierce the overlying muscles in series along the midaxillary line (**C**). In the superficial fascia those derived from each of the lower intercostal nerves divide into anterior and posterior divisions which supply a long oblique strip of skin. This extends downwards and forwards round the body wall between the area supplied by the anterior cutaneous branch in front and that supplied by the corresponding dorsal ramus behind (**205B**). Complete oblique semicircular strips of skin are thus innervated by branches of single spinal nerves and are called dermatomes.

The lateral branches of the subcostal and iliohypogastric nerves do not innervate abdominal skin. They enter the superficial fascia just above the anterior part of the iliac crest (**C**) and descend to supply skin areas below the anterior superior iliac spine.

DIRECT INGUINAL HERNIA IN TRANSVERSE SECTION

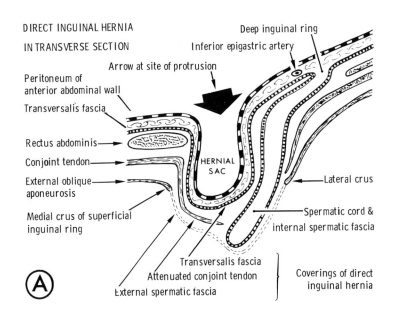

Deep inguinal ring

Inferior epigastric artery

Arrow at site of protrusion

Peritoneum of anterior abdominal wall

Transversalis fascia

Rectus abdominis

Conjoint tendon

External oblique aponeurosis

Medial crus of superficial inguinal ring

HERNIAL SAC

Lateral crus

Spermatic cord & internal spermatic fascia

Transversalis fascia
Attenuated conjoint tendon
External spermatic fascia

Coverings of direct inguinal hernia

(A)

NERVES OF ANTERIOR & LATERAL ABDOMINAL WALLS GENERAL PLAN

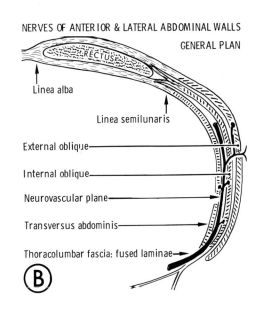

RECTUS

Linea alba

Linea semilunaris

External oblique

Internal oblique

Neurovascular plane

Transversus abdominis

Thoracolumbar fascia: fused laminae

(B)

CUTANEOUS NERVES: DERMATOMES

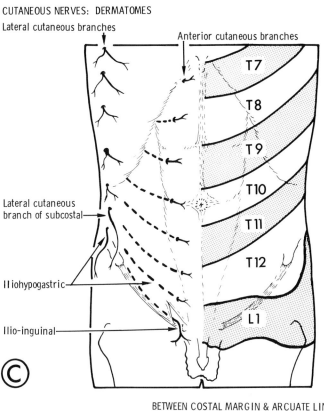

Lateral cutaneous branches

Anterior cutaneous branches

T7
T8
T9
T10
T11
T12
L1

Lateral cutaneous branch of subcostal

Iliohypogastric

Ilio-inguinal

(C)

ARRANGEMENT AT COSTAL MARGIN

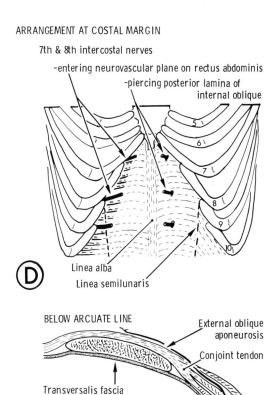

7th & 8th intercostal nerves

—entering neurovascular plane on rectus abdominis

—piercing posterior lamina of internal oblique

5
6
7
8
9
10

Linea alba

Linea semilunaris

(D)

BETWEEN COSTAL MARGIN & ARCUATE LINE

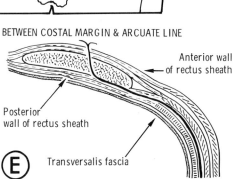

Anterior wall of rectus sheath

Posterior wall of rectus sheath

Transversalis fascia

(E)

BELOW ARCUATE LINE

External oblique aponeurosis

Conjoint tendon

Transversalis fascia

Iliohypogastric (L1)

(F)

Innervation of the anterior abdominal muscles reflects the courses of the nerves described above.

1. All the nerves lie between internal oblique and transversus abdominis and all contribute to the nerve supply of both muscles.
2. Rectus abdominis is supplied by the lower intercostal and subcostal nerves which traverse it (**215E**), but not by the iliohypogastric and ilio-inguinal nerves which do not come into contact with the muscle (**215F**).
3. The external oblique is supplied mainly by the lateral branches of the lower intercostal nerves, which are in close relationship to its outer surface, but not by the lateral branches of the subcostal and iliohypogastric nerves which descend into the thigh.

The vessels of the anterior and lateral abdominal walls

The deep vessels consist of two groups which anastomose with each other in the region of the rectus sheath.

1. Numerous branches of the lumbar and lower intercostal arteries, accompanied by veins, encircle the abdominal wall in the neurovascular plane, in close association with the nerves described above. They are not of individual importance.
2. On the other hand the exact anatomical courses of the superior and inferior epigastric arteries with their venae comitantes are surgically important.

The superior epigastric artery arises as a terminal branch of the internal thoracic artery (**139A**). It immediately passes downwards, between the sternal and costal origins of the diaphragm and over the upper borders of transversus abdominis and the posterior lamina of the internal oblique aponeurosis, into the rectus sheath (**A**). It lies first behind the rectus abdominis and then continues downwards within the upper quarter of the muscle.

The inferior epigastric artery, which is considerably larger than the superior epigastric, arises from the external iliac artery. It crosses the posterior wall of the inguinal canal and continues upwards and medially deep to the transversalis fascia, first behind the conjoint tendon and then behind the lower quarter of rectus abdominis (**211C**). At this point it pierces the transversalis fascia and, passing in front of the arcuate line, runs upwards in the rectus sheath (**A**). At first it lies on the posterior surface of rectus abdominis but then continues upwards in the substance of the muscle to anastomose with the superior epigastric midway between the xiphoid process and the umbilicus (**A**). The epigastric veins drain into the internal thoracic and external iliac veins.

The superficial vessels are arranged in two sets which anastomose at about the level of the umbilicus. The tissues above the umbilicus are supplied by the lateral thoracic branch of the axillary artery (**509A**), while those below the umbilicus receive the superficial epigastric branch of the femoral artery which runs upwards over the inguinal ligament (**335C**). The veins which accompany these arteries (**B**) drain into the axillary vein and the great saphenous vein (**373A**). The anastomosis between these two sets of veins, known as the thoraco-epigastric anastomosis, may allow the establishment of a collateral venous circulation if the external iliac vein is blocked.

Surface anatomy of the abdomen

The majority of structures in the abdominal cavity cannot be located distinctly through the anterior abdominal wall because of their soft consistency. Consequently, their position is usually defined by their relationship to a number of bony points which can be easily distinguished through the overlying skin. Palpate on your own body the several bony points which are indicated in **C**.

The umbilicus is also used in some instances as a landmark, but it has to be recognised that it has the disadvantage that its position is not exactly the same in all individuals. In particular it tends to be at a lower level in infants, the middle-aged, the elderly and the obese than it is in muscular young adults.

It helps in the definition of the position of abdominal structures to divide the abdomen into a number of regions. This can be done in two ways.

In **D** the projections of four planes on the anterior abdominal wall are shown. These planes divide the abdomen into nine regions. Each lateral plane is sagittal and traverses both the midpoint of the clavicle and the midpoint of the inguinal ligament. The transpyloric plane is horizontal and lies midway between the suprasternal notch and the upper border of the pubic symphysis. The transtubercular plane is also horizontal and passes through the tubercles of the iliac crests (**C**). The vertebral levels of these two horizontal lines are shown (**D**). Note the names given to the nine regions which are demarcated by the four planes.

In the alternative method, which is often used in clinical practice, the abdomen is simply divided into four quadrants by the median plane and a horizontal plane through the umbilicus.

Thus the base of the vermiform appendix can be described as being situated either in the right iliac region or in the right lower abdominal quadrant.

RECTUS SHEATH: ARTERIES

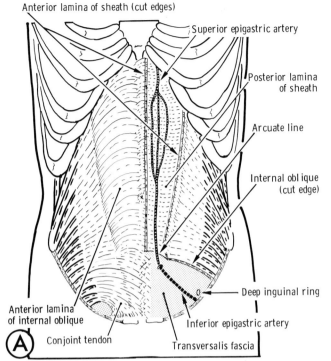

Anterior lamina of sheath (cut edges)

Superior epigastric artery

Posterior lamina of sheath

Arcuate line

Internal oblique (cut edge)

Deep inguinal ring

Inferior epigastric artery

Transversalis fascia

Anterior lamina of internal oblique

Conjoint tendon

(A)

ANTERIOR ABDOMINAL WALL: SUPERFICIAL VEINS

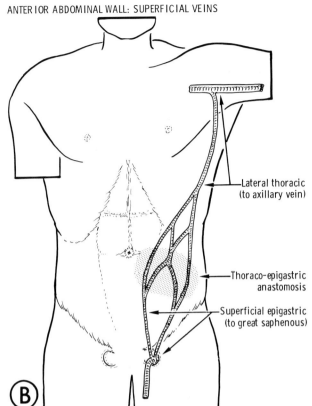

Lateral thoracic (to axillary vein)

Thoraco-epigastric anastomosis

Superficial epigastric (to great saphenous)

(B)

ABDOMEN: PALPABLE BONY POINTS

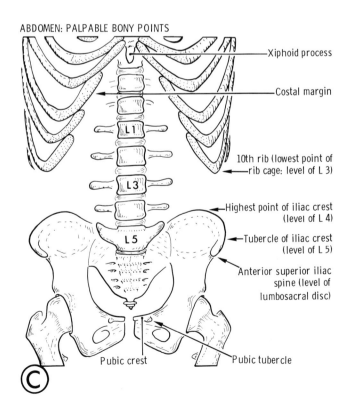

Xiphoid process

Costal margin

L 1

L 3

L 5

10th rib (lowest point of rib cage: level of L 3)

Highest point of iliac crest (level of L 4)

Tubercle of iliac crest (level of L 5)

Anterior superior iliac spine (level of lumbosacral disc)

Pubic crest

Pubic tubercle

(C)

ABDOMINAL CAVITY: PLANES & REGIONS

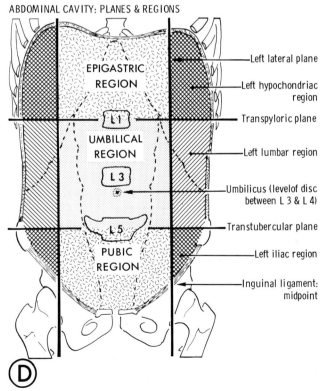

EPIGASTRIC REGION

L 1

UMBILICAL REGION

L 3

L 5

PUBIC REGION

Left lateral plane

Left hypochondriac region

Transpyloric plane

Left lumbar region

Umbilicus (level of disc between L 3 & L 4)

Transtubercular plane

Left iliac region

Inguinal ligament: midpoint

(D)

217

Abdominal incisions

An incision through the abdominal wall for the exposure of a structure in the abdominal cavity should, if possible, have certain basic characteristics.

1. It should give good access to the operation area.
2. It should avoid division of nerves where possible. However, because of the multiple nerve supply of abdominal muscles and the overlap of adjacent abdominal dermatomes, division of a single nerve usually causes no detectable paralysis or anaesthesia.
3. It should divide vascular tissues such as muscle which heal readily, rather than avascular tissues such as the linea alba which heal less firmly.
4. Where possible it should divide tissue layers parallel to the common stress trajectories, so as to avoid postoperative tension across the incision. Thus skin is preferably divided along a skin crease and muscles and aponeuroses are best split along the line of their fibres.
5. An incision should be so placed that it can be safely extended if necessary.

The more common abdominal incisions are listed below.

A paramedian incision passes through the rectus sheath (**A**), and it is helpful to revise the structure of the sheath, with particular attention to the relationship of the tendinous intersections to the anterior and posterior walls, the presence of transversus abdominis muscle fibres in the upper part of the posterior wall of the sheath, and the direct relationship of rectus abdominis to the transversalis fascia in the lower part of the sheath.

The anterior wall of the sheath is divided longitudinally. The medial margin of rectus abdominis is then freed from the sheath so that the muscle can be displaced laterally exposing the posterior wall of the sheath. As the intercostal nerves reach the rectus from its lateral side they are not damaged by this manoeuvre. The posterior wall of the sheath, the transversalis fascia, extraperitoneal tissue and peritoneum are then incised longitudinally.

In closure of such an incision, the layers behind rectus abdominis are sutured, the muscle is allowed to return to its normal position, and the anterior wall of the sheath and finally the skin and superficial fascia are sutured.

A midline incision traverses the several layers of the abdominal wall along the line of the linea alba. It has the advantage of being a quick and comparatively bloodless route into the abdominal cavity, but it heals less firmly than most other incisions, and the scar is more likely to stretch as time passes than a paramedian incision.

A gridiron incision is frequently used for operations in the right iliac region including that of appendicectomy. The skin, superficial fascia and external oblique muscle are divided in the line of the fibres of that muscle, the incision being centred over McBurney's point which is situated one-third of the distance from the anterior superior iliac spine to the umbilicus (**B**). The internal oblique and transversus abdominis muscles are split in the lines of their fibres (**C**). The transversalis fascia and peritoneum are then opened. After the operation is completed, the peritoneum and skin require suturing, but the muscle layers return naturally to their original state and healing is firm.

An incision in the loin is obliquely placed so that its posterior end is over the tip of the twelfth rib and its anterior end is as far forward as the surgeon requires (**D, E**). The muscles, thoracolumbar fascia and transversalis fascia are divided in the line of the skin incision. On the other hand, the peritoneum is stripped forwards off the posterior abdominal wall to expose the kidney or, at a lower level, the ureter or other posteriorly-placed structures (**E**).

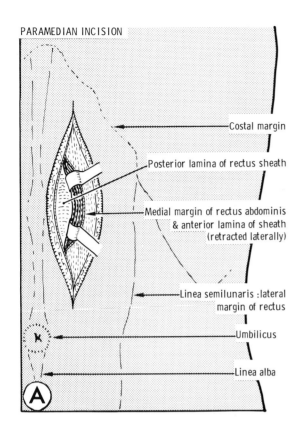

PARAMEDIAN INCISION

- Costal margin
- Posterior lamina of rectus sheath
- Medial margin of rectus abdominis & anterior lamina of sheath (retracted laterally)
- Linea semilunaris : lateral margin of rectus
- Umbilicus
- Linea alba

(A)

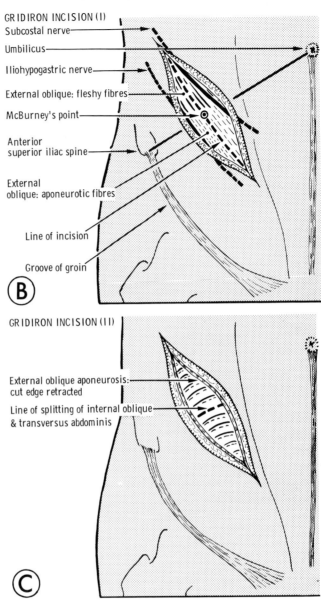

GRIDIRON INCISION (I)

- Subcostal nerve
- Umbilicus
- Iliohypogastric nerve
- External oblique: fleshy fibres
- McBurney's point
- Anterior superior iliac spine
- External oblique: aponeurotic fibres
- Line of incision
- Groove of groin

(B)

GRIDIRON INCISION (II)

- External oblique aponeurosis: cut edge retracted
- Line of splitting of internal oblique & transversus abdominis

(C)

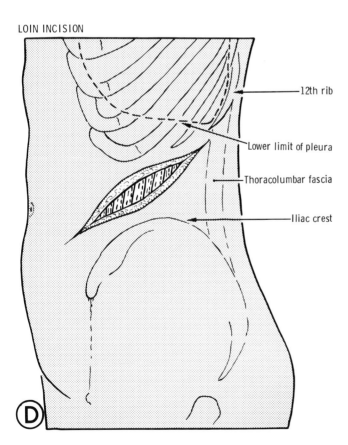

LOIN INCISION

- 12th rib
- Lower limit of pleura
- Thoracolumbar fascia
- Iliac crest

(D)

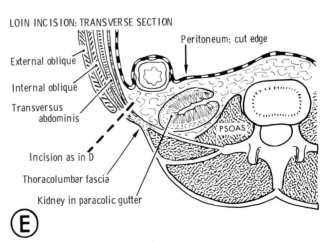

LOIN INCISION: TRANSVERSE SECTION

- Peritoneum: cut edge
- External oblique
- Internal oblique
- Transversus abdominis
- Incision as in D
- Thoracolumbar fascia
- Kidney in paracolic gutter
- PSOAS

(E)

GENERAL MORPHOLOGY OF THE VISCERA OF THE ABDOMINAL CAVITY PROPER

The kidneys, ureters and suprarenal glands are paired viscera. The spleen, the gastro-intestinal tract and the glands secreting into it, are single, unpaired structures. This section considers their shape, appearance and general position but not their exact positions of their relations.

The kidneys

Each kidney is a large, solid, bean-shaped viscus which lies against the upper part of the posterior abdominal wall (**A**). It has anterior and posterior surfaces, a convex lateral border, a concave medial border, and upper and lower poles.

The medial part of the kidney encloses a large cavity, the renal sinus, which opens through a hilus at the middle of the medial border (**B**). The wall of the sinus exhibits some fifteen conical elevations called the renal papillae. The orifices of the ducts of Bellini, through which urine leaves the kidney substance, can be seen with a magnifying glass on the surface of these papillae (**B**).

A thin, readily-detachable fibrous capsule covers the surface of the kidney, and lines the free parts of the walls of the renal sinus (**B**).

Congenital absence of one kidney occurs about once in every 2500 individuals.

The ureters

Each ureter is a muscular tube which passes down the posterior abdominal wall from the kidney, in the abdominal cavity proper, to the urinary bladder in the pelvic cavity (**A**).

The wall of the ureter contains a large amount of plain muscle, and, at operation, peristaltic contractions can sometimes be seen passing down it. These peristaltic contractions help to distinguish the ureters from other structures of similar size and position, whose normal appearances may be distorted by disease.

The greater part of the ureter has a uniform lumen, about the diameter of a match head. However, at its upper end it runs close to the lower part of the medial border of the kidney, and then turns laterally through the hilus into the renal sinus, expanding as it goes (**A**, **C**). This funnel-shaped segment is called the renal pelvis. Within the sinus,

the pelvis divides into two or three major calyces, and these divide in turn into some ten or so minor calyces. Each minor calyx is attached to the wall of the sinus so that one or two renal papillae project into its lumen (**C**).

In 3–4% of individuals there are two ureters (double ureter) on one or both sides. Most frequently, these join just short of their junction with the bladder, but they may open into the bladder separately.

The suprarenal glands

These endocrine glands are coarsely granular in texture and consist of two functionally distinct parts, namely a central medulla and a peripheral cortex (**D**). Each gland lies above the corresponding kidney, against the posterior fibres of the diaphragm. (**A**) Both are thin, with anterior and posterior surfaces and a peripheral margin, but they differ in shape and position (**A**). The right gland is roughly triangular. The left gland is shaped like an inverted comma.

The spleen

This is a firm but friable, purplish-red organ about the size of an adult fist. It lies in the upper left abdominal quadrant, deep to the lower ribs (**225A**). Functionally, it is concerned both with the lymphatic system and with the control of the circulating erythrocyte population.

It has two surfaces named diaphragmatic and visceral. These are separated by anterior and posterior ends and by an inferior border and a characteristically notched superior border (**E**). The diaphragmatic surface is smoothly convex. The visceral surface (**E**) is marked, in the fixed cadaver, by a number of gently concave impressions because of its close relationship with neighbouring viscera. In the centre of this surface is the hilus, a long fissure, through which large blood vessels enter and leave the spleen.

The gastro-intestinal tract

The oesophagus, having passed through the lower part of the neck and the thorax, enters the abdominal cavity through the oesophageal opening in the diaphragm (**201B**).

KIDNEYS & SUPRARENAL GLANDS

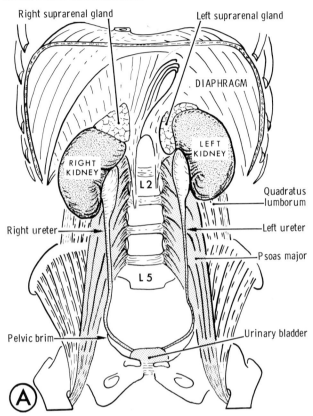

Right suprarenal gland

Left suprarenal gland

DIAPHRAGM

LEFT KIDNEY

RIGHT KIDNEY

L 2

Right ureter

Left ureter

Quadratus lumborum

Psoas major

L 5

Pelvic brim

Urinary bladder

Ⓐ

KIDNEY: LONGITUDINAL SECTION

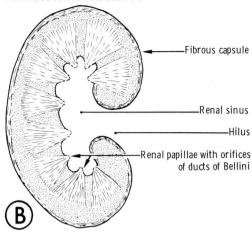

Fibrous capsule

Renal sinus

Hilus

Renal papillae with orifices of ducts of Bellini

Ⓑ

PELVIS OF URETER

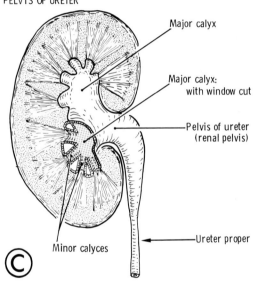

Major calyx

Major calyx: with window cut

Pelvis of ureter (renal pelvis)

Minor calyces

Ureter proper

Ⓒ

SUPRARENAL GLAND: VERTICAL SECTION

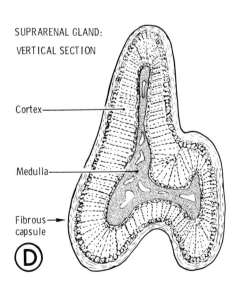

Cortex

Medulla

Fibrous capsule

Ⓓ

SPLEEN

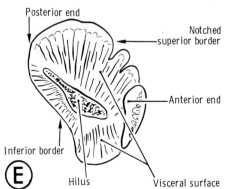

Posterior end

Notched superior border

Anterior end

Inferior border

Hilus

Visceral surface

Ⓔ

From that point the abdominal oesophagus passes down and to the left for 1.0–1.5 cm before it joins the stomach at the cardiac orifice of that viscus (**A, C**).

The muscular coat of this part of the gut consists solely of plain muscle. This is arranged as inner circular and outer longitudinal layers. Both are directly continuous with correspondingly disposed muscle fibres on the stomach wall, and there is no anatomical sphincter between the two viscera. In the absence of a sphincter it is possible that regurgitation from a full stomach is prevented by the pressure of the distended stomach fundus (see below) against the adjacent oesophagus (**A, B**).

The stomach is separated from the posterior abdominal wall by part of the serous cavity of the abdomen. Consequently, it has a considerable degree of mobility and may vary greatly in shape, size and position. However, what may be regarded as an average shape is shown in **A, B, C**.

The continuity of the stomach with the oesophagus at the cardiac orifice is easily identified (**C**). Its continuity with the duodenum at the pyloric orifice is less obvious. It is indicated visually by a slight circumferential sulcus on the surface of the viscus, and by the prepyloric vein which runs vertically across its anterior surface (**B**). At operation, it is most easily identified by palpating the junction between the very thick muscle wall of the terminal part of the stomach (**C**) and the thinner wall of the duodenum.

The viscus has anterior and posterior surfaces and two curved borders, which are traditionally named the greater and lesser curvatures (**B**). The lesser curvature is acutely angulated at its most dependent point, forming the angular notch, while opposite this feature, the greater curvature exhibits a complementary bulge (**B**).

The stomach is customarily divided into three parts. Observe the limits of the parts known as the fundus, the body and the pyloric part in **B**.

The plain muscle fibres of the stomach wall are arranged in two layers. The outer layer contains longitudinal fibres, the inner circular and a few oblique fibres. The direct continuity of both layers with correspondingly disposed fibres in the wall of the oesophagus has been noted. Traced downwards and to the right the longitudinal fibres are continuous with those of the duodenum. On the other hand, the circular layer gradually thickens through the pyloric part of the stomach and forms the thick pyloric sphincter just short of the pyloric orifice. The sphincter is demarcated from the circular muscle of the duodenum by a fibrous partition (**C**).

The small intestine runs from the stomach to the large intestine and consists of three parts, the duodenum, the jejunum and the ileum.

The duodenum, except for its first 2 cm, is fixed against the posterior abdominal wall. It consists of four parts of different lengths, set at approximately right angles to one another (**D**). The second part receives the secretions of the liver and the pancreas through the bile duct and the main and accessory pancreatic ducts (**229D**).

The jejuno-ileal segment of the small intestine is about 5 m long. Its beginning at the duodenojejunal junction (**E**) and its end at the ileocolic junction (**E**) are both fixed to the posterior abdominal wall. Between these two points the gut is freely movable within the abdominal cavity. Indeed, in the living subject peristaltic contractions in its wall, which are greatest after a meal, continually alter its position.

The jejunum is defined as the upper two-fifths and the ileum as the lower three-fifths of the jejuno-ileal segment, but there is no obvious demarcation between the two parts and in practice jejunum and ileum are used as general rather than exact terms.

The calibre of the small intestine as a whole gradually diminishes along its length. The diameter is about 4.5 cm at the beginning of the duodenum and 3.5 cm at the end of the ileum.

The plain muscle fibres of its muscular coat are arranged as uniformly disposed, outer longitudinal and inner circular layers. At the ileocoecal orifice the circular layer is slightly thickened to form a sphincter muscle which controls the passage of material from the small into the large intestine. Its mucous membrane is thrown into permanent circumferentially-orientated folds (circular folds). The folds begin about half way along the first part of the duodenum, and reach a maximum size in the terminal part of the duodenum and the upper half of the jejunum (**F**). Thereafter, the folds diminish and are almost non-existent in the lower half of the ileum (**F**). As a result of this distribution of the circular folds, the wall of the jejunum feels thicker on palpation than that of the ileum. The constantly changing position of the jejuno-ileal part of the small intestine in the abdominal cavity may make it difficult for a surgeon to tell by inspection through a small incision whether a particular loop of the bowel is jejunal or ileal. The thickness of the gut wall is one of the factors on which his decision is based.

In about 2% of the population a tubular offshoot of similar calibre to the rest of the small intestine, and about 4 cm in length, arises from the ileum rather less than a metre from the ileocolic junction. It may end freely or be attached to the umbilicus by a fibrous cord. This congenital malformation is known as a Meckel's diverticulum. It is sometimes affected by inflammatory changes which produce symptoms similar to those of appendicitis.

STOMACH: POSITION

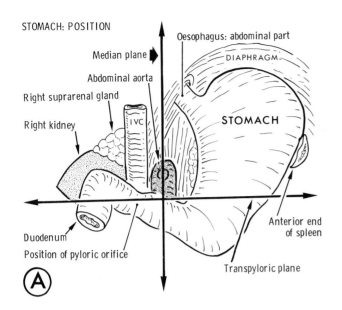

Median plane
Abdominal aorta
Right suprarenal gland
Right kidney
IVC
Oesophagus: abdominal part
DIAPHRAGM
STOMACH
Anterior end of spleen
Duodenum
Position of pyloric orifice
Transpyloric plane

A

STOMACH: PARTS

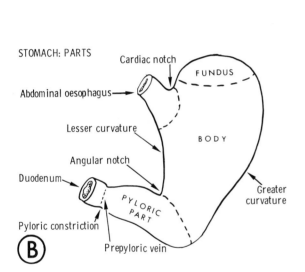

Cardiac notch
FUNDUS
Abdominal oesophagus
Lesser curvature
Angular notch
BODY
Duodenum
Pyloric constriction
PYLORIC PART
Prepyloric vein
Greater curvature

B

STOMACH: INTERIOR

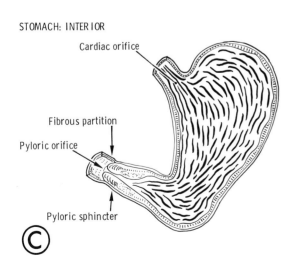

Cardiac orifice
Fibrous partition
Pyloric orifice
Pyloric sphincter

C

DUODENUM

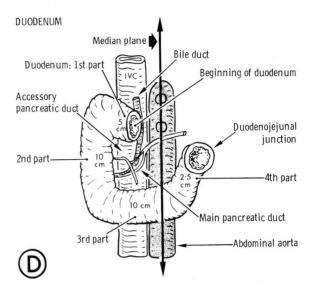

Median plane
Duodenum: 1st part
IVC
Bile duct
Beginning of duodenum
Accessory pancreatic duct
5 cm
2nd part
10 cm
Duodenojejunal junction
2·5 cm
4th part
Main pancreatic duct
3rd part
10 cm
Abdominal aorta

D

JEJUNO-ILEAL SEGMENT

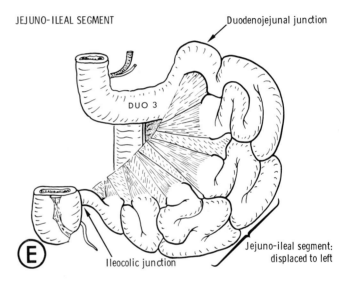

Duodenojejunal junction
DUO 3
Ileocolic junction
Jejuno-ileal segment: displaced to left

E

JEJUNUM & ILEUM: DIFFERENCES

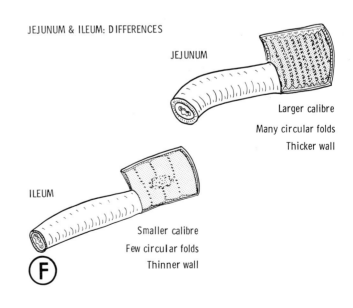

JEJUNUM
Larger calibre
Many circular folds
Thicker wall

ILEUM
Smaller calibre
Few circular folds
Thinner wall

F

223

The large intestine is only about a quarter of the length of the small intestine. It consists of several parts, and the names of these parts and their average lengths are indicated in **A**. That diagram also shows the parts which are fixed to the posterior abdominal wall (stippled) and those which are freely mobile in the abdominal cavity.

Some of the more important features of this part of the gut are listed below.

1. The caecum is a blind pouch which lies in the right iliac fossa and is continuous with the ascending colon opposite the ileocolic junction (**A**).
2. The vermiform appendix is a tubular diverticulum of the caecum of variable length arising from the upper part of its posteromedial wall (**A**).
3. The ascending colon extends up the right side of the posterior abdominal wall onto the anterior aspect of the right kidney (**A**).
4. The ascending and transverse colons are continuous at a right angle bend in front of the right kidney and just below the liver. The bend is consequently named the right or hepatic flexure (**A**).
5. The transverse colon crosses the abdominal cavity proper from right to left passing in front of the second part of the duodenum (**A**).
6. The flexure between the transverse and descending colons in front of the left kidney is much more acute and considerably higher than the left flexure. It is named the left colic flexure or, because of its proximity to the spleen, the splenic flexure (**A**).
7. The descending colon runs downwards on the left side of the posterior abdominal wall into the left iliac fossa and turns medially at its lower end. It becomes directly continuous with the sigmoid (pelvic) colon at the pelvic brim (**A**).
8. The terminal parts of the large intestine consist of the pelvic colon and rectum, both of which lie in the pelvic cavity, and the anal canal, which is situated in the perineum.
9. Clinicians sometimes use the general terms right colon and left colon, largely because, of the two regions, the left is much more frequently affected by both inflammatory and neoplastic conditions.
10. In general the muscular coat of the large intestine becomes progressively thicker in a proximodistal direction as the bowel contents become more solid. It is characteristic of this muscular coat of the abdominal part of the large intestine, but not in the pelvic cavity or perineum, that, although the circular fibres are uniformly disposed, the longitudinal fibres are aggregated into three longitudinal bands called the taeniae coli. Because the taeniae are shorter than the colon itself, the colonic wall is puckered into a series of sacculations or haustrations (**A**). Traced proximally, the three taeniae pass onto the wall of the caecum, one anteriorly and two posteriorly. They converge on the base of the vermiform appendix and thereafter form a uniform longitudinal muscle layer along the length of the appendix. This relationship may be of considerable assistance in finding the appendix at operation if the viscus is obscured as a result of inflammation.

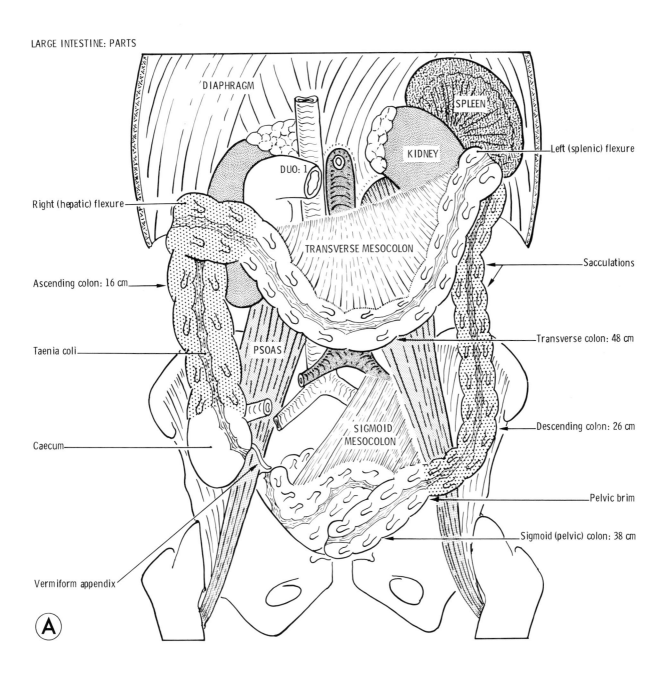

DIAPHRAGM

SPLEEN

KIDNEY

DUO: 1

Left (splenic) flexure

Right (hepatic) flexure

TRANSVERSE MESOCOLON

Sacculations

Ascending colon: 16 cm

Transverse colon: 48 cm

Taenia coli

PSOAS

Descending colon: 26 cm

SIGMOID MESOCOLON

Caecum

Pelvic brim

Sigmoid (pelvic) colon: 38 cm

Vermiform appendix

Ⓐ

The liver

The liver is a large gland which, being of soft consistency and surrounded by only a thin capsule, is easily lacerated by external violence.

Amongst other functions, it secretes bile through a system of ducts into the second part of the duodenum.

It lies within the concavity of the diaphragm, mainly in the upper right abdominal quadrant but extending to a lesser extent across the median plane into the upper left quadrant (**C**). It is relatively a good deal larger in the infant than in the adult.

The viscus is approximately conical, its base facing to the right and its apex to the left. It has four surfaces. The superior, anterior and right surfaces are moulded against the under surface of the diaphragm and are consequently convex, and smoothly continuous with one another (**A**). The posterior surface (**B**) is deeply concave where it crosses the median prominence of the lumbar part of the diaphragm (**E**) while the inferior surface faces downwards and backwards. The inferior surface is separated from the anterior and right surfaces by a thin sharp inferior border (**B**). On the other hand, although the right part of the border separating the inferior and posterior surfaces is clearly defined by neighbouring features, its left part is to be regarded as notional (**B**).

Examine the central parts of the posterior and inferior surfaces of the liver (**B**, **E**) and observe the following features.

1. The sharply depressed, oval area on the inferior surface, through which blood vessels enter the liver and the bile ducts leave it (**E**). This is the porta hepatis and the following two features diverge from its left end.
2. The ligamentum teres runs forwards across the inferior surface and border, and thereafter continues downwards close to the anterior abdominal wall to reach the umbilicus (**E**, **A**). It is a solid fibrous cord formed by obliteration of the umbilical vein soon after birth (**211**). However, even in the adult it is accompanied by minute veins, called the para-umbilical veins, which are of clinical importance (**252**).
3. The fissure for the ligamentum venosum runs upwards across the posterior surface of the liver (**B**). It bites deeply into the liver substance, first forwards and then to the right (**D**). Note the L-like relationship of this fissure on the posterior surface to the porta hepatis on the inferior surface (**B**, **E**). In the depth of the fissure lies a second fibrous cord, the ligamentum venosum. This is formed by the obliteration of the ductus venosus, a large vessel which shunts blood past the liver from the umbilical vein to the inferior vena cava during much of foetal life (**253D**).

4. The gall bladder is grey-blue in life, but in the cadaver it becomes stained green by the bile it contains. It is a pear-shaped sac, the main part or body lying against the inferior surface of the liver (**E**). The narrow neck passes into the right end of the porta hepatis and the fundus projects forwards just beyond the inferior border (**A**).
5. A deep, wide and vertically-disposed groove is situated on the posterior surface of the liver. It contains the upper part of the inferior vena cava and is named accordingly (**B**, **D**). The numerous hepatic veins, by which blood leaves the liver, run through the wall of the groove to open into the vena cava (**233A**).

The liver is customarily divided into a number of named regions which are defined below. It has to be stressed that these regions are purely convenient morphological entities which have no distinct functional significance. The physiological lobes of the liver will be discussed later (**254**).

1. The lines of the ligamentum teres and ligamentum venosum traditionally demarcate a large right lobe from a small left lobe (**B**, **E**).
2. The term quadrate lobe refers to that part of the inferior surface of the right lobe which is bounded by the porta hepatis, the gall bladder, the ligamentum teres and the inferior margin of the liver (**E**).
3. The term caudate lobe refers to the convex part of the posterior surface of the right lobe which is situated between the fissure for the ligamentum venosum and the groove for the inferior vena cava (**B**, **D**). Note in **D** that, because of the depth and orientation of the fissure for the ligamentum venosum, the caudate lobe has anterior and left surfaces as well as a posterior surface.
4. The caudate process is a narrow ridge running transversely across the inferior surface of the right lobe between the porta hepatis in front and the lower end of the groove for the inferior vena cava behind (**B**). Note in particular the L-shaped continuity of the caudate lobe on the posterior surface of the liver and the caudate process on the inferior surface.

It is a useful exercise, at this time, to study the sagittal section of the liver shown in **229A** and to note the interrelationship of the several features which it traverses.

Much of the inferior surface and some of the posterior surface of the liver are closely related to other abdominal viscera. In life the softer substance of the liver is moulded by these relationships, and when the liver is fixed in the cadaver, this moulding becomes permanent and is seen as a number of concave impressions. The positions of these impressions should be studied in **B**, **E**.

LIVER: ANTERIOR SURFACE

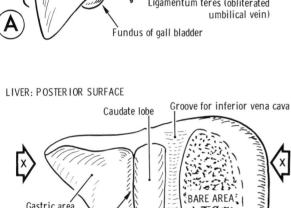

Base

RIGHT LOBE

LEFT LOBE

Apex

Inferior border

Ligamentum teres (obliterated umbilical vein)

Fundus of gall bladder

A

LIVER: POSTERIOR SURFACE

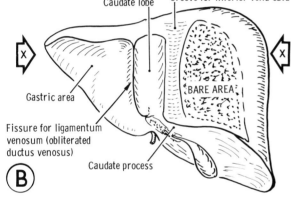

Caudate lobe

Groove for inferior vena cava

X

Gastric area

BARE AREA

X

Fissure for ligamentum venosum (obliterated ductus venosus)

Caudate process

B

LIVER: SURFACE PROJECTION

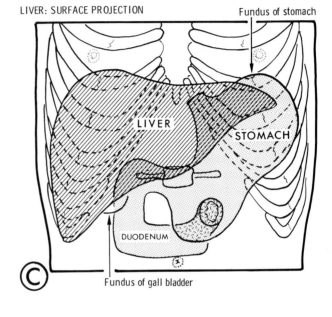

Fundus of stomach

LIVER

STOMACH

DUODENUM

Fundus of gall bladder

C

LIVER: SECTIONED AT X-X ABOVE

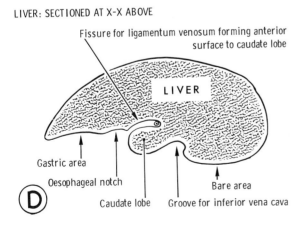

Fissure for ligamentum venosum forming anterior surface to caudate lobe

LIVER

Gastric area

Oesophageal notch

Caudate lobe

Groove for inferior vena cava

Bare area

D

LIVER: INFERIOR SURFACE

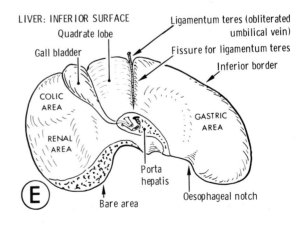

Quadrate lobe

Gall bladder

Ligamentum teres (obliterated umbilical vein)

Fissure for ligamentum teres

Inferior border

COLIC AREA

RENAL AREA

GASTRIC AREA

Porta hepatis

Bare area

Oesophageal notch

E

The pancreas

The pancreas is a large gland of soft granular texture which lies obliquely across the central convexity of the posterior abdominal wall from the left to the right kidney (**B**). The left end is at an appreciably higher level than the right. The gland is customarily divided into several parts as indicated in **B**. Note particularly the following features.

1. The uncinate process is part of the head and projects to the left in front of the abdominal aorta below the neck and body.
2. The neck is so named because it is thinner from before backwards than the body. This cannot be seen when the gland is viewed from in front.
3. The tail of the gland turns forwards from the anterior surface of the left kidney to reach the hilus of the spleen (**239E**).

The pancreas consists of two types of glandular tissue. The islets of Langerhans which are diffusely scattered throughout the gland are endocrine in nature. The greater part of the gland is exocrine, and secretes digestive enzymes into the second part of the duodenum through a duct system.

The excretory ducts of the liver and pancreas

These two duct systems differ greatly in their length outside the viscera they drain. The bile ducts have a long extrahepatic course whereas the pancreatic ducts are almost entirely contained within the pancreas.

In the case of the liver, right and left hepatic ducts issue through the porta hepatis (**C**). They are very short and unite, near the right end of the porta hepatis, to form the common hepatic duct. This runs downwards from the liver and has a length of about 3 cm. The position of the gall bladder and the relationship of its neck to the right end of the porta hepatis has been described already (**226**). In this situation the neck becomes continuous with the cystic duct which passes downwards and somewhat to the left in an increasingly close association with the common hepatic duct. The cystic duct eventually joins the common hepatic duct to form the bile duct.

The bile duct is about 7 cm long. It runs in a continuous curve downwards and to the right, behind the first part of the duodenum and the head of the pancreas (**C, D**) before entering the second part of the duodenum in common with the main pancreatic duct (see below).

The exocrine part of the pancreas excretes through a main and an accessory duct, both of which receive tributaries in herring-bone fashion throughout their lengths.

The main duct traverses the gland from left to right, sinking abruptly to a lower level as it enters the head (**D**). Within that part it inclines backwards to the posterior surface of the gland where it lies immediately below the bile duct (see above). The two ducts reach the posteromedial aspect of the middle of the second part of the duodenum, and pass through the muscular coat into the submucosa. Here they unite to form a short common channel named the hepatopancreatic ampulla (**C, D**). The constricted end of the ampulla opens on the summit of a mucosal eminence called the major duodenal papilla (**D**).

An accessory pancreatic duct begins in the lower part of the head of the pancreas. It runs upwards and to the right in front of the main duct, with which it usually communicates, to open into the upper part of the second part of the duodenum on the summit of the minor duodenal papilla (**D**).

In the wall of the gall bladder the mucous layer is surrounded by a fibromuscular coat in which fibrous tissue is mixed with smooth muscle fibres. Except at their termination the large biliary ducts contain considerably less smooth muscle; indeed such fibres appear to be almost or entirely absent in most individuals. At the terminations of the bile duct and main pancreatic duct, and in the region of the hepatopancreatic ampulla, the situation is different. In all subjects an involuntary sphincter surrounds the terminal part of the bile duct (sphincter choledochus), and sphincter muscles around the main pancreatic duct and the ampulla are present in a proportion of individuals.

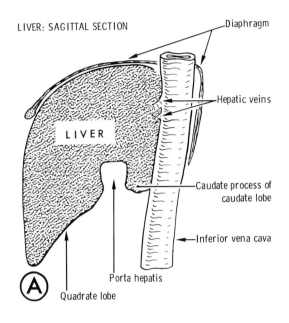

LIVER: SAGITTAL SECTION

Diaphragm

Hepatic veins

LIVER

Caudate process of
caudate lobe

Inferior vena cava

Porta hepatis

A

Quadrate lobe

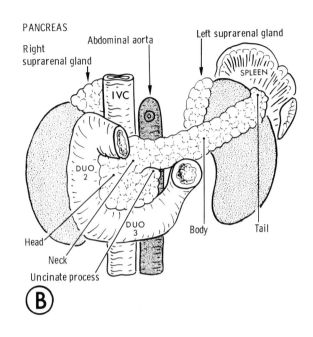

PANCREAS

Right
suprarenal gland

Abdominal aorta

Left suprarenal gland

IVC

SPLEEN

DUO
2

DUO
3

Body

Tail

Head

Neck

Uncinate process

B

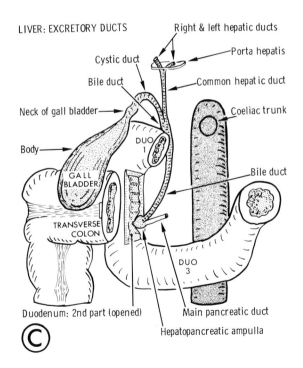

LIVER: EXCRETORY DUCTS

Right & left hepatic ducts

Cystic duct

Porta hepatis

Bile duct

Common hepatic duct

Neck of gall bladder

Coeliac trunk

DUO
1

Body

GALL
BLADDER

Bile duct

TRANSVERSE
COLON

DUO
3

Duodenum: 2nd part (opened)

Main pancreatic duct

Hepatopancreatic ampulla

C

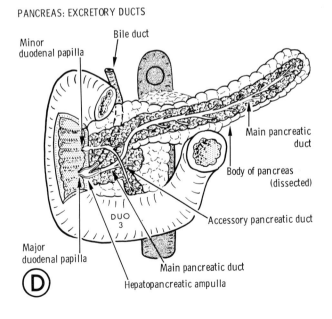

PANCREAS: EXCRETORY DUCTS

Minor
duodenal papilla

Bile duct

Main pancreatic
duct

Body of pancreas
(dissected)

Accessory pancreatic duct

DUO
3

Major
duodenal papilla

Main pancreatic duct

Hepatopancreatic ampulla

D

Foregut, midgut and hindgut

During early foetal life the digestive tube lies entirely in the midline and consists of three segments named the foregut, the midgut and the hindgut (**A**).

The arrangement of the definitive digestive tract is, of course, much more complex and certain glands, particularly the liver and pancreas, have developed as outgrowths from it. But it can still be divided into three parts which have been derived from the primitive segments (**B**).

Because the blood supply, lymph drainage and nerve supply of these three definitive parts of the gut and the glands developed from it follow distinctive pathways, it is important that their composition, shown in **B** should be memorised. Note particularly that, although the greater part of the pancreas is formed as an outgrowth from the foregut, the lower part of the head including the uncinate process is derived from the midgut.

The visceral arteries

The viscera of the abdominal cavity proper are supplied by three sets of paired branches, and three unpaired branches, of the abdominal aorta (**C**).

The paired and unpaired branches are to be regarded as distinct arterial systems which supply different groups of viscera and do not anastomose appreciably with one another.

The paired branches supply the paired viscera, namely, the suprarenal glands, kidneys and ureters. It is convenient to note here that similar paired branches of the abdominal aorta also supply the gonads, because, although neither the testes nor the ovaries are definitively situated in the abdominal cavity proper, both originally develop in that region.

The three unpaired branches supply the unpaired viscera, namely, the gastro-intestinal tract, liver, pancreas and spleen. Developmentally, these are the arteries of the foregut (coeliac artery), midgut (superior mesenteric artery) and hindgut (inferior mesenteric artery) and it is helpful to appreciate that when development is complete they are still distributed strictly to those parts of the gut derived from the three primitive segments (**A, C**).

The visceral branches of the abdominal aorta, together with the phrenic and lumbar arteries which are distributed to the body wall, are shown in **C**. Note the names of the vessels, the order in which they arise and the relationship of their origins to the lumbar vertebral bodies.

Because numerous large branches arise in the region of L1 the aorta suddenly narrows beyond that level. In the thorax the arch of the aorta also narrows suddenly immediately beyond the origin of the three large arteries to

the head, neck and upper limbs. The parts of the aorta just distal to these two constrictions are the most common sites of aortic aneurysm.

The venous drainage of the viscera

It has been seen that the paired and unpaired viscera are supplied by territorially distinct, paired and unpaired branches of the abdominal aorta. The venous drainages of these two groups of viscera are even more distinct.

Systemic veins

The inferior vena cava, which is the main systemic vein in the abdominal cavity proper, does not drain directly any part of the gastrointestinal tract. Its tributaries can be divided into three groups (**D**).

1. The phrenic and lumbar veins which drain much of the deep tissues of the abdominal wall.
2. The veins draining the paired abdominal viscera, that is the suprarenal glands, kidneys, ureters, and gonads. Note that the right suprarenal and gonadal veins drain directly into the vena cava, whereas the corresponding veins on the left side drain into the vena cava indirectly, through the left renal vein.
3. The hepatic veins enter the upper part of the vena cava carrying the blood from the liver sinusoids (see below).

Portal venous system

The portal venous system (**233A**) transports all the venous blood from the gastro-intestinal tract, liver, pancreas and spleen, that is, those viscera supplied by the unpaired branches of the abdominal aorta. Veins from these viscera converge on the large portal vein. This passes upwards and divides into right and left branches which enter the substance of the liver through the porta hepatis. In the liver these branches divide into progressively smaller vessels which finally open into the capillary-like liver sinusoids. The sinusoids converge on the hepatic veins which open into the inferior vena cava as it lies in the groove on the posterior surface of the liver.

Thus in the portal system, the blood passes through two sets of exchange vessels, namely, the capillaries in the viscera which the system drains and the hepatic sinusoids.

Unlike most veins neither the portal vein nor its tributaries have valves.

Physiologically the portal venous system carries much of the nutrient material absorbed from the gut to the liver, where it is extracted from the blood and metabolised.

DIGESTIVE TUBE:
DEVELOPMENTAL SEGMENTS (I)

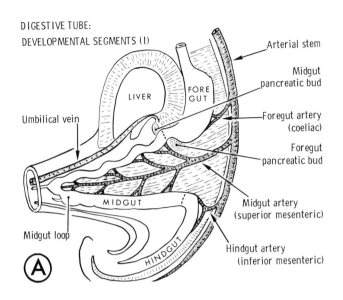

Arterial stem

Midgut pancreatic bud

Foregut artery (coeliac)

Foregut pancreatic bud

Midgut artery (superior mesenteric)

Hindgut artery (inferior mesenteric)

LIVER

FORE GUT

MIDGUT

HINDGUT

Umbilical vein

Midgut loop

(A)

DIGESTIVE TUBE:
DEVELOPMENTAL SEGMENTS (II)

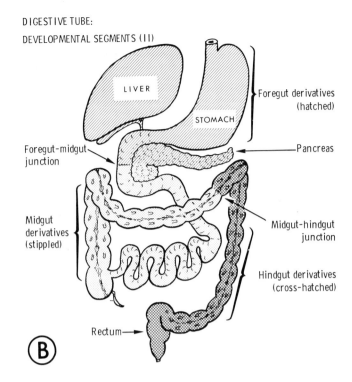

LIVER

STOMACH

Foregut derivatives (hatched)

Pancreas

Foregut-midgut junction

Midgut derivatives (stippled)

Midgut-hindgut junction

Hindgut derivatives (cross-hatched)

Rectum

(B)

ABDOMINAL AORTA

PARIETAL BRANCHES

VISCERAL BRANCHES

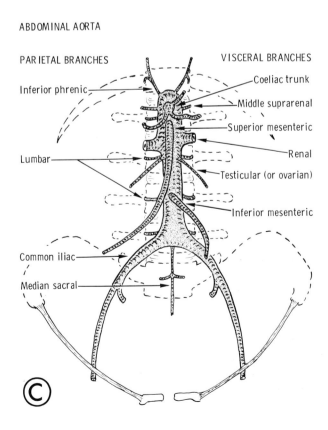

Inferior phrenic

Lumbar

Common iliac

Median sacral

Coeliac trunk

Middle suprarenal

Superior mesenteric

Renal

Testicular (or ovarian)

Inferior mesenteric

(C)

VENOUS DRAINAGE: SYSTEMIC

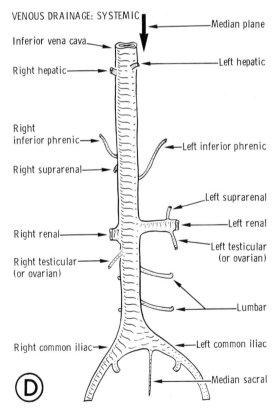

Median plane

Inferior vena cava

Right hepatic

Left hepatic

Right inferior phrenic

Left inferior phrenic

Right suprarenal

Left suprarenal

Left renal

Right renal

Left testicular (or ovarian)

Right testicular (or ovarian)

Lumbar

Right common iliac

Left common iliac

Median sacral

(D)

In large measure the portal and systemic venous systems in the abdomen are quite separate from each other until the junction of the hepatic veins with the inferior vena cava, but at a few sites, called portosystemic anastomoses, the terminal radicles of the two systems are in continuity.

In certain conditions the flow of blood from the portal system through the liver to the inferior vena cava may be obstructed, either by obstruction of the hepatic sinusoidal blood flow as a result of liver disease (e.g. hepatic cirrhosis) or by thrombosis in the portal vein itself or some of its tributaries. In these circumstances the pressure in the portal system rises (portal hypertension), plasma leaks through the walls of the portal vessels into the peritoneal cavity (ascites) and at the same time the obstructed blood leaks back to the systemic veins through the portosystemic anastomoses causing dilatation and varicosity of the anastomotic channels. Haemorrhage may occur from some of these distended vessels, especially those in the wall of the abdominal oesophagus (**252**).

One form of surgical treatment of portal obstruction is by joining the divided portal vein to the side of the inferior vena cava (**A**) below the liver (portacaval shunt), or by joining tributaries of these major vessels such as the splenic vein and the left renal vein (splenorenal shunt) (**237C**).

General features of the peritoneum

The peritoneum is a serous membrane which forms a complicated sac within the abdomen. The free surface of the membrane is formed by a single layer of flattened mesothelial cells. In life it is covered by a thin layer of fluid and consequently appears smooth and glistening.

Part of the peritoneum lines the deep aspect of the abdominal fascial envelope (**B, C**) and constitutes the parietal peritoneum. In other regions viscera are interposed between the peritoneum and the posterior wall of the fascial envelope, in what is described as a retroperitoneal position (**B**). In other regions again, viscera invaginate the wall of the peritoneal cavity—usually the posterior wall—so that they are suspended from the body wall by two closely related layers of peritoneum known as a mesentery (**B**). The peritoneum which covers viscera and that which forms mesenteries is called the visceral peritoneum.

It is very important, from a clinical point of view, to recognise that the sensory nerve supplies of parietal and visceral peritoneum differ both in the courses they follow and in the nature of the stimuli which give rise to the conscious appreciation of pain. The sensory fibres from parietal peritoneum run in the somatic nerves of the abdominal wall. They respond to the same kind of stimuli as cutaneous sensory fibres, but what is more important, the pain which these stimuli, including inflammation,

cause is accurately localised in consciousness to the position of the stimulus. On the other hand viscera and visceral peritoneum are innervated by visceral afferent fibres. These follow autonomic nerve pathways and they respond only to stretching and to pathological processes such as inflammation (**120**). Furthermore the impulses caused by such stimuli produce conscious pain which is not usually localised to the position of the affected tissue.

In the pelvic cavity and the lower part of the abdominal cavity proper there is only one peritoneal sac (**B**). This also extends into the uppermost part of the abdominal cavity, but in that region it is separated from the posterior abdominal wall by another, smaller sac (**C**). The two sacs, known as the greater sac and the lesser sac (alternatively the omental bursa) are in direct communication through a small aperture, placed a little to the right of the midline, and named the epiploic foramen (alternatively the foramen of Winslow) (**C**).

A large part of the stomach and the first 2 cm of the duodenum are situated between the two sacs (**C**). Consequently these viscera are, in a sense, attached to the body wall, on either side, by closely related parts of the posterior wall of the greater sac and the anterior wall of the lesser sac. These regions of peritoneum, which are somewhat similar to mesenteries, are named omenta or peritoneal ligaments (**C**). Together with the peritoneum covering the stomach and duodenum they form another part of the visceral peritoneum.

The following general features of the peritoneum should be clearly understood before its detailed disposition is considered.

1. Normally the visceral peritoneum is separated from the parietal peritoneum only by a very thin film of fluid, so that the peritoneal cavity is extremely narrow. However, because it greatly facilitates understanding of the peritoneum, it is an accepted anatomical convention to show the peritoneal sacs in diagrams as widely patent cavities (**B, C**).
2. Except for the fluid film mentioned above, no structure lies inside the peritoneal cavity. The viscera, and the vessels and nerves associated with them, all lie outside the cavity although, in many situations, they invaginate one of its walls (**B**).
3. The vessels and nerves which are associated with suspended viscera (**B**) can only reach them by passing between the two layers of peritoneum forming the corresponding mesenteries, omenta or ligaments.
4. The function of peritoneum is the same as that of other serous membranes, such as pleura and pericardium. It allows large changes in the shape and size of viscera and in their positions within the abdominal cavity.

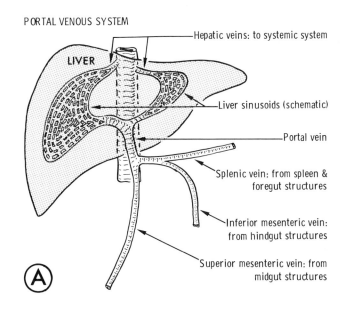

PORTAL VENOUS SYSTEM

- Hepatic veins: to systemic system
- LIVER
- Liver sinusoids (schematic)
- Portal vein
- Splenic vein: from spleen & foregut structures
- Inferior mesenteric vein: from hindgut structures
- Superior mesenteric vein: from midgut structures

Ⓐ

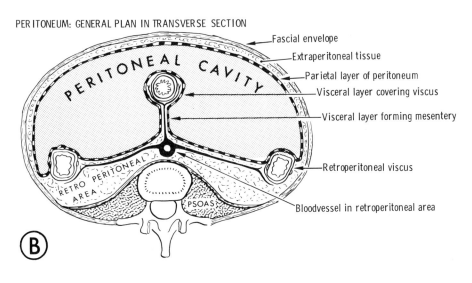

PERITONEUM: GENERAL PLAN IN TRANSVERSE SECTION

- Fascial envelope
- Extraperitoneal tissue
- Parietal layer of peritoneum
- Visceral layer covering viscus
- Visceral layer forming mesentery
- Retroperitoneal viscus
- Bloodvessel in retroperitoneal area

PERITONEAL CAVITY

RETRO PERITONEAL AREA

PSOAS

Ⓑ

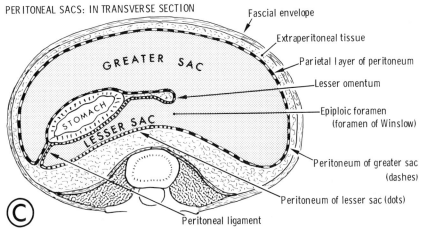

PERITONEAL SACS: IN TRANSVERSE SECTION

- Fascial envelope
- Extraperitoneal tissue
- Parietal layer of peritoneum
- Lesser omentum
- Epiploic foramen (foramen of Winslow)
- Peritoneum of greater sac (dashes)
- Peritoneum of lesser sac (dots)
- Peritoneal ligament

GREATER SAC

STOMACH

LESSER SAC

Ⓒ

5. At operation, or in the dissecting room, it is not uncommon to find fibrous bands joining adjacent areas of visceral peritoneum, or areas of visceral and parietal peritoneum. These are the end result of inflammation and are called adhesions. Much less commonly, however, bands of a congenital nature may be found. If any of these structures press against part of the bowel they may cause obstruction and require surgical division.

DETAILED ANATOMY OF THE UPPER PART OF THE ABDOMINAL CAVITY PROPER

The general features of the viscera, blood vessels and peritoneum of this region have been described, and it is now time to consider the exact dispositions of these structures and the manner in which they are related to one another. These relationships, together, comprise a complex three-dimensional pattern, most of which is admittedly difficult to visualise when it is first studied.

The retroperitoneal structures

The kidneys are retroperitoneal viscera which lie on either side on the posterior abdominal wall (**A, B, C, D**).

The renal hila are about 5 cm from the median plane, and at about the level of the intervertebral disc between L1 and L2 (**A, D**), but the left kidney is slightly higher and more medial than the right. Because of the central prominence of the posterior abdominal wall, formed by the lumbar vertebral bodies, the psoas major muscles and the crura of the diaphragm, the transverse axes of the kidneys are oblique (**B**). Observe that, consequently, the aspects of the kidney described as the anterior and posterior surfaces are in fact obliquely orientated.

Each kidney is sourrounded by a mass of perirenal fat, which is enclosed in turn by a condensed plane of connective tissue called the renal fascia.

It is accepted anatomical convention that in diagrams which include the kidney, the perirenal fat and the renal fascia are usually omitted, and the viscera are shown as if they were directly related to neighbouring structures.

Bearing in mind the presence of the perirenal fat and renal fascia, observe the following features.

1. The manner in which the kidney is related, posteriorly, to the posterior part of the diaphragm, the medial and lateral arcuate ligaments, the twelfth rib, the psoas major and quadratus lumborum muscles, the thoracolumbar fascia and the subcostal, iliohypogastric and ilioinguinal nerves (**A**). The relationship to the twelfth rib is particularly important because a severe blow may drive the bone into the kidney.

2. The manner in which the diaphragm separates the kidney from the posterior part of the costodiaphragmatic recess of the pleural cavity (**D**).
3. The presence in some individuals of a triangular deficiency between the lumbar and costal parts of the diaphragm (**200**). In such circumstances the kidney is in very close relationship with the pleura, which may be injured during surgical mobilisation of the kidney.

The ureters lie partly in the abdominal cavity proper and partly in the pelvic cavity. On each side, the renal pelvis (**221C**) emerges through the hilus of the kidney, and the ureter proper then runs vertically downwards on the psoas major muscle, crossing the genitofemoral nerve from lateral to medial side (**A, C**). It lies anterior to the tips of the lumbar transverse processes, a feature which is important in its radiological examination (**D**).

The renal arteries are large vessels which run laterally from the sides of the aorta opposite the L1–2 intervertebral disc (**C**). Because of the slightly asymmetrical positions of the aorta and the two kidneys, the right renal artery is rather longer than the left. Each artery crosses the crus of the diaphragm and, as it approaches the hilus of the kidney, it divides into numerous branches. The highest of these turns upwards to reach the suprarenal gland, while the lowest turns downwards to supply the upper part of the ureter. The other branches pass through the renal hilus into the sinus of the kidney and enter the kidney substance between the minor calyces. The majority of these branches pass in front of the renal pelvis but, because the pelvis is usually opened from behind in the removal of a stone, it is important to be aware that one branch usually curls over the upper margin of the pelvis on to its posterior aspect.

In a third of the population, additional renal arteries are present below, or less commonly above, the main vessel. These usually arise from the aorta, and usually enter the kidney substance below or above the hilus without entering the renal sinus. It is important that the possible presence of such aberrant renal arteries should be borne in mind when the vascular pedicle of the kidney is being isolated and tied during the removal of a kidney.

KIDNEY: POSTERIOR RELATIONS

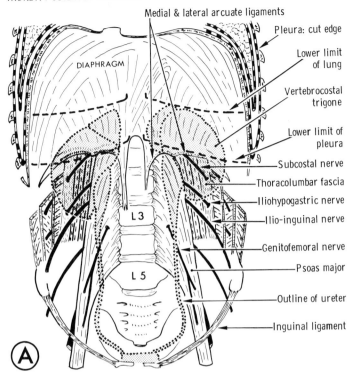

Medial & lateral arcuate ligaments
DIAPHRAGM
Pleura: cut edge
Lower limit of lung
Vertebrocostal trigone
Lower limit of pleura
Subcostal nerve
Thoracolumbar fascia
Iliohypogastric nerve
Ilio-inguinal nerve
Genitofemoral nerve
Psoas major
Outline of ureter
Inguinal ligament
L 3
L 5
Ⓐ

KIDNEYS: IN TRANSVERSE SECTION

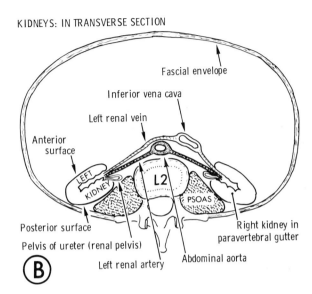

Fascial envelope
Inferior vena cava
Left renal vein
Anterior surface
LEFT KIDNEY
L 2
PSOAS
Posterior surface
Pelvis of ureter (renal pelvis)
Left renal artery
Abdominal aorta
Right kidney in paravertebral gutter
Ⓑ

KIDNEYS & SUPRARENAL GLANDS: ARTERIES

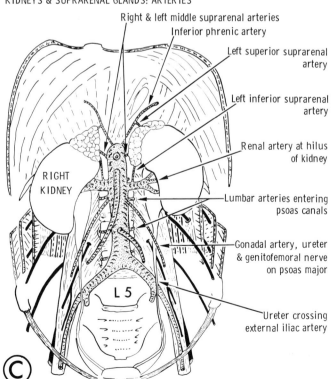

Right & left middle suprarenal arteries
Inferior phrenic artery
Left superior suprarenal artery
Left inferior suprarenal artery
Renal artery at hilus of kidney
RIGHT KIDNEY
Lumbar arteries entering psoas canals
Gonadal artery, ureter & genitofemoral nerve on psoas major
Ureter crossing external iliac artery
L 5
Ⓒ

KIDNEYS & URETERS: SKELETAL RELATIONSHIP

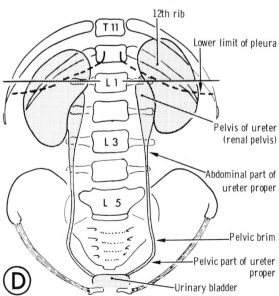

12th rib
Lower limit of pleura
T 11
L 1
L 3
L 5
Pelvis of ureter (renal pelvis)
Abdominal part of ureter proper
Pelvic brim
Pelvic part of ureter proper
Urinary bladder
Ⓓ

The suprarenal glands are also paired retroperitoneal structures. Their shapes and their relationships to the corresponding kidneys have been considered. Each is embedded with the kidney in the perirenal fat, but it is important to note that the amount of fat separating the two viscera is quite considerable so that there is no real danger of injuring a suprarenal gland during the mobilisation and removal of a kidney.

Posteriorly, each gland is related to the posterior part of the diaphragm which separates it from the costodiaphragmatic pleural recess (**A, B**).

Three suprarenal arteries provide the gland with a very profuse blood supply which is relatively immune to interruption by vascular accidents (**B**).

1. The superior suprarenal artery is a branch of the phrenic.
2. The middle suprarenal artery arises directly from the aorta.
3. The inferior suprarenal artery is a branch of the renal.

The gonadal arteries arise from the anterior aspect of the aorta at the level of the second lumbar vertebral body, and the first part of their course is the same in both sexes. They pass downwards and somewhat laterally on the psoas major muscle, crossing the ureter and giving branches to it. The upper part of the ureter is thus supplied by both the renal and gonadal arteries (**A**).

The inferior vena cava and its tributaries have been considered in general terms already (**231D**). Observe now (**A, B**) that in the middle part of its course the vessel lies in front of the medial half or so of the right suprarenal gland and also passes in front of the right phrenic, right middle suprarenal, right renal and right lumbar arteries. In contrast, the right gonadal artery usually passes in front of the vena cava.

The renal vein (**A, B, C, D**) is formed, on either side, by the convergence of numerous tributaries in the renal sinus. It emerges through the kidney hilus, in front of the renal artery and the renal pelvis. The two veins are wide vessels of very different lengths. The right is only about 1 cm long: this tends to make its ligature, during nephrectomy, technically difficult (**A**). The left is about four times as long (**A, B**). After passing to the right in front of the corresponding artery, it crosses in front of the aorta. Note how the superior mesenteric artery arises just above that part of the vein, and immediately turns downwards and a little to the right across its anterior aspect (**A**).

Recall that, although the right suprarenal and right gonadal veins drain directly into the inferior vena cava, on the left side the corresponding vessels drain from above and below into the left renal vein (**A, B**).

The portal vein is a large unpaired vessel which receives the venous blood from the unpaired abdominal viscera—the gastro-intestinal tract, pancreas and spleen (**230**). It begins directly in front of the junction of the left renal vein with the inferior vena cava (**C**). From that point

it ascends to the liver but it is convenient, at this stage, to consider only the initial part of the vessel. In **C** it is consequently shown cut off after only a short part of its course.

The portal vein is formed by the confluence of the superior mesenteric and splenic veins, and a major tributary of the splenic vessel is the inferior mesenteric vein (**C**).

The superior mesenteric vein, in the terminal part of its course, ascends on the right side of the corresponding artery (**C**).

The splenic vein begins at the hilus of the spleen, and draws its initial tributaries from the stomach. In then passes backwards to the anterior surface of the left kidney (**C**). This early part of its course will be considered later. The vein passes to the right in front of the left kidney and its hilus, the left renal vein and the superior mesenteric artery, to join the superior mesenteric vein (**C**).

The inferior mesenteric vein passes up the posterior abdominal wall and curves gently to the right before joining the splenic vein. Notice its relationship to the left gonadal vein which also runs upwards on the posterior abdominal wall before joining the left renal vein (**C**).

The bile duct (**228**) is picked up in **C** as it descends from the liver on the anterior surface of the lower part of the portal vein. From there it sweeps, in a continuous curve, downwards and to the right passing in front of the inferior vena cava and the right renal vein (**C**). It ends by opening into the second part of the duodenum.

The pancreas (**228**) lies predominantly against the highly vascular region on the posterior abdominal wall between the two kidneys. In this region it crosses the median prominence of the lumbar vertebral bodies and the psoas major muscles and is consequently convex forwards. Observe the relationships of the several parts of the pancreas in **D** and **239A**.

1. The greater part of the head of the pancreas lies in front of the inferior vena cava, the right renal vein, and the bile duct. Its right margin abuts against the right kidney. From the lower part of its left margin, the uncinate process extends to the left between the aorta, behind, and the superior mesenteric vessels, in front.
2. The neck of the pancreas lies in front of the terminal part of the superior mesenteric vein and the beginning of the portal vein. Its posterior surface is consequently smooth, and thread-like veins pass from it into the portal vein.
3. The body extends to the left and slightly upwards. It lies in front of the splenic vein and its inferior mesenteric tributary, the left renal vein and the terminations of its suprarenal and gonadal tributaries, the superior mesenteric artery, the lowest part of the left suprarenal gland and the hilus and part of the anterior surface of the left kidney.

KIDNEYS & SUPRARENAL GLANDS: VEINS

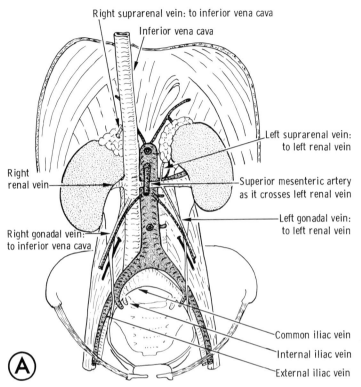

Right suprarenal vein: to inferior vena cava

Inferior vena cava

Left suprarenal vein: to left renal vein

Superior mesenteric artery as it crosses left renal vein

Right renal vein

Left gonadal vein: to left renal vein

Right gonadal vein: to inferior vena cava

Common iliac vein

Internal iliac vein

External iliac vein

(A)

INFERIOR VENA CAVA: POSTERIOR RELATIONS

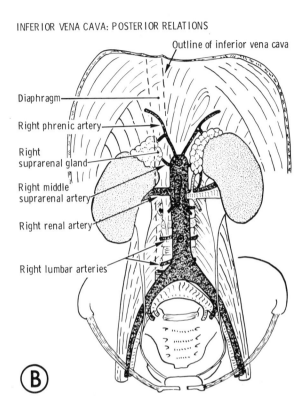

Outline of inferior vena cava

Diaphragm

Right phrenic artery

Right suprarenal gland

Right middle suprarenal artery

Right renal artery

Right lumbar arteries

(B)

PORTAL VEIN: FORMATION

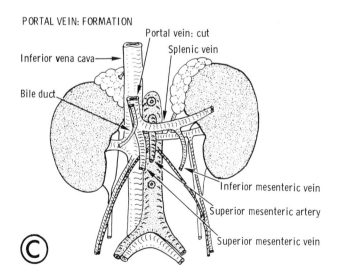

Portal vein: cut

Splenic vein

Inferior vena cava

Bile duct

Inferior mesenteric vein

Superior mesenteric artery

Superior mesenteric vein

(C)

PANCREAS: POSTERIOR RELATIONS

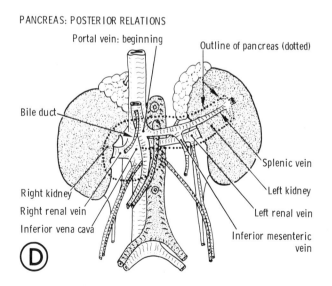

Portal vein: beginning

Outline of pancreas (dotted)

Bile duct

Right kidney

Right renal vein

Inferior vena cava

Splenic vein

Left kidney

Left renal vein

Inferior mesenteric vein

(D)

237

4. The tail of the pancreas turns forwards from about the middle of the anterior surface of the left kidney and eventually, as will be seen later, reaches the hilus of the spleen (**E**). It has the splenic vein on its left side. In **237D** the tail of the pancreas and the terminal part of the splenic vein have been removed.

The coeliac artery (**A**) is the highest of the three unpaired branches of the abdominal aorta and is distributed to the derivatives of the foetal foregut plus the spleen. It passes directly forwards for about 1.5 cm, immediately above the upper margin of the body of the pancreas, and then divides into three large branches. These are the hepatic, splenic and left gastric arteries. The three diverge across the posterior abdominal wall, rather like the spokes of a wheel, and will be considered later.

The duodenum (**222**) is closely related throughout its course to the head and neck of the pancreas. Examine the position and relations of its four parts (**A**).

1. The first part begins at the pylorus at the vertebral level of the lower part of L1, a little to the right of the midline and in front of the upper border of the neck of the pancreas (but separated from it in its first 2 cm or so by part of the peritoneal cavity, as will be seen later). The portal vein, as it runs upwards from behind the neck of the pancreas, passes behind this part of the duodenum.

2. The second part of the duodenum runs downwards, resting directly on the adjacent parts of the right kidney and the head of the pancreas and finally on the upper part of the right ureter. Recall its association with the hepatopancreatic ampulla and the accessory pancreatic duct (**228**). This part of the duodenum is readily separated from the kidney, but is firmly held to the pancreas by the bile and pancreatic ducts.

3. The third part passes to the left along the lower border of the head of the pancreas and its uncinate process at the vertebral level of L3. Note its direct posterior relationship to the right ureter, the right psoas major muscle, the right gonadal vessels, the inferior vena cava and the origin of the inferior mesenteric artery from the abdominal aorta. Observe, also, how the superior mesenteric vessels cross the anterior aspect of this part of the duodenum. This part of the gut is sandwiched between these mesenteric vessels and the aorta, and in some individuals this appears to cause a degree of obstruction to the onward passage of duodenal contents.

4. The short fourth segment of the duodenum ascends in front of the left border of the aorta to the lower border of the body of the pancreas. There it turns abruptly forwards at the duodenojejunal junction.

Note that, whereas the inferior mesenteric artery arises behind the third part of the duodenum, the inferior mesenteric vein passes up the posterior abdominal wall, just to the left of the fourth part. The vein is therefore a valuable guide to the duodenojejunal junction at operation.

The lesser peritoneal sac (omental bursa)

It has been seen (**232**) that the peritoneal cavity consists of two compartments called, simply from their respective sizes, the greater and lesser sacs. The greater sac extends the whole length of the abdominal cavity, from the diaphragm above to the pelvic diaphragm below. In contrast, the lesser sac is confined to the upper part of the abdominal cavity proper, where it lies behind the greater sac and communicates with it through the epiploic foramen (foramen of Winslow). This opening lies a little to the right of the median plane, is directed from right to left, and admits two or three fingers.

From the epiploic foramen a channel of the same calibre, named the aditus of the lesser sac, passes to the left for about 3 cm (**B, C**). Beyond the aditus, the sac abruptly opens out to its full vertical extent. It has extensive anterior and posterior walls, which are practically in contact with each other (though in diagrams it is conventional to show the cavity widely patent) and narrow margins.

To understand the disposition of the lesser sac it is important to appreciate that it consists of a fixed and two free parts.

The posterior wall of the fixed part directly covers parts of the posterior abdominal wall and certain retroperitoneal structures which lie directly upon it. Examine the extent of the 'translucent' posterior wall of this part (**B**) and note the structures which lie directly behind it.

The aditus is situated in front of the segment of the inferior vena cava between the first part of the duodenum and the liver. To the left of the aditus the peritoneum covers the upper medial quadrant of the left kidney, the left suprarenal gland, the body, neck and upper left quadrant of the head of the pancreas, the upper part of the abdominal aorta and its several branches, and part of the diaphragm.

The two free parts of the lesser sac extend respectively to the left and downwards (**C, D, E**). In these regions the posterior wall of the sac is in contact with neither the posterior abdominal wall nor retroperitoneal structures (**D, E**). The position of the left free part is evident in the transverse section in **E**. Note that it lies in front of the spleen and the tail of the pancreas.

The position of the lower free part is apparent in **D**. Visualise in **D** and **B** that it lies in front of the region of the duodenojejunal junction, parts of the superior mesenteric vessels and the lower medial quadrant of the left kidney.

DUODENUM & PANCREAS

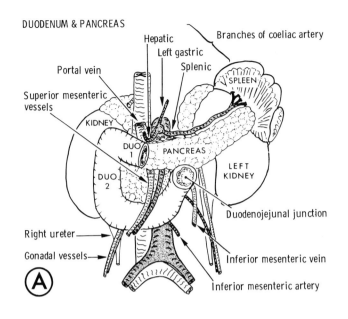

Portal vein
Hepatic
Left gastric
Splenic
Branches of coeliac artery
Superior mesenteric vessels
KIDNEY
SPLEEN
DUO 1
PANCREAS
DUO 2
LEFT KIDNEY
Right ureter
Gonadal vessels
Duodenojejunal junction
Inferior mesenteric vein
Inferior mesenteric artery

(A)

LESSER PERITONEAL SAC (OMENTAL BURSA): FIXED PART

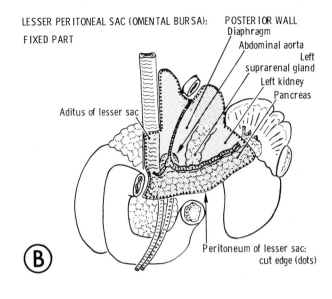

POSTERIOR WALL
Diaphragm
Abdominal aorta
Left suprarenal gland
Left kidney
Pancreas
Aditus of lesser sac
Peritoneum of lesser sac: cut edge (dots)

(B)

LESSER PERITONEAL SAC: FIXED & FREE PARTS

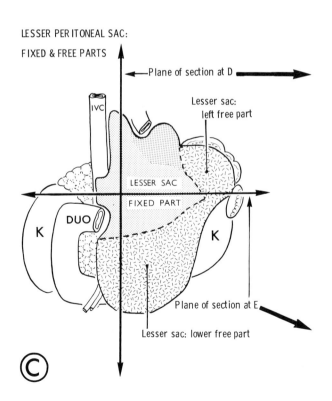

Plane of section at D
IVC
Lesser sac: left free part
LESSER SAC FIXED PART
K
DUO
K
Plane of section at E
Lesser sac: lower free part

(C)

LESSER PERITONEAL SAC: MEDIAN SECTION

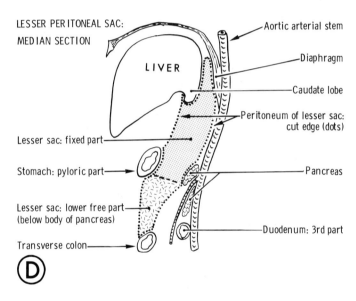

Aortic arterial stem
LIVER
Diaphragm
Caudate lobe
Peritoneum of lesser sac: cut edge (dots)
Lesser sac: fixed part
Stomach: pyloric part
Pancreas
Lesser sac: lower free part (below body of pancreas)
Duodenum: 3rd part
Transverse colon

(D)

LESSER PERITONEAL SAC: TRANSVERSE SECTION

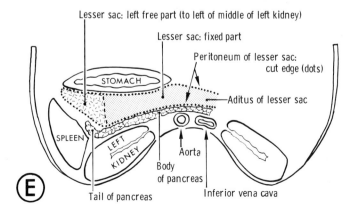

Lesser sac: left free part (to left of middle of left kidney)
Lesser sac: fixed part
Peritoneum of lesser sac: cut edge (dots)
STOMACH
Aditus of lesser sac
SPLEEN
LEFT KIDNEY
Aorta
Body of pancreas
Inferior vena cava
Tail of pancreas

(E)

239

The positions of the oesophagus, stomach and duodenum and their relations to the lesser sac

In **A**, **B** the continuity of oesophagus, stomach and duodenum has been completed. Observe the relationship of these parts to the lesser sac, and note that the oesophagus and the stomach fundus lie above the lesser sac, the body and the pyloric part of the stomach and the first 2 cm of the duodenum lie in front of it, while the rest of the duodenum is situated to the right of and below the sac.

The variability of the exaçt position of the stomach has been noted already. Its average relationship to the body wall is shown in **E**. The oesophagus, the cardiac orifice and the fundus are situated in the left hypochondrium, the greater part of the body of the stomach and the pyloric part lie in the epigastric and umbilical regions, while the pylorus is placed on the transpyloric plane, to the right of the midline.

The position of the transverse colon and its relation to the lesser sac

The transverse colon extends across the abdominal cavity between the right and left colic flexures. Observe (**B**) that the right flexure lies against the anterior surface of the right kidney, that the first few centimetres of the transverse colon pass to the left in contact with the anterior surface of the second part of the duodenum, and that the left flexure is placed on the lower part of the left margin of the left kidney. Between the second part of the duodenum and the left flexure, the transverse colon is free of the posterior abdominal wall and follows a course which is convex forwards and downwards. All but the right few centimetres of this free part of the transverse colon abuts against the inferior margin of the lower free part of the lesser sac (**B**, **239D**).

The position of the spleen and its relation to the lesser sac

The spleen (**220**) lies far back in the left hypochondrium with its posterior end some 4 cm from the median plane and its anterior end, somewhat lower, over the midaxillary line.

Although the viscus moves considerably with respiration, it is not normally palpable below the thoracic cage even in deep inspiration. However, in certain diseases the spleen becomes enlarged so that its superior margin moves downwards and forwards and becomes palpable below the right costal margin. The notch characteristic of the superior border (**221D**), is helpful in differentiating an enlarged spleen from other abdominal masses.

Its convex, posterolateral diaphragmatic surface fits snugly against the posterior part of the diaphragm (**C**, **D**). It is related, through that muscle, to the costodiaphragmatic recess of the left pleura and the inferior margin of the left lung and, further back still, to the posterior parts of the ninth, tenth and eleventh ribs (**C**, **D**). These ribs may severely damage the spleen in injuries to the lower left thorax.

The three facets of the visceral surface (**C**) are related respectively to the upper lateral part of the anterior surface of the left kidney (**239E**), to the posterior surface of the stomach (**239E**) and to the left colic flexure (**B**). The long hilus of the spleen (**221E**) lies against the posterior wall of the left free part of the lesser sac between kidney and stomach (**239E**). The tail of the pancreas, with the splenic vein, passes from the kidney to the hilus of the spleen in contact with this peritoneal layer (**C**).

The position of the liver and its relation to the lesser sac

The gross surface features of the liver have been considered (**226**). Now observe the general position of the viscus in the uppermost part of the abdominal cavity (**E**). The superior surface and base rest against the under surface of the diaphragm. The right and left parts of the anterior surface are also related to the diaphragm, but the central part of this surface lies against the infrasternal part of the anterior abdominal wall. Note how the right part of the liver is related through the diaphragm to the right pleura and lung (**E**), and how the central and left parts are related through the diaphragm to the heart and pericardium (**E**).

Although, because of its relationship to the diaphragm, the position of the liver alters with respiration, its position does not change significantly in quiet breathing. Its boundaries are defined by percussion. Heavy percussion at successively lower levels over the anterior chest wall indicates the upper limit of the viscus, as a change from the resonance of the lung to the dull note of the solid liver, along a line which runs from fifth rib in the right lateral line to the sixth rib in the left lateral line. Lighter percussion over the right costal margin and the epigastrium shows the inferior margin of the liver as a change from liver dullness to intestinal resonance. The margin is coincident with the right costal margin as far as the right ninth costal cartilage, and then passes obliquely across the epigastrium to the left eighth costal cartilage (**E**).

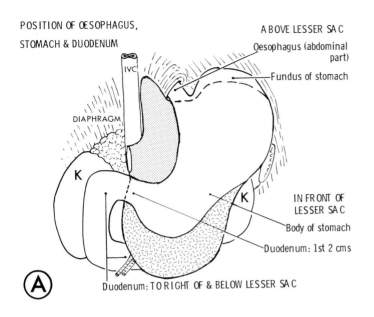

POSITION OF OESOPHAGUS,
STOMACH & DUODENUM

ABOVE LESSER SAC

Oesophagus (abdominal part)

Fundus of stomach

IVC

DIAPHRAGM

K

K

IN FRONT OF LESSER SAC

Body of stomach

Duodenum: 1st 2 cms

Duodenum: TO RIGHT OF & BELOW LESSER SAC

(A)

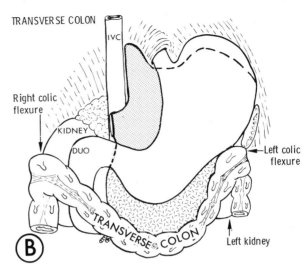

TRANSVERSE COLON

IVC

Right colic flexure

KIDNEY

DUO

Left colic flexure

TRANSVERSE COLON

Left kidney

(B)

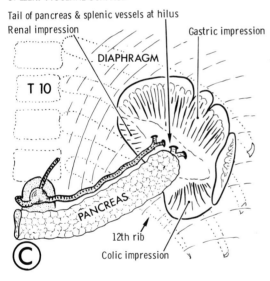

SPLEEN: VISCERAL SURFACE

Tail of pancreas & splenic vessels at hilus
Renal impression

Gastric impression

DIAPHRAGM

T 10

PANCREAS

12th rib

Colic impression

(C)

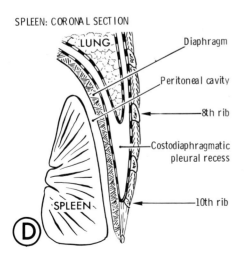

SPLEEN: CORONAL SECTION

LUNG

Diaphragm

Peritoneal cavity

8th rib

Costodiaphragmatic pleural recess

10th rib

SPLEEN

(D)

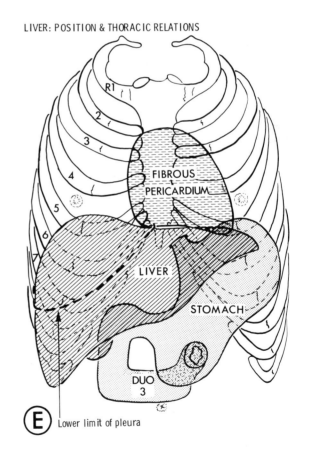

LIVER: POSITION & THORACIC RELATIONS

R1

2

3

4

5

6

FIBROUS
PERICARDIUM

LIVER

STOMACH

DUO
3

(E)   Lower limit of pleura

The location of areas of abnormal tissue within the liver can be defined by a liver scan because the cells in these areas do not perform the functions of normal liver cells. A radioactive material which is taken up by normal liver cells is injected intravenously and its distribution, and therefore the position of normal liver tissue, is determined by use of a scintillation scanner.

The relations of neither the posterior nor the inferior surface of the liver can be seen when the intact and undisturbed viscus is viewed from in front. However in **A**, which shows the outline of the posterior surface of the liver, the relations of that surface can be visualised. Thus the right half or so of the surface is related to the diaphragm, the inferior vena cava and the upper part of the right suprarenal gland, and it is to be noted that these are direct relationships in the sense that no peritoneum intervenes. The left half or so of the same surface is related to the uppermost region of the fixed part of the lesser sac, the abdominal oesophagus and the upper part of the stomach, but, as will be seen later (**245C**), is separated from these structures by the greater peritoneal sac.

The relations of the inferior surface of the liver can be visualised if one imagines that that surface has been tilted upwards as in **B**. Thus in **C** the tilted and foreshortened inferior surface is visible and the normal position of its inferior margin is indicated by an interrupted line. Observe in **C** and in **D** that the caudate process on the inferior surface is directly related to the roof of the aditus of the lesser sac whereas other parts of the inferior surface are separated by the greater peritoneal sac (see below) from the following parts:

1. the lower right quadrant of the right suprarenal gland
2. the upper part of the right kidney
3. the right colic flexure
4. part of the anterior wall of the lesser sac
5. the first and second parts of the duodenum
6. part of the body of the stomach

The relationship of the liver to the lesser peritoneal sac is very important and is conveniently considered intially in two parts. As has been noted in **C** and **D**, the roof of the aditus is related to the caudate process, so that the anterior wall of the aditus passes downwards from the posterior margin of the porta hepatis, while the posterior wall runs downwards on the anterior surface of the inferior vena cava. Similarly, it can be seen in the horizontal section in **E** that the right margin of the lesser sac above the aditus is moulded against all aspects of the caudate lobe. As a consequence of this relationship, the posterior wall of the lesser sac passes to the left from the left margin of the inferior vena cava, while the anterior wall passes to the left from the depth of the fissure for the ligamentum venosum.

These two zones of relationship between the liver and the lesser sac are continuous, the caudate process and caudate lobe on the liver being continuous and the roof of the aditus and the upper part of the right border of the lesser sac being similarly continuous. This continuity can be seen in **F**, in which the inferior surface of the liver has been tilted upwards again but in which, in addition, the left lobe of the liver has been removed by a sagittal section through the viscus from its anterior surface to the depth of fissure for the ligamentum venosum (**G**). It will be seen from this consideration that the anterior wall of the lesser sac (including the aditus) is attached to (i.e. comes into contact with) the liver along a continuous L-shaped line formed by the posterior margin of the porta hepatis and the deepest part of the fissure for the ligamentum venosum (**F**).

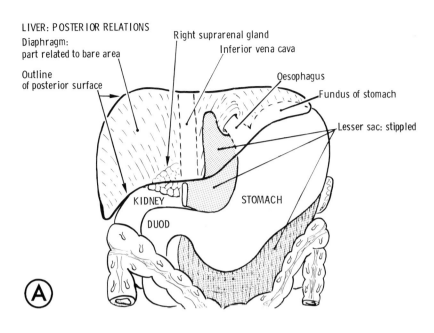

LIVER: POSTERIOR RELATIONS

Diaphragm:
part related to bare area

Right suprarenal gland

Inferior vena cava

Oesophagus

Fundus of stomach

Outline
of posterior surface

Lesser sac: stippled

KIDNEY

STOMACH

DUOD

(A)

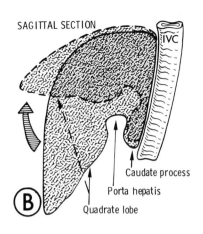

SAGITTAL SECTION

IVC

Caudate process

Porta hepatis

Quadrate lobe

(B)

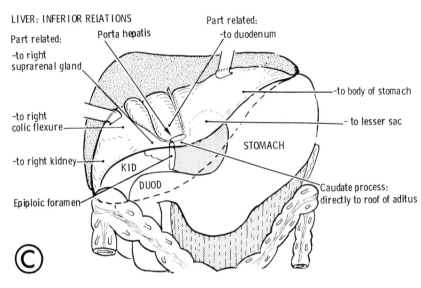

LIVER: INFERIOR RELATIONS

Part related:
-to right
suprarenal gland

Porta hepatis

Part related:
-to duodenum

-to body of stomach

- to lesser sac

-to right
colic flexure

STOMACH

-to right kidney

KID

DUOD

Epiploic foramen

Caudate process:
directly to roof of aditus

(C)

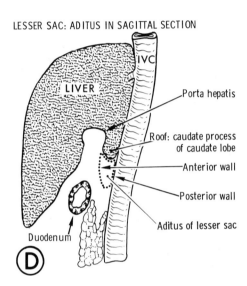

LESSER SAC: ADITUS IN SAGITTAL SECTION

IVC

LIVER

Porta hepatis

Roof: caudate process
of caudate lobe

Anterior wall

Posterior wall

Duodenum

Aditus of lesser sac

(D)

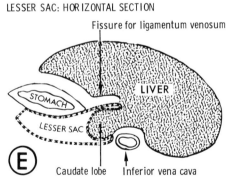

LESSER SAC: HORIZONTAL SECTION

Fissure for ligamentum venosum

STOMACH

LIVER

LESSER SAC

Caudate lobe

Inferior vena cava

(E)

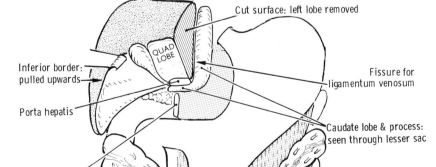

LIVER: INFERIOR SURFACE (LEFT LOBE REMOVED)

Cut surface: left lobe removed

QUAD
LOBE

Inferior border:
pulled upwards

Fissure for
ligamentum venosum

Porta hepatis

Caudate lobe & process:
seen through lesser sac

Epiploic foramen

(F)

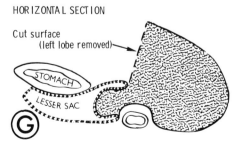

HORIZONTAL SECTION

Cut surface
(left lobe removed)

STOMACH

LESSER SAC

(G)

243

The greater peritoneal sac

Relationship to the liver

The liver invaginates the upper posterior part of the greater sac so that a large part of its surface is covered by greater sac peritoneum. Because the ligamentum teres, or its precursor the umbilical vein, extends from the inferior margin of the liver to the umbilicus the invagination is triradiate in form. The liver is thus 'suspended' from the diaphragm and anterior abdominal wall by three peritoneal ligaments which are continuous with one another.

In front the anterior and superior surfaces of the liver are attached to the diaphragm and anterior abdominal wall by the two layers of greater sac peritoneum which constitute the falciform ligament (**A**, **B**). The parietal line of attachment of this ligament is in the median plane, whereas the hepatic line of attachment is a little to the right. Below, the two layers of ligament are continuous, and this free margin encloses the ligamentum teres. Anteriorly and above, the two layers separate and pass left and right on the diaphragm and anterior abdominal wall (**D**). Posteriorly, the two layers again separate and pass left and right on to the superior and anterior surfaces of the liver.

Posteriorly the liver is attached to the diaphragm by two peritoneal ligaments. The lines along which the layers of these ligaments are reflected off the liver surface are shown in **C** and the lines along which they are attached to the diaphragm are shown in **E**. In the case of the ligament associated with the right lobe the two peritoneal layers are separated throughout most of their extent by a wide triangular bare area of liver surface which is attached to the diaphragm by connective tissue, but to the right they become continuous with each other. The wide part of the ligament is called the coronary ligament and the narrow part the right triangular ligament.

The two layers of greater sac peritoneum reflected off the left lobe of the liver are closely approximated throughout their extent and become continuous to the left. They constitute the left triangular ligament (**C**).

Between the posterior layer of the left triangular ligament and the inferior layer of the coronary ligament a continuous sheet of greater sac peritoneum leaves the liver surface and passes downwards from the anterior margin of the porta hepatis (**C**) and to the left from the deepest part of the fissure for the ligamentum venosum (**D**). Note that, as it leaves the liver, this layer is in contact with the anterior wall of the upper right part of the lesser sac (**C**, **D**).

Relationship to other upper abdominal structures

Figure **E** shows the upper abdominal viscera and the lesser sac of peritoneum. In addition, the lines of reflection of greater sac peritoneum from the posterior surface of the liver are shown as interrupted lines above and to the right, and the outline of the greater omentum is similarly indicated below. The greater omentum is a peritoneal fold consisting of two layers of greater sac peritoneum which are suspended from the left three-quarters or so of the transverse colon. It will be considered in detail later.

The relationship of the posterior wall of the greater peritoneal sac to the upper abdominal viscera and to the lesser sac is now to be considered by studying its disposition in the several sagittal and transverse sections shown in **247B–L**. Their positions are shown in **247A** which is an unlabelled duplicate of **E**.

The lesser omentum (**247D**, **247E**, **247J**, **247K**) is a double sheet of peritoneum which extends from the liver to the stomach and the first part of the duodenum. Its anterior layer is part of the posterior wall of the greater sac and its posterior layer part of the anterior wall of the lesser sac. Its hepatic attachment—that is, the line along which its two layers reach the liver and part company from each other—is L-shaped. Below it encloses the porta hepatis (**247D**), while above it runs along the floor of the fissure for the ligamentum venosum (**247J**). The gastro-intestinal attachment is along the whole of the lesser curvature of the stomach and the upper margin of the first 2 cm of the duodenum (**247D**, **247E**, **247J**, **247K**). To the right the omentum has a free margin where the anterior and posterior layers are continuous (**247K**). This extends from the right limit of the porta hepatis to the first part of the duodenum in front of the epiploic foramen. Above, between the cardiac orifice of the stomach and the upper end of the fissure for the ligamentum venosum, the omentum is attached to the diaphragm (**247E**). Here the posterior layer is reflected downwards on to the posterior abdominal wall as the posterior wall of the lesser sac, while the anterior layer turns forwards towards the left lobe of the liver where it becomes the posterior layer of the left triangular ligament.

The abdominal oesophagus (**247F**) is covered anteriorly by greater sac peritoneum which reaches it from the anterior surface of the body of the stomach. It eventually passes on to the diaphragm and then on to the left lobe of the liver as the posterior layer of the left triangular ligament. Note the relationship of the oesophagus to the posterior surface of the left lobe of the liver, and that the two structures are separated by a recess of the greater sac. Posteriorly, the oesophagus lies directly on the diaphragm.

LIVER FROM IN FRONT: PERITONEAL CONNEXIONS

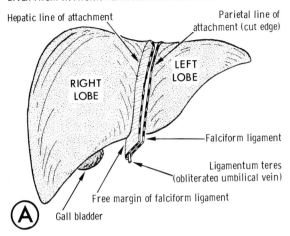

Hepatic line of attachment

Parietal line of attachment (cut edge)

RIGHT LOBE

LEFT LOBE

Falciform ligament

Ligamentum teres (obliterated umbilical vein)

Free margin of falciform ligament

Gall bladder

Ⓐ

FALCIFORM LIGAMENT

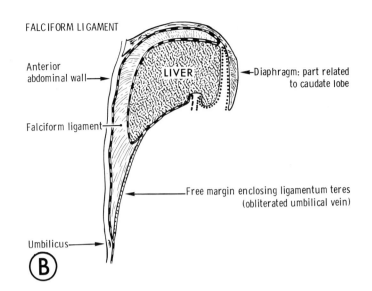

Anterior abdominal wall

LIVER

Diaphragm: part related to caudate lobe

Falciform ligament

Free margin enclosing ligamentum teres (obliterated umbilical vein)

Umbilicus

Ⓑ

LIVER FROM BEHIND: PERITONEAL CONNEXIONS

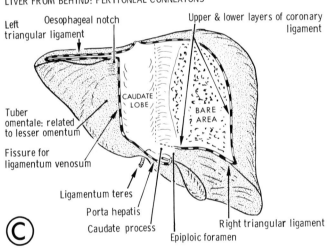

Left triangular ligament

Oesophageal notch

Upper & lower layers of coronary ligament

CAUDATE LOBE

BARE AREA

Tuber omentale: related to lesser omentum

Fissure for ligamentum venosum

Ligamentum teres

Porta hepatis

Caudate process

Epiploic foramen

Right triangular ligament

Ⓒ

UPPER ABDOMINAL VISCERA

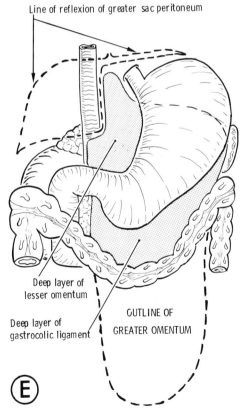

Line of reflexion of greater sac peritoneum

Deep layer of lesser omentum

Deep layer of gastrocolic ligament

OUTLINE OF GREATER OMENTUM

Ⓔ

LIVER: HORIZONTAL SECTION: PERITONEAL CONNEXIONS

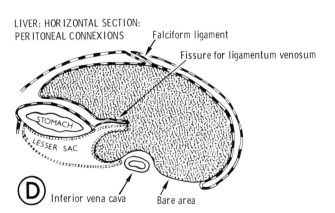

Falciform ligament

Fissure for ligamentum venosum

STOMACH

LESSER SAC

Inferior vena cava

Bare area

Ⓓ

The fundus of the stomach is covered by greater sac peritoneum on both its anterior and posterior surfaces (**G**).

The gastrophrenic ligament (**G, J**) consists of an upper layer of greater sac peritoneum and a lower layer which is part of the upper margin of the lesser sac. It passes backwards from the fundus of the stomach to the diaphragm. Here the upper layer ascends and eventually becomes continuous with the posterior layer of the left triangular ligament, while the lower layer turns downwards as the posterior wall of the greater sac. Note the route (arrowed) by which this ligament can be approached.

The spleen and its ligaments. This viscus is closely associated with two peritoneal layers which, in general, pass forwards and to the left from the middle of the anterior surface of the left kidney and the junction of the body and tail of the pancreas to the greater curvature of the stomach (**K**). The right layer is the posterior wall of the left free part of the lesser sac and its middle part is in contact with the hilus of the spleen (**221E**). The left layer is greater sac peritoneum, which approaches the region from the lateral and posterior abdominal walls and across the upper lateral quadrant of the anterior surface of the left kidney. It then passes forwards and to the left to the greater curvature of the stomach, but between kidney and stomach it is invaginated to the left by the spleen so that it covers all aspects of the viscus except the region of the hilus. In front of and behind the hilus of the spleen the peritoneum of the greater and lesser sacs are in contact and constitute the gastrosplenic and lienorenal ligaments respectively.

The gastrosplenic ligament (**K**) is so orientated that it intervenes between the posterior surface of the stomach and the gastric impression on the visceral surface of the spleen.

The lienorenal ligament is unique amongst peritoneal ligaments in containing a viscus. The tail of the pancreas passes forwards and laterally between its two layers of peritoneum and terminates by making direct contact with the hilus of the spleen (**K**). It is evident that the latter relationship differs in kind from the other visceral relations of the spleen.

The left colic flexure and the upper part of the descending colon (**L**) lie directly against the lower left quadrant of the left kidney but are covered on all but their posterior aspects by greater sac peritoneum. The upper surface of the flexure is separated from the colic impression on the spleen by part of the greater sac of peritoneum (**H**).

The gastrocolic ligament (**F, L**) joins the greater curvature of the stomach and the first 2 cm of the duodenum to the upper aspect of the transverse colon from the left colic flexure as far as the lower part of the right border of the lesser sac. It consists of the posterior wall of the greater sac in contact with the anterior wall of the lesser sac. To the right the two layers separate (**L**), the posterior layer turning to the left on the head and body of the pancreas while the anterior layer continues to the right across the upper right quadrant of the pancreatic head. To the left it is directly continuous with the two peritoneal layers of the lienorenal and gastrosplenic ligaments which in turn are continuous above with the gastrophrenic ligament. It is important to appreciate this continuity of the several ligaments which leave the greater curvature and posterior aspect of the stomach.

The transverse mesocolon (**D, F**) extends downwards and forwards from the posterior abdominal wall and the body and head of the pancreas to the transverse colon between the left colic flexure and the second part of the duodenum. It consists of two parts. To the right of the lesser sac (**D**) it is short and consists of two layers of greater sac peritoneum. Below it envelops the colon while above the two layers reach the middle of the pancreatic head and separate, the anterior layer passing upwards and the posterior layer downwards. Throughout the rest of its extent (**E, F, G**) the posterior layer of the mesocolon is greater sac peritoneum passing from the lower border of the body of the pancreas to the colon while the anterior layer is the posterior wall of the lower free part of the lesser sac passing between the same two viscera.

Note that at operation the lesser sac can be opened to allow examination of the posterior surface of the body of the stomach and the structures which lie behind the fixed part of the lesser sac, by making an opening either through the gastrocolic ligament or through the main left part of the transverse mesocolon. The overhang of the lesser omentum by the left lobe of the liver make that a less attractive approach.

The greater omentum (**E, F, G**). The two sheets of greater sac peritoneum which approach the transverse colon as the anterior layer of the gastrocolic ligament and the posterior layer of the transverse mesocolon are projected downwards for a variable distance from the inferior margin of the colon as a two-layered fold, which although thin in children usually contains a considerable amount of fat between its layers in adults. This is the greater omentum. It hangs downwards, rather like an apron in front of the coils of small intestine and is continually moved into different positions by peristaltic contractions in those parts of the gut. When an abdominal viscus such as the appendix or gallbladder becomes inflamed, part of the greater omentum often adheres to it, and tends to isolate the inflammatory focus from the rest of the peritoneal cavity. It should be noted that at operation the greater omentum must be displaced upwards before the inferior aspect of the transverse mesocolon can be reached.

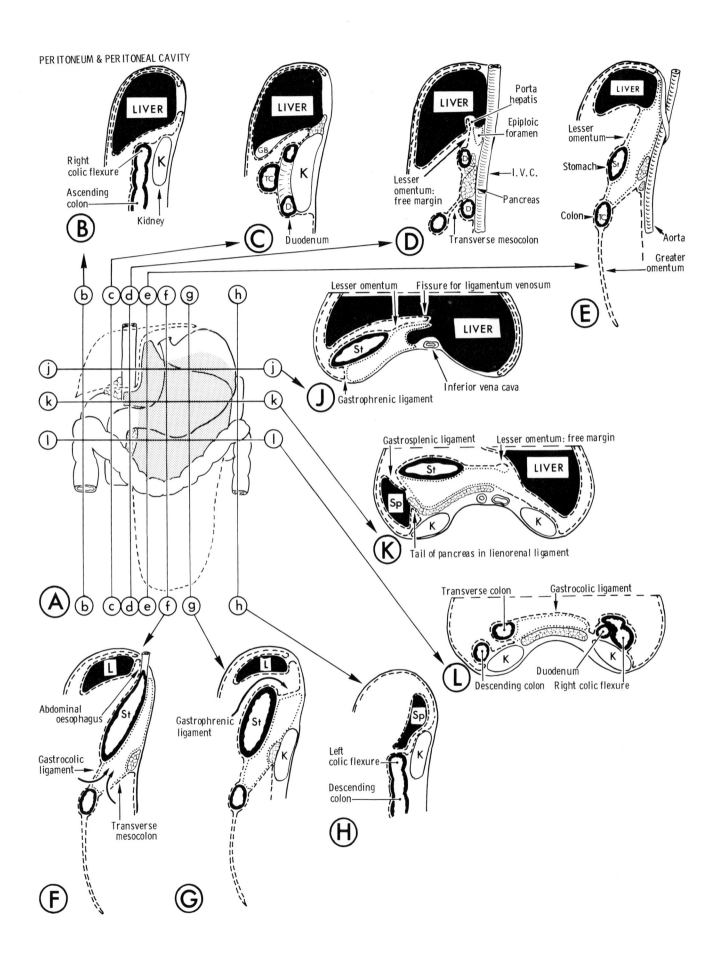

B

Right colic flexure
Ascending colon
Kidney
K

C
GB
TC
K
D
Duodenum

D
Porta hepatis
Epiploic foramen
I.V.C.
Lesser omentum: free margin
Pancreas
Transverse mesocolon

E
Lesser omentum
Stomach
St
Colon
TC
Aorta
Greater omentum

J
Lesser omentum
Fissure for ligamentum venosum
St
LIVER
Inferior vena cava
Gastrophrenic ligament

K
Gastrosplenic ligament
Lesser omentum: free margin
St
LIVER
Sp
K
K
Tail of pancreas in lienorenal ligament

L
Transverse colon
Gastrocolic ligament
K
K
Duodenum
Descending colon
Right colic flexure

A
b c d e f g h
j j
k k
l l

F
L
Abdominal oesophagus
St
Gastrocolic ligament
Transverse mesocolon

G
L
St
Gastrophrenic ligament
K

H
Left colic flexure
Descending colon
Sp
K

The subphrenic spaces are two deep peritoneal recesses which lie between the liver and the diaphragm and are separated by the falciform ligament. The left space overlies the anterior and superior surfaces of the left lobe of the liver and is limited posteriorly by the anterior layer of the left triangular ligament. The right space covers the anterior, superior and right surfaces of the liver and is limited behind by the upper layer of the coronary and right triangular ligaments. Both spaces are surgically important because infections in the peritoneal cavity may become walled off as local abscesses within them. The right space has an additional importance in relation to liver biopsy.

The diagnosis of liver diseases sometimes requires percutaneous biopsy of the viscus. A core of liver tissue is obtained by suction through a small-bore needle. The needle is introduced through the right eighth or ninth intercostal space in the midaxillary line, and passed horizontally with a slight backward inclination so as to avoid the porta hepatis. It can be seen (**B**) that the needle, having passed through the muscles of the chest wall, traverses the costodiaphragmatic pleural recess, the diaphragm and the right subphrenic peritoneal space. Consequently pneumothorax, haemothorax, peritonitis and intra-abdominal haemorrhage are all possible hazards of the procedure.

The subhepatic spaces are two peritoneal recesses which lie below and behind the liver. The left subhepatic space is the lesser peritoneal sac and its position and relations have been considered already. The right space (**247B, C**), often known alternatively as the hepatorenal or Morison's pouch, is a deep narrow recess. Its anterior wall is formed by the inferior surface of the right lobe of the liver and the gall bladder while its posterior wall is that area of greater sac peritoneum which covers part of the diaphragm, the lower part of the right suprarenal gland, the upper part of the

right kidney, parts of the first and second parts of the duodenum and the left colic flexure and the right end of the transverse colon. Note that this space is continuous to the right with the right subdiaphragmatic space and to the left, through the epiploic foramen, with the left subhepatic space (lesser sac). As the right subhepatic space is one of the lowest parts of the peritoneal cavity when a patient lies supine, peritoneal infections may result in a localised abscess forming within it.

The peritoneal and other anterior relations of the kidneys are summarised in **C** and **D**.

The peritoneal relations of the pancreas are summarised in **E**. Note the lines of attachment of the two parts of the transverse mesocolon, and the gastrocolic ligament. The tail of the pancreas has been removed at its junction with the body but its peritoneal relations as it extends through the lienorenal ligament have already been noted in **247K**.

Hiatus herniae. Herniae of abdominal viscera occasionally occur through the diaphragm. The majority occur in middle age at the oesophageal hiatus and are known as hiatus herniae. The more common 'sliding' type is illustrated in **F** and the 'rolling' type in **G**.

In the normal, as has been noted (**222**), there is a functional sphincter mechanism between the stomach and the oesophagus which appears to be due to pressure on the abdominal oesophagus by the gastric fundus.

In a sliding hernia the normal relationship of fundus and oesophagus is lost and reflux of gastric contents occurs, especially when the patient is lying supine. It is this reflux which gives rise to most of the symptoms of the condition.

In a rolling hernia the normal relationship of the oesophagus and stomach fundus is retained, and the symptoms based on reflux are correspondingly much less marked.

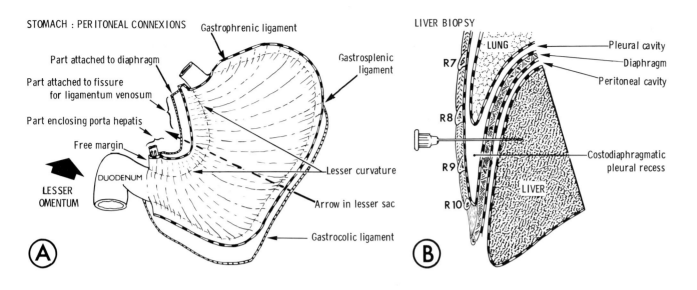

STOMACH : PERITONEAL CONNEXIONS

Gastrophrenic ligament

Part attached to diaphragm

Part attached to fissure for ligamentum venosum

Part enclosing porta hepatis

Free margin

DUODENUM

LESSER OMENTUM

Gastrosplenic ligament

Lesser curvature

Arrow in lesser sac

Gastrocolic ligament

(A)

LIVER BIOPSY

LUNG

R7

R8

R9

R10

LIVER

Pleural cavity

Diaphragm

Peritoneal cavity

Costodiaphragmatic pleural recess

(B)

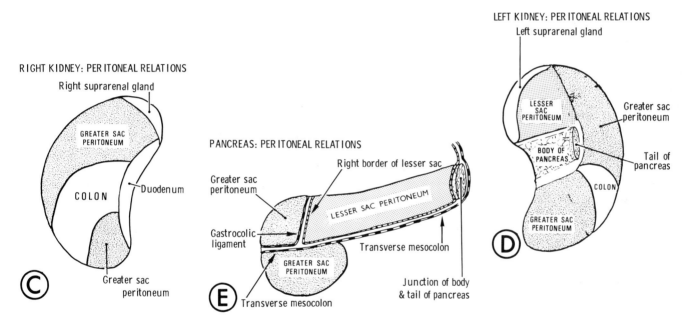

RIGHT KIDNEY: PERITONEAL RELATIONS

Right suprarenal gland

GREATER SAC PERITONEUM

COLON

Duodenum

Greater sac peritoneum

(C)

PANCREAS: PERITONEAL RELATIONS

Greater sac peritoneum

Gastrocolic ligament

GREATER SAC PERITONEUM

Transverse mesocolon

Right border of lesser sac

LESSER SAC PERITONEUM

Transverse mesocolon

Junction of body & tail of pancreas

(E)

LEFT KIDNEY: PERITONEAL RELATIONS

Left suprarenal gland

LESSER SAC PERITONEUM

BODY OF PANCREAS

GREATER SAC PERITONEUM

Greater sac peritoneum

Tail of pancreas

COLON

(D)

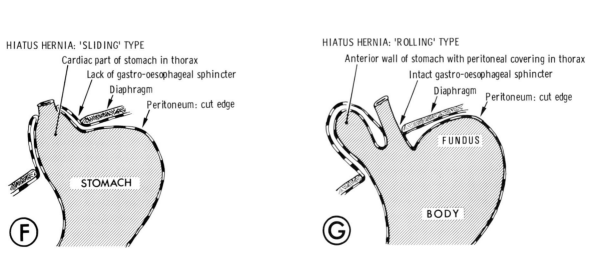

HIATUS HERNIA: 'SLIDING' TYPE

Cardiac part of stomach in thorax

Lack of gastro-oesophageal sphincter

Diaphragm

Peritoneum: cut edge

STOMACH

(F)

HIATUS HERNIA: 'ROLLING' TYPE

Anterior wall of stomach with peritoneal covering in thorax

Intact gastro-oesophageal sphincter

Diaphragm

Peritoneum: cut edge

FUNDUS

BODY

(G)

The coeliac artery and its branches

Recall that the coeliac artery is the highest of the three unpaired ventral branches of the abdominal aorta, and that its branches are distributed to the spleen, liver and pancreas, and to those parts of the gastrointestinal tract which are derived from the foetal foregut, that is from the oesophageal hiatus to the middle of the second part of the duodenum (**230**).

This large artery arises opposite the upper border of the first lumbar vertebral body (**231C**) and runs forwards for about 1 cm between the crura of the diaphragm and immediately above the body of the pancreas (**A**). There it abuts against the posterior wall of the lesser peritoneal sac and divides abruptly into three large but unequal branches.

It is useful to bear in mind that in general, each of these branches follows a C-shaped course, running first behind the lesser sac, then round one of its borders, and finally in front of the sac to reach the viscera it supplies. It should also be remembered that because lesser sac peritoneum forms one layer of a number of peritoneal ligaments in the upper part of the abdomen (see above), many parts of the branches of the coeliac artery are contained between the layers of these ligaments.

The left gastric artery

The left gastric artery, the smallest of the three large branches, passes upwards and to the left behind the lesser sac, and then turns forwards over its upper border, just to the right of the cardiac orifice of the stomach (**A, B**). Here it gives off several branches which supply the abdominal part of the oesophagus. Thereafter the artery turns downwards in front of the lesser sac, and therefore between the two layers of the lesser omentum (**B**), and runs downwards and to the right along the upper two thirds of the lesser curvature of the stomach. It ends by anastomosing with the right gastric artery (see below).

The splenic artery

The splenic artery is the largest of the three branches, and follows a characteristically sinuous course to the left behind the lesser sac (**A**). Note the relationships of this part of the vessel to the pancreas, the left suprarenal gland and the left kidney (**A**). It gives off numerous branches to the pancreas. The artery now turns forwards from the anterior surface of the left kidney to the hilus of the spleen, lying immediately above the tail of the pancreas and between the two layers of the lienorenal ligament (**C**). At the hilus it divides into several large branches which enter the spleen, and other

branches which supply the stomach. The latter run towards the stomach initially between the layers of the gastrosplenic ligament (**C**) which, it will be recalled, is continuous above with the gastrophrenic ligament and below with the gastrocolic ligament.

Several short gastric arteries extend upwards through the continuous gastrosplenic and gastrophrenic ligaments to reach the posterior aspect of the fundus of the stomach (**B**).

The left gastro-epiploic artery passes to the right through the continuous gastrosplenic and gastrocolic ligaments a short distance below the greater curvature of the stomach (**B**); there it anastomoses with the right gastro-epiploic artery (see below).

The common hepatic artery

The common hepatic artery passes to the right and emerges from behind the lower part of the right border of the lesser sac, just above the neck of the pancreas (**A**). Here it lies behind the first part of the duodenum, and gives off its large gastroduodenal branch (**B**). Beyond the origin of this branch it is known simply as the hepatic artery. This turns upwards and passes, with the portal vein and bile duct, through the interval between the duodenum and the floor of the aditus to the lesser sac (**B**) to lie in front of the aditus and therefore between the layers of the lesser omentum, close to its right free margin (**247D**). It ascends through the omentum and divides into right and left branches which enter the liver through the porta hepatis (**256**). In its course it gives off the following branches.

The gastroduodenal artery arises as the common hepatic emerges from behind the lesser sac (**B**) and runs downwards between the first part of the duodenum and the pancreas. This position of the artery is important, for an ulcer on the posterior wall of the duodenum may eventually erode the vessel and cause massive vomiting of blood (haematemesis). Below the duodenum the gastroduodenal artery divides into the following two diverging branches.

The superior pancreaticoduodenal (**B**) passes to the right and supplies the duodenum as far as the hepatopancreatic ampulla, the terminal part of the bile duct and the upper half of the head of the pancreas.

The right gastro-epiploic artery turns to the left in front of the lesser sac (**B**) and between the layers of the gastrocolic ligament. In this ligament it becomes directly continuous with the left gastro-epiploic branch of the splenic without the intervention of a capillary bed (**B**). This gastro-epiploic arterial arch supplies the lower half of the greater curvature of the stomach. It also gives off numerous branches (**D**) which pass vertically downwards through the gastrocolic ligament and in front of the transverse colon to reach and supply the greater omentum.

COELIAC ARTERY: BRANCHES BEHIND LESSER SAC

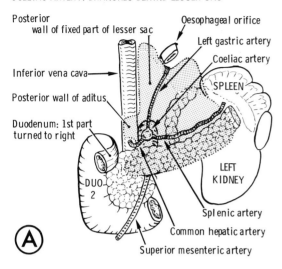

Posterior wall of fixed part of lesser sac

Oesophageal orifice

Left gastric artery

Coeliac artery

Inferior vena cava

Posterior wall of aditus

SPLEEN

Duodenum: 1st part turned to right

DUO 2

LEFT KIDNEY

Splenic artery

Common hepatic artery

Superior mesenteric artery

(A)

COELIAC ARTERY: BRANCHES IN FRONT OF LESSER SAC

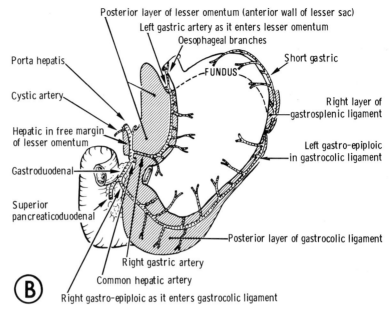

Posterior layer of lesser omentum (anterior wall of lesser sac)

Left gastric artery as it enters lesser omentum

Oesophageal branches

Short gastric

FUNDUS

Porta hepatis

Cystic artery

Hepatic in free margin of lesser omentum

Right layer of gastrosplenic ligament

Left gastro-epiploic in gastrocolic ligament

Gastroduodenal

Superior pancreaticoduodenal

Posterior layer of gastrocolic ligament

Right gastric artery

Common hepatic artery

Right gastro-epiploic as it enters gastrocolic ligament

(B)

SPLENIC ARTERY IN TRANSVERSE SECTION

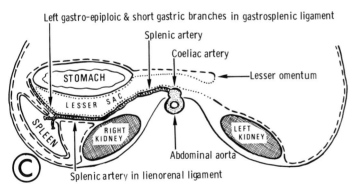

Left gastro-epiploic & short gastric branches in gastrosplenic ligament

Splenic artery

Coeliac artery

STOMACH

Lesser omentum

LESSER SAC

SPLEEN

RIGHT KIDNEY

LEFT KIDNEY

Abdominal aorta

(C)

Splenic artery in lienorenal ligament

GASTRO-EPIPLOIC ARTERIAL ARCH

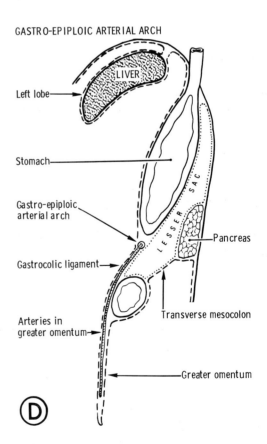

Left lobe

LIVER

Stomach

Gastro-epiploic arterial arch

Gastrocolic ligament

Arteries in greater omentum

LESSER SAC

Pancreas

Transverse mesocolon

Greater omentum

(D)

The right gastric branch of the hepatic artery arises as soon as the latter enters the lesser omentum. It is usually small and passes to the left between the two layers of the omentum to form a directly continuous arterial arch with the left gastric artery. This gastric arterial arch supplies the lesser curvature of the stomach (**251B**).

The cystic artery is a branch of the right division of the hepatic artery which supplies the gall bladder. It is considered later (**256**).

The portal vein and its tributaries of origin

It has already been noted that the large portal vein is formed between the neck of the pancreas and the left margin of the inferior vena cava (**236**). Emerging from behind the pancreas it runs upwards behind the first part of the duodenum (**A, B**) where it is situated behind the continuity of the common hepatic and hepatic arteries. As it rises above the duodenum it passes in front of the aditus of the lesser sac, which separates it from the inferior vena cava, and thus comes to lie between the two layers of the lesser omentum (**B, C**). It continues upwards close to the right free margin of the omentum and behind the hepatic artery before dividing into short right and left branches. These enter the liver through the porta hepatis. The tributaries of the portal vein can now be considered.

The superior mesenteric vein

The distal part of this vessel will be considered later but note now that its upper part crosses the third part of the duodenum and the uncinate process of the pancreas covered by greater sac peritoneum (**A, C**). It then passes between the neck of the pancreas and the left edge of the inferior vena cava to the formation of the portal vein.

The right gastro-epiploic vein courses to the right between the layers of the gastrocolic ligament and, turning round the right border of the lesser sac (**C**), joins the upper part of the superior mesenteric vein.

The splenic vein

This is formed at the hilus of the spleen by the confluence of large vessels issuing from that viscus. It passes backwards through the lienorenal ligament on the left side of the tail of the pancreas to the anterior surface of the left kidney (**237D**). There it turns to the right and runs behind the body of the pancreas (**A**), along the course described previously, to the origin of the portal vein. Note the levels of the splenic artery and vein on the posterior abdominal wall (**A**). The vein drains the body and tail of the pancreas through numerous small vessels and also receives the following additional tributaries.

The short gastric and left gastro-epiploic veins drain the fundus and left part of the stomach. They follow the courses of the corresponding arteries (**251B**) and join the splenic vein at the hilus of the spleen.

The inferior mesenteric vein has a long course up the left side of the posterior abdominal wall, most of which will be considered later. The upper part of the vessel sweeps upwards and to the right between the posterior abdominal wall and its covering greater sac peritoneum, passing close to the left side of the fourth part of the duodenum (**A**). It finally passes deep to the body of the pancreas to join the splenic vein.

Direct portal tributaries

The left gastric vein follows the corresponding artery from the lesser curvature of the stomach to the region of the coeliac artery (**C, A**). Thereafter it accompanies the common hepatic artery and, emerging with that vessel from behind the lesser sac, joins the portal vein at the upper border of the neck of the pancreas.

As it passes over the upper border of the lesser sac, this vein receives tributaries from the abdominal part of the oesophagus (**C**). These anastomose with the veins which drain the thoracic part of the oesophagus into the azygos venous system. This is one of the portosystemic anastomoses which become grossly dilated and varicose when there is obstruction to the portal blood stream (**232**). Because they lie in the submucous tissue, such dilated veins are frequently ruptured, giving rise to gross haemorrhage and subsequent vomiting of blood.

The right gastric vein accompanies the right gastric artery and joins the portal immediately above the first part of the duodenum (**C**).

The veins of the gall bladder do not join, as might be expected, to form a single cystic vein. Instead, they run directly into the adjacent liver substance to join intrahepatic branches of the portal vein.

The para-umbilical veins are small vessels which pass from the umbilicus, in close association with the ligamentum teres within the falciform ligament, to join the left branch of the portal vein (**D**). At the umbilicus they anastomose with systemic veins in the anterior abdominal wall. In portal obstruction this portosystemic anastomosis may also become dilated so that varicose veins appear beneath the skin around the umbilicus.

In the foetus the left branch of the portal vein is connected to the placenta by the umbilical vein and to the inferior vena cava by the ductus venosus which short-circuits much of the placental blood past the liver. At birth these vessels become obliterated and replaced by the fibrous ligamentum teres and ligamentum venosum (**D**). These remain attached to the wall of the left branch of the portal vein.

PORTAL VEIN

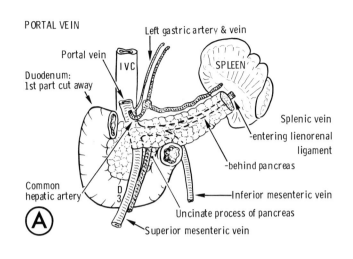

Left gastric artery & vein

Portal vein

Duodenum: 1st part cut away

IVC

SPLEEN

Splenic vein
-entering lienorenal ligament
-behind pancreas

Common hepatic artery

D 3

Inferior mesenteric vein

Uncinate process of pancreas

Superior mesenteric vein

(A)

PORTAL VEIN: IN VERTICAL SECTION

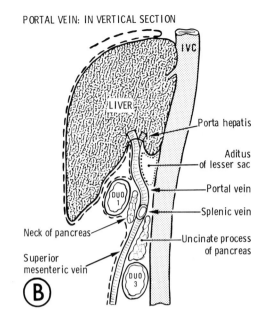

IVC

LIVER

Porta hepatis

Aditus of lesser sac

Portal vein

Splenic vein

DUO 1

Neck of pancreas

Uncinate process of pancreas

Superior mesenteric vein

DUO 3

(B)

PORTAL VEIN: TRIBUTARIES

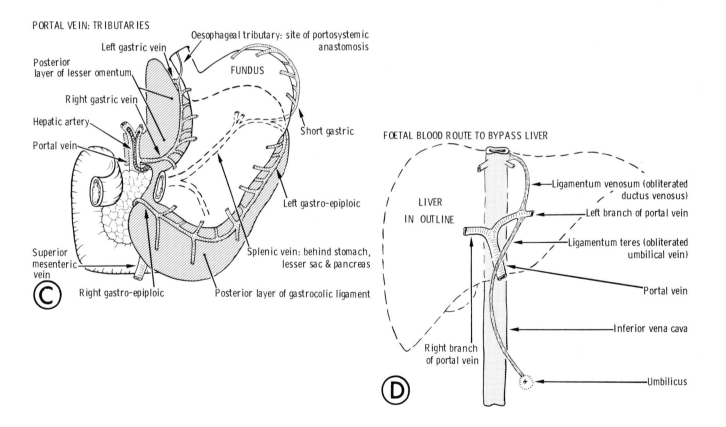

Left gastric vein

Oesophageal tributary: site of portosystemic anastomosis

FUNDUS

Posterior layer of lesser omentum

Right gastric vein

Hepatic artery

Portal vein

Short gastric

Left gastro-epiploic

Superior mesenteric vein

Right gastro-epiploic

Splenic vein: behind stomach, lesser sac & pancreas

Posterior layer of gastrocolic ligament

(C)

FOETAL BLOOD ROUTE TO BYPASS LIVER

LIVER IN OUTLINE

Ligamentum venosum (obliterated ductus venosus)

Left branch of portal vein

Ligamentum teres (obliterated umbilical vein)

Portal vein

Inferior vena cava

Right branch of portal vein

Umbilicus

(D)

Trans-splenic portal venography

The spleen is enlarged in patients with hepatic cirrhosis and portal hypertension (**232**). Advantage is taken of this to demonstrate the portal venous circulation by percutaneous trans-splenic portal venography (injection of a radio-opaque medium into the splenic pulp). The extent of the splenic enlargement is assessed by percussion and the optimal site for insertion of the needle is usually through the eighth or ninth left intercostal space in the midaxillary line. Note that this procedure involves the passage of the needle through the costodiaphragmatic recess of the pleural cavity, the diaphragm and the greater peritoneal sac before it reaches the spleen (**A**).

The vascular architecture of the liver

Both the portal vein, which carries about 80% of the blood to the liver, and the hepatic artery, which carries the other 20%, divide into right and left branches below the porta hepatis. Within the liver the primary branches of the hepatic artery divide dichotomously into vessels which are distributed to specific segments of the viscus, which do not correspond to the topographical lobes which have been described previously (**226**).

The vascular right and left lobes are demarcated by a plane passing forwards from the groove for the inferior vena cava to the gall bladder bed (**B**). The right lobe consists of anterior and posterior segments (**B**). The left vascular lobe is divisible into a medial segment, which includes the topographical quadrate and caudate lobes, and a lateral segment which is more or less coextensive with the topographical left lobe.

The venous drainage through the hepatic veins into the inferior vena cava does not follow the same segmental pattern. The left lateral segment is drained by one hepatic vein but all other segments are drained by more than one vessel.

The biliary ducts

Bile is carried away from the liver by the right and left hepatic ducts, which emerge from the porta hepatis (**C**). These ducts are short and unite almost immediately to form the common hepatic duct near the right end of the porta. This structure descends between the two layers of the lesser omentum lying at its right free margin, to the right of the hepatic artery and in front of the portal vein.

The gall bladder lies on the inferior surface of the liver along the right edge of the quadrate lobe. Its free surface is covered by greater sac peritoneum and is in relation, through the right subhepatic space (**248**), with the first and second parts of the duodenum and the right end of the transverse colon. In front, the blind fundus projects slightly beyond the inferior margin of the liver and is in contact with the anterior abdominal wall at the junction of the lateral margin of right rectus abdominis (linea semilunaris) and the right ninth costal cartilage. Behind and above, the narrow neck lies just to the right of the porta hepatis and becomes continuous with the cystic duct which turns downwards into the lesser omentum on the right side of the common hepatic duct. Cystic duct and common hepatic duct join, usually about 3 cm below the porta hepatis, to form the bile duct.

The bile duct continues downwards in the lesser omentum still at the right free margin, to the right of the hepatic artery and in front of the portal vein, until it disappears behind the first part of the duodenum. The terminal part of its course has already been considered (**229C, 229D**).

SPLENIC INJECTION FOR PORTAL VENOGRAPHY

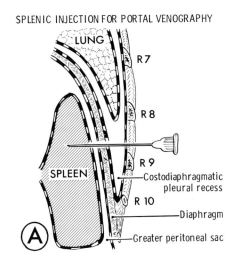

LUNG

R 7

R 8

R 9

R 10

SPLEEN

Costodiaphragmatic pleural recess

Diaphragm

Greater peritoneal sac

(A)

LIVER: VASCULAR ARCHITECTURE

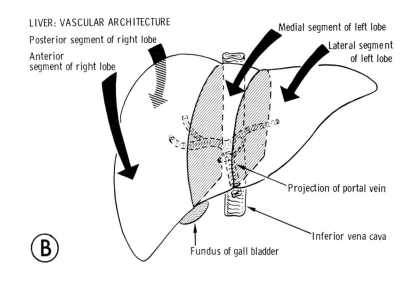

Posterior segment of right lobe

Anterior segment of right lobe

Medial segment of left lobe

Lateral segment of left lobe

Projection of portal vein

Inferior vena cava

Fundus of gall bladder

(B)

THE BILIARY DUCTS

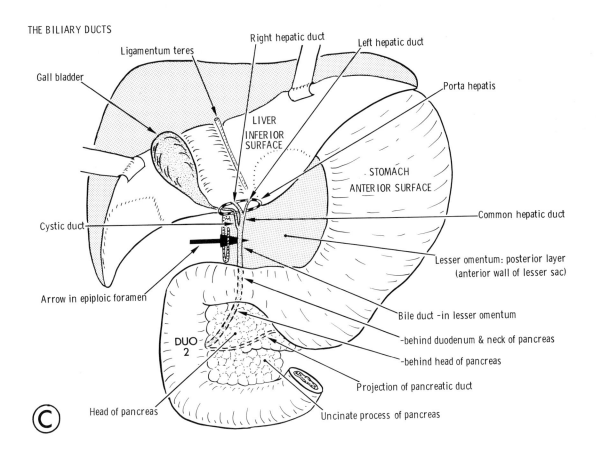

Ligamentum teres

Gall bladder

Right hepatic duct

Left hepatic duct

Porta hepatis

LIVER INFERIOR SURFACE

STOMACH ANTERIOR SURFACE

Common hepatic duct

Cystic duct

Lesser omentum: posterior layer (anterior wall of lesser sac)

Arrow in epiploic foramen

Bile duct -in lesser omentum

-behind duodenum & neck of pancreas

-behind head of pancreas

DUO 2

Projection of pancreatic duct

Head of pancreas

Uncinate process of pancreas

(C)

The structures in the right free margin of the lesser omentum

A group of very important structures lie within the omentum, close to its right free margin and in front of the epiploic foramen. These are the portal vein (**237C**), the hepatic artery (**251B**) and the biliary ducts (**255C**), namely the two hepatic ducts, the common hepatic duct, the cystic duct and the bile duct. As operations in this region are common, the interrelationship of these three sets of structures is important. Study carefully the normal relationships which are present in the majority of the population (**A**) and observe the more common of the many unusual arrangements which may be encountered at operation (**B, C, D, E, F, G**).

1. Normally, the right branch of the hepatic artery passes from left to right behind the common hepatic duct and in front of the portal vein. In some individuals it passes in front of the duct and is then more vulnerable to injury at operation (**B**).
2. The cystic artery usually arises from the right branch of the hepatic artery and runs behind and above the cystic duct. Occasionally the vessel arises from the left branch of the hepatic artery and passes to the right in front of the common hepatic duct (**C**). Rarely there are two cystic arteries.
3. Abnormal vessels may either replace or augment the usual right and left branches of the hepatic artery. An abnormal left hepatic usually springs from the left gastric artery and runs to the porta hepatis through the lesser omentum (**D**). An abnormal right hepatic may arise from the superior mesenteric artery behind the pancreas and pass upwards through the lesser omentum behind the portal vein (**E**).
4. Although the cystic duct usually joins the common hepatic duct a short distance below the porta hepatis (**A**), a junction at a considerably lower level is not uncommon. The two ducts then run for some distance in close proximity (**F**) and both may be included in the one ligature during removal of the gall bladder.
5. In some individuals the cystic duct crosses in front or behind the common hepatic duct and joins its left margin (**G**).

LESSER OMENTUM: CONTENTS

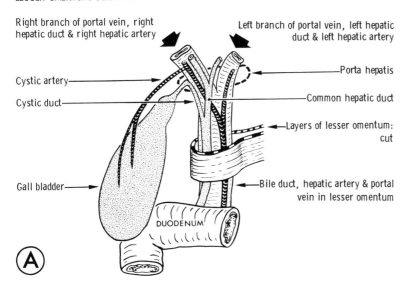

Right branch of portal vein, right hepatic duct & right hepatic artery

Left branch of portal vein, left hepatic duct & left hepatic artery

Porta hepatis

Cystic artery

Cystic duct

Common hepatic duct

Layers of lesser omentum: cut

Gall bladder

Bile duct, hepatic artery & portal vein in lesser omentum

DUODENUM

Ⓐ

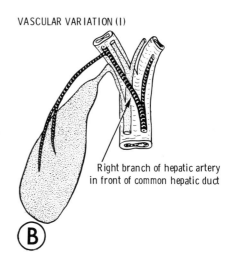

VASCULAR VARIATION (I)

Right branch of hepatic artery in front of common hepatic duct

Ⓑ

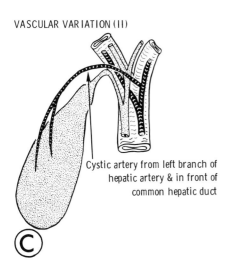

VASCULAR VARIATION (II)

Cystic artery from left branch of hepatic artery & in front of common hepatic duct

Ⓒ

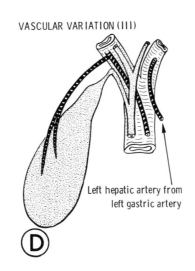

VASCULAR VARIATION (III)

Left hepatic artery from left gastric artery

Ⓓ

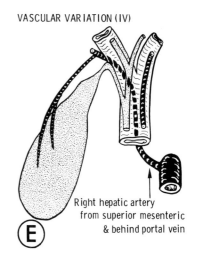

VASCULAR VARIATION (IV)

Right hepatic artery from superior mesenteric & behind portal vein

Ⓔ

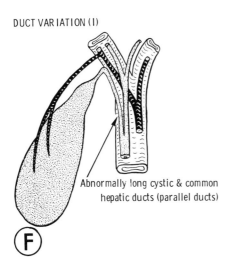

DUCT VARIATION (I)

Abnormally long cystic & common hepatic ducts (parallel ducts)

Ⓕ

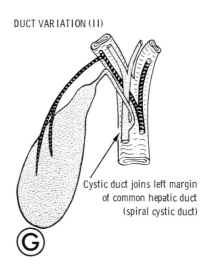

DUCT VARIATION (II)

Cystic duct joins left margin of common hepatic duct (spiral cystic duct)

Ⓖ

DETAILED ANATOMY OF THE LOWER PART OF THE ABDOMINAL CAVITY PROPER

This section deals with the lower part of the abdominal cavity proper, between the root of the transverse mesocolon above and the inguinal ligaments and the pelvic brim below.

It is helpful to revise the muscles which form the posterior wall of the region (**201B**), and the major blood vessels (**231**), and the branches of the lumbar nerve plexus (**205C**).

The region is lined by three concentric tissue layers. The outermost consists of the relevant parts of the general fascial envelope of the abdomen. Internal to that is a layer of fatty areolar extraperitoneal tissue, and this is lined in turn by greater sac peritoneum.

On both sides of the body, two diverticula arise from the fascial lining of the lower part of the region and extend out of the abdominal cavity. The internal spermatic fascia, which arises from the deep inguinal ring and forms the deepest fascial layer of the spermatic cord, has been considered already (**210**). The other diverticulum passes downwards behind the medial half of the inguinal ligament into the upper part of the anterior aspect of the thigh. This is the femoral sheath (**333, 335**).

The femoral sheath will be considered more fully with the lower limb, but it should be noted now that it is divided by two sagittal septa into medial, intermediate and lateral compartments. The lumen of each diverticulum is, of necessity, continuous above with the abdominal extraperitoneal tissue, whereas the peritoneum simply extends as a sheet across their orifices.

It is convenient to consider here the relationships of a number of abdominal structures to these fascial diverticula and to observe how these relationships are determined by the tissue layer they occupy in the abdomen.

The external iliac vessels lie in the abdominal extraperitoneal tissue. Thus, traced downwards, the artery leaves the abdomen by passing behind the midpoint of the inguinal ligament into the lateral compartment of the femoral sheath where it becomes the femoral artery (**B**). Similarly, the femoral vein ascends from the middle compartment of the sheath into the abdomen where it becomes the external iliac vein.

The genitofemoral nerve emerges from the anterior surface of the psoas major muscle, passes through the psoas fascia and divides, in the extraperitoneal tissue, into genital and femoral branches. Because they are situated in this layer both branches are in a position to enter the diverticula of the abdominal fascial envelope described above. The genital branch passes through the deep inguinal ring into the spermatic cord (**A, 213A**). The femoral branch passes into the lateral compartment of the femoral sheath on the lateral side of the external iliac artery (**A, 331C**).

The lateral branches of the lumbar plexus all lie outside the abdominal fascial envelope and consequently none can enter the diverticula of that envelope. In particular the femoral nerve enters the lower limb by passing behind the inguinal ligament just lateral to and outside the femoral sheath (**C**). The lateral cutaneous nerve of the thigh enters the thigh by passing behind the lateral end of the inguinal ligament (**C, 331C**).

The gonadal arteries have already been noted as paired branches arising from the front of the aorta behind the third part of the duodenum, and running downwards and laterally onto psoas major, the artery of the right side usually crossing in front of the inferior vena cava (**237A**).

Observe in **A** that, on the psoas muscles, the arteries are closely associated with, but anterior to, the genitofemoral nerve, being situated in the extraperitoneal tissue. In the male (**213A**) the testicular artery eventually turns forwards from psoas and enters the internal spermatic fascia by traversing the deep inguinal ring. In the female the ovarian artery turns medially over the external iliac vessels to enter the pelvic cavity (**281A**).

The gonadal veins initially follow the courses of the corresponding arteries, usually as a plexus of several vessels, which later become reduced to single veins on either side. Observe in (**A**) that in the upper part of their courses the veins diverge from the corresponding arteries, the right ending in the inferior vena cava, and the left, at a higher level, in the left renal vein (**237A**).

The ductus deferens (**211D, 213A**) leaves the spermatic cord by passing through the deep inguinal ring into the abdominal extraperitoneal tissue. Here it turns medially and backwards and passes over the external iliac vessels into the pelvic cavity (**A**).

The round ligament of the uterus follows a similar abdominal course to that of the ductus deferens, but of course in the reverse direction.

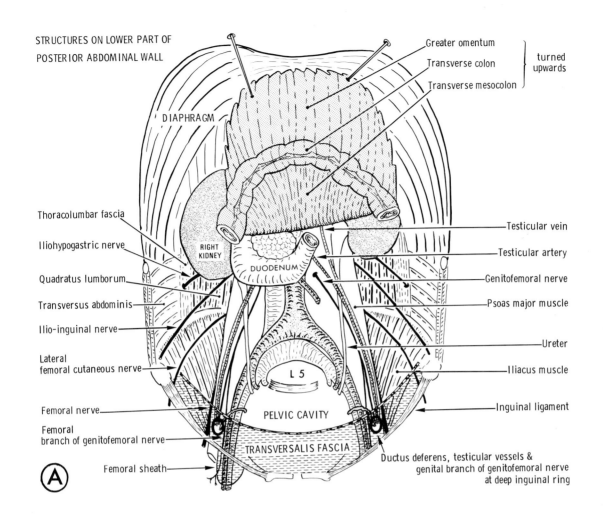

STRUCTURES ON LOWER PART OF
POSTERIOR ABDOMINAL WALL

Greater omentum
Transverse colon   turned
Transverse mesocolon upwards

DIAPHRAGM

Thoracolumbar fascia

Iliohypogastric nerve

Quadratus lumborum

Transversus abdominis

Ilio-inguinal nerve

Lateral
femoral cutaneous nerve

Femoral nerve

Femoral
branch of genitofemoral nerve

Femoral sheath

RIGHT KIDNEY

DUODENUM

L 5

PELVIC CAVITY

TRANSVERSALIS FASCIA

Testicular vein

Testicular artery

Genitofemoral nerve

Psoas major muscle

Ureter

Iliacus muscle

Inguinal ligament

Ductus deferens, testicular vessels &
genital branch of genitofemoral nerve
at deep inguinal ring

(A)

FEMORAL SHEATH: SAGITTAL SECTION

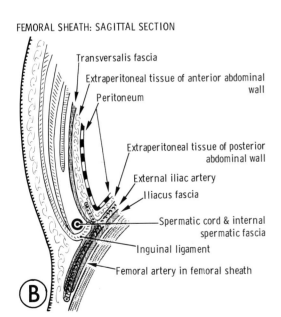

Transversalis fascia

Extraperitoneal tissue of anterior abdominal wall

Peritoneum

Extraperitoneal tissue of posterior abdominal wall

External iliac artery

Iliacus fascia

Spermatic cord & internal spermatic fascia

Inguinal ligament

Femoral artery in femoral sheath

(B)

FEMORAL SHEATH: ABDOMINAL ASPECT

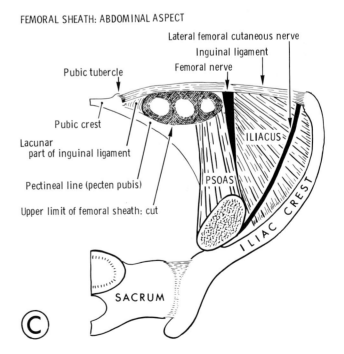

Lateral femoral cutaneous nerve
Inguinal ligament
Femoral nerve

Pubic tubercle

Pubic crest

Lacunar
part of inguinal ligament

Pectineal line (pecten pubis)

Upper limit of femoral sheath: cut

ILIACUS

PSOAS

ILIAC CREST

SACRUM

(C)

259

The ureters

The positions and relations of the upper parts of the ureters have been described previously (**221A**). The right ureter enters the region under consideration from behind the third part of the duodenum. The left ureter appears from behind the body of the pancreas and the root of the transverse mesocolon (**A**). Thereafter, each ureter passes downwards on the anterior aspect of the corresponding psoas major. In its course it moves obliquely from the lateral to the medial side of the genitofemoral nerve and the gonadal vessels, passing anterior to the nerve and posterior to the vessels. Traced downwards, it crosses in front of the medial border of psoas major and the bifurcation of the common iliac artery, before turning downwards over the brim of the pelvis into the pelvic cavity. The blood supply to this part of the ureter is derived from the gonadal vessels. From a radiological point of view it is important to note that, as it descends, the ureter lies some distance in front of the tips of the lumbar transverse processes and in front of the sacroiliac joint at the level of the lumbosacral disc.

The caecum and the ascending colon

Revise the form and structure of the caecum (**225A**), and note (**A**) that it lies in the right iliac fossa. This part of the large bowel is usually completely invested by peritoneum, so that it is comparatively mobile and may even be found as a content of an inguinal hernia. Behind, the deep retrocaecal peritoneal pouch separates it from the iliopsoas fascia (**B**) which in turn separates the pouch from the iliacus, the lateral border of psoas major and the lateral femoral cutaneous nerve (**A**).

The ascending colon rises from the right iliac fossa through the right lumbar region. Observe in **A** the several structures which lie behind it. Unlike the caecum, the ascending colon in most individuals is covered by peritoneum only over its anterior, medial and lateral aspects (**C**). A deep peritoneal-lined paracolic gutter extends backwards between it and the lateral abdominal wall (**C**) and is continuous above with the right subphrenic space.

Anteriorly both the caecum and ascending colon, because of their large size, are usually in contact with the anterior abdominal wall, but the relationship is variable and some coils of small intestine or part of the greater omentum may intervene.

Over the ascending colon, but not usually on the caecum, the peritoneum exhibits a number of fat-filled pouches known as appendices epiploicae.

The descending colon

This segment of the colon runs downwards from the left colic flexure through the left lumbar region into the left iliac fossa. There it turns medially over the psoas major muscle and the external iliac vessels to the brim of the pelvis, where it becomes the sigmoid (pelvic) colon (**A**). Throughout its course its posterior surface is related to the structures shown in **A**. Peritoneum, exhibiting appendices epiploicae, covers it anteriorly, medially and laterally (**C**). The descending colon is a good deal narrower than the ascending colon and caecum. Consequently, coils of small intestine usually intervene between it and the anterior abdominal wall, and the left paracolic gutter is shallower than the right (**C**).

The mesentery

Over the quadrangular area (**D**) between the right and left parts of the colon and the root of the transverse mesocolon and the pelvic brim, peritoneum covers the posterior abdominal wall and the structures which lie upon it, except along an oblique line where it is carried forwards as a two-layered mesentery which encloses and suspends the jejunum and ileum which have already been described (**C**). The root of the mesentery, as this line of reflection is called, is slightly convex to the left and extends downwards and to the right from the duodenojejunal junction to the ileocolic junction. Study in **D** the structures which it crosses in its course.

The measurement of the mesentery, from root to bowel, diminishes from a central maximum of about 20 cm to zero at either end. The root of the mesentery is about 15 cm long while the intestinal border is nearly 6 m. Because of the disparity between these two measurements, the intestinal border is elaborately pleated, and jejunum and ileum are intricately coiled in the lower part of the abdominal cavity. Fatty areolar tissue occupies the interval between the two layers of the mesentery but is considerably more abundant in the lower than the upper part.

POSITIONS OF CAECUM, ASCENDING COLON & DESCENDING COLON

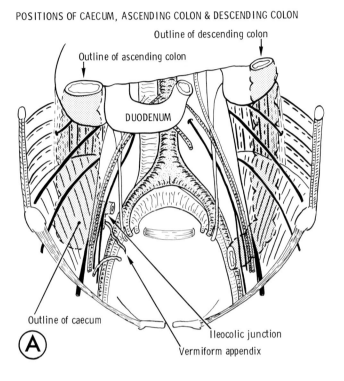

Outline of descending colon

Outline of ascending colon

DUODENUM

Outline of caecum

Ileocolic junction

Vermiform appendix

(A)

CAECUM & ASCENDING COLON: SAGITTAL SECTION

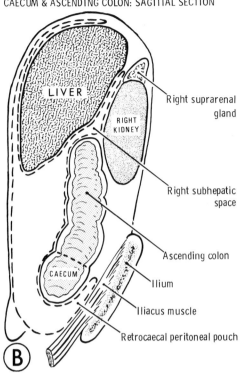

LIVER

RIGHT KIDNEY

Right suprarenal gland

Right subhepatic space

Ascending colon

Ilium

Iliacus muscle

Retrocaecal peritoneal pouch

CAECUM

(B)

ASCENDING & DESCENDING COLON: HORIZONTAL SECTION

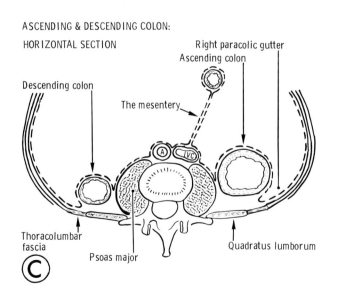

Right paracolic gutter
Ascending colon

Descending colon

The mesentery

Thoracolumbar fascia

Psoas major

Quadratus lumborum

(C)

ROOT OF THE MESENTERY

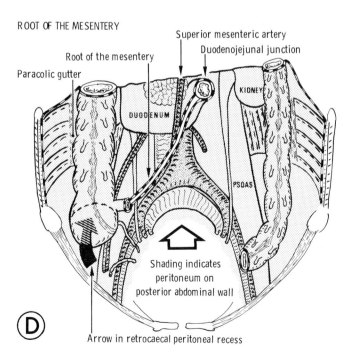

Root of the mesentery

Superior mesenteric artery

Duodenojejunal junction

Paracolic gutter

DUODENUM

KIDNEY

PSOAS

Shading indicates peritoneum on posterior abdominal wall

Arrow in retrocaecal peritoneal recess

(D)

The vermiform appendix and the meso-appendix

The form of the appendix and its attachment to the posteromedial aspect of the caecum just below the ileocolic junction have been described already (**225A**). The position of its base (i.e. its attachment to the caecum) is constant and lies deep to what is traditionally known as McBurney's point (**219B**). This is situated at the junction of the lateral and middle thirds of the line joining the anterior superior iliac spine to the umbilicus. The position of the rest of the appendix varies. In about two-thirds of individuals it lies in the retrocaecal pouch, in which it may be rather difficult to locate through an anterior abdominal wall incision. In nearly another third of individuals the appendix is long and extends medially over the pelvic brim into the pelvic cavity.

The appendix is enclosed in a peritoneal meso-appendix which is an extension of the left layer of the lowest part of the mesentery of the small intestine (**A**). This relationship is most easily visualised in a section traversing ileum, mesentery, appendix and meso-appendix (**B**).

The superior mesenteric artery

Recall that the artery arises as a single ventral branch of the aorta at the level of L1. And that it immediately turns downwards in front of the left renal vein and behind the splenic vein and the body of the pancreas (**237D**). At the lower border of the pancreas the artery passes behind the root of the transverse mesocolon (**C**) and continues downwards over the uncinate process of the pancreas and the third part of the duodenum (**C**). In this situation it lies a short distance to the right of the mesentery but then inclines into the root of that structure (**C**). It ends in the lower part of the root by joining one of its own branches (**C**).

The branches of the artery supply those parts of the intestine derived from the foetal midgut (**231B**) but it is to be noted that the branches do not arise in the same order as the parts of the midgut they supply. They can be considered conveniently in four groups.

The middle colic artery, which is the first branch, supplies the right three-quarters of the transverse colon which is developmentally the terminal part of the midgut. It arises at the lower border of the body of the pancreas and passes into the transverse mesocolon (**C**). Near the transverse colon it divides into right and left divisions which run in corresponding directions a short distance from the gut. Note that, on either side of the stem of the artery, the transverse mesocolon is almost avascular so that an opening can be made through it, into the lesser sac, when this is surgically necessary.

The inferior pancreaticoduodenal artery arises at the upper border of the third part of the duodenum. It runs to the right, immediately deep to the peritoneum, to supply the lower part of the head of the pancreas and the duodenum as far as the hepatopancreatic ampulla (**C**), where it anastomoses with the superior pancreaticoduodenal vessel which is derived from the coeliac artery (**251B**). Note that this branch supplies the part of the duodenum which is the initial part of the midgut.

An ileocolic and usually, though not constantly, a *right colic branch* arise from the right side of the superior mesenteric artery. They diverge to the right immediately behind the area of peritoneum which lies in the interval between the root of the mesentery and the right colon (**C**). The right colic artery divides near the right colic flexure into ascending and descending divisions (**C**). The ileocolic vessel divides close to the ileocolic junction into superior and inferior divisions. The adjacent divisions of the middle colic, right colic and ileocolic vessels join directly, without intervening capillaries, to form a marginal artery from which slender branches are distributed to the colon (**C**). The inferior division of the ileocolic turns to the left into the lower part of the root of the mesentery, where it becomes directly continuous with the stem of the superior mesenteric artery. Its branches supply the caecum, the terminal part of the ileum and the vermiform appendix (**C**). Note that the appendicular branch runs in the free margin of the meso-appendix and sends small branches to the appendix (**A**).

The jejunal and ileal branches are fifteen or so large vessels which supply the whole of the jejunum and ileum except the terminal metre or so. The upper three or four run a short distance to the left before reaching the mesentery (**C**). As the vessels run between the layers of the mesentery they are at first parallel to one another, but at some distance from the bowel they undergo repeated divisions and anastomoses to form a series of arterial arcades as shown in **D**. The number of arcades is greatest in the longest middle part of the mesentery. The terminal arcades form a continuous scalloped arterial channel from which twigs are distributed to either side of the gut.

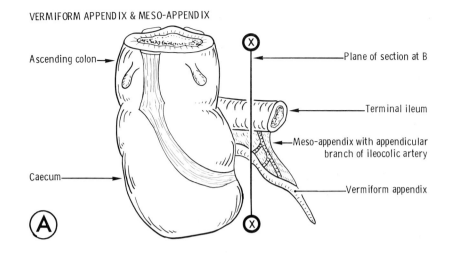

VERMIFORM APPENDIX & MESO-APPENDIX

Ascending colon

Plane of section at B

Terminal ileum

Meso-appendix with appendicular branch of ileocolic artery

Caecum

Vermiform appendix

Ⓐ

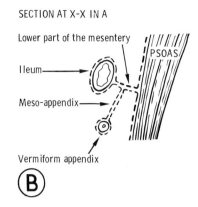

SECTION AT X-X IN A

Lower part of the mesentery

Ileum

PSOAS

Meso-appendix

Vermiform appendix

Ⓑ

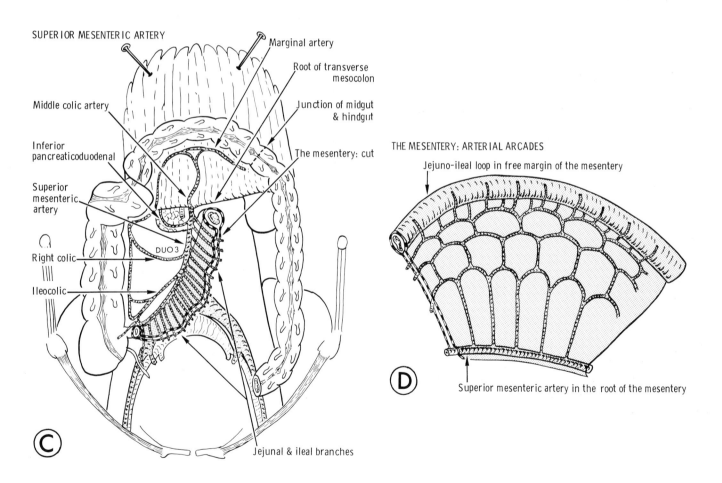

SUPERIOR MESENTERIC ARTERY

Marginal artery

Root of transverse mesocolon

Junction of midgut & hindgut

Middle colic artery

Inferior pancreaticoduodenal

The mesentery: cut

Superior mesenteric artery

THE MESENTERY: ARTERIAL ARCADES

Jejuno-ileal loop in free margin of the mesentery

Right colic

DUO 3

Ileocolic

Jejunal & ileal branches

Superior mesenteric artery in the root of the mesentery

Ⓒ

Ⓓ

The superior mesenteric vein

This large vein drains the region of the intestine supplied by the superior mesenteric artery into the portal venous system. It always lies on the right side of the artery and joins the splenic vein behind the neck of the pancreas (**253A**). It receives tributaries corresponding to the branches of the artery and also, unexpectedly, the right gastro-epiploic vein. The right colic and ileocolic anastomose to a small degree with systemic veins on the posterior abdominal wall. In portal venous obstruction these anastomoses become dilated and varicose, and allow leakage of some portal blood into the systemic system.

The inferior mesenteric artery

This vessel is considerably smaller than the superior mesenteric artery. Through its various branches it supplies those parts of the bowel developed from the hindgut (**231B**). It is a single ventral branch of the abdominal aorta (**231C**) which arises at about the level of L3, either behind or immediately below the third part of the duodenum (**A**). It runs downwards and to the left behind the peritoneum and as it approaches the left common iliac artery it divides abruptly into its terminal branches. It should be noted that whereas the superior mesenteric artery crosses the right ureter, the inferior mesenteric divides on the medial side of the left ureter.

   The left colic artery passes to the left towards the descending colon immediately behind the peritoneum, crossing the structures on the anterior surface of the left psoas including the ureter (**A, 235C**). It then divides into ascending and descending divisions. The former follows the colon upwards onto the left kidney and into the left end of the transverse mesocolon, where it joins directly the left division of the middle colic artery (**263C**) and forms a free anastomosis between the inferior and superior mesenteric arteries (**A**).

   The upper two or three sigmoid branches run downwards and laterally across the ureter on the lateral side of the left common iliac artery (**A**). Near the lower part of the descending colon each divides into ascending and descending divisions. The adjacent divisions of the upper sigmoid and left colic arteries join directly to form a continuous marginal artery, from which the descending colon and the left quarter of the transverse colon are supplied. It is important to note that the continuity of this marginal artery with the middle colic branch of the superior mesenteric artery is usually sufficient to maintain the viability of the descending colon should it be necessary to divide the main trunk of the inferior mesenteric artery.

   The lower sigmoid and superior rectal branches are considered in the section dealing with the pelvic cavity (**269A**). It may be noted now however (**A**) that the superior rectal artery enters the pelvic cavity by passing over the left common iliac vessels some distance to the medial side of the left ureter.

The inferior mesenteric vein

This major tributary of the portal venous system is formed by the coalescence of the superior rectal, sigmoid, and left colic veins. Notice that whereas the superior mesenteric vein lies on the right side and is almost coextensive with the corresponding artery (**237D**), the inferior mesenteric vein runs on the left side of its artery and ascends to a much higher level (**A**). The vein passes upwards on psoas major, skirts the left side of the duodenojejunal junction and curves to the right behind the body of the pancreas to join the splenic vein (**253A**). It has some degree of anastomosis with systemic veins on the posterior abdominal wall, which become varicose in portal venous obstruction. Observe that the inferior mesenteric vein runs parallel to and medial to the left gonadal vein which also passes behind the pancreas but joins the left renal vein (**237D**).

THE PELVIC PART OF THE ABDOMINAL CAVITY

The features of the osteoligamentous pelvis have been considered (**196**). Recall that the pelvic brim demarcates the region of the false pelvis, which contributes to the walls of the abdominal cavity proper, from the true pelvis which contributes to the walls of both the pelvic part of the abdominal cavity and the perineum.

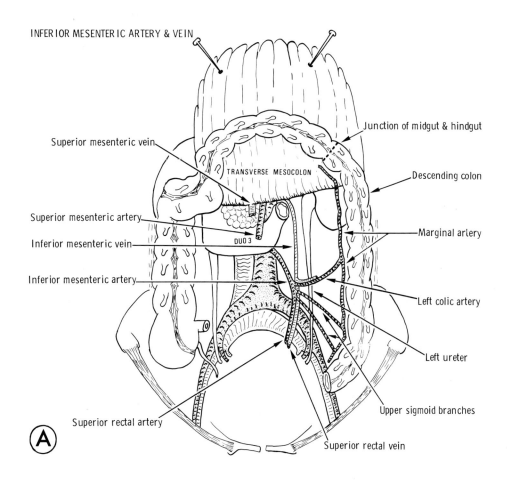

INFERIOR MESENTERIC ARTERY & VEIN

Junction of midgut & hindgut

Superior mesenteric vein

TRANSVERSE MESOCOLON

Descending colon

Superior mesenteric artery

DUO 3

Inferior mesenteric vein

Marginal artery

Inferior mesenteric artery

Left colic artery

Left ureter

Superior rectal artery

Upper sigmoid branches

Superior rectal vein

(A)

Note again the sacrotuberous and sacrospinous ligaments and the obturator membrane. Observe in the median section through the osteoligamentous pelvis (**A**) the three apertures in the lateral wall of the true pelvis, namely the greater and lesser sciatic foramina and the obturator canal. All lead into the tissues of the lower limb. Three muscles are closely applied to the inner aspect of the true pelvis.

Obturator internus arises from the area of bone and membrane indicated in **A**. Its muscle fibres converge backwards and downwards, and its tendon turns at right angles to its original plane through the lesser sciatic foramen into the buttock (**B**). The free surface of the muscle is covered by a thick layer of fascia which will be seen later to be of importance.

Piriformis originates from the anterior surface of the second, third, and fourth segments of the sacrum, between and lateral to the pelvic sacral foramina (**9B**). It runs laterally through the greater sciatic foramen into the buttock (**B, 339A**).

Coccygeus lies on the deep aspect of the sacrospinous ligament and has the same bony attachments (**B**). Its upper border is parallel to, but a little separate from, the lower border of piriformis.

This muscle-lined true pelvis is divided, albeit incompletely, into its two constituent compartments by the bowl-shaped pelvic diaphragm. This is shown diagrammatically in **C**. The compartment above the diaphragm is the pelvic part of the abdominal cavity—or more briefly the pelvic cavity—while that below the diaphragm is the perineum.

The pelvic diaphragm

This consists of the thin, sheet-like, left and right levator ani muscles. Each muscle arises from a linear origin on the side wall of the true pelvis (**B**). The line begins on the back of the body of the pubis, 1 cm or so from the median plane, and ends behind on the medial aspect of the ischial spine. Between these two bony attachments the muscle arises from the thick fascia covering obturator internus (**C**). Each muscle is convex downwards and its fibres run downwards, backwards and medially to reach the midline. The anterior borders of the two muscles are separated by a gap, limited in front by the back of the pubic symphysis, while the posterior borders are contiguous with the lower margins of the coccygeus muscles (**D, E**).

Three groups of fibres can be recognised in the levatores ani.

1. The anterior fibres intermingle with those of the opposite side in a median fibromuscular mass called the perineal body (central tendon of the perineum) (**D, E**). It is important to note that this is much thicker than the levator ani muscles, and, indeed, extends downwards to be attached to the perineal skin (**C**).

2. Behind the perineal body the rectum, in the pelvic cavity, is continuous with the anal canal in the perineum (**D**). The middle fibres of the levator ani muscles sweep backwards across the right and left aspects of this anorectal junction and become directly continuous behind it (**E**). These fibres are usually distinguished by the name puborectalis.

3. The posterior fibres of the levator ani muscles intermingle in a second median fibromuscular mass called the anococcygeal raphé (ligament) (**D**) which is attached to the coccyx behind and to the perineal skin below (**E**).

The pelvic cavity

Because of the bowl-shaped form of the pelvic diaphragm, the walls of the pelvic cavity blend gradually into one another (**D**). The anterior wall is very short and consists of the upper half of the pubic symphysis and the pubic bodies. In contrast the posterior wall is long and curved and is formed by the sacrum and coccyx with the piriformis and coccygeus muscles. The lateral walls are formed largely by those parts of the obturator internus muscles which lie above the origins of the levator ani muscles. The floor is the pelvic diaphragm including its two median fibromuscular masses.

Above, the pelvic cavity is in broad continuity with the abdominal cavity proper at the level of the pelvic brim. Three apertures lead from the cavity into the adjacent region. The greater sciatic foramen and the obturator canal lead laterally into the lower limb, while the central gap in the anterior part of the pelvic diaphragm leads downwards into the perineum (**E**). Note particularly (**B**) that the lesser sciatic foramen, which was noted above as an aperture in the wall of the true pelvis, lies below the origin of levator ani and consequently is situated in the perineum and not in the pelvic cavity.

The spinal nerves of the pelvic cavity

The spinal nerves which lie in the pelvic cavity are mainly passing through that region on their way to supply structures in the lower limb. They lie directly against the bones and muscles forming the walls of the cavity.

1. *The obturator nerve*, which is a branch of the lumbar plexus (**205C**), is formed by the union of branches from the ventral rami of L2, 3 and 4 in the substance of psoas major in the abdominal cavity proper. It emerges from the medial surface of that muscle and crosses the brim of the pelvis deep to the common iliac vessels (**269B**). The nerve then passes forwards and downwards between the uppermost part of

OSTEOLIGAMENTOUS PELVIS: MEDIAN SECTION

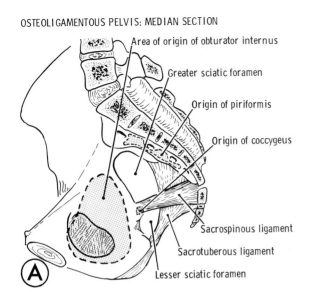

Area of origin of obturator internus
Greater sciatic foramen
Origin of piriformis
Origin of coccygeus
Sacrospinous ligament
Sacrotuberous ligament
Lesser sciatic foramen

(A)

MUSCLES OF PELVIS

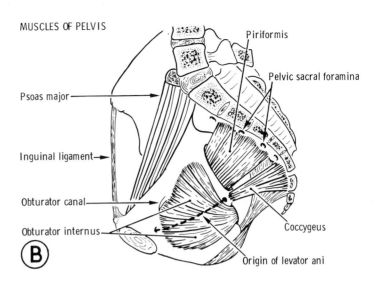

Piriformis
Pelvic sacral foramina
Psoas major
Inguinal ligament
Obturator canal
Obturator internus
Coccygeus
Origin of levator ani

(B)

PELVIS: CORONAL SECTION

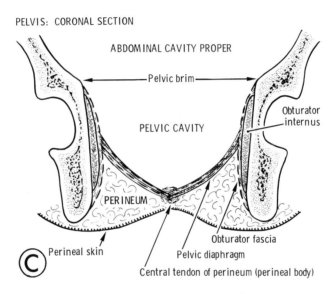

ABDOMINAL CAVITY PROPER
Pelvic brim
Obturator internus
PELVIC CAVITY
PERINEUM
Perineal skin
Obturator fascia
Pelvic diaphragm
Central tendon of perineum (perineal body)

(C)

PELVIC DIAPHRAGM

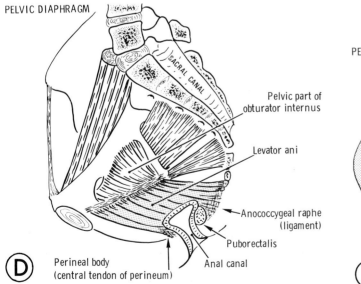

SACRAL CANAL
Pelvic part of obturator internus
Levator ani
Anococcygeal raphe (ligament)
Puborectalis
Anal canal
Perineal body (central tendon of perineum)

(D)

PELVIC DIAPHRAGM: FROM BELOW

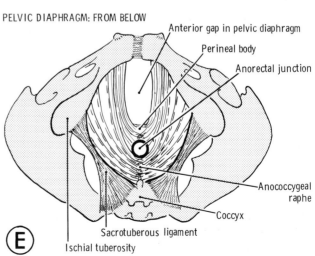

Anterior gap in pelvic diaphragm
Perineal body
Anorectal junction
Anococcygeal raphe
Coccyx
Sacrotuberous ligament
Ischial tuberosity

(E)

267

obturator internus and its fascia to reach the obturator canal (**B**). It traverses the canal into the tissues of the lower limb (**329A**).

2. *The sacral plexus* is formed by the convergence of a number of roots across the surface of piriformis to form a thick trunk in the region of the greater sciatic foramen. The lower division of the ventral ramus of L4 emerges from psoas above the obturator nerve and deep to the common iliac vessels (**A**). The ventral ramus of L5 passes laterally through the lumbosacral intervertebral foramen, turns forwards over the upper surface of the lateral part of the sacrum, and then inclines downwards in front of the sacro-iliac joint. These two elements unite to form a large nerve, called the lumbosacral trunk (**A, B**). The ventral rami of S1, 2 and 3 appear through the corresponding pelvic sacral foramina (**A**). Note the diminishing sizes of these nerves from above down. The ventral ramus of S4 emerges through the fourth pelvic sacral foramen and divides into an ascending division which joins the sacral plexus and a descending division (**A**). Fine branches of these roots of the sacral plexus innervate piriformis, coccygeus, and levator ani. The plexus itself passes through the greater sciatic foramen and supplies branches to the muscles and skin of the lower limb (**339A**).

3. *The coccygeal plexus* is very small. The descending division of S4 passes downwards on coccygeus (**A**). The ventral rami of S5 and the coccygeal nerve emerge through the fibrous posterior wall of the sacral canal (**9C**) and turn forwards through coccygeus onto its pelvic surface (**A**). These three nerves join to form the two loops of the coccygeal plexus (**A**). The plexus gives off cutaneous branches which pass back through coccygeus and supply an area of perineal skin in front of the coccyx (**291D, 291E**).

The internal iliac artery

This is a stout vessel, only about 2 cm long, which descends from the bifurcation of the common iliac artery at the brim of the pelvis to the upper border of the greater sciatic foramen (**A, B**). Here it divides into a large number of visceral and parietal branches (**B**) which lie internal to the spinal nerves described above. The visceral branches supply all the pelvic viscera in both sexes, apart from the pelvic colon and the greater part of the rectum; they will be considered later in relation to the viscera themselves.

The parietal branches are distributed to two regions. Observe the large branches which pass to the lower limb, namely, the obturator artery, which lies below the obturator nerve and traverses the obturator canal (**B**), the superior gluteal artery, which passes laterally through the upper part of the greater sciatic foramen above piriformis,

and the inferior gluteal and internal pudendal arteries which pass downwards and disappear, with the greater part of the sacral plexus, through the lower part of the greater sciatic foramen (**B**). The other parietal branches are in series with the spinal branches of the lumbar and intercostal arteries and enter the vertebral canal through the lumbosacral intervertebral foramen and the pelvic sacral foramina (**B**).

The internal iliac vein

Veins accompany all the branches of the internal iliac artery, and coalesce to form the internal iliac vein immediately behind the termination of the artery. It ascends in front of the sacro-iliac joint to join the external iliac vein (**A**). All these vessels belong to the systemic venous system.

The median sacral vessels

Note the origin and course of the artery in **A**. It is accompanied by venae comitantes which drain into the left common iliac vein.

The pelvic viscera

The genital and urinary viscera in the pelvic cavity differ in the male and female sexes. On the other hand, the pelvic (sigmoid) colon and rectum, which form the pelvic part of the large intestine, are the same in the male and female, apart, of course, from their relations. In the lower part of the pelvic cavity the pelvic viscera are embedded in, and separated from the pelvic walls by, a mass of fatty areolar tissue called the pelvic fascia. This is continuous with the extraperitoneal tissue of the abdomen. The upper parts of the viscera, on the other hand, are clothed in various ways by peritoneum, which is continuous with the greater sac peritoneum of the abdominal cavity proper.

The pelvic colon

The beginning and end of the pelvic colon are both retroperitoneal. The beginning lies over the left external iliac vessels, while the end is in the midline, in front of the third piece of the sacrum. Between these points the colon is suspended from the body wall by a mesentery, the pelvic (sigmoid) mesocolon. The root of this mesocolon is in the form of an inverted V, the apex of the V overlying the bifurcation of the common iliac artery and therefore over the left ureter as it passes over the pelvic brim (**A**). Note the positions and relations of the lateral and medial limbs of the mesocolon root by comparison of the two sides of **A**.

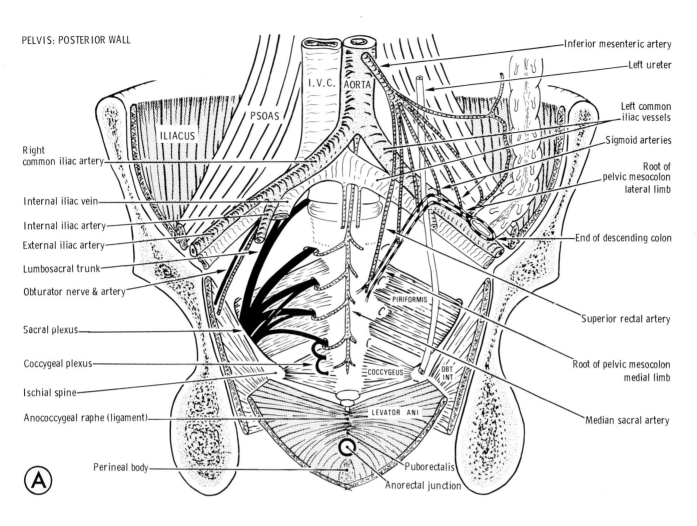

PELVIS: POSTERIOR WALL

Inferior mesenteric artery

Left ureter

Left common iliac vessels

Sigmoid arteries

Root of pelvic mesocolon lateral limb

I.V.C. AORTA

PSOAS

ILIACUS

Right common iliac artery

Internal iliac vein

Internal iliac artery

External iliac artery

Lumbosacral trunk

Obturator nerve & artery

Sacral plexus

Coccygeal plexus

Ischial spine

Anococcygeal raphe (ligament)

Perineal body

PIRIFORMIS

OBT INT

COCCYGEUS

LEVATOR ANI

Puborectalis

Anorectal junction

End of descending colon

Superior rectal artery

Root of pelvic mesocolon medial limb

Median sacral artery

(A)

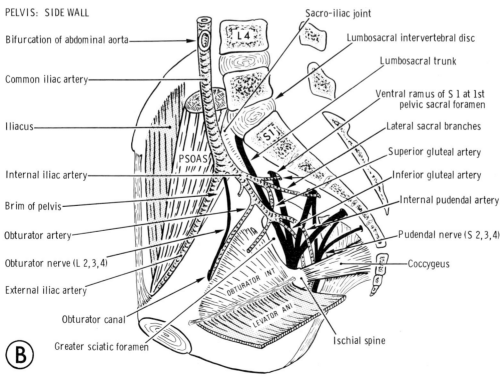

PELVIS: SIDE WALL

Bifurcation of abdominal aorta

Common iliac artery

Iliacus

Internal iliac artery

Brim of pelvis

Obturator artery

Obturator nerve (L 2,3,4)

External iliac artery

Obturator canal

Greater sciatic foramen

Sacro-iliac joint

Lumbosacral intervertebral disc

Lumbosacral trunk

Ventral ramus of S 1 at 1st pelvic sacral foramen

Lateral sacral branches

Superior gluteal artery

Inferior gluteal artery

Internal pudendal artery

Pudendal nerve (S 2,3,4)

Coccygeus

Ischial spine

L4

S1

PSOAS

OBTURATOR INT

LEVATOR ANI

(B)

269

The lower sigmoid branches of the inferior mesenteric artery reach and supply the sigmoid colon through the sigmoid mesocolon. The lower sigmoid veins accompany the arteries and drain into the inferior mesenteric vein. They are consequently part of the portal venous system (**264**).

The rectum

The rectum is about 12 cm long and extends in close contact with the continuously concave posterior wall and floor of the pelvic cavity to the anorectal junction (**A**). This sagittal or sacral curvature is associated with a number of side to side flexures.

Unlike the rest of the large intestine the rectum has no taeniae coli, its longitudinal muscle fibres being spread uniformly around its circumference, and a number of semi-circular folds, consisting of mucous membrane and circular muscle fibres, protrude into its lumen. Above, the lumen is equal to that of the sigmoid colon but in its lower third it abruptly expands, forming the ampulla (**A, B**).

Observe the posterior relations of the rectum in the outline drawing of **B**. Note particularly the pelvic parts of the sympathetic trunks which have not yet been described (**293B**).

The superior rectal artery, which is the terminal branch of the inferior mesenteric artery, is the principal artery of the rectum. It enters the pelvic cavity over the left common iliac artery medial to the left ureter and the apex of the root of the pelvic mesocolon (**269A**). On the wall of the rectum the artery divides first into left and right branches, and subsequently into a large number of vessels which are evenly distributed around the circumference. This blood supply is augmented to a minor extent by the middle rectal branch of the internal iliac artery and the median sacral artery. Veins accompany these arteries and the superior rectal vein, having left the pelvic cavity to the left of the artery, joins the inferior mesenteric vein as a tributary of the portal system.

The genito-urinary viscera of the male pelvic cavity

The prostate

The prostate gland is a firm structure in which a stroma of fibrous tissue and plain muscle fibres enclose numerous glandular follicles which open into the urethra through 20 or so long ducts. The stroma is condensed over the surface of the gland to form a thin firmly-adherent capsule.

The gland is rather conical in form and about 3 cm in length. The base measures about 4 cm transversely and 2 cm anteroposteriorly, and is directed upwards in structural continuity with the neck of the urinary bladder (**A, D**). The apex points downwards through the gap

between the anterior borders of the levator ani muscles immediately in front of the perineal body (**A**). A number of surfaces are usually described though they are not sharply demarcated from one another. The anterior surface lies about 2 cm behind the pubic symphysis (**A**), while the inferolateral surfaces are related to the pelvic surfaces of the levator ani muscles (**D**). The posterior surface is closely related to the ampulla of the rectum (**A**) so that the size and regularity of the gland can be assessed in life by rectal examination.

The prostate is separated from all these relations by pelvic fascia which is of considerable importance in operations on the gland. The fascia is described below (**274**).

The prostate is traversed by a number of tubular structures.

The prostatic urethra passes vertically downwards through the gland considerably nearer its anterior than its posterior aspect (**A**). A number of features lie on its posterior wall (**C**) and can be seen through a urethroscope. The median urethral crest separates two prostatic sinuses into which the prostatic glands open. The colliculus seminalis (verumontanum) is an expansion on the middle of the crest.

The ejaculatory ducts enter the gland on either side of the midline at the junction of the base and posterior surface (**273C**) and run downwards and medially to open into the urethra on the surface of the colliculus seminalis (**C**).

It is convenient to recognise different regions in the prostate although they are not sharply demarcated from one another. The isthmus is the region in front of the urethra; it contains comparatively few glandular elements. The median lobe is the pyramidal zone which lies between the ejaculatory ducts and the upper half of the prostatic urethra. The rest of the gland constitutes the left and right lobes.

The gland remains small during childhood, but enlarges rapidly at puberty, doubling its size within about a year. It then remains about the same size until middle age, when there is a further, though much more gradual, enlargement which may give rise to disorders of micturition.

The male urinary bladder

The empty adult bladder is a hollow muscular viscus which lies entirely within the pelvic cavity (**A**). Its shape is a three-sided cone with rounded-off borders. The apex is placed just behind the upper border of the pubic symphysis and is continuous with a fibrous cord, the urachus, which extends up the deep aspect of the transversalis fascia to the umbilicus (**A**). Rarely the urachus has a lumen which is continuous with that of the bladder. The base faces backwards towards the rectal ampulla (**A**) although, as will be seen later, other viscera intervene. The inferolateral surfaces fit against the bowl of the levator ani muscles below the level of the obturator nerves, while the superior

RECTUM, PROSTATE & URINARY BLADDER:
SAGITTAL SECTION

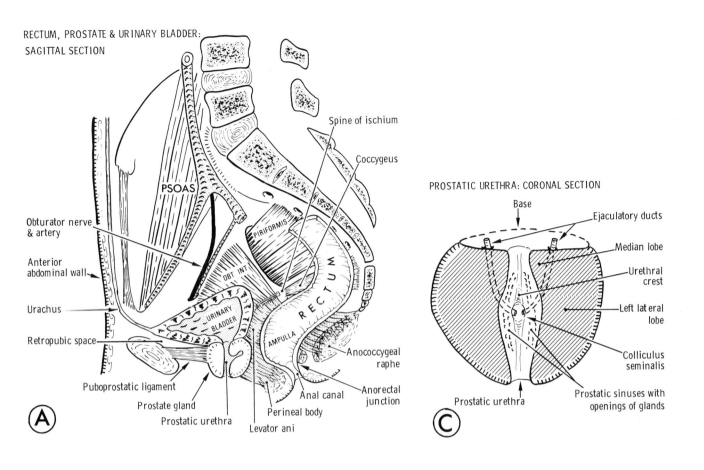

Spine of ischium

Coccygeus

Obturator nerve & artery

Anterior abdominal wall

Urachus

Retropubic space

PSOAS

PIRIFORMIS

OBT INT

URINARY BLADDER

RECTUM

AMPULLA

Puboprostatic ligament

Prostate gland

Prostatic urethra

Anal canal

Perineal body

Levator ani

Anococcygeal raphe

Anorectal junction

PROSTATIC URETHRA: CORONAL SECTION

Base

Ejaculatory ducts

Median lobe

Urethral crest

Left lateral lobe

Colliculus seminalis

Prostatic sinuses with openings of glands

Prostatic urethra

RECTUM: POSTERIOR RELATIONS

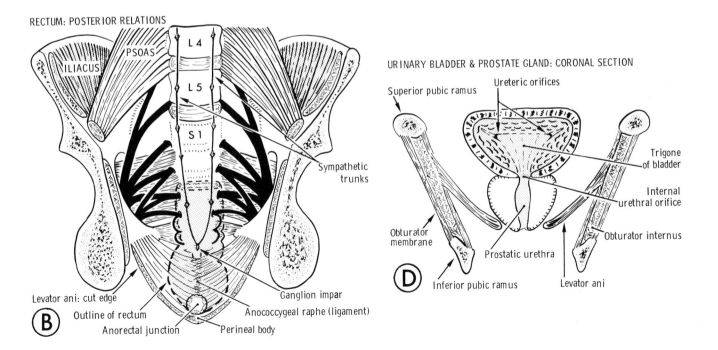

PSOAS

ILIACUS

L 4

L 5

S 1

Sympathetic trunks

Levator ani: cut edge

Outline of rectum

Anorectal junction

Perineal body

Ganglion impar

Anococcygeal raphe (ligament)

URINARY BLADDER & PROSTATE GLAND: CORONAL SECTION

Superior pubic ramus

Ureteric orifices

Trigone of bladder

Internal urethral orifice

Obturator internus

Obturator membrane

Inferior pubic ramus

Prostatic urethra

Levator ani

surface is directly upwards towards the abdominal cavity proper. The inferior angle of the bladder is, as it were, bevelled off, and is structurally continuous with the base of the prostate. Here the lumen of the bladder opens through the internal urethral orifice into the prostatic urethra (**271A, 271D**).

The muscular wall—often called collectively the detrusor muscle—consists of three layers of plain muscle fibres: an outer longitudinal layer, a middle circular layer and an inner layer consisting of a meshwork of interlacing bundles. When the outflow of urine is chronically obstructed, this trabeculation of the inner layer becomes progressively more pronounced.

There is a considerable concentration of muscle and elastic fibres around the internal urethral orifice at the neck of the bladder. This has usually been interpreted as a concentration of circular muscle fibres forming a sphincter vesicae which controls the escape of urine into the urethra. There is now evidence that there is in fact no muscular sphincter vesicae. The internal urethral orifice seems to be surrounded by circularly disposed elastic fibres which normally keep it closed, while fibres of the longitudinal muscle coat are inserted radially into the mucosa around the orifice and pull it open when the detrusor contracts with sufficient force.

The mucous membrane which lines the bladder is loosely attached over most of the muscle wall so that when the viscus is empty it is thrown into folds. However, over an area called the trigone, mucosa and muscle are firmly adherent, and the former is permanently smooth. The trigone (**B, 271D**) has its apex at the internal urethral orifice while its base is formed by the slight ridge between the ureteric orifices. It lines the posterior part of the neck and the greater part of the base of the bladder. It should be noted that the most anterior part of the trigone overlies the median lobe of the prostate, and may be elevated by enlargement of that part of the prostate so that it obstructs the passage of urine into the urethra.

If the bladder is distended by the introduction of 300–450 ml of water through an instrument known as a cystoscope, previously passed into it through the urethra, all the features described above can be seen and abnormalities and disease processes can be noted.

The male ureters

Having crossed the brim of the pelvis over the bifurcation of the common iliac artery (**261A**), each ureter passes downwards and backwards (in the erect posture),

immediately internal to the muscles, nerves and arteries of the pelvic wall (**269B**), until it lies on the spine of the ischium at the lower border of the greater sciatic foramen (**A**). Here it bends sharply forwards and reaches the lateral angle of the base of the bladder (**A, C**), which it pierces obliquely in a forward and medial direction (**B**). The slit-like ureteric orifices are situated at the lateral angles of the trigone (**B**). The oblique passage of the ureters through the bladder wall produces the ureteric folds of mucous membrane just lateral to each ureteric orifice, and prevents reflux of urine by a rise in intravesical pressure through the compression of the anterior against the posterior walls.

The ureteric orifices can be viewed directly during cystoscopy (see above). Fine catheters can be introduced through the cystoscope into the orifices and passed up the ureters. By this procedure urine can be collected from each kidney, or radio-opaque material can be injected to allow radiographic visualisation of the ureter and pelvis. The normal capacity of the renal pelvis in the adult is 7–10 ml.

The ductus deferens

It will be recalled that, on either side of the body, the ductus is a tube with a thick muscular wall and a narrow lumen which has already been traced from its origin at the tail of the epididymis, through the spermatic cord to the deep inguinal ring (**211D, 213A**). Here it hooks medially round the inferior epigastric artery and, crossing the external iliac vessels and the brim of the pelvis (**A**), runs backwards and a little downwards, internal to the muscles, nerves and arteries of the pelvic wall, to the lateral angle of the urinary bladder (**A**). At this point it turns medially across the upper surface of the terminal part of the corresponding ureter, and immediately inclines downwards and slightly medially in the interval between the base of the bladder and the ampulla of the rectum (**C**). This segment of the duct is thin-walled and dilated (the ampulla) except for its termination, which is again narrow.

The seminal vesicles

The paired seminal vesicles are almond-shaped bodies about 5 cm long, each of which lies obliquely lateral to the ampulla of one ductus deferens, behind the base of the bladder and in front of the ampulla of the rectum (**C**). Despite its solid appearance each vesicle is, in fact, a tube about 12 cm long, with blind diverticula, which is wound into coils held together by fibrous tissue.

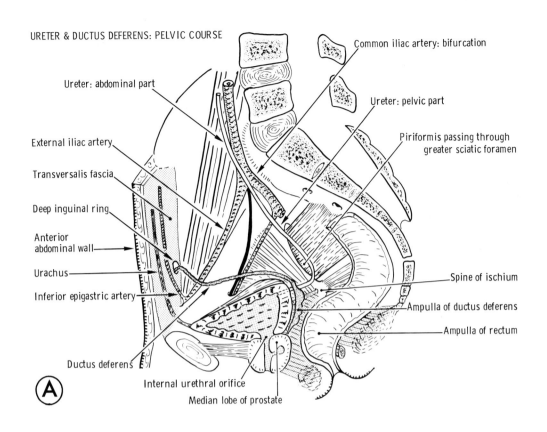

URETER & DUCTUS DEFERENS: PELVIC COURSE

Ureter: abdominal part

Common iliac artery: bifurcation

Ureter: pelvic part

External iliac artery

Piriformis passing through greater sciatic foramen

Transversalis fascia

Deep inguinal ring

Anterior abdominal wall

Urachus

Inferior epigastric artery

Spine of ischium

Ampulla of ductus deferens

Ampulla of rectum

Ductus deferens

Internal urethral orifice

Median lobe of prostate

(A)

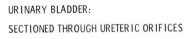

URINARY BLADDER:

SECTIONED THROUGH URETERIC ORIFICES

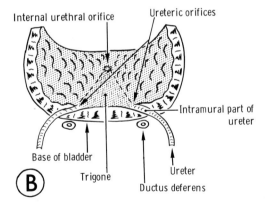

Internal urethral orifice

Ureteric orifices

Intramural part of ureter

Base of bladder

Trigone

Ureter

Ductus deferens

(B)

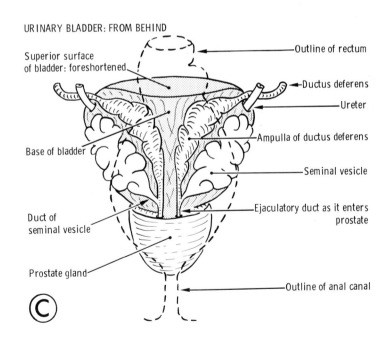

URINARY BLADDER: FROM BEHIND

Superior surface of bladder: foreshortened

Outline of rectum

Ductus deferens

Ureter

Base of bladder

Ampulla of ductus deferens

Seminal vesicle

Ejaculatory duct as it enters prostate

Duct of seminal vesicle

Prostate gland

Outline of anal canal

(C)

The ejaculatory ducts

The narrow ejaculatory ducts are formed on either side, a short distance from the median plane, by the coalescence of ductus deferens and seminal vesicle in the groove between the bladder and prostate (**273C**). As has been seen, they pass downwards and forwards through the substance of the prostate gland to open into the middle of the prostatic urethra on the colliculus seminalis (**271C**). Surgical removal of the prostate therefore necessarily divides the ejaculatory ducts.

The fascia of the male pelvic cavity

The muscles and bones which comprise the walls of the pelvic cavity are lined by a thin dense layer of fascia which is part of the fascial envelope of the whole abdominal cavity.

Internal to this is fatty areolar tissue which is continuous above with the extraperitoneal tissue of the abdominal cavity proper. In the upper part of the pelvic cavity, above the level of the empty urinary bladder, this extraperitoneal tissue is comparatively thin and envelops the ductus deferens, the ureter and the upper two-thirds of the rectum. On the other hand, in the lower part of the cavity, the tissue is generally thicker and occupies the whole interval between the viscera and the pelvic walls. It contains the arteries and veins associated with the viscera. Although this fascia is a continuous zone of tissue, it is conveniently described as distinct regions, and it will be seen that some parts are denser and more fibrous than others.

1. The wedge-shaped spaces between the lateral aspects of the rectal ampulla and the levator ani muscles are occupied by the loose pelvirectal fascia (**B**).
2. The fascia which surrounds all free aspects of the prostate is known collectively as the prostatic sheath. Note the distinction between the sheath and the capsule of the prostate. The anterior part of the sheath in the interval between prostate and pubic symphysis (**A**), and the lateral parts of the sheath between the gland and the levator ani muscles (**D**), are of loose texture and are traversed by the thin walled veins of the prostatic venous plexuses. These plexuses, which are important factors in many operations on the prostate, are continuous in front with the single deep dorsal vein of the penis (**A, C**) and drain upwards and backwards across the side walls of the pelvic cavity into the internal iliac veins. The puboprostatic ligaments are bilateral bands of dense fibrous tissue which anchor the vesicoprostatic junction to the pubic bones (**C**). In contrast, the posterior part of the sheath is thin and dense in consistency and practically avascular (**A**). It separates the prostate from the rectal ampulla and merges below with the perineal body.
3. Above the level of the puboprostatic ligaments, the anterior margin of the urinary bladder and the back of the pubic symphysis are separated by the retropubic space occupied by loose areolar tissue (**A**).
4. Thinner layers of this tissue, permeated by the vesical venous plexuses, extend backwards between the inferolateral surfaces of the bladder and the pelvic diaphragm (**C**). These plexuses are continuous below with the prostatic plexuses and drain, like them, into the internal iliac veins.
5. The dense and avascular posterior part of the prostatic sheath continues upwards between the rectal ampulla behind, and the base of the bladder, the ampullae of the deferent ducts and the seminal vesicles in front. The zone is known as the rectovesical fascia (**A**).

The visceral branches of the internal iliac artery in the male

In the male three visceral branches arise from the internal iliac artery.

The superior vesical artery

This vessel runs downwards and forwards in the extraperitoneal tissue on the pelvic side wall (**E**) lying deep to the ureter and the ductus deferens. It supplies branches to both these structures and continues to the upper part of the bladder.

The artery has one very unusual feature. A solid fibrous cord arises from its wall close to its origin (**E**). This passes forwards just below the pelvic brim and extends upwards and a little medially on the deep aspect of the transversalis fascia on the anterior abdominal wall to the umbilicus. It is known alternatively as the obliterated umbilical artery or the medial umbilical ligament.

In the foetus, the abdominal aorta divides into two umbilical arteries which pass through the pelvic cavity and up the anterior abdominal wall to reach the placenta through the umbilical cord (**175D**). The greater part of each artery becomes obliterated soon after birth, but the proximal parts persist as the common iliac and internal iliac arteries and the proximal parts of the superior vesical arteries.

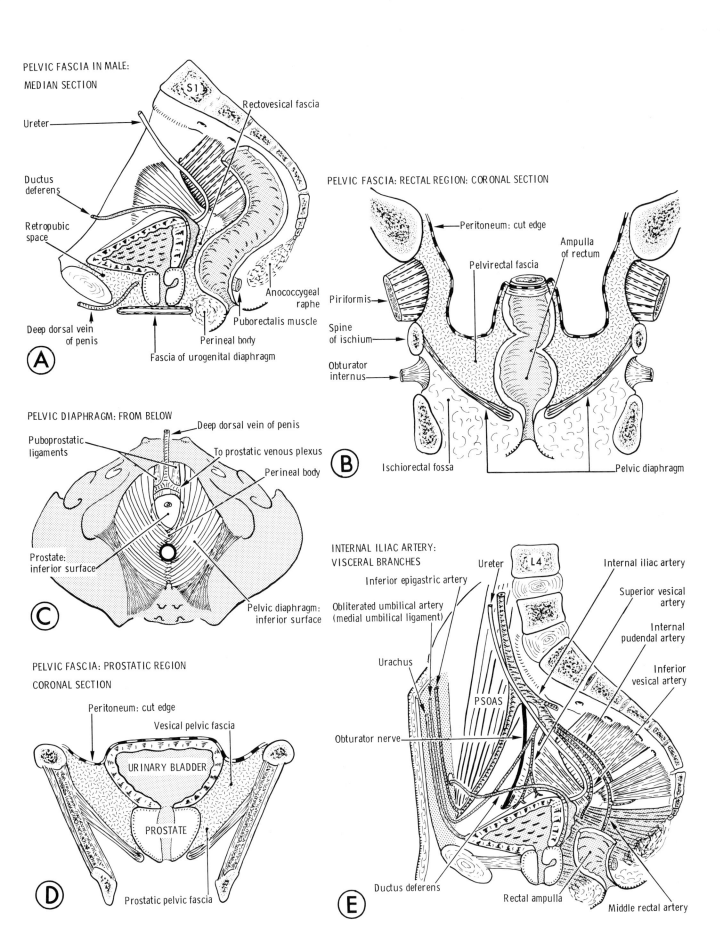

PELVIC FASCIA IN MALE:
MEDIAN SECTION

Ureter

Ductus
deferens

Retropubic
space

Deep dorsal vein
of penis

Rectovesical fascia

Anococcygeal
raphe

Puborectalis muscle

Perineal body

Fascia of urogenital diaphragm

(A)

PELVIC FASCIA: RECTAL REGION: CORONAL SECTION

Peritoneum: cut edge

Ampulla
of rectum

Pelvirectal fascia

Piriformis

Spine
of ischium

Obturator
internus

Ischiorectal fossa

Pelvic diaphragm

(B)

PELVIC DIAPHRAGM: FROM BELOW

Deep dorsal vein of penis

Puboprostatic
ligaments

To prostatic venous plexus

Perineal body

Prostate:
inferior surface

Pelvic diaphragm:
inferior surface

(C)

PELVIC FASCIA: PROSTATIC REGION
CORONAL SECTION

Peritoneum: cut edge

Vesical pelvic fascia

URINARY BLADDER

PROSTATE

Prostatic pelvic fascia

(D)

INTERNAL ILIAC ARTERY:
VISCERAL BRANCHES

Ureter

Inferior epigastric artery

Obliterated umbilical artery
(medial umbilical ligament)

Urachus

Obturator nerve

Ductus deferens

Internal iliac artery

Superior vesical
artery

Internal
pudendal artery

Inferior
vesical artery

PSOAS

Rectal ampulla

Middle rectal artery

(E)

The inferior vesical artery

This vessel passes downwards at a lower level. It supplies the prostate and lower part of the bladder, the seminal vesicles and the terminal parts of the ductus deferens and ureter (**275E**). It should be recalled that the ureter as a whole receives its blood supply from a number of successive sources, namely the renal, gonadal, superior vesical and inferior vesical arteries.

The middle rectal artery

This small vessel frequently arises from the inferior vesical artery. It passes medially through the pelvirectal fascia and augments the blood supply of the lowest part of the rectum by the superior rectal artery.

The peritoneum in the male pelvic cavity

The reflection of peritoneum in the upper left part of the pelvic cavity to form the sigmoid mesocolon has already been described (**269A**). Below that level peritoneum covers the sides and front of the upper two-thirds of the rectum (**A**) and sweeps away from that viscus, on either side, to cover the greater part of the posterior and lateral pelvic walls and all the structures which lie on them (**B**). At the upper part of the rectal ampulla the peritoneum turns laterally over the regions of pelvirectal fascia (**275B**) and forwards over the upper limit of the rectovesical fascia to the base of the bladder at the level of the ureters (**B**). The serous membrane then covers the uppermost part of the bladder base before sweeping forwards over its superior surface to reach the anterior abdominal wall. The slight recess between the bladder and the rectum is the rectovesical pouch, which is the most dependent part of the peritoneal cavity in the sitting posture. Infective fluid thus tends to collect in this region and may become walled off by adhesions to form a pelvic abscess.

The female pelvic viscera

The sigmoid colon and rectum

The sigmoid colon and the upper two-thirds of the rectum in the female are exactly similar to the same structures in the male which have been described already (**268, 270**).

The lower one-third of the rectum is identical in the two sexes except for its anterior relations which will be considered later (**279A**).

The urinary bladder

The positions and relations of the apex and inferolateral surfaces of the urinary bladder, the entrance of the ureters into the bladder, and the characters of the muscular wall and the lining mucosa are the same in the two sexes. However in the female there is, of course, no prostate gland and the inferior angle is not bevelled off. The urethra descends from the inferior angle of the bladder and passes through the anterior gap in the pelvic diaphragm into the perineum (**C**). The relations of the base of the bladder in the female are quite different from those already described in the male and will be considered later.

The female pelvic genital viscera

The female genital viscera are illustrated diagrammatically in **C**, **D**. Observe the general positions and shapes of the paired ovaries and uterine tubes, and the single uterus and vagina, and note that some of these viscera have distinctly named parts.

The vagina and uterus

The vagina is a muscular tube lined by non-keratinised stratified squamous epithelium. Although it is open to the exterior its lumen is normally occluded by apposition of its walls, but it is convenient in diagrams to show the lumen as patent (**C, D**). Its lower part lies in the perineum, immediately in front of the perineal body, and will be considered in the section of that region. Its upper part extends upwards and backwards through the anterior gap in the pelvic diaphragm (**267E**) into the pelvic cavity. Here it is placed between the base of the bladder and the urethra in front, and the ampulla of the rectum behind. Ultimately it rises to its vault above the level of the superior surface of the empty bladder (**C**).

The cervix of the uterus is barrel-shaped and is inserted at right angles through the supravesical part of the anterior vaginal wall so that it consists of supravaginal and vaginal halves (**C, D**). The cervical canal opens into the vaginal lumen through the external os, and becomes continuous with the lumen of the body of the uterus at the internal os. The protrusion of the vaginal cervix creates recesses of the vaginal cavity on its four aspects, known as the posterior, the anterior, and the two lateral vaginal fornices (**C, D**).

The body and fundus of the uterus lie almost horizontally above the urinary bladder so that their surfaces are superior and inferior. The long axis of body and fundus lie at a slight angle to that of the cervix, this relationship being known as anteflexion (**C**). The almost orthogonal normal relationship of the uterus as a whole to the vagina is called anteversion (**C**).

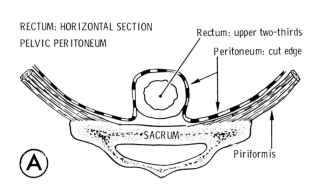

RECTUM: HORIZONTAL SECTION
PELVIC PERITONEUM

Rectum: upper two-thirds

Peritoneum: cut edge

SACRUM

Piriformis

Ⓐ

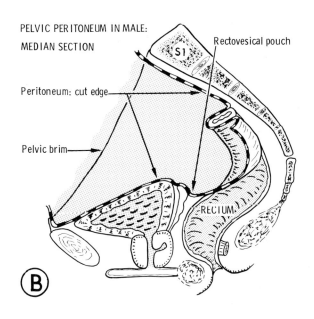

PELVIC PERITONEUM IN MALE:
MEDIAN SECTION

S1

Rectovesical pouch

Peritoneum: cut edge

Pelvic brim

RECTUM

Ⓑ

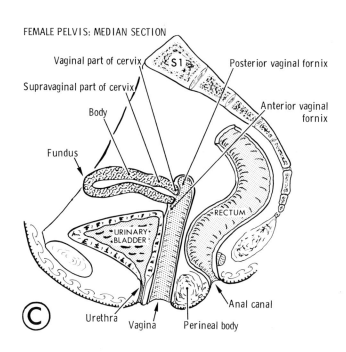

FEMALE PELVIS: MEDIAN SECTION

Vaginal part of cervix

S1

Supravaginal part of cervix

Body

Fundus

Posterior vaginal fornix

Anterior vaginal fornix

RECTUM

URINARY BLADDER

Urethra   Vagina   Perineal body

Anal canal

Ⓒ

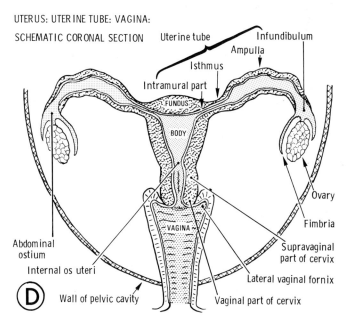

UTERUS: UTERINE TUBE: VAGINA:
SCHEMATIC CORONAL SECTION

Uterine tube

Infundibulum

Ampulla

Isthmus

Intramural part

FUNDUS

BODY

Abdominal ostium

Internal os uteri

Wall of pelvic cavity

VAGINA

Ovary

Fimbria

Supravaginal part of cervix

Lateral vaginal fornix

Vaginal part of cervix

Ⓓ

The pelvic fascia in the female

In the female, loose connective tissue separates the bladder from the pubic symphysis (retropubic space) and from the levator ani muscles (**A**) as it does in the male, and this continues downwards around the urethra where it is comparable, though very much less vascular, than the anterior and lateral parts of the prostatic sheath (**275A, 275D**). Lateral to the rectal ampulla lie wedge-shaped areas of pelvirectal fascia similar to those seen in the male.

Most of the anterior wall of the pelvic part of the vagina is very intimately related to the bladder and urethra, little fascia intervening (**A**). Posteriorly, the lower half of the pelvic vagina is separated from the rectal ampulla by a dense and avascular layer of rectovaginal fascia which is continuous below with the perineal body (compare with the rectovesical fascia in the male) (**A**). Laterally the whole pelvic vagina plus the supravaginal cervix is separated from the levator ani muscles by an extensive zone of loose fascia which is called the parametrium (**B**). It is to be particularly noted that, as the ureters run forwards from the ischial spines to the lateral angles of the bladder, they traverse this tissue lying only a short distance above the lateral vaginal fornices and lateral to the supravaginal cervix (**B**).

The pelvic peritoneum in the female

The disposition of the peritoneum in relation to the sigmoid colon, the upper two-thirds of the rectum, and the superior surface of the urinary bladder are the same in male and female.

The peritoneum in the central part of the female pelvic cavity is most conveniently considered, initially, in the median plane (**A**). Trace the peritoneum as it turns sharply forwards from the posterior margin of the superior surface of the bladder to reach the uterus at the junction of cervix and body. Then follow the membrane over the inferior and superior surfaces of the body and fundus of the uterus and over the upper surface of the supravaginal cervix. Finally observe the peritoneum passing from the cervix over the posterior vaginal fornix, and the vault and the upper quarter of the posterior wall of the vagina, before turning upwards onto the anterior surface of the rectum. Note particularly the following features.

1. The upper surface of the supravaginal cervix is covered by peritoneum, but the lower surface is in direct contact with the urinary bladder.

2. The deep peritoneal recess known as the uterovesical pouch (**A**).
3. The deeper peritoneal recess which passes downwards between the uterus and vagina in front, and the rectum behind. It is variously named the rectovaginal or the recto-uterine pouch. Traditionally it is called the pouch of Douglas, particularly in clinical parlance. This recess is the most dependent part of the peritoneal cavity in the female and, as in the rectovesical pouch in the male, infected fluid may be walled off in this region by adhesions, forming a pelvic abscess.

The layers of peritoneum which cover the upper and lower surfaces of the uterus leave the lateral margins of the viscus in close apposition and pass across the pelvic cavity to reach its lateral walls, where they separate from one another. These folds of peritoneum form a more or less horizontal partition across the pelvic cavity, and are known as the broad ligaments (**B**). Each ligament has a free anterior margin at which its two peritoneal layers are continuous, while behind, the two layers separate over the parametrium, the lower layer turning forwards and the upper layer continuing backwards (**C**). Each broad ligament contains a number of structures which are described below.

The uterine tubes

These are paired muscular tubes, lined by mucous membrane, which pass laterally on either side from the junction of the body and fundus of the uterus. Recall the morphologically distinct parts of the tubes which have already been noted (**277D**). Each uterine tube lies within the medial three-quarters of the corresponding broad ligament, close to its free anterior margin (**B**). At the lateral end of the tube the infundibulum and fimbriae turn backwards and pierce the upper peritoneal layer of the broad ligament so that, while their outer aspects are covered by peritoneum, their inner aspects face into the peritoneal cavity and are covered by mucous membrane (**C**). The opening between the ampulla and infundibulum, which is called the abdominal ostium, establishes continuity between the general peritoneal cavity and the lumina of the uterine tube, uterus and vagina. It is of the greatest importance to note, therefore, that whereas the peritoneal cavity in the male is a completely closed sac, in the female it is open to the exterior, and is consequently more exposed to infections.

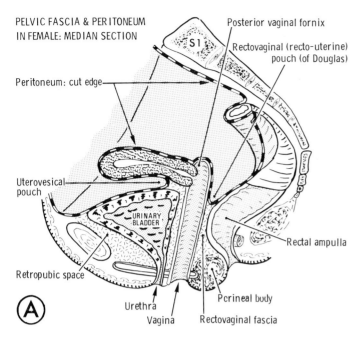

PELVIC FASCIA & PERITONEUM
IN FEMALE: MEDIAN SECTION

Posterior vaginal fornix

Rectovaginal (recto-uterine)
pouch (of Douglas)

Peritoneum: cut edge

Uterovesical
pouch

URINARY
BLADDER

Retropubic space

Rectal ampulla

Urethra

Perineal body

Vagina

Rectovaginal fascia

Ⓐ

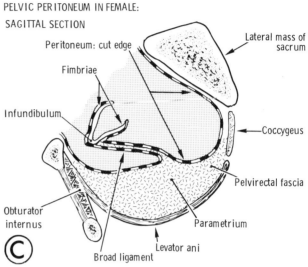

PELVIC PERITONEUM IN FEMALE:
SAGITTAL SECTION

Peritoneum: cut edge

Fimbriae

Infundibulum

Obturator
internus

Broad ligament

Lateral mass of
sacrum

Coccygeus

Pelvirectal fascia

Parametrium

Levator ani

Ⓒ

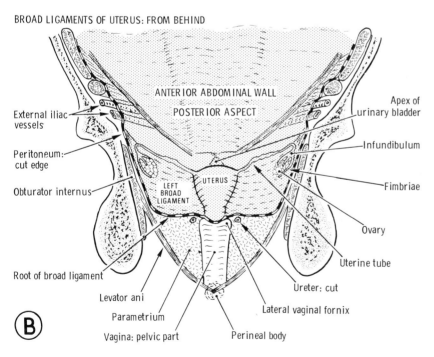

BROAD LIGAMENTS OF UTERUS: FROM BEHIND

ANTERIOR ABDOMINAL WALL
POSTERIOR ASPECT

External iliac
vessels

Peritoneum:
cut edge

Obturator internus

LEFT
BROAD
LIGAMENT

UTERUS

Apex of
urinary bladder

Infundibulum

Fimbriae

Ovary

Uterine tube

Root of broad ligament

Levator ani

Parametrium

Vagina: pelvic part

Perineal body

Lateral vaginal fornix

Ureter: cut

Ⓑ

The ovaries

The paired ovaries are solid almond-shaped structures with upper and lower poles and medial and lateral surfaces (**A**). Each is suspended in the pelvic cavity by a short mesentery or mesovarium in the form of a tube of peritoneum derived from the upper layer of the broad ligament behind and below the infundibulum (**B**).

The glistening peritoneum of the mesovarium encloses the anterior part of the ovary, but the posterior part of the viscus is covered by dull greyish cubical epithelium. This is the germinal epithelium, through which ova are shed on rupture of ovarian follicles during the reproductive phase of life. The shed ova pass a short distance across the peritoneal cavity, and through the abdominal ostium into the uterine tube (**A**).

The lateral surface of the ovary rests against the peritoneum on the lateral pelvic wall, while its upper pole is closely related to the several fimbriae of the infundibulum of the uterine tube. Its lower pole is attached to the uterus just behind the uterine tube by the fibromuscular ligament of the ovary which lies within the broad ligament (**A**).

The round ligaments of the uterus

These are another pair of fibromuscular bands within the broad ligaments. Each passes laterally from the uterus just in front of the uterine tube and leaves the broad ligament and the pelvic cavity by crossing the external iliac vessels (**A**). Here it hooks round the lateral side of the inferior epigastric artery, and, passing through the deep inguinal ring, traverses the inguinal canal to become fixed to the dense fibrous tissue comprising the major labium (**A, C**).

The blood vessels of the female pelvis

The majority of the pelvic blood vessels are the same in the two sexes. This is true of the following.

1. The parietal branches of the internal iliac artery.
2. The lower sigmoid and superior rectal branches of the inferior mesenteric artery.
3. The superior vesical branch of the internal iliac artery, including its obliterated umbilical branch.

On the other hand there are three paired visceral arteries which are peculiar to the female.

The vaginal artery replaces the inferior vesical branch in the male. It arises from the internal iliac and passes downwards and medially through the parametrium and divides into branches which are distributed to the vagina and the base of the bladder (**A, C**).

The uterine artery is a large and important vessel which runs a C-shaped course. It arises from the internal iliac. The initial part of the vessel runs medially through the parametrium, just below the root of the broad ligament, until it reaches the lateral aspect of the supravaginal cervix (**A, C**). In this part of its course it crosses close above the terminal part of the ureter (**C**). As the uterine artery must be tied and divided when the uterus is surgically removed (hysterectomy), this relationship is one of the greatest significance. In this region the vessel gives off descending branches which anastomose profusely in the vaginal wall with those of the vaginal arteries. The artery now turns forwards within the broad ligament along the lateral border of the uterus to which it supplies numerous branches (**C**). Reaching the uterine tube it turns laterally alongside this structure, still within the broad ligament (**A, C**). The artery ends in the mesovarium by anastomosing with the ovarian artery. Both the artery and its accompanying vein are tortuous and this is probably associated with the great elongation and enlargement which both undergo in pregnancy.

The ovarian artery is the female homologue of the testicular artery. Its origin and its relations as it passes downwards on psoas major have been considered already (**237A, 259A**). Some 2 cm above the inguinal ligament it turns medially over the external iliac vessels and comes into relationship with the round ligament of the uterus (**A, C**). The artery then enters the broad ligament and subsequently the mesovarium to supply the ovary and anastomose freely with the uterine artery. The asymmetry of the ovarian veins has been noted previously (**259A**). Recall that while that on the right joins the inferior vena cava directly, that on the left passes up the posterior abdominal wall, lateral to the inferior mesenteric vein, to join the left renal vein (**237D**).

Variations in the position of some pelvic viscera

1. The descriptions of the urinary bladder given above (**270, 276**) apply to the empty viscus in the adult. When the adult bladder is distended its margins are obliterated and it becomes ovoid in form. The positions of its base and neck do not change, but its apex moves upwards through the loose extraperitoneal tissue of the lower part of the anterior abdominal wall, so that it can be regarded as stripping the peritoneum off the transversalis fascia (**D**). The viscus is thus much more exposed to injury when it is distended than when it is empty, and may be ruptured by a blow on the lower part of the abdominal wall. Moreover if the bladder is distended through a catheter in the anaesthetised patient, it can be entered through a median suprapubic incision without disturbing the peritoneum.

OVARY & ROUND LIGAMENT

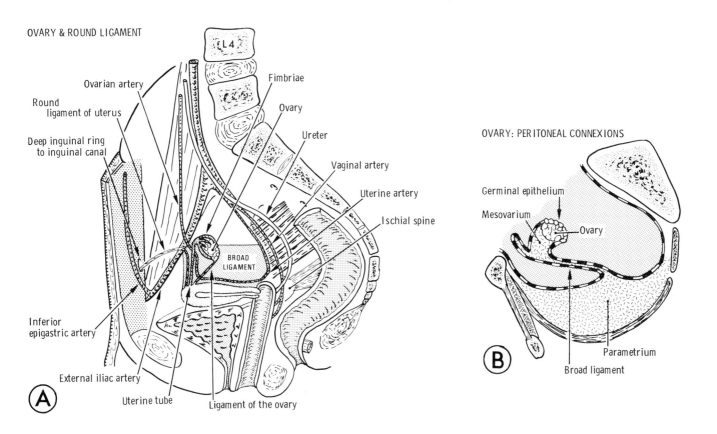

L4

Ovarian artery

Round
ligament of uterus

Deep inguinal ring
to inguinal canal

Fimbriae

Ovary

Ureter

Vaginal artery

Uterine artery

Ischial spine

BROAD
LIGAMENT

Inferior
epigastric artery

External iliac artery

Uterine tube

Ligament of the ovary

A

OVARY: PERITONEAL CONNEXIONS

Germinal epithelium

Mesovarium

Ovary

Parametrium

Broad ligament

B

FEMALE PELVIS: BLOODVESSELS

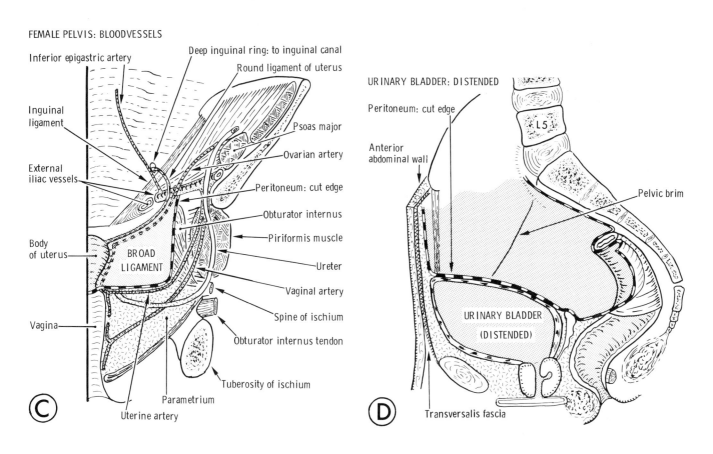

Inferior epigastric artery

Deep inguinal ring: to inguinal canal

Round ligament of uterus

Inguinal
ligament

Psoas major

Ovarian artery

External
iliac vessels

Peritoneum: cut edge

Obturator internus

Piriformis muscle

Body
of uterus

BROAD
LIGAMENT

Ureter

Vaginal artery

Spine of ischium

Vagina

Obturator internus tendon

Tuberosity of ischium

Parametrium

Uterine artery

C

URINARY BLADDER: DISTENDED

Peritoneum: cut edge

L5

Anterior
abdominal wall

Pelvic brim

URINARY BLADDER
(DISTENDED)

Transversalis fascia

D

281

At birth the pelvic cavity is disproportionately small compared to the abdominal cavity proper. As a result the greater part of the urinary bladder lies above the pelvic brim and in direct contact with the transversalis fascia of the lower two-thirds of the infra-umbilical part of the abdominal wall. The organ sinks slowly to a lower level, but does not achieve its adult position until about puberty. Thus incisions through the lower part of the abdominal wall in children may damage the bladder and fail to open into the peritoneal cavity.

2. The uterus is also somewhat higher in the infant than in the adult, and the cervix is larger than the body. The adult position and form are achieved before puberty. The position of the adult non-gravid uterus is influenced by the degree of distension of the bladder. When the bladder is empty the uterus lies horizontally on its upper surface, whereas when the bladder is distended the uterus is forced upwards into a more vertical orientation.

In some individuals the normal anteversion of the uterus on the vagina (**277C**) may be replaced by a relationship known as retroversion, in which the fundus and body of the uterus are turned backwards into the rectovaginal peritoneal pouch (**279A**).

During pregnancy the uterus becomes enormously enlarged, reaching into the epigastric region of the abdominal cavity proper in the eighth month.

3. Like the urinary bladder and the uterus, the ovary lies at a higher level in infancy than in the adult. At birth it is above the pelvic brim and does not sink to its adult position until near puberty.

THE PERINEUM

This is the lowest compartment of the trunk, which is situated below the pelvic diaphragm. It differs from the thorax and abdomen in having no serous cavity. On the contrary, the region is occupied by connective tissues of varying densities, which are traversed by the terminal part of the intestinal, urinary and genital tracts.

The roof of the perineum is the pelvic diaphragm (**A**). Through the gap in the diaphragm bordered by the anterior margins of the levator ani muscles, the pubic symphysis and the perineal body (central tendon of the perineum), the perineum is continuous with the pelvic cavity. The walls of the region, which are more or less vertical, are formed by those parts of the bones, muscles and ligaments of the true pelvis which are below the lines of origin of the levator ani muscles. Observe these structures carefully (**B**), and pay particular attention to the lesser sciatic foramen. Note that this foramen connects the perineum with the lower limb, whereas the greater sciatic foramen connects the lower limb with the pelvic part of the abdominal cavity. The lesser sciatic foramen and the gap in the pelvic diaphragm (**A**) are the main routes through which vessels and nerves enter or leave the perineum. The space surrounded by the inferior margin of the perineal walls (**A**, **B**) is often described as the pelvic outlet, because during the birth process, the infant's body must pass out through this osteoligamentous ring. However, it must be appreciated that the term refers, not to the outlet from the pelvic part of the abdominal cavity, but to the outlet from that part of the true bony pelvis which is the perineum. The area of skin which forms the perineal floor covers the pelvic outlet. It extends from the pubic symphysis to the coccyx, and continues on either side on to the medial aspects of the thighs.

This perineum is approximately diamond-shaped (**A**) and it is evident in coronal sections (**C**) that, because the pelvic diaphragm is bowl-shaped and the perineal skin more or less flat, the lateral parts of the region are much deeper than the central part.

On both anatomical and clinical grounds it is reasonable to divide the perineum into several compartments. The primary division is into an anal triangle behind and a urogenital triangle in front, by a coronal plane which traverses the perineal body and the anterior limits of the ischial tuberosities (**A**).

The urogenital triangle

The urogenital triangle is comprised of a number of spaces. The deep perineal pouch is a closed space with a thin fascial roof and a much thicker floor called the perineal membrane (inferior fascia of the urogenital diaphragm). Both fascial layers are attached on either side to the ischiopubic rami (**D**). Anteriorly, they are fused a short distance behind the pubic symphysis (**E**). Posteriorly they also fuse and are incorporated centrally in the perineal body (**E**). The central part of the roof of the pouch lies immediately below the anterior gap in the pelvic diaphragm (**D**) and therefore immediately below the pelvic cavity. Lateral to this, it is related to the anterior margins of the levator ani muscles (**D**). Still further laterally, it forms the floor of a loose connective tissue space bordered medially by levator ani and laterally by obturator internus (**D**). It will be seen later that these spaces are continuous posteriorly with the ischiorectal fossae of the anal triangles.

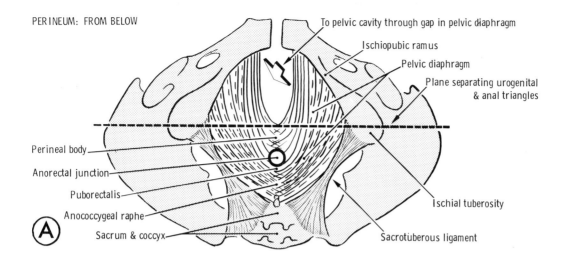

PERINEUM: FROM BELOW

To pelvic cavity through gap in pelvic diaphragm
Ischiopubic ramus
Pelvic diaphragm
Plane separating urogenital & anal triangles
Perineal body
Anorectal junction
Puborectalis
Anococcygeal raphe
Sacrum & coccyx
Ischial tuberosity
Sacrotuberous ligament

Ⓐ

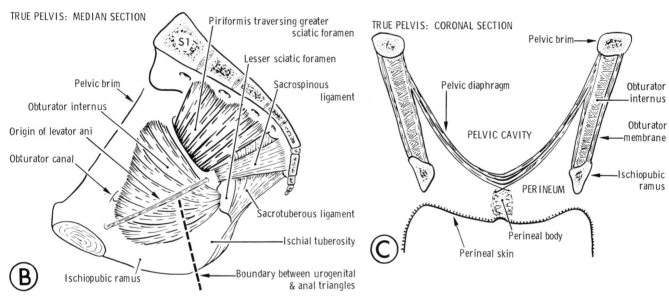

TRUE PELVIS: MEDIAN SECTION

S1
Piriformis traversing greater sciatic foramen
Lesser sciatic foramen
Sacrospinous ligament
Pelvic brim
Obturator internus
Origin of levator ani
Obturator canal
Sacrotuberous ligament
Ischial tuberosity
Ischiopubic ramus
Boundary between urogenital & anal triangles

Ⓑ

TRUE PELVIS: CORONAL SECTION

Pelvic brim
Pelvic diaphragm
PELVIC CAVITY
Obturator internus
Obturator membrane
Ischiopubic ramus
PERINEUM
Perineal body
Perineal skin

Ⓒ

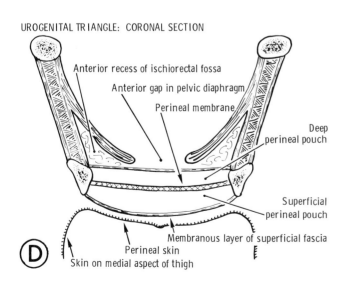

UROGENITAL TRIANGLE: CORONAL SECTION

Anterior recess of ischiorectal fossa
Anterior gap in pelvic diaphragm
Perineal membrane
Deep perineal pouch
Superficial perineal pouch
Membranous layer of superficial fascia
Perineal skin
Skin on medial aspect of thigh

Ⓓ

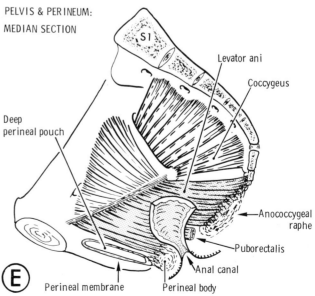

PELVIS & PERINEUM: MEDIAN SECTION

S1
Levator ani
Coccygeus
Deep perineal pouch
Anococcygeal raphe
Puborectalis
Anal canal
Perineal membrane
Perineal body

Ⓔ

The superficial fascia of the urogenital triangle is a continuation of the same layer on the abdominal wall and, like it, consists of superficial fatty and deeper membranous layers. The membranous layer is attached laterally to the inferior margins of the ischiopubic rami (**283E**). Posteriorly it fuses with the perineal membrane, and centrally with the perineal body (**A**). Anteriorly it envelops the external gentialia and ascends in front of the pubic symphysis on to the anterior abdominal wall (**A**). The loose connective tissue space between this membranous layer of the superficial fascia and the perineal membrane is the superficial perineal pouch. Observe that, whereas the deep perineal pouch is closed in all directions, the superficial pouch has no anterior wall, and that its anterior part is continuous through the interval between the deep pouch and the pubic symphysis, and then through the anterior gap in the pelvic diaphragm with the pelvic cavity (**A**).

The anal triangle

The anal triangle consists of two extensive fascial spaces named the ischiorectal fossae which are largely, though not completely, separated by a series of midline structures which extend from the pelvic diaphragm to the perineal skin (**A, B**). From before backwards these are the perineal body, the anal canal and the anococcygeal raphé. Note that, both immediately in front of and behind the anal canal, the barrier between the two fossae is weaker than elsewhere, so that an abscess in one fossa may extend across the midline into the other.

Each ischiorectal fossa is wedge-shaped (**C**). The lateral wall is also the lateral wall of the anal triangle. Observe its composition in **D**. The medial wall consists of an upper part formed by a levator ani muscle and a lower part formed by the perineal body, anal canal and anococcygeal raphé (**B, C**). Behind, these walls meet. Anteriorly, the superficial part of the fossa is limited by the fused posterior walls of the deep and superficial perineal pouches (**B**). The deepest part of the fossa, as has been seen, is continued forwards into the urogenital triangle, above the deep perineal pouch, as the anterior recess (**B, 283D**). The floor of the fossa is discussed in the section on anal musculature later on this page.

The pudendal canal is a tunnel which runs forwards in the fascia on obturator internus on the lateral wall of the ischiorectal fossa. It begins at the lesser sciatic foramen and lies deeply in the perineum, some 4 cm above the margin of the ischial tuberosity. It contains the internal pudendal artery, and its venae comitantes, and the pudendal nerve (**D**). The artery is a branch of the internal iliac which leaves the pelvic cavity through the lower part of the greater sciatic foramen, crosses the outer surface of the ischial spine in the buttock and enters the perineum through the lesser sciatic foramen. The nerve arises from the sacral plexus at the lower border of the greater sciatic foramen and follows the artery into the perineum. It draws its somatic fibres from the ventral rami of S2, 3 and 4. The artery and nerve supply the majority of the structures in the perineum.

The anal canal

The anorectal junction is situated, by definition, at the level of the pelvic diaphragm, so that the rectum lies in the pelvic cavity and the anal canal in the perineum (**C, E**). The canal is about 4 cm long and passes downwards and backwards to the anus (**A**). This orifice lies in the cleft between the buttocks some 4 cm in front of the coccyx. The skin immediately around it is pigmented and radially wrinkled.

Developmentally, the upper half of the anal canal is derived from the hindgut and the lower half from a depression on the skin surface. The two halves are separated in early development by the anal membrane, which normally breaks down during the third month of pregnancy. Occasionally this process fails and the child is born with an imperforate anus which demands immediate surgical correction.

The anal mucous membrane (**E**) exhibits some 10 longitudinal ridges, the anal columns, in the upper half of the canal. The lower extremities of the columns are joined by crescentic folds (anal valves) with small recesses (anal sinuses) above them. The circular marking round the middle of the anal canal formed by the anal valves in series is called the pectinate line. It is said to mark the position of the anal membrane (see above). Above the pectinate line, the mucosa is plum coloured and covered by columnar epithelium like that of the rectum, a transitional zone immediately below the line is bluish white, while the lowest part of the canal is lined by true skin.

The anal musculature is a complex arrangement of both involuntary and voluntary sphincter muscles.

1. The involuntary elements are downward continuations of the inner circular and outer longitudinal layers of plain muscle in the wall of the rectum (**E**). The circular layer becomes noticeably thicker as it crosses the anorectal junction and continues along the anal canal to the level of the transitional mucosal zone. This constitutes the internal anal sphincter. It is an involuntary muscle which relaxes automatically in response to the stimulus of faeces in the rectum (**298**). The longitudinal muscle of the rectum undergoes an unusual change in character at the anorectal junction to a tubular fibro-elastic lamina which continues along the anal canal outside the internal sphincter. Below, it divides into a number of radiating divisions. One of these is attached to the mucosa of the lowest part of the canal and retracts this tissue after it has been protruded somewhat through the anus during defaecation (**E**). Others are attached to the peri-anal

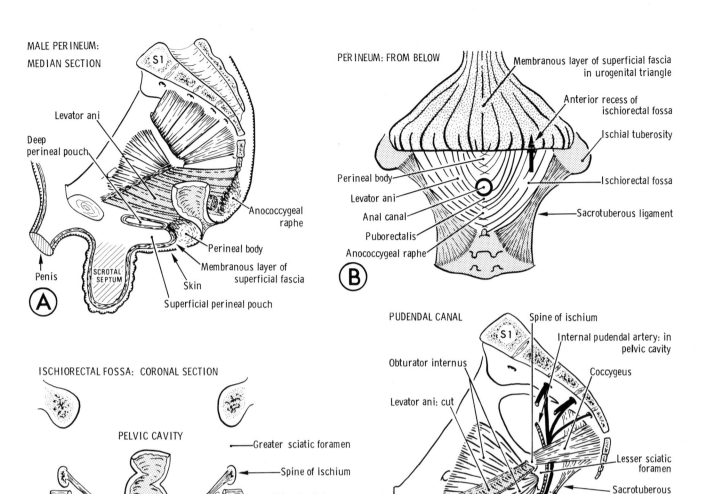

MALE PERINEUM:
MEDIAN SECTION

Levator ani

Deep
perineal pouch

S1

Anococcygeal
raphe

Penis

Perineal body

SCROTAL
SEPTUM

Membranous layer of
superficial fascia

Skin

Superficial perineal pouch

Ⓐ

PERINEUM: FROM BELOW

Membranous layer of superficial fascia
in urogenital triangle

Anterior recess of
ischiorectal fossa

Ischial tuberosity

Perineal body

Levator ani

Anal canal

Puborectalis

Anococcygeal raphe

Ischiorectal fossa

Sacrotuberous ligament

Ⓑ

ISCHIORECTAL FOSSA: CORONAL SECTION

PELVIC CAVITY

Greater sciatic foramen

Spine of ischium

Obturator internus

Sacrotuberous ligament

Anal canal

Levator ani

Ischiorectal fossa

Ⓒ

PUDENDAL CANAL

Spine of ischium

S1

Internal pudendal artery: in
pelvic cavity

Obturator internus

Coccygeus

Levator ani: cut

Lesser sciatic
foramen

Sacrotuberous
ligament

Pudendal nerve

Internal pudendal artery:
in perineum

Ischial tuberosity

Anterior limit of lateral wall
of ischiorectal fossa

Ⓓ

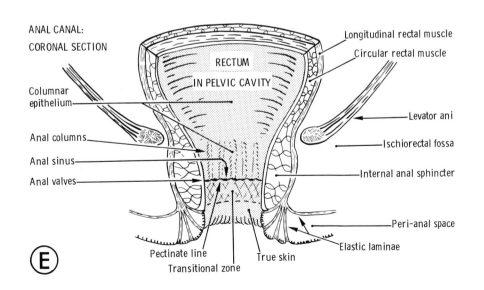

ANAL CANAL:
CORONAL SECTION

Longitudinal rectal muscle

Circular rectal muscle

RECTUM
IN PELVIC CAVITY

Columnar
epithelium

Anal columns

Anal sinus

Anal valves

Levator ani

Ischiorectal fossa

Internal anal sphincter

Peri-anal space

Elastic laminae

Pectinate line

Transitional zone

True skin

Ⓔ

skin and maintain it in a wrinkled state which allows stretching during defaecation. The most peripheral division radiates laterally on either side forming the floors of the ischiorectal fossae. This layer tends to delay the extension of an ischiorectal abscess towards the perineal skin for a considerable time. Between it and the perineal skin is the peri-anal space in which the connective tissue is of a looser texture. Peri-anal abscesses point on the overlying skin within a few days.

2. The main voluntary muscle is the external anal sphincter (**A**) which is described in three parts, although this individuality is not always clear. The subcutaneous part encircles the lowest part of the anal canal below the level of the internal sphincter and is traversed by the cutaneous divisions of the longitudinal elastic lamina of the anal canal (see above). The superficial part surrounds the middle half of the canal while the deep part is related to its upper quarter. It has been noted previously (**266**) that puborectalis fibres of the pelvic diaphragm form a sling round the lateral and posterior aspects of the anorectal junction. It acts as a sphincter only in so far as its contraction accentuates the angulation of that part of the gut. In contrast to the internal sphincter, these voluntary sphincter muscles can be consciously contracted so as to prevent defaecation when that process is stimulated by the presence of faeces in the rectum. Alternatively, if the circumstances are suitable, they can be voluntarily relaxed so that the process can proceed. Division or paralysis of the voluntary sphincters are very serious conditions because, with only the internal sphincter operative, there is faecal incontinence, in which periodic evacuation of the bowel occurs automatically (**298**).

The blood vessels of the anal canal reflect its bipartite development. The upper half, above the pectinate line, is supplied by the slender terminal branches of the superior rectal artery which run distally in the submucous tissue of the anal columns. The lower half is supplied by the inferior rectal branches of the internal pudendal artery (**B**) which run medially across the ischiorectal fossae from the pudendal canals (**285D**). The two sets of branches anastomose in the region of the pectinate line. It is perhaps worth stressing that the inferior rectal artery does not supply any part of the rectum!

The venous drainage corresponds to the arterial supply. The anastomotic vessels between the superior and inferior rectal veins quite frequently become varicose and bulge the covering mucosa into the lumen of the anal canal. The varicosities may lie above or below the pectinate line and are known in these situations as internal or external haemorrhoids respectively. As the superior rectal vein is a tributary of the portal venous system, while the inferior rectal vein is systemic, the venous anastomosis in the anal wall is portosystemic in nature. Haemorrhoids can therefore be a consequence of portal obstruction, but it is important to appreciate that in the very great majority of cases there is no portal abnormality and the varicosities appear to be due to the fact that they lie at the lowest point of the valveless portal system.

The nerve supply of the anal canal is also derived from two sources. The internal anal sphincter is innervated by autonomic fibres while sensory impulses from the mucous membrane above the pectinate line are conducted along visceral sensory nerve fibres which follow autonomic pathways. The autonomic and visceral sensory pathways associated with the anal canal are discussed more fully later.

The inferior rectal branch of the pudendal nerve arises in the pudendal canal (**285D**) and crosses the ischiorectal fossa in company with the inferior rectal vessels (**B**). Its somatic motor fibres innervate the external anal sphincter. Its somatic sensory fibres convey sensation from the anal mucosa below the pectinate line and from the skin around the anus. The somatic sensory fibres from the lower part of the canal, unlike the visceral sensory fibres from the upper half, respond to the same general stimuli as skin, such as injury, temperature and touch. Because of the pattern of innervation of the anal canal, lesions involving the mucous membrane below the pectinate line, such as anal fissure, are very painful and are associated with reflex spasm of the external sphincter, which tends to increase the pain during and after defaecation.

The contents of the urogenital triangle in the male

The deep perineal pouch contains the following structures (**B**).

1. *The membranous part of the urethra* is continuous with the prostatic urethra through the roof of the pouch and with the penile urethra through the perineal membrane (**289F**). This short segment is the narrowest and least distensible part of the urethra apart from the external urethral orifice.

2. *The voluntary sphincter urethrae muscle* surrounds the membranous urethra. It is innervated from the pudendal nerve. Contrast this with the involuntary sphincter mechanism at the internal urethral orifice (**272**).

3. *The two bulbo-urethral glands*, which are each about the size of a pea, are embedded in the sphincter urethrae on either side of the urethra (**B**). They produce a small part of the seminal fluid. The single ducts of the glands pierce the perineal membrane and open into the penile urethra.

4. *The pudendal nerve* enters the pouch from the pudendal canal (**285D**) and runs forwards along its bony lateral wall (**B**). It supplies the membranous urethra and its sphincter muscle and then passes through the perineal membrane as the dorsal nerve of the penis (**B, 289A**).

ANAL SPHINCTERS

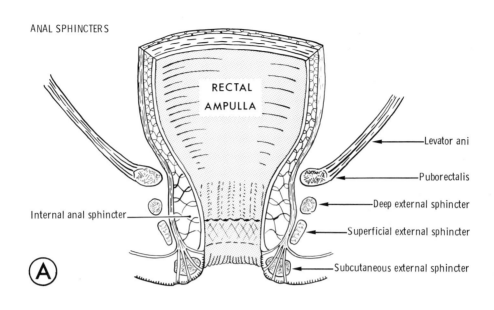

RECTAL AMPULLA

Levator ani

Puborectalis

Deep external sphincter

Internal anal sphincter

Superficial external sphincter

Subcutaneous external sphincter

(A)

MALE PERINEUM: DEEP PERINEAL POUCH:
MEMBRANOUS SUPERFICIAL FASCIA & PERINEAL MEMBRANE
REMOVED FROM UROGENITAL TRIANGLE

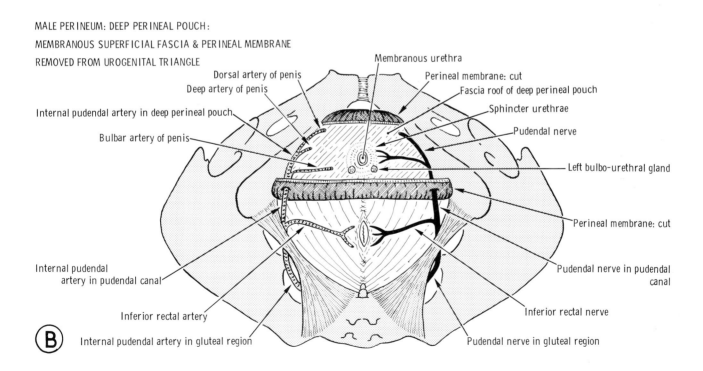

Dorsal artery of penis

Deep artery of penis

Membranous urethra

Perineal membrane: cut

Fascia roof of deep perineal pouch

Internal pudendal artery in deep perineal pouch

Sphincter urethrae

Bulbar artery of penis

Pudendal nerve

Left bulbo-urethral gland

Perineal membrane: cut

Internal pudendal artery in pudendal canal

Pudendal nerve in pudendal canal

Inferior rectal artery

Inferior rectal nerve

Internal pudendal artery in gluteal region

Pudendal nerve in gluteal region

(B)

5. The internal pudendal artery follows the pudendal nerve into the deep pouch (**287B**). It ends as three penile branches, bulbar, deep and dorsal, all of which pierce the perineal membrane to reach the penis in the superficial pouch (**A**). The artery is accompanied by small venae comitantes but it is important to note that these veins do not drain the tissues of the penis.

The superficial perineal pouch contains the fixed part of the penis, and the arteries and nerves associated with it. Recall that this pouch has no structural anterior wall (**285A**). Its anterior limit is arbitrarily regarded as being situated below the pubic symphysis and beyond this it is directly continuous with the scrotum, which has been described already (**208**), and the free part of the penis.

The penis

The penis consists of three masses of erectile tissue, each composed of a continuous labyrinth of blood spaces embedded in a tough framework of collagenous elastic, and plain muscle fibres. In the superficial perineal pouch (**A**), the two tapering corpora cavernosa lie against the ischiopubic rami and gradually converge and come into contact below the pubic symphysis. The single corpus spongiosum is situated in the midline, attached to the under surface of the perineal membrane. Behind, it ends in an expansion called the bulb of the penis, while anteriorly it comes to lie in the ventral groove between the corpora cavernosa (**A**).

The free part of the penis is described as having ventral and dorsal surfaces (**B**). Except at its anterior end, it is formed by the same three erectile masses noted below the pubic symphysis. The corpora cavernosa end bluntly some distance short of the end of the penis (**C, D**). On the other hand the corpus spongiosum expands anteriorly into the conical glans penis which covers the ends of the corpora cavernosa and projects beyond them as the corona glandis (**C**). To just short of this corona, the erectile masses are loosely invested by the membranous layer of the superficial fascia and a layer of thin skin (**D**). Anteriorly, the skin and fascia are firmly attached to the erectile tissue of the glans. Between these two regions the skin forms a tubular fold called the prepuce or foreskin, which ensheaths the glans and is attached to its ventral aspect by a median frenulum (**D, E**).

The arteries of the penis are branches of the internal pudendal artery which pierce the perineal membrane. The bulbar arteries supply the corpus spongiosum (**A**) and the deep arteries the corpora cavernosa (**A, B**). The dorsal arteries pass forwards on the dorsal aspects of the corpora cavernosa, between the erectile tissue and the membranous layer of fascia, and supply branches to both the corpora cavernosa and the skin (**A, B**).

The venous drainage of the penis is through two dorsal veins both of which lie in the median plane (**B**). The superficial dorsal vein, which is situated between the membranous fascial layer and the skin, drains these superficial tissues into one or both great saphenous veins (**335C**) in the upper part of the anterior aspect of the thigh. The deep dorsal vein which runs backwards between the two dorsal arteries, and in the same tissue plane, drains the erectile tissues. It continues backwards in the midline below the pubic symphysis, and then passes upwards, first between the symphysis and the deep perineal pouch, and subsequently through the anterior gap in the pelvic diaphragm (**F**). Entering the pelvic fascia it divides and becomes continuous with the two prostatic venous plexuses (**274**).

The skin of the free part of the penis derives its nerve supply from two sources. The proximal part is innervated by terminal branches of the ilio-inguinal nerve (L1). The rest of the penile skin is supplied by the dorsal nerves of the penis (S2). These begin as terminal branches of the pudendal nerves in the deep perineal pouch, pierce the perineal membrane and continue forwards on the dorsal aspects of the corpora cavernosa, deep to the membranous layer of the superficial fascia. Observe the positions of the vessels and nerves on the dorsum of the penis in **B**.

The penile or spongy part of the urethra enters the penile bulb through the perineal membrane as a continuation of the membranous urethra (**F**). Observe the following features.

1. It traverses the corpus spongiosum in the median plane, to the external urethral orifice which is the narrowest part of the whole urethra.
2. It exhibits two dilatations along its course known as the intrabulbar and navicular fossae.
3. Numerous blind pit-like recesses or lacunae extend backwards from the urethral lumen, and may obstruct the passage of a catheter or urethral instrument. The largest lacuna arises from the dorsal wall of the navicular fossa.
4. The male urethra as a whole is S-shaped when the free part of the penis is flaccid and dependent (**F**). When this part is held at right angles to the abdominal wall, the urethra follows a single curve between the spongy and membranous parts. It is then most readily traversed by an instrument of J-shaped form.

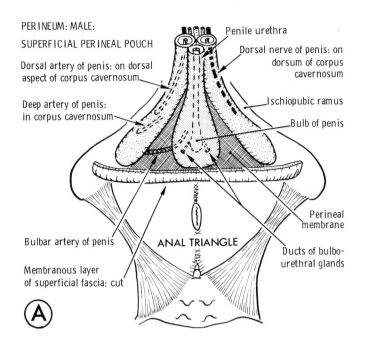

PERINEUM: MALE:
SUPERFICIAL PERINEAL POUCH

Dorsal artery of penis: on dorsal aspect of corpus cavernosum

Deep artery of penis: in corpus cavernosum

Penile urethra

Dorsal nerve of penis: on dorsum of corpus cavernosum

Ischiopubic ramus

Bulb of penis

Bulbar artery of penis

Membranous layer of superficial fascia: cut

ANAL TRIANGLE

Perineal membrane

Ducts of bulbo-urethral glands

(A)

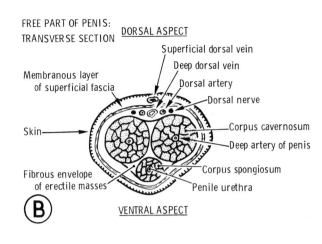

FREE PART OF PENIS:
TRANSVERSE SECTION   DORSAL ASPECT

Superficial dorsal vein
Deep dorsal vein
Dorsal artery
Dorsal nerve

Membranous layer of superficial fascia

Skin

Corpus cavernosum
Deep artery of penis

Corpus spongiosum

Fibrous envelope of erectile masses

Penile urethra

(B)   VENTRAL ASPECT

FREE PART OF PENIS: HORIZONTAL
LONGITUDINAL SECTION

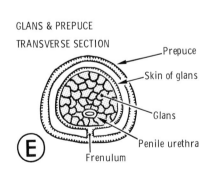

Loose areolar tissue
Skin
Membranous layer of superficial fascia

Glans penis
Skin of glans
Prepuce

Corpora cavernosa

(D)

FREE PART OF PENIS: ERECTILE MASSES

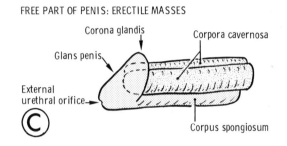

Corona glandis
Glans penis
External urethral orifice

Corpora cavernosa

Corpus spongiosum

(C)

GLANS & PREPUCE
TRANSVERSE SECTION

Prepuce
Skin of glans
Glans
Penile urethra
Frenulum

(E)

PENIS & UROGENITAL TRIANGLE:
MEDIAN SECTION

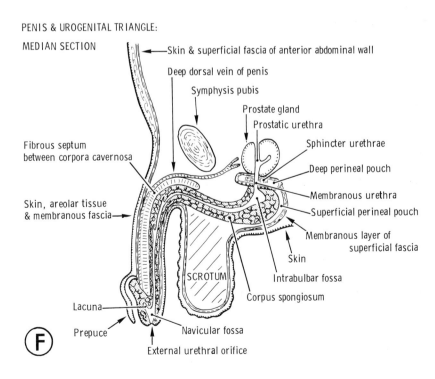

Skin & superficial fascia of anterior abdominal wall
Deep dorsal vein of penis
Symphysis pubis
Prostate gland
Prostatic urethra
Sphincter urethrae
Deep perineal pouch
Membranous urethra
Superficial perineal pouch
Membranous layer of superficial fascia
Skin
Intrabulbar fossa
Corpus spongiosum

Fibrous septum between corpora cavernosa

Skin, areolar tissue & membranous fascia

SCROTUM

Lacuna
Prepuce
Navicular fossa
External urethral orifice

(F)

The contents of the urogenital triangle in the female

The main viscera in this region are the urethra, the vagina, the erectile tissue of the clitoris and the greater vestibular glands.

The urethra and vagina enter the region from the pelvic cavity (**277C**) by passing through the anterior gap in the pelvic diaphragm and following a straight course downwards and somewhat forwards to the exterior (**A**).

Not only is the female urethra straight, it is also shorter, wider and more distensible than the male urethra. Consequently, an instrument such as a cystoscope (**272**) is more easily passed in the female than in the male.

The deep perineal pouch (**A**) is traversed by the vagina and the urethra. In this part of its course the urethra is surrounded by the voluntary sphincter urethrae muscle.

The superficial perineal pouch (**B**) contains the terminal parts of the vagina and urethra and the erectile bodies of the clitoris. The latter are similar to, though much smaller than, those of the penis. The bulbs of the vestibule lie on the under surface of the perineal membrane on either side of the vagina. They expand behind, but taper anteriorly and fuse in front of the urethral orifice. The two convergent corpora cavernosa are attached to the perineal membrane and the inferior pubic rami, and fuse below and behind the pubic symphysis to form the clitoris. The free part of the clitoris turns downwards and backwards for a short distance in front of the urethral orifice and ends in a rounded tubercle, the glans clitoridis (**A**, **B**, **C**).

The two greater vestibular glands are about the size of peas, and lie deep to the posterior ends of the bulbs of the vestibule (**B**). Their ducts open into the vestibule of the vagina (**C**) (see below). These ducts may become blocked so that the glands undergo cystic enlargement (Bartholin's cysts).

The urogenital triangle in the female is supplied by branches of the internal pudendal artery and pudendal nerve, which are essentially similar to, though smaller than, those in the male.

The vulva

The surface features of the female urogenital triangle are described collectively as the vulva and are illustrated in **C**. Observe the following features.

1. The thick outer skin folds, the labia majora, which overlie the corpora cavernosa. They are composed of fatty fibrous tissue and are covered on their lateral surface by hairs. The two folds are continuous anteriorly in the mons pubis.
2. The thinner labia minora which overlie the bulbs of the vestibule. Each divides anteriorly into two parts.

The lateral folds are continuous anterior to the clitoris, forming a hood or prepuce. The medial folds are attached to the posterior surface of the clitoris forming a frenulum.
3. The vestibule of the vagina is the depression bordered by the labia minora. It exhibits in its floor the external urethral orifice and the vaginal orifice, with the openings of the greater vestibular ducts on either side of it.
4. The hymen is an anular mucosal fold of variable individual shape, which partially closes the vaginal orifice in the virgin state, but is ruptured during the first intercourse.

The innervation of the perineal skin

Four nerves or groups of nerves innervate this area of skin (**D**).

1. The anococcygeal nerves arise from the coccygeal plexus (S4, 5, **C**) within the pelvic cavity and reach the perineum by piercing the coccygeus muscle and the sacrospinous and sacrotuberous ligaments.
2. The perineal branch of the posterior cutaneous nerve of the thigh (**341B**) (S1, 2, 3) turns medially over the ischial tuberosity and helps to supply the central part of the perineum.
3. Cutaneous branches of the pudendal nerve (S2, 3, 4) supply or contribute to the supply of the greater part of the perineum.
4. Branches arising from the ilio-inguinal nerve (L1), as it traverses the superficial inguinal ring, supply the skin over the dorsum and sides of the root of the penis and the adjacent part of the lateral aspects of the scrotum in the male, and the skin over the anterior ends of the labia majora and the mons pubis in the female.

The segmental innervation of the area which is shown in **E** should be compared with the distribution of the individual nerves (**D**). Note particularly the following points.

1. The break in the sequence of the spinal segments represented, between L1 and S2.
2. The sequence of segmental areas from S2 anteriorly to the coccygeal segment posteriorly.
3. Local anaesthetic injected through the sacral hiatus into the lower part of the sacral canal diffuses upwards as far as, or a little beyond, the lower limit of the spinal dura (S2) and anaesthetises all the perineal skin except that innervated from L1 (sacral anaesthesia or caudal analgesia).

PERINEUM: FEMALE:
MEDIAN SECTION

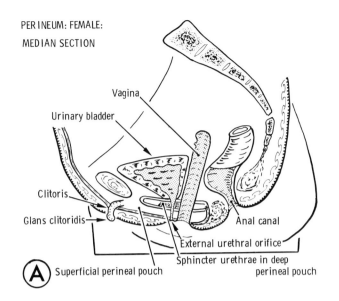

Vagina

Urinary bladder

Clitoris

Glans clitoridis

Anal canal

External urethral orifice

Sphincter urethrae in deep
perineal pouch

(A) Superficial perineal pouch

SUPERFICIAL PERINEAL
POUCH: FEMALE

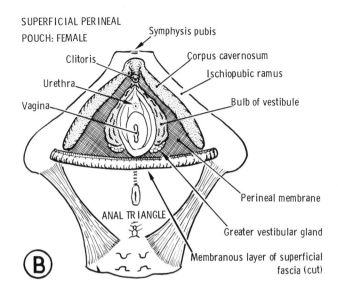

Symphysis pubis

Clitoris

Corpus cavernosum

Urethra

Ischiopubic ramus

Vagina

Bulb of vestibule

ANAL TRIANGLE

Perineal membrane

Greater vestibular gland

Membranous layer of superficial
fascia (cut)

(B)

THE VULVA

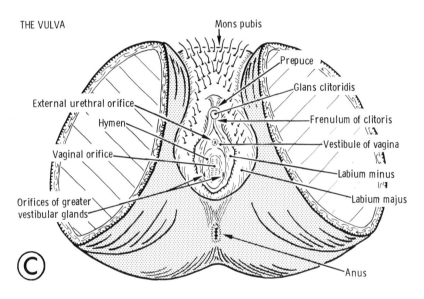

Mons pubis

Prepuce

Glans clitoridis

External urethral orifice

Frenulum of clitoris

Hymen

Vestibule of vagina

Vaginal orifice

Labium minus

Labium majus

Orifices of greater
vestibular glands

Anus

(C)

MALE PERINEUM FROM BELOW:
SKIN INNERVATION

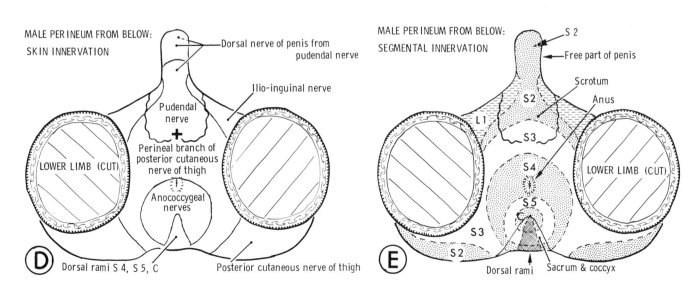

Dorsal nerve of penis from
pudendal nerve

Ilio-inguinal nerve

Pudendal
nerve

LOWER LIMB (CUT)

Perineal branch of
posterior cutaneous
nerve of thigh

Anococcygeal
nerves

(D) Dorsal rami S 4, S 5, C

Posterior cutaneous nerve of thigh

MALE PERINEUM FROM BELOW:
SEGMENTAL INNERVATION

S 2

Free part of penis

Scrotum

S2

Anus

L 1

S3

S 4

LOWER LIMB (CUT)

S 5

S 3

S 2

(E)

Dorsal rami

Sacrum & coccyx

INNERVATION OF ABDOMINAL VISCERA

The pathways followed by the abdominal and perineal sympathetic, parasympathetic and visceral afferent impulses all traverse central autonomic plexuses and their branch plexuses (**A**).

The central autonomic plexuses

A single plexus extends continuously along the front of the abdominal aorta, the fifth lumbar vertebral body, the lumbosacral intervertebral disc and the uppermost part of the sacrum, and is customarily divided into coeliac, inferior mesenteric and superior hypogastric plexuses. Observe the positions of these parts (**A**) and in particular the association of the coeliac plexus with the roots of both the coeliac and superior mesenteric arteries.

About halfway down the sacrum the single plexus divides into the paired inferior hypogastric plexuses which pass downwards and then forwards across the pelvic floor on either side of the midline pelvic viscera (**A**).

Branch plexuses arise from these central plexuses. Most pass along the visceral arterial branches of the aorta and are named accordingly, e.g. hepatic and gonadal plexuses. Others continue forwards from the inferior hypogastric plexuses and are named according to the viscera with which they are associated, e.g. vesical, prostatic and uterovaginal plexuses.

The abdominal and perineal sympathetic pathways

The preganglionic sympathetic fibres concerned with the innervation of these regions (and some other regions) arise from cells in the lateral cell columns in the T5–L2 spinal segments. They follow the usual route of preganglionic sympathetic fibres to the corresponding ganglia on the sympathetic trunk (**117B–D**). Note that whereas the thoracic white rami are short and pass medially (**B**), the lumbar white rami are longer and pass forwards through the psoas canals (**C**).

The relevant parts of the sympathetic trunks

The relevant parts of the sympathetic trunks are shown in **B**. The thoracic parts each carry the seven or eight lower thoracic ganglia, the lumbar parts usually four and the sacral parts five.

Observe the relationships of the trunks to the following structures.

1. The heads of the ribs in the lower part of the thorax.
2. The medial arcuate ligament.
3. The lumbar vertebral bodies and intervertebral discs, the psoas canals, the inferior vena cava or the aorta, and the common iliac vessels in the lumbar region.
4. The pelvic surface of the sacrum, medial to the pelvic sacral foramina.
5. The pelvic surface of the coccyx where the two trunks end in the single ganglion impar.

When the preganglionic sympathetic fibres reach this part of the sympathetic trunk through the white rami communicantes T5–L2, many descend so that a quota is received by each ganglion. These fibres may end their course in the sympathetic trunk in one of two ways. Some synapse with postganglionic sympathetic cells in the ganglia, and the fibres of these cells leave the trunk in the grey rami communicantes. Others leave the ganglia, without synapsing, in medial branches which pass medially to some part of the central autonomic plexuses.

Grey rami comunicantes join the ventral rami of all the spinal nerves. In the thoracic and sacral regions they are short and pass laterally (**B**), whereas in the lumbar region they are longer and pass backwards through the psoas canals (**C**). These postganglionic fibres pass through both the ventral and dorsal rami of the spinal nerves and supply the blood vessels, sweat glands and arrectores pilorum muscles in the somatic areas to which the nerves are distributed. The total area includes the lower part of the thoracic wall, the abdominal wall and perineum, and the whole of the lower limbs.

The medial branches of the sympathetic trunk ganglia concerned with the innervation of the abdomen and perineum are shown in **A, B**. Observe the parts of the central autonomic plexuses to which each passes (**118**). The greater and lesser splanchnic nerves enter the abdomen by piercing the crura of the diaphragm, while the least splanchnic nerves pass behind the medial arcuate ligaments medial to the sympathetic trunks (**A**).

In the central autonomic plexuses the preganglionic sympathetic fibres in the medial branches of the sympathetic trunks synapse with postganglionic cells whose fibres pass through branch plexuses to the abdominal, pelvic and perineal viscera. In general these fibres are vasoconstrictor to the vessels with which they become associated. It is held by some that they are also inhibitory to the general musculature of the hollow abdominal and perineal viscera and excitatory to their sphincters, but this is not certain.

ABDOMINAL CENTRAL AUTONOMIC PLEXUSES

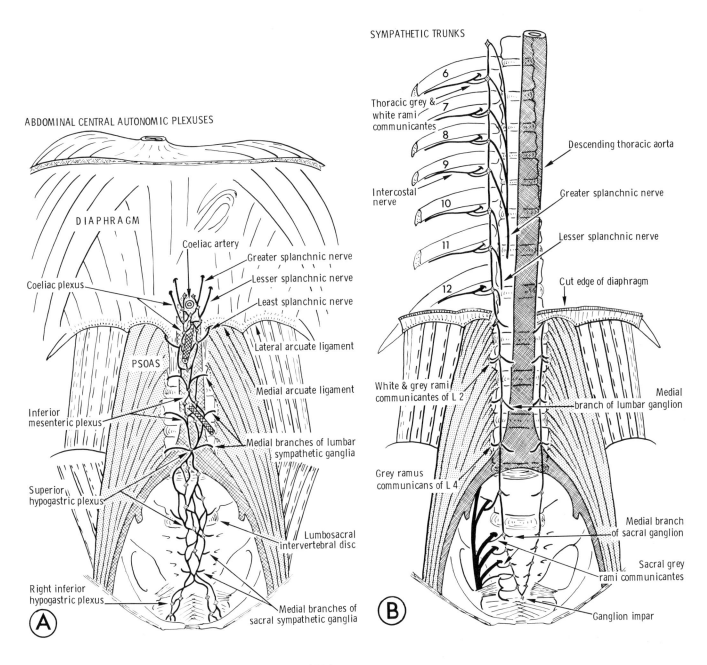

DIAPHRAGM

Coeliac artery
Greater splanchnic nerve
Lesser splanchnic nerve
Least splanchnic nerve
Coeliac plexus
Lateral arcuate ligament
PSOAS
Medial arcuate ligament
Inferior mesenteric plexus
Medial branches of lumbar sympathetic ganglia
Superior hypogastric plexus
Lumbosacral intervertebral disc
Right inferior hypogastric plexus
Medial branches of sacral sympathetic ganglia

(A)

SYMPATHETIC TRUNKS

6
Thoracic grey & white rami communicantes
7
8
9
Intercostal nerve
10
11
12

Descending thoracic aorta
Greater splanchnic nerve
Lesser splanchnic nerve
Cut edge of diaphragm

White & grey rami communicantes of L 2
Medial branch of lumbar ganglion
Grey ramus communicans of L 4
Medial branch of sacral ganglion
Sacral grey rami communicantes
Ganglion impar

(B)

SYMPATHETIC TRUNKS: TRANSVERSE SECTION AT L 2

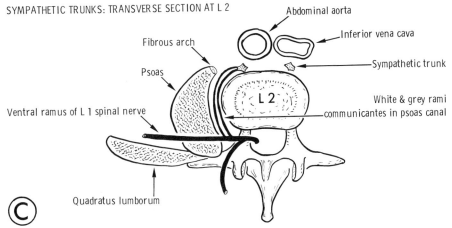

Abdominal aorta
Inferior vena cava
Fibrous arch
Sympathetic trunk
Psoas
Ventral ramus of L 1 spinal nerve
White & grey rami communicantes in psoas canal
L 2
Quadratus lumborum

(C)

The abdominal parasympathetic pathways

Parasympathetic fibres enter the abdomen by two routes.

The anterior and posterior vagal trunks, formed by the re-aggregation of preganglionic vagal fibres in the lower part of the oesophageal plexus, traverse the oesophageal opening in the diaphragm. The anterior trunk lies on the anterior surface of the abdominal oesophagus, and divides into branches which pass to the anterior aspect of the body and fundus of the stomach, and, through the lesser omentum, to the porta hepatis, the pyloric part of the stomach and the proximal half of the duodenum. The posterior trunk runs downwards a short distance from the posterior surface of the oesophagus and divides into branches to the posterior aspect of the body and fundus of the stomach, and a coeliac branch which runs alongside the proximal part of the left gastric artery, behind the lesser peritoneal sac, to the coeliac plexus.

The gastric branches relay in the myenteric and submucous plexuses in the walls of the stomach and upper half of the duodenum.

The fibres of the coeliac branch pass through the coeliac plexus (**A**) without relaying and continue through the peri-arterial branch plexuses around the superior mesenteric artery to all parts of the midgut intestine. The preganglionic fibres finally synapse with the cells of the nerve plexuses in the intestinal wall. In general the short postganglionic fibres are excitatory to the intestinal musculature and inhibitory to the ileocolic sphincter (**222**).

The sacral outflow of preganglionic parasympathetic fibres arises from cells in the lateral grey column in the S2 and S3 spinal segments. Passing through the ventral roots of the corresponding spinal nerves, they leave the ventral rami of these nerves in the pelvic cavity as the pelvic splanchnic nerves (**B**). These ramify in the hypogastric plexuses which they pass through without relay.

Some of the fibres ascend through the superior hypogastric plexus into the inferior mesenteric plexus, and thereafter pass along the inferior mesenteric artery and its branches to reach the hindgut part of the intestine. Reaching the gut these fibres synapse with the cells of the plexuses in the intestinal wall. These fibres are excitatory to the intestinal musculature and inhibitory to the internal anal sphincter.

Other fibres descend into the vesical, prostatic, or uterovaginal plexuses, and relay in these plexuses or in the walls of the pelvic viscera. The short postganglionic fibres are excitatory to the muscles in the walls of the pelvic viscera and vasodilatory to the arteries of the penis.

The visceral afferent pathways

The visceral afferent nerve fibres which run from the abdominal and pelvic viscera to the central nervous system are arranged in two functional groups which convey sensations of pain and visceral distension respectively. Both groups of fibres arise from pseudo-unipolar nerve cells situated either in spinal ganglia (the dorsal root ganglia of spinal nerves) or in the ganglia of the vagus nerve.

Pain fibres follow closely the sympathetic outflow pathways already described. Leaving a viscus such as the splenic flexure of the colon which is taken as an example in **C** they run in the peri-arterial autonomic branch plexus associated with the artery supplying the viscus to reach the corresponding part of the central autonomic plexus. They then run to the sympathetic trunk through one of its medial branches and ascend to the ganglion corresponding to the spinal segment in which they will ultimately end. They pass through the corresponding white ramus communicans to the ventral ramus of the corresponding spinal nerve and reach their cells of origin in the spinal ganglion. The central processes of these cells continue into the spinal cord. Because they traverse white rami communicantes and medial branches of the sympathetic trunk the pain fibres from all abdominal and perineal viscera end in the spinal cord segments T5–L2 inclusive. Pain associated with a visceral lesion is usually projected (referred) to an area of the body surface which both reflects the embryological position of the viscus and derives its cutaneous innervation from those spinal segments which receive the visceral afferent pain fibres. Thus, pain impulses stimulated by inflammation of the vermiform appendix enter the T9, 10 and 11 segments of the spinal cord. In the early stages of development the midgut, from which the appendix develops, is a midline structure. Consequently, even in the adult, the pain is felt in the midline at the level of the umbilicus which is innervated by somatic sensory fibres from T10. It is only when the inflammation spreads from the appendix to the adjacent parietal peritoneum, which is innervated by somatic sensory fibres, that pain moves to the situation of the appendix in the right iliac region.

In the same way the splenic flexure of the colon is also a midline structure in the early stages of development and its visceral afferent pain fibres enter the T12 and L1 spinal segments. Pain caused by a lesion of this part of the gut is thus experienced in the midline of the suprapubic region (**C**).

In contrast to the association of pain fibres with sympathetic fibres, distension fibres follow the parasympathetic pathways and enter the central nervous system either in the S2 and 3 spinal segments or in the brain stem through the vagus nerves. Their cells of origin are situated either in the spinal ganglia of S2 and 3 or in the ganglia on the upper cervical part of the vagus nerves. The distension pathway from the hepatic flexure of the colon is shown as an example in **D**.

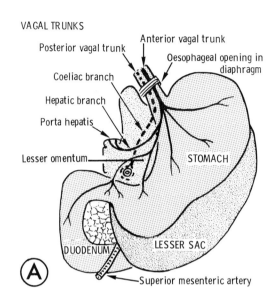

VAGAL TRUNKS

Posterior vagal trunk
Anterior vagal trunk
Oesophageal opening in diaphragm
Coeliac branch
Hepatic branch
Porta hepatis
Lesser omentum
STOMACH
DUODENUM
LESSER SAC
Superior mesenteric artery

A

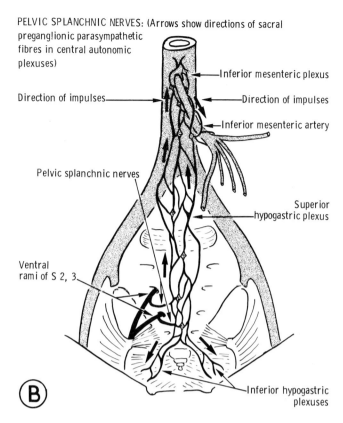

PELVIC SPLANCHNIC NERVES: (Arrows show directions of sacral preganglionic parasympathetic fibres in central autonomic plexuses)

Inferior mesenteric plexus
Direction of impulses
Direction of impulses
Inferior mesenteric artery
Pelvic splanchnic nerves
Superior hypogastric plexus
Ventral rami of S 2, 3
Inferior hypogastric plexuses

B

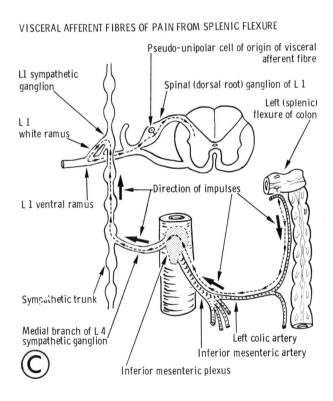

VISCERAL AFFERENT FIBRES OF PAIN FROM SPLENIC FLEXURE

Pseudo-unipolar cell of origin of visceral afferent fibre
Spinal (dorsal root) ganglion of L 1
L1 sympathetic ganglion
Left (splenic) flexure of colon
L 1 white ramus
L 1 ventral ramus
Direction of impulses
Sympathetic trunk
Medial branch of L 4 sympathetic ganglion
Left colic artery
Inferior mesenteric artery
Inferior mesenteric plexus

C

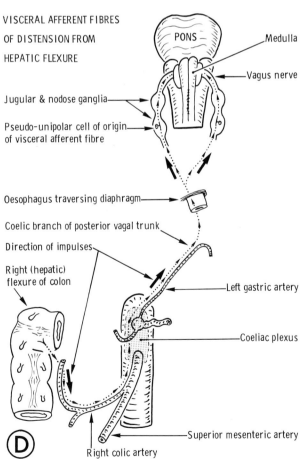

VISCERAL AFFERENT FIBRES OF DISTENSION FROM HEPATIC FLEXURE

PONS
Medulla
Vagus nerve
Jugular & nodose ganglia
Pseudo-unipolar cell of origin of visceral afferent fibre
Oesophagus traversing diaphragm
Coelic branch of posterior vagal trunk
Direction of impulses
Right (hepatic) flexure of colon
Left gastric artery
Coeliac plexus
Superior mesenteric artery
Right colic artery

D

The innervation of the stomach

The parasympathetic and sympathetic pathways to the stomach and the two visceral afferent pathways which are associated with them are shown diagrammatically in **A** and **B**.

Muscular activity in the stomach wall is in the form of peristaltic waves which originate in a pace-setter situated near the upper part of the greater curvature, and spread by direct electric conduction from muscle cell to muscle cell, to the antrum and pylorus. The lumen of the pylorus is normally open, and in these circumstances duodenal contents may regurgitate into the stomach when the pressure difference between the two compartments is suitable. The lumen is closed when a peristaltic wave passes along the antrum and pylorus and moves a small amount of stomach content ahead of it into the duodenum. In this sense the antrum and pylorus may be regarded as a peristaltic pump. Efferent parasympathetic impulses arriving at the stomach, through the vagal trunks (**A**), increase this autonomous peristaltic muscular activity and the efficacy of the pyloric pump, and therefore the rate of stomach emptying. This parasympathetic effect is itself increased reflexly by distension of the stomach, which increases the rate of impulses in the visceral afferent fibres in the vagal trunks (**A**).

Parasympathetic stimulation also greatly increases the activity of the acid-secreting cells of the stomach mucosa.

Vagotomy is an operation in which the anterior and posterior vagal trunks are divided, or alternatively selected branches of these trunks are divided. The operation reduces acid secretion in the stomach and is commonly employed as a treatment of peptic ulcer. Because it of itself also tends to prolong gastric emptying time by decreasing gastric peristalsis, the operation is usually combined with some additional surgical procedure which facilitates emptying of the stomach.

Sympathetic stimulation appears to have little direct effect on either the muscle or glands of the stomach. The great majority of sympathetic fibres passing towards the stomach (**B**) are vasomotor and control the rate of blood flow throughout the stomach wall. Changes in the vascularity of the gastric mucosa may in turn affect its rate of secretion.

Pain caused by lesions of the stomach is conveyed along those visceral afferent fibres which follow sympathetic pathways and have their pseudo-unipolar cells of origin in the spinal ganglia of the seventh and eighth thoracic nerves (**B**). The pain is referred to the skin area innervated by somatic afferent fibres associated with the same spinal segments, that is in the epigastrium. This is so even when, as in many individuals, the stomach extends downwards into the lower part of the abdominal cavity proper and the lesion is well below the epigastric region.

Nerves of the gall bladder and bile ducts

The bile produced by the liver is prevented from entering the duodenum, between successive phases of digestion, by tonic contraction of the sphincter choledochus (**228**) and is consequently diverted into the gall bladder through the cystic duct. Here it is concentrated about tenfold.

The presence of food, particularly fat, in the duodenum causes the liberation of hormones which cause contraction of the bladder wall and relaxation of the bile duct sphincter, and thus release bile into the duodenum. Some work suggests that these changes are augmented by stimulation of the gall bladder musculature and inhibition of the sphincter choledochus by vagal fibres, which pass through the posterior vagal trunk, the coeliac plexus and the hepatic peri-arterial plexus.

The visceral afferent fibres which convey pain impulses from the gall bladder and bile ducts follow sympathetic pathways and traverse the hepatic peri-arterial plexus, the coeliac plexus and the greater splanchnic nerve, and reach the spinal segments T7–9. The pain is referred to the somatic area innervated by somatic afferent fibres associated with the same segments. Thus 'pure' biliary pain is felt in the midline in the epigastrium (**C**).

However, pain due to a lesion of the biliary tract can also be experienced in other situations (**C**). If inflammation extends from the fundus of the gall bladder to the adjacent parietal peritoneum on the anterior abdominal wall, pain is transmitted through the somatic afferent fibres innervating that peritoneum and is felt in the upper right abdominal quadrant just below the right ninth costal cartilage. Furthermore, if inflammation of the gall bladder causes irritation of the diaphragm, impulses pass through the phrenic nerve to the C4 segment and pain is referred to the region of the right shoulder, which is innervated by somatic afferent fibres from the same spinal segment through the supraclavicular nerve (**401C**).

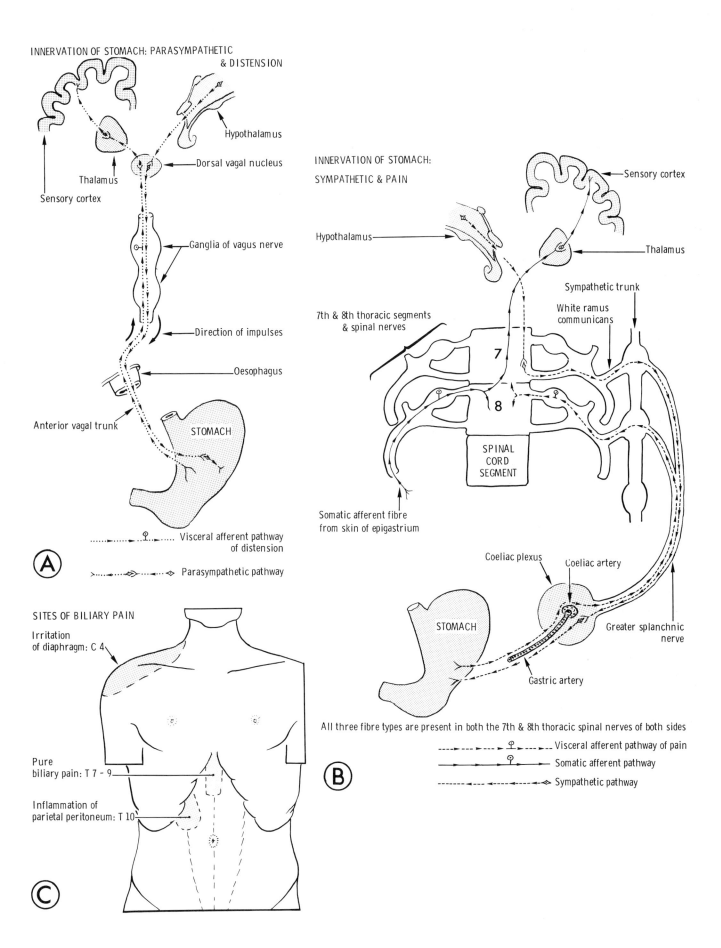

INNERVATION OF STOMACH: PARASYMPATHETIC & DISTENSION

Hypothalamus

Dorsal vagal nucleus

Thalamus

Sensory cortex

Ganglia of vagus nerve

Direction of impulses

Oesophagus

Anterior vagal trunk

STOMACH

— — — ⚓ Visceral afferent pathway of distension

— — — ◇ Parasympathetic pathway

(A)

INNERVATION OF STOMACH: SYMPATHETIC & PAIN

Sensory cortex

Hypothalamus

Thalamus

Sympathetic trunk

White ramus communicans

7th & 8th thoracic segments & spinal nerves

7

8

SPINAL CORD SEGMENT

Somatic afferent fibre from skin of epigastrium

Coeliac plexus

Coeliac artery

STOMACH

Greater splanchnic nerve

Gastric artery

All three fibre types are present in both the 7th & 8th thoracic spinal nerves of both sides

— — — ⚓ Visceral afferent pathway of pain

— — — Somatic afferent pathway

— — — ◇ Sympathetic pathway

(B)

SITES OF BILIARY PAIN

Irritation of diaphragm: C 4

Pure biliary pain: T 7 – 9

Inflammation of parietal peritoneum: T 10

(C)

297

The innervation of the rectum and anal canal

The nerve supply of these regions is summarised below.

1. The parasympathetic pathway originating from the spinal segments S2 and 3 follows the route shown in **A**.

    Parasympathetic stimulation causes peristaltic contractions of the rectal wall and inhibition of the internal anal sphincter.
2. The sympathetic pathway arises from the spinal cord from the L1 and 2 segments and passes along the route indicated in **B**. The traditional view is that postganglionic sympathetic fibres inhibit the rectal musculature and excite contraction of the internal anal sphincter. However, bilateral removal of the lumbar sympathetic trunks has no long-term effects on anorectal function, and it now seems probable that the sympathetic supply to the rectum and anal canal is largely vasomotor.
3. As far as the rectum and anal canal are concerned the pudendal nerve (S2, 3, 4) carries somatic motor fibres to the voluntary external anal sphincter and somatic afferent fibres conveying cutaneous sensation from the lining membrane of the lower half of the anal canal (**C**).
4. Visceral afferent fibres which convey impulses concerned with the sensation of rectal distension follow the parasympathetic pathway to the spinal segments S2 and 3 (**A**). Thereafter, these impulses ascend to the brain and are consciously appreciated.
5. Visceral afferent fibres which convey impulses concerned with pain from the rectum and the upper half of the anal canal follow the sympathetic pathways to the spinal segments L1 and 2 (**B**). The pain is referred to the skin area which is supplied with somatic afferent fibres from the same spinal segments, namely, the suprapubic region (**B**).

Defaecation

Between successive acts of defaecation the rectum is empty and the internal and external anal sphincters are tonically contracted.

When faeces are driven into the rectum by colonic peristalsis, impulses pass along the visceral afferent distension fibres and cause a number of effects.

1. Through ascending spinal pathways they promote conscious appreciation of rectal distension and the desire to defaecate (**A**).
2. Through a local reflex in the sacral segments of the cord, they excite impulses in the parasympathetic fibres passing from S2 and 3 to the involuntary muscle of the rectum and anal canal, producing peristaltic contraction of the rectum and relaxation of the internal anal sphincter (**A**).
3. Through another reflex arc at the same level they inhibit the somatic efferent neurons of the pudendal nerve in S2, 3 and 4 (**A**, **C**) and consequently cause relaxation of the voluntary external anal sphincter.

If circumstances are convenient for defaecation, the intra-abdominal pressure is raised and the faeces are voided. On the other hand if defaecation must be postponed, the reflex relaxation of the external anal sphincter (see 3 above) is overcome by cerebral stimulation of the muscle through the corticospinal tracts (**C**).

After transection of the spinal cord above the sacral region, the sacral defaecation reflexes are preserved but conscious appreciation of rectal distension (**A**) and the ability of voluntary contraction of the external sphincter (**C**) are both lost. Consequently a periodic reflex defaecation occurs of which the patient is unaware.

INNERVATION OF RECTUM & ANAL CANAL:
PARASYMPATHETIC PATHWAY:
VISCERAL AFFERENT PATHWAY (DISTENSION)

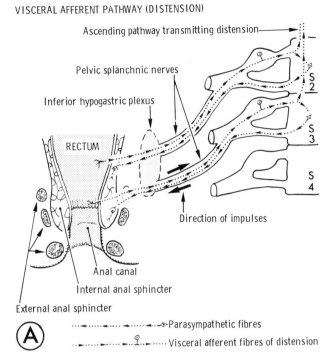

Ascending pathway transmitting distension

Pelvic splanchnic nerves

Inferior hypogastric plexus

RECTUM

S2

S3

S4

Direction of impulses

Anal canal

Internal anal sphincter

External anal sphincter

(A)

········► Parasympathetic fibres

·····🔑····· Visceral afferent fibres of distension

INNERVATION OF RECTUM & ANAL CANAL:
SOMATIC AFFERENT & EFFERENT PATHWAYS

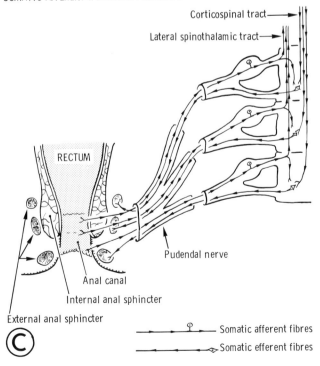

Corticospinal tract

Lateral spinothalamic tract

RECTUM

Pudendal nerve

Anal canal

Internal anal sphincter

External anal sphincter

(C)

——🔑— Somatic afferent fibres

——◆ Somatic efferent fibres

INNERVATION OF RECTUM & ANAL CANAL:
SYMPATHETIC PATHWAY:
VISCERAL AFFERENT PATHWAY (PAIN)

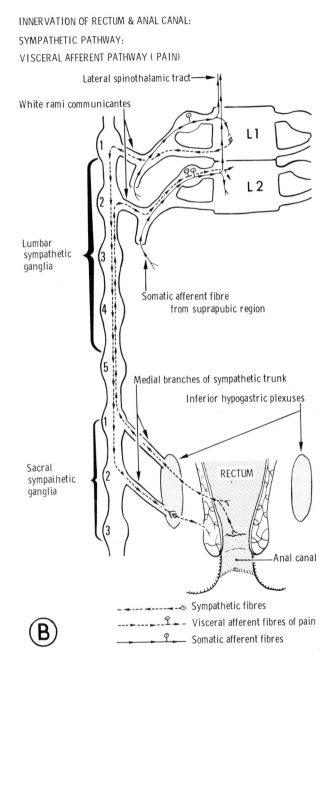

Lateral spinothalamic tract

White rami communicantes

L1

L2

1

2

Lumbar sympathetic ganglia

3

4

Somatic afferent fibre from suprapubic region

5

Medial branches of sympathetic trunk

Inferior hypogastric plexuses

1

RECTUM

Sacral sympathetic ganglia

2

3

Anal canal

(B)

——◇ Sympathetic fibres

——🔑— Visceral afferent fibres of pain

——🔑— Somatic afferent fibres

299

The innervation of the bladder

The nerve pathways involved in the innervation of the bladder and sphincter urethrae are summarised below.

1. The parasympathetic pathway originates in the spinal segments S2 and 3, and follows the route to the bladder wall shown in **A**. Stimulation of the parasympathetic nerves produces contraction of the detrusor muscle.
2. The sympathetic pathway arises in the spinal segments T11–L2 and follows the route indicated in **B**. It is now probable that these sympathetic fibres are concerned solely with control of the blood vessels associated with the bladder.
3. Somatic motor fibres arise in the spinal segments S2, 3 and 4 and pass through the pudendal nerve to innervate the sphincter urethrae (**C**). They can be stimulated from the motor cortex through the corticospinal tracts.
4. Sensations of bladder distension are conveyed along the parasympathetic pathways to the spinal segments S2 and 3 (**A**). Some of their branches ascend through the spinal cord and are responsible for the sensation of distension reaching consciousness (**A**). Other branches form reflex arcs with preganglionic parasympathetic cells in the same segments (**A**). And others again establish inhibitory connections with the somatic motor neurons in the same region of the spinal cord (**C**).
5. Impulses produced by painful stimuli in the bladder traverse the sympathetic route to the spinal segments T10–L2 as shown in **B**. The pain is referred to the abdominal parietes innervated by somatic afferent fibres associated with the same segments, and transmitted to consciousness through the lateral spinothalamic tracts (**B**).

Micturition

The act of micturition is considered here on the basis of the concept that an aggregation of detrusor muscle fibres are inserted radially to the mucosa of the internal urethral orifice so that this orifice is automatically closed by elastic fibres when the detrusor muscle is relaxed, and opened by its contraction (**272**).

In a normal adult, when the bladder is empty or near empty the detrusor muscle is relaxed and the internal urethral orifice closed. The sphincter urethrae is tonically contracted and cannot be voluntarily relaxed although the power of its contraction can be voluntarily increased.

When the contents of the bladder exceed about 300 ml, impulses are transmitted along the distension afferent fibres (**A**) and their impulses have several effects. They reach consciousness through ascending spinal pathways. They cause reflex stimulation of the parasympathetic supply to the bladder and thereby cause contraction of the detrusor muscle, with consequent compression of the bladder contents and opening of the internal urethral orifice. Through other branches they inhibit the impulses traversing the motor neurons of the pudendal nerve to the sphincter urethrae (**C**) so that the muscle relaxes and micturition proceeds.

Micturition can be prevented by cerebral inhibition of the reflex arcs in the sacral spinal segments and by voluntary contraction of the sphincter urethrae motivated through the corticospinal tracts (**C**). The control over micturition which develops during early childhood depends on the establishment of this voluntary inhibition.

After transection of the spinal cord above the S2 level, the sacral reflexes involved in micturition are isolated from higher centres. Consequently, the patient cannot appreciate bladder distension and cannot inhibit relaxation of the sphincter urethrae. But, as the reflexes themselves are intact, the bladder empties automatically every few hours much as it does in infants (automatic reflex bladder).

Destruction of the sacral segments of the spinal cord produces a flaccid paralysis of the detrusor and sphincter urethrae muscles, and divides the visceral afferent distension pathway. Because of the paralysis of the detrusor the internal urethral orifice cannot be actively dilated. As a result the bladder becomes filled by urine until, at an abnormally large capacity, passive stretching of the bladder wall opens the internal orifice and thus allows a continuous dribbling incontinence.

INNERVATION OF URINARY BLADDER & URETHRA:
PARASYMPATHETIC PATHWAY:
VISCERAL AFFERENT PATHWAY (DISTENSION)

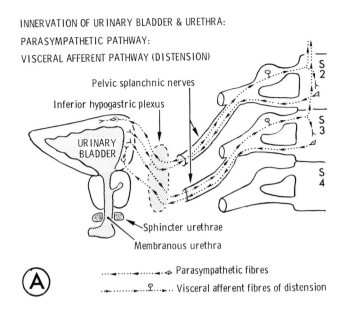

Pelvic splanchnic nerves

Inferior hypogastric plexus

URINARY BLADDER

S 2

S 3

S 4

Sphincter urethrae

Membranous urethra

- - - · · · - - ⊶ Parasympathetic fibres

- - - · · · 🖣 · · · - Visceral afferent fibres of distension

(A)

INNERVATION OF URINARY BLADDER:
SYMPATHETIC PATHWAY:
VISCERAL AFFERENT PATHWAY (PAIN)

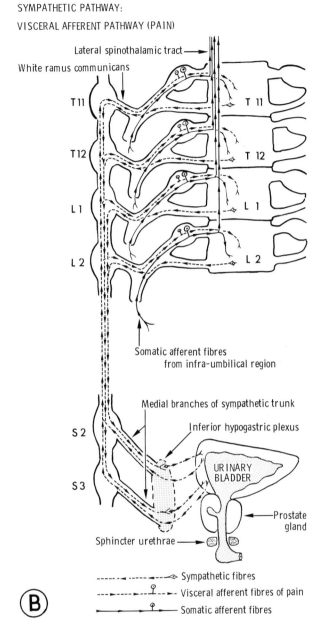

Lateral spinothalamic tract →

White ramus communicans

T 11

T 12

L 1

L 2

T 11

T 12

L 1

L 2

Somatic afferent fibres
from infra-umbilical region

Medial branches of sympathetic trunk

Inferior hypogastric plexus

S 2

S 3

URINARY BLADDER

Sphincter urethrae →

Prostate gland

- - - - - ◁ Sympathetic fibres

- - - 🖣 - - Visceral afferent fibres of pain

———— 🖢 —— Somatic afferent fibres

(B)

INNERVATION OF URINARY BLADDER:
SOMATIC EFFERENT PATHWAY

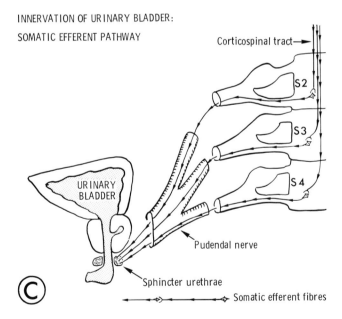

Corticospinal tract →

S2

S3

S 4

URINARY BLADDER

Pudendal nerve

Sphincter urethrae

- - - -⟫- - - -⟫ Somatic efferent fibres

(C)

THE LYMPHATIC DRAINAGE OF ABDOMINAL AND PERINEAL STRUCTURES

It is wise to recall, at the outset, that in the abdomen and perineum, as in other regions of the body, the lymphatic vessels usually, but not always, follow the blood vessels of the part, and predominantly drain external or internal surface tissues. Thus in these regions profuse lymphatic plexuses are associated with the skin, the peritoneum and subperitoneal tissues and the mucosa of hollow viscera. Apart from these tissues some lymphatic vessels originate in the substance of the liver, between and around the renal tubules, and within the testes and epididymides. It is notable that, although the spleen contains a large amount of lymphoid tissue as the white pulp, lymphatic vessels are absent from the parenchyma of the viscus, and are present only immediately below its peritoneal covering.

Most of the lymph in the abdominal vessels has the same composition and the same colourless appearance as lymph in other regions of the body. However, the lymph derived from the mucosa of the small intestine appears milky because it contains minute particles of fat, called chylomicra. It is known as chyle, and the vessels which transmit it as lacteals.

The lymph pathways in the abdomen are joined by those from the lower limbs and perineum and, after passing through numerous lymph nodes, end, with a few exceptions, in the expanded lower end of the thoracic duct. As this expansion receives chyle from the small intestine, as well as clear lymph from other regions, it is called the cisterna chyli.

The cisterna chyli

This thin-walled, elongated sac, which is about 6 cm long, is situated in the oblique aortic opening on the diaphragm in front of the first two lumbar vertebral bodies. It lies on the right side of the abdominal aorta and is normally overlapped and hidden by the right crus of the diaphragm. In this situation it is very deeply placed, being covered anteriorly by many of the retroperitoneal vessels and viscera of the upper part of the abdominal cavity proper. To appreciate these anterior relations of the cisterna chyli compare **A** with **B** and **C**.

The central abdominal lymph nodes

Observe the longitudinal chains of interconnected groups of lymph nodes which lie alongside the major blood vessels (**B**). Note the following features.

1. The external iliac nodes receive lymph from the inguinal nodes in the upper part of the thigh which drain the lower limb, the skin of the lower part of the abdominal wall, the skin of the perineum including that of the penis and scrotum, the lining membranes of the lower half of the anal canal and the vestibule of the vagina.
2. The internal iliac nodes drain most of the pelvic viscera including, in part, the rectum.
3. The lateral aortic nodes receive efferents from the viscera supplied by lateral paired branches of the aorta including the kidney, suprarenal glands, ureter, testis and ovary. They drain into the cisterna chyli through an inconstant number of lumbar trunks.
4. The pre-aortic nodes receive lymph from the gastro-intestinal tract and drain through one or more intestinal trunks into the cisterna chyli.

The lymphatic drainage of the viscera

The stomach. The lymphatic drainage of the stomach is of especial surgical importance, because of the frequency of malignant disease in that viscus. The lymphatic vessels follow the courses of the gastric arteries to the coeliac group of pre-aortic nodes, passing through small peripheral groups on their way. It will be found helpful to revise the relationship of these arteries to the lesser peritoneal sac. The lymphatic vessels are arranged in three main streams.

1. From most of the lesser curvature (**C**) the vessels pass upwards in the lesser omentum, through the lower left gastric nodes. They then turn over the upper border of the lesser sac through the paracardial nodes. Finally, they run downwards and to the right behind the lesser sac through the upper left gastric nodes to the coeliac nodes.
2. From the fundus and the upper part of the greater curvature (**D**), the vessels pass through the gastrosplenic ligament to the hilus of the spleen and thereafter to the anterior surface of the left kidney. They then travel to the right along the splenic artery behind the lesser sac, and through the pancreaticosplenic nodes to the coeliac nodes.
3. From the right part of the greater curvature and the pylorus (**C**), the lymph vessels pass to the right in the gastrocolic ligament through the right gastro-epiploic nodes. They then turn upwards along the gastroduodenal artery, through the pyloric nodes, and finally run to the left behind the lesser sac, along the common hepatic artery, through the hepatic nodes, to the coeliac group.

From the coeliac nodes the lymph is carried through an intestinal trunk (**B**) to the cisterna chyli and thus to the thoracic duct.

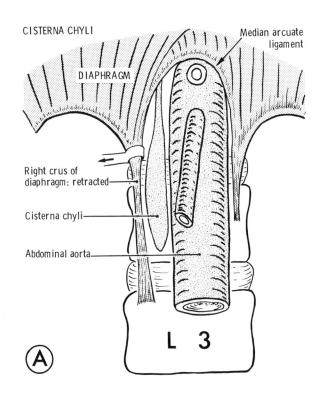

CISTERNA CHYLI

DIAPHRAGM

Median arcuate ligament

Right crus of diaphragm: retracted

Cisterna chyli

Abdominal aorta

L 3

Ⓐ

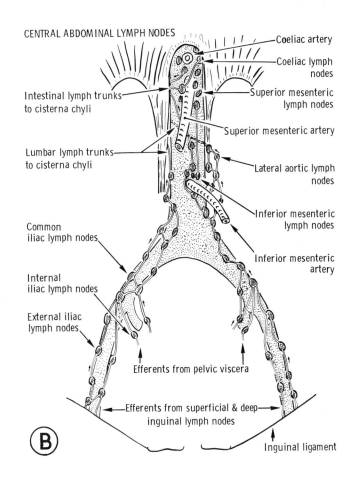

CENTRAL ABDOMINAL LYMPH NODES

Coeliac artery

Coeliac lymph nodes

Intestinal lymph trunks to cisterna chyli

Superior mesenteric lymph nodes

Superior mesenteric artery

Lumbar lymph trunks to cisterna chyli

Lateral aortic lymph nodes

Inferior mesenteric lymph nodes

Common iliac lymph nodes

Inferior mesenteric artery

Internal iliac lymph nodes

External iliac lymph nodes

Efferents from pelvic viscera

Efferents from superficial & deep inguinal lymph nodes

Inguinal ligament

Ⓑ

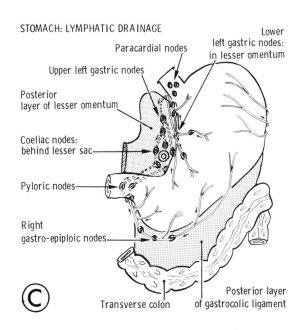

STOMACH: LYMPHATIC DRAINAGE

Lower left gastric nodes: in lesser omentum

Paracardial nodes

Upper left gastric nodes

Posterior layer of lesser omentum

Coeliac nodes: behind lesser sac

Pyloric nodes

Right gastro-epiploic nodes

Transverse colon

Posterior layer of gastrocolic ligament

Ⓒ

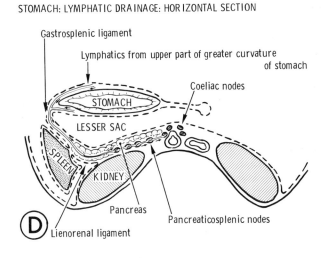

STOMACH: LYMPHATIC DRAINAGE: HORIZONTAL SECTION

Gastrosplenic ligament

Lymphatics from upper part of greater curvature of stomach

Coeliac nodes

STOMACH

LESSER SAC

SPLEEN

KIDNEY

Pancreas

Pancreaticosplenic nodes

Lienorenal ligament

Ⓓ

303

The liver. Two main streams of lymph vessels leave the liver (**A**). One drains the posterior surface and the upper and posterior parts of the parenchyma, and follows the inferior vena cava through the diaphragm to the right lateral diaphragmatic nodes around the termination of that vessel. The other drains the subserous vessels from the superior, anterior, and inferior aspects of the viscus, and the lower part of the parenchyma. These vessels converge on the porta hepatis, and follow the hepatic artery through the right free margin of the lesser omentum and behind the lesser peritoneal sac to the coeliac nodes.

The jejunum and ileum. The lymph vessels commence as blind central lacteals in the intestinal villi, into which fat is absorbed (see above). These join larger vessels which pass through the mesentery to its root, interrupted in passage by a hundred or so mesenteric nodes (**B**). At the root of the mesentery, the vessels from the mesentery follow the superior mesenteric artery to the group of nodes around its origin, and so to the coeliac group and the cisterna chyli.

The terminal ileum and the midgut parts of the colon. The lymph vessels follow the appropriate branches of the superior mesenteric artery to the superior mesenteric nodes (see above). In passage they are interrupted by small paracolic nodes close to the gut, and intermediate nodes around the stems of the ileocolic, right colic and middle colic arteries (**B**).

Removal of a malignant growth involves the simultaneous removal of as much as possible of the lymphatic vessels and nodes into which the area of the growth drains. And, since these lymphatic structures are usually intimately associated with blood vessels, it is often necessary to remove these blood vessels and consequently the whole area of tissue which they supply. Thus removal of a malignant growth in the ascending colon may call for removal of the ileocolic and right colic vessels, and consequently excision of the right part of the transverse colon, the ascending colon, the caecum and appendix and the terminal metre of the ileum. The stumps of the ileum and transverse colon are then anastomosed.

The descending and sigmoid colons. The lymph vessels are interrupted, like those of the proximal colon, by paracolic and intermediate nodes as they follow the appropriate arteries to the inferior mesenteric group of pre-aortic nodes (**B**). It should be noted that although some of the efferents of this group traverse higher pre-aortic nodes and intestinal trunks to reach the cisterna chyli, many others reach this destination through the lateral aortic nodes and lumbar trunks (**303B**).

The rectum and upper half of the anal canal. These regions have a common drainage through lymph vessels which connect with pararectal nodes lying along the wall of the rectum. The efferents follow the superior and middle rectal arteries (**C**) to reach the inferior mesenteric and common iliac nodes respectively.

The lower half of the anal canal. The lymphatic drainage of this region is of special surgical importance. Unlike the lymph vessels draining most regions, those associated with the lower half of the anal canal do not follow the artery of the part (the inferior rectal branch of the internal pudendal). On the contrary, they course forwards and laterally, deep to the perineal skin, to end in the superficial inguinal nodes (**C**).

The testis and epididymis. The lymph vessels follow the testicular artery, through the spermatic cord and up the posterior abdominal wall, to the lateral aortic nodes at the origin of that vessel at the level of L2 (**D**). Thus, although the testis and epididymis do not lie in the abdominal cavity, nodal secondaries from malignant growths arising in them tend to appear first high up the posterior abdominal wall, where they may be difficult to palpate.

The kidney. The lymph vessels from the kidney drain into the upper lateral aortic nodes.

The pelvic genito-urinary viscera. Most of the pelvic viscera in both sexes are drained by lymph vessels which pass to the external and internal iliac lymph nodes. The exceptions are the rectum (see above) and the ovary and uterine tube, which drain mainly along the ovarian vessels to the lateral aortic nodes high on the posterior abdominal wall (**D**).

Lymphatic drainage of the skin

In the lymphatic drainage of the abdominal skin there is a watershed about the level of the umbilicus. From below this level, lymphatics from all aspects of the abdominal wall converge on the superficial inguinal group of nodes (**D**); from above it, vessels pass upwards and laterally round the lateral margin of pectoralis major to reach the axillary nodes (**513A**).

The lymphatics from the skin of the perineum pass forwards and then laterally into the superficial inguinal nodes (**D**). It should be noted particularly that this catchment area includes the following regions.

1. The mucosa of the anal canal below the pectinate line, which thus has a markedly different lymphatic drainage from the upper half of the canal (see above).
2. The vestibule of the vagina which thus again drains along a course distinct from that from the vagina above the hymen (see above).
3. The skin of the scrotum and penis. The skin of the scrotum and the testis and epididymis thus have distinct drainage routes, and it follows that secondaries resulting from primary growths in these closely related tissues occur in completely different sites.

LIVER: LYMPHATIC DRAINAGE

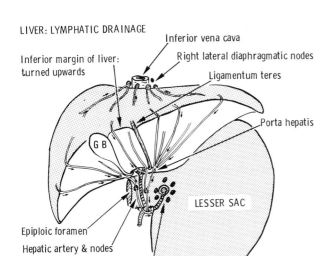

Inferior margin of liver: turned upwards
Inferior vena cava
Right lateral diaphragmatic nodes
Ligamentum teres
Porta hepatis
G B
LESSER SAC
Epiploic foramen
Hepatic artery & nodes
Coeliac artery & nodes: behind lesser sac
A

JEJUNUM, ILEUM & COLON: LYMPHATIC DRAINAGE

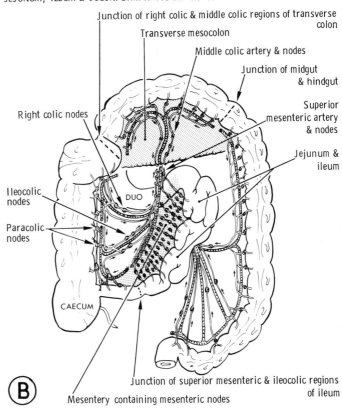

Junction of right colic & middle colic regions of transverse colon
Transverse mesocolon
Middle colic artery & nodes
Junction of midgut & hindgut
Superior mesenteric artery & nodes
Right colic nodes
Jejunum & ileum
Ileocolic nodes
DUO
Paracolic nodes
CAECUM
Junction of superior mesenteric & ileocolic regions of ileum
Mesentery containing mesenteric nodes
B

RECTUM & ANAL CANAL LYMPHATIC DRAINAGE

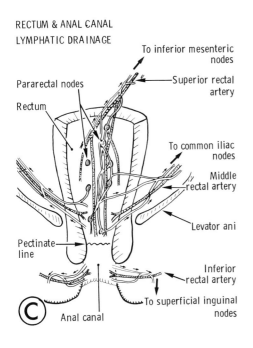

To inferior mesenteric nodes
Superior rectal artery
Pararectal nodes
Rectum
To common iliac nodes
Middle rectal artery
Levator ani
Pectinate line
Inferior rectal artery
Anal canal
To superficial inguinal nodes
C

TESTIS, SCROTUM & OVARY: LYMPHATIC DRAINAGE

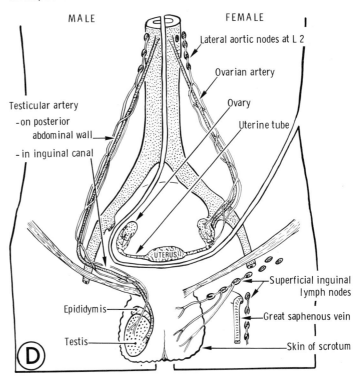

MALE
FEMALE
Lateral aortic nodes at L 2
Ovarian artery
Ovary
Testicular artery
-on posterior abdominal wall
Uterine tube
- in inguinal canal
UTERUS
Superficial inguinal lymph nodes
Epididymis
Great saphenous vein
Testis
Skin of scrotum
D

EXAMINATION OF ABDOMINAL VISCERA IN THE LIVING SUBJECT

Radiographic examination

To demonstrate abdominal organs by X-rays, a means has to be found of producing a contrast between the organ being examined and the other viscera. This is done by introducing, in various ways, an agent containing an element opaque to X-rays which appears white on the viewing screen or radiograph. In examination of the oesophagus, stomach, duodenum and upper jejunum the agent is barium sulphate and is swallowed. The radiologist watches the 'barium meal' passing through oesophagus and stomach and duodenum on an X-ray screen, and so assesses function as well as form. By tilting the patient in various positions the fundus of the stomach can be filled, and by pressing on the stomach the radiologist can outline details of the mucosa (**A**). If the 'meal' is allowed to pass through the small intestine and then the large intestine and studied at intervals, the examination is called a 'follow through', and shows the small bowel (**B**) and finally the colon. Examinaton of the colon is more precisely done by introducing a thinner preparation of barium sulphate via a nozzle into the rectum until the whole colon, and usually the terminal ileum, are filled. This is a 'barium enema' examination. After the enema fluid has been run out of the bowel again via the nozzle, air can be passed in to distend the colon to show mucosal abnormalities such as small ulcers or polyps. This is called a 'double contrast enema' because air produces a dark interior shadow against the white wall (**C**).

BARIUM MEAL

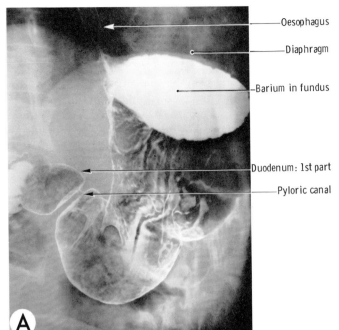

Oesophagus

Diaphragm

Barium in fundus

Duodenum: 1st part

Pyloric canal

A

JEJUNUM & ILEUM: BARIUM FOLLOW THROUGH

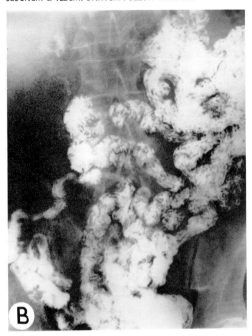

B

BARIUM ENEMA

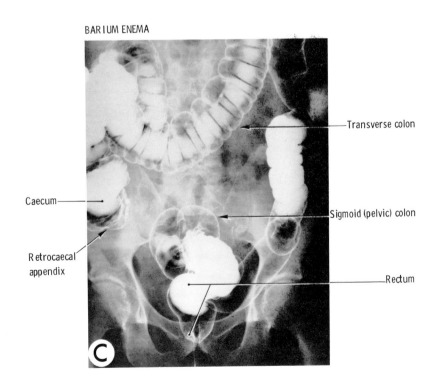

Transverse colon

Caecum

Sigmoid (pelvic) colon

Retrocaecal
appendix

Rectum

C

Gall bladder function is demonstrated by giving the patient tablets of an iodine-containing substance by mouth. These are absorbed by the gut, excreted into the liver, and concentrated in the gall bladder with the bile. Twelve hours later a 'fatty meal' of about 50 ml of arachis oil is given by mouth. This stimulates the flow of bile into the duodenum so that the gall bladder, if normal, contracts. Failure of concentration of the bile due to inflammation of the gall bladder wall, will show on the radiograph, as will any gallstones (**A**). The biliary system can also be demonstrated by percutaneous cholangiography where sterile radio-opaque material is injected directly into an intrahepatic bile duct via a needle passed under X-ray control through the skin.

An iodine containing radio-opaque substance is also used in radiographic examination of the urinary system. It is injected into the median cubital vein (**531**) and is excreted from the blood stream by the kidneys (intravenous pyelogram). Its excretion by the kidneys into the ureters and urinary bladder (**B**) may indicate not only abnormalities of form but also of function in the urinary tract. The retention of an appreciable amount of radio-opaque material in the bladder after micturition indicates obstruction at the bladder neck.

Ultrasound examination

Organs of different densities reflect high frequency sound waves to different degrees, so that an ultrasound source passed along the skin surface can be linked to a visual representation of the underlying viscus. Size, shape, and density of content of many organs can be shown by this method, and abnormalities diagnosed. The method has the great practical virtue of requiring no particular patient preparation, being comfortable and quick, and requiring no injection into the patient's body with the risks this involves. The gall bladder, for example, can be demonstrated by this method as well as by radiography (**C**).

Direct inspection

Direct inspection of the inside of the upper and lower gastro-intestinal tract now complements contrast radiography of these organs by oesophago-gastro-duodenoscopy and colonoscopy respectively. The instruments are flexible and fibre-light illuminated. A very fine calibre flexible wire tube with jaws on its tip activated by an opening and closing device can be passed along the scope and small portions of mucosa or of suspicious ulcers can be removed, and withdrawn for examination by a pathologist (biopsy). Through a gastroscope the orifices of the bile and pancreatic ducts in the duodenum can be directly inspected and even cannulated if desired. Biopsies are also taken via a colonoscope. Before any of these examinations is carried out, the gastro-intestinal tract must be completely empty of any material which might cause confusion in diagnosis.

Radioactive scanning

A substance containing a radio-active element which a particular organ will concentrate can be injected intravenously in a suitably safe dose. A scanner can later be passed over the organ involved, when the amount of radioactivity given off can be relayed to a visual representation. This diagnostic method is more suitable for detecting degrees of over- or under-activity of an organ, rather than its shape *per se*.

CHOLECYSTOGRAM

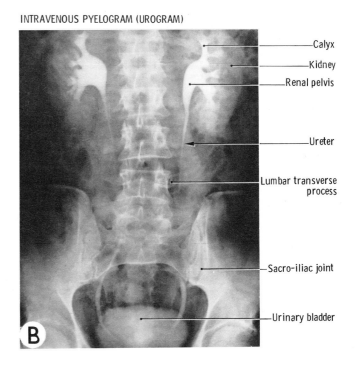

— 12th rib

Common
hepatic duct

— Cystic duct

— Bile duct

— Gall bladder

INTRAVENOUS PYELOGRAM (UROGRAM)

— Calyx
— Kidney
— Renal pelvis

— Ureter

— Lumbar transverse
process

— Sacro-iliac joint

— Urinary bladder

A

B

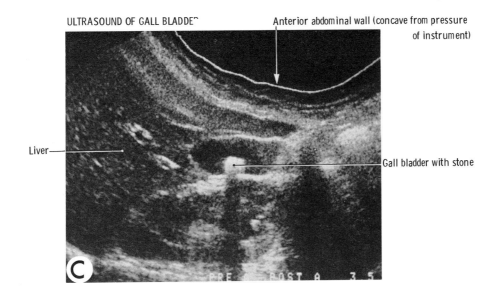

ULTRASOUND OF GALL BLADDER

Anterior abdominal wall (concave from pressure
of instrument)

Liver—

Gall bladder with stone

C

CHAPTER 5

The lower limb

INTRODUCTION

In colloquial speech the whole of this region is called the leg, but in anatomical nomenclature that word is restricted to the region between the knee and ankle joints. The part distal to the ankle joint is the foot. That between the knee and the trunk is the thigh, and this may be taken as including the gluteal region or buttock which lies behind and above the hip joint (**A**).

In many ways the anatomical organisation of the upper and lower limbs is similar, but this similarity is modified in almost every region by the very different functions which the two limbs must serve. On occasion the lower limb, like the upper, may move freely through space in relationship to the trunk, as when a footballer kicks a ball or when the free limb swings forwards in walking. More frequently, the muscles and joints of the lower limb operate when the foot is on the ground, in one of those weight-bearing actions such as standing, walking and running which make up, collectively, a large part of everyday activity. In these circumstances, much of the muscular activity of the part is concerned, not with the production of movements, but with the prevention of those movements which body weight continually tends to produce, and which, if permitted, would impair the maintenance of the erect posture.

PARTS OF LOWER LIMB

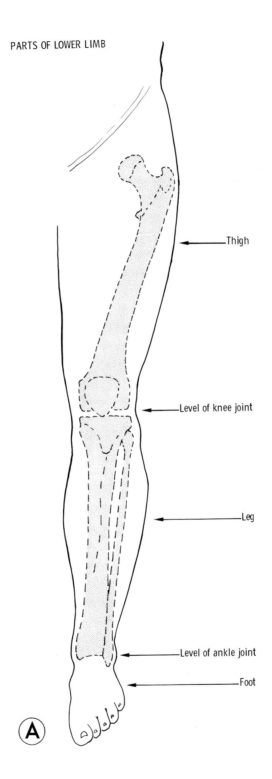

Thigh

Level of knee joint

Leg

Level of ankle joint

Foot

Ⓐ

THE THIGH AND BUTTOCK

The osteoligamentous pelvis

Revise the bony features and ligaments which are visible on the outer aspect of the osteoligamentous pelvis (**A**).

Although many of the structures in the thigh are attached to the outer aspect of the osteoligamentous pelvis, others originate within the abdominal, pelvic and perineal compartments of the trunk and traverse one of several apertures to reach the lower limb. Re-examine the positions, names and boundaries of these apertures.

The acetabulum

Identify the deep concavity of the acetabulum on the central part of the outer surface of the hip bone (**A**). It faces downwards and forwards as well as laterally, and articulates with the spherical head of the femur at the hip joint. Recall that the acetabulum is contributed to by all three primary centres of ossification in the hip bone (**195C**), and that in childhood its iliac, ischial and pubic components are separated by a triradiate strip of cartilage (**B**). This tissue does not begin to ossify until 12 years, and consolidation of the acetabulum is not achieved until after puberty.

Examine the detailed form of the acetabulum (**A, C, D**). The peripheral, smooth, lunate surface, which is covered in life by articular cartilage, surrounds the depressed region of the acetabular fossa and notch which are rough and non-articular. Notice in a dried bone and in **D** the very thin bone which separates the fossa and notch from the pelvic cavity, and compare this with the much thicker parts of the hip bone which underlie the weight-bearing lunate surface.

A circular fibrocartilaginous labrum (**C, D**) is attached to the bone immediately outside the lunate surface, and bridges the acetabular notch, converting it into a tunnel. This tunnel gives passage to the small artery which runs in the ligament of the head of the femur (**317E**). The labrum appreciably deepens the acetabulum and, because of its shape (**D**), grips the head of the femur in its socket and thereby contributes to the stability of the hip joint.

The femur

Study the shape of the femur and identify the following features.

1. The head, neck, shaft and expanded lower end (**E, F**). Note in particular the inclinations of the shaft and neck (**E**). The shaft is inclined upwards and laterally at about 10° to the sagittal plane. This allows the knees to come into contact despite the separation of the upper ends of the femoral shafts by the femoral necks and pelvis. Because of the greater width of the pelvis in the female, the inclination of the shaft is somewhat more pronounced in that sex. The neck forms an angle of about 125° with the shaft. Diminution of this angle is called coxa vara and accentuation coxa valga.

2. The medial and lateral condyles which project backwards from the lower end of the bone, and the deep intercondylar fossa (notch) which separates them (**F**).

3. The medial and lateral epicondyles situated near the centres of the outer surface of the medial and lateral condyles, and the deep pit a short distance below the lateral epicondyle (**F**).

4. The greater and lesser trochanters at the upper end of the shaft, and the intertrochanteric line and crest which join the trochanters across the anterior and posterior aspects of the bone (**F, G**).

5. The bony markings on the posterior aspect of the shaft (**F**). The middle third of this aspect exhibits a prominent ridge named the linea aspera. Above, the linea aspera divides into the gluteal tuberosity and spiral line, which diverge upwards to the region of the intertrochanteric crest. Below, the linea aspera divides into two fine supracondylar lines which bound the triangular popliteal surface. The medial supracondylar line ends below in the prominent adductor tubercle (**E, F**).

Much of the femur is deeply situated among the muscles of the thigh and cannot be readily felt in the living subject. But confirm on your own limb that the upper part of the lateral surface of the shaft and the greater trochanter are readily palpable, and that, in the region of the knee joint, the patellar facet, the outer margins of the femoral condyles, the medial and lateral epicondyles and the adductor tubercle can all be made out without difficulty.

The articular surfaces of the femur

Examine the form and extent of the upper and lower articular surfaces (**G, H**). The upper articular cartilage covers the spherical head of the femur except over the deep pit on its medial aspect (**G**). During childhood and adolescence the circumference of this cartilage merges with that of the related cartilaginous growth plate except above, where a narrow non-articular strip of bone, marked by vascular foramina, intervenes (**G**).

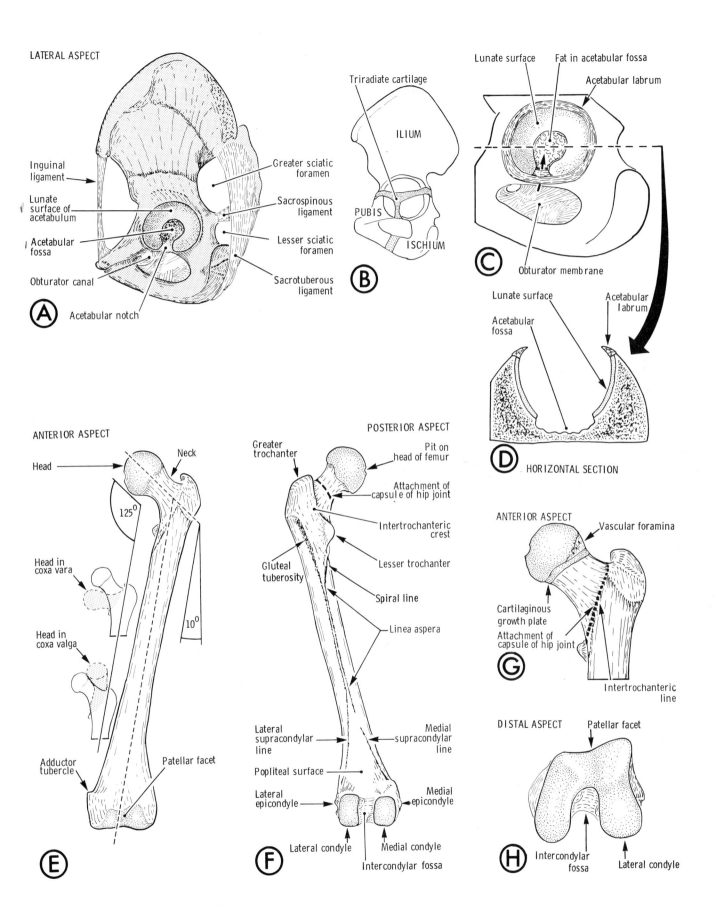

LATERAL ASPECT

Inguinal ligament

Lunate surface of acetabulum

Acetabular fossa

Obturator canal

Acetabular notch

Greater sciatic foramen

Sacrospinous ligament

Lesser sciatic foramen

Sacrotuberous ligament

(A)

Triradiate cartilage

ILIUM

PUBIS

ISCHIUM

(B)

Lunate surface

Fat in acetabular fossa

Acetabular labrum

Obturator membrane

(C)

Lunate surface

Acetabular fossa

Acetabular labrum

(D) HORIZONTAL SECTION

ANTERIOR ASPECT

Head

Neck

125°

Head in coxa vara

Head in coxa valga

10°

Adductor tubercle

Patellar facet

(E)

POSTERIOR ASPECT

Greater trochanter

Pit on head of femur

Attachment of capsule of hip joint

Intertrochanteric crest

Lesser trochanter

Gluteal tuberosity

Spiral line

Linea aspera

Lateral supracondylar line

Medial supracondylar line

Popliteal surface

Lateral epicondyle

Medial epicondyle

Lateral condyle

Medial condyle

Intercondylar fossa

(F)

ANTERIOR ASPECT

Vascular foramina

Cartilaginous growth plate

Attachment of capsule of hip joint

Intertrochanteric line

(G)

DISTAL ASPECT

Patellar facet

Intercondylar fossa

Lateral condyle

(H)

The importance of this relationship is concerned with the blood supply of the femoral head (**315G**).

At the lower end of the femur, articular cartilage covers a U-shaped area (**315H**). The limbs of the U are the condylar facets. These extend over the inferior and posterior, and, to a small extent, the superior aspects of the femoral condyles, and are convex from side to side. The central part of the U-shaped area, called the patellar facet (**315E, 315H**) covers the distal and anterior aspects of the bone end and is deeply grooved from above, downwards and backwards. The lateral lip of this groove is considerably more prominent than the medial.

The development of the femur

Although the distinction between shaft and neck is clear in the adult femur, it must be remembered that both parts belong to the diaphysis and that both are ossified by extension of the one primary centre of ossification, which appears in the shaft some 7 weeks after conception. At birth (**A**) two growth plates separate a bony shaft from upper and lower cartilaginous epiphyses, and the lesser trochanter is represented by a cartilage nodule on the upper part of the shaft. The lower epiphysis includes the whole of both condyles and is ossified from a secondary centre appearing shortly before birth (**A**).

Elongation of the diaphysis in the *shaft axis* proceeds uninterruptedly at the lower growth plate until the plate is obliterated at 20 years. In the upper epiphysis secondary centres appear in the head at 1 year and in the greater trochanter at 4 years (**C**). Elongation of the diaphysis in the *shaft axis* occurs at the central and lateral thirds of the upper growth plate, but only during the first four years of life (**B**). Thereafter, cartilage proliferation in the central third of the plate ceases, and ossification proceeds through the static tissue to establish a definitive upper bony limit between the head and the greater trochanter (**C**). At the same time the lateral third of the growth plate becomes quiescent so that, although it persists until 20 years, it makes no further contribution to diaphysial elongation (**D**). In contrast, in the medial part of the growth plate, cartilage proliferation occurs continually until about 20 years of age, causing elongation of the diaphysis along the *neck axis* throughout that period.

A secondary centre appears in the cartilaginous lesser trochanter at about 12 years (**D**). It forms a traction epiphysis which fuses with the shaft at about 20 years.

Displacement of an epiphysis in relation to the diaphysis of a long bone is not uncommon: separation of the lower humeral epiphysis by a fall on the elbow is an example. At the upper end of the femur an unusual kind of displacement of the head on the neck (slipped upper femoral epiphysis) sometimes occurs at puberty without any history of significant injury. The displacement of the head is often bilateral and occurs gradually, in a predominantly backward direction.

The hip joint

This ball and socket joint is formed by the articulation of the head of the femur (**315E**) and the acetabulum (**315A**). These surfaces are joined by the ligament of the head of the femur, which extends obliquely across the joint cavity from that part of the acetabular labrum which bridges the acetabular notch (**315A**), to the pit on the femoral head (**315F**).

The acetabular fossa is occupied by fat, and this tissue and the ligament of the femoral head are enclosed by a funnel-shaped tube of synovial membrane (**E**).

The fibrous capsule of the joint is a thick and very strong sleeve of fibrous tissue. On the medial side it is attached to the acetabular labrum and the bone just wide of the acetabulum. Its lateral attachment to the femur (**F, G**) is of particular importance and should be studied carefully. Note that, because of the position of this attachment, the surface of the femoral neck is entirely intracapsular except for the lateral half or so of its posterior aspect. The fibres of the capsule are spirally disposed (**G**), the anterior fibres inclining downwards and laterally, and the posterior fibres upwards and laterally, so that all become taut when the joint is extended (i.e. when the lower end of the femur moves backwards), and slack when it is flexed.

Synovial membrane lines the deep aspect of the fibrous capsule and is reflected from it on to the intracapsular part of the neck of the femur, which it covers as far as the femoral articular surface (interrupted line in **E**).

Movements and stability of the hip joint

Largely because the acetabulum is much deeper than the glenoid fossa of the scapula, movement at the hip joint is less free than at the shoulder. Despite the fact that the hip joint is of the ball and socket type, and is consequently capable of movement in all directions, it is convenient to name certain cardinal movements. Flexion involves forward movement of the femur on the pelvis or of the pelvis on the femur: extension is the opposite movement. Adduction and abduction are self-explanatory. Medial and lateral rotation of the thigh around its own long axis are named, as usual, according to the direction and displacement of the anterior aspect of the limb.

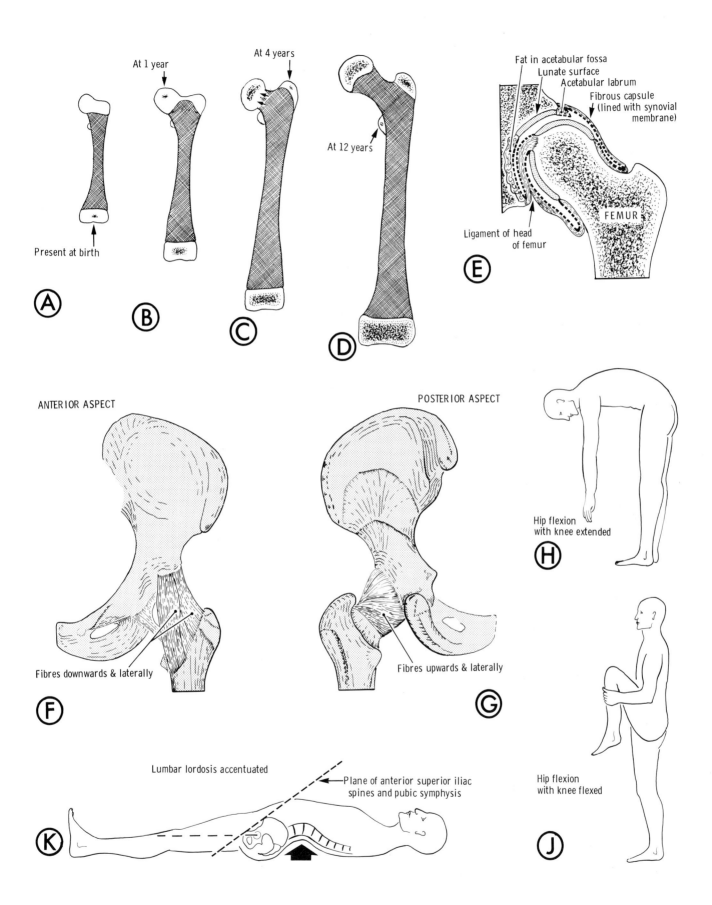

At 1 year

At 4 years

At 12 years

Present at birth

Ⓐ Ⓑ Ⓒ Ⓓ

Fat in acetabular fossa
Lunate surface
Acetabular labrum
Fibrous capsule
(lined with synovial membrane)

FEMUR

Ligament of head of femur

Ⓔ

ANTERIOR ASPECT

POSTERIOR ASPECT

Fibres downwards & laterally

Fibres upwards & laterally

Ⓕ Ⓖ

Hip flexion with knee extended

Ⓗ

Lumbar lordosis accentuated

Plane of anterior superior iliac spines and pubic symphysis

Ⓚ

Hip flexion with knee flexed

Ⓙ

317

Except for flexion and extension, these movements seldom reach their limits in normal activity. Note in your own limb how the position of the knee joint influences the limitation of flexion at the hip. When the knee is extended, as in bending to touch the toes (**317H**), flexion of the hip is limited at an angle which varies considerably in different people, by tension in muscles which run from the pelvis through the posterior compartment of the thigh to the leg bones (the hamstrings). On the other hand when the knee is flexed, flexion at the hip is limited only by contact of the thigh with the anterior abdominal wall (**317J**). Extension at the hip is limited rather abruptly, a few degrees beyond alignment of thigh and trunk, by the sudden tightening of the spirally disposed fibres of the fibrous capsule. It is worth stressing that, in the living subject, the relationship of thigh and trunk when the hip joint is fully extended is partly dependent on the position of the pelvis, which in turn is dependent on the degree of flexion or extension of the lumbar vertebral column. If the lumbar column is strongly extended the pelvis rotates, so that its upper part moves anteriorly and its lower part posteriorly, as is shown by the plane passing through the anterior superior iliac spines and the pubic symphysis (**317K**). When this position is adopted by a supine patient the thigh will lie flat on the bed even if there is a considerable reduction in the normal range of extension at the hip joint, and the joint abnormality may not be recognised.

Dislocation of the hip joint

Congenital dislocation of the hip joint may be present at birth, or develop in infancy, owing to a malformation of the acetabulum. The rim of bone which normally surrounds the socket and gives it its depth is poorly developed, so that the acetabulum is no more than a shallow depression. As a result, muscle tension or body weight displaces the head of the femur upwards on to the outer surface of the ilium, so that the limb is considerably shortened.

Traumatic dislocation of the joint in an adult is only produced by very considerable force. It usually results from a force acting along the femoral shaft, when the hip is flexed and adducted, so that the fibrous capsule is slack and the head of the femur is only partially supported by the posterior lip of the acetabulum.

Thus if the front seat passenger in a car is sitting cross-legged (hip joint flexed and adducted), and the lower end of the femur is driven against the dashboard, the hip joint may be dislocated.

The blood supply of the head and neck of the femur

In most growing long bones a metaphysis is supplied by large vessels which enter it from surrounding muscles through correspondingly large foramina, and to a much smaller extent by the nutrient artery, which enters the bone at some distance from the metaphysial region. The epiphysis derives its vessels from the fibrous capsule of the related joint which is wholly or partly attached to it (**B**).

Because of the complete attachment of the hip capsule to the femoral diaphysis, and the consequent intracapsular position of the upper metaphysis and growth plate of the femur, the usual vascular pattern is considerably modified (**A**). Note in particular the following features.

1. The artery which runs within the ligament of the femoral head. It reaches the ligament by traversing the acetabular notch and supplies the lower medial part of the head.
2. The vessels which arise in the upper part of the hip capsule and run medially on the upper surface of the neck, between bone and synovial membrane. In a young person these eventually cross the upper margin of the growth plate and traverse the foramina between it and the articular cartilage (**A**) to supply the upper and lateral parts of the head.
3. Other vessels which arise in the hip capsule and run medially beneath the synovial membrane on all aspects of the neck before entering the large metaphysial foramina. Only one example of this group of vessels is shown in **A**. In a young person these vessels are separated from the femoral head by a growth plate, and consequently supply only the neck of the bone. In an adult the growth plate has been obliterated and appreciable anastomosis has been established between the epiphysial and metaphysial vessels. But despite this change the routes by which arteries approach the bone and the points at which they enter it remain unchanged.

In a number of circumstances one or more of these vessels may be torn or obstructed, so that the blood supply to the head or neck of the femur, or to both, may be reduced, or entirely cut off. The bone then dies. The condition is named 'avascular necrosis', and it is evident that it may result from either an intracapsular fracture of the neck of the femur or a dislocation of the hip joint.

Sometimes in children of about 5 or 6 years avascular necrosis of the femoral head occurs without a history of severe injury. This condition, known as Perthes disease, is presumably due to some abnormality of the circulation within the head of the femur, but the nature and cause of the abnormality are unknown.

The knee joint

This large and complex synovial joint is formed by the articulation of the lower end of the femur (**315H**) and the upper end of the tibia (**F**). Although the fibula gives attachment to the fibular collateral ligament of the joint, it is not directly involved.

HEAD & NECK OF FEMUR: BLOOD SUPPLY

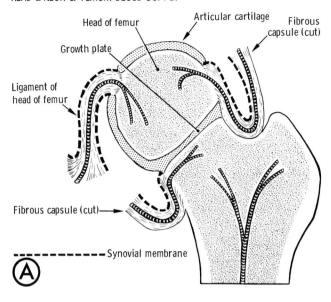

Head of femur

Articular cartilage

Fibrous capsule (cut)

Growth plate

Ligament of head of femur

Fibrous capsule (cut)

Synovial membrane

(A)

BLOOD SUPPLY: METAPHYSIAL AND EPIPHYSIAL

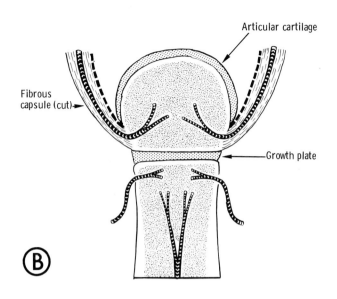

Articular cartilage

Fibrous capsule (cut)

Growth plate

(B)

LEG BONES (PROXIMAL): ANTERIOR ASPECT

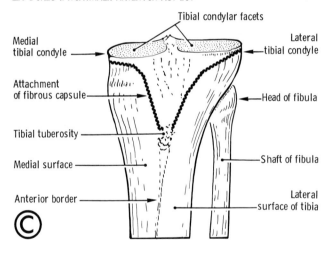

Tibial condylar facets

Medial tibial condyle

Lateral tibial condyle

Attachment of fibrous capsule

Head of fibula

Tibial tuberosity

Medial surface

Shaft of fibula

Anterior border

Lateral surface of tibia

(C)

LEG BONES (PROXIMAL): POSTERIOR ASPECT

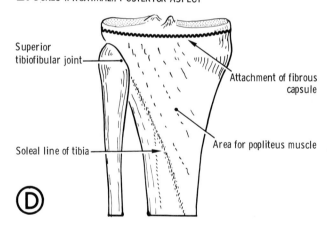

Superior tibiofibular joint

Attachment of fibrous capsule

Soleal line of tibia

Area for popliteus muscle

(D)

LEG BONES (PROXIMAL): LATERAL ASPECT

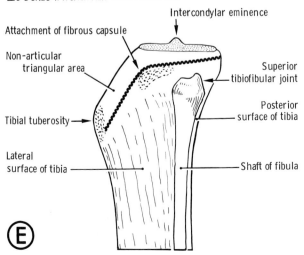

Intercondylar eminence

Attachment of fibrous capsule

Non-articular triangular area

Superior tibiofibular joint

Posterior surface of tibia

Tibial tuberosity

Lateral surface of tibia

Shaft of fibula

(E)

LEG BONES (PROXIMAL): SUPERIOR ASPECT

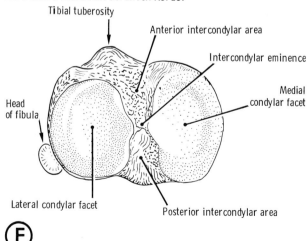

Tibial tuberosity

Anterior intercondylar area

Intercondylar eminence

Medial condylar facet

Head of fibula

Lateral condylar facet

Posterior intercondylar area

(F)

Because of the normal upward and lateral obliquity of the shaft of the femur, the shafts of the two articulating bones are not aligned in the extended limb. The angle is about 190° in the male and somewhat greater in the female.

The upper end of the tibia and fibula

Examine the anterior (**319C**), posterior (**319D**), lateral (**319E**) and superior (**319F**) aspects of the leg bones, and note the following features.

1. The transverse expansion of the upper end of the tibia to form the ill-defined medial and lateral condyles.
2. The different outlines of the gently concave cartilage facets on the upper surfaces of the two condyles, the medial facet being oval and the lateral facet circular. These facets articulate with the condylar facets on the femur.
3. The separation of the tibial condylar facets by an hour-glass shaped nonarticular zone, which is divisible into a central intercondylar eminence and triangular anterior and posterior intercondylar areas.
4. The tuberosity of the tibia at the upper end of the sharp anterior border of the shaft, and the triangular area of bone which slopes upwards and backwards from the tuberosity to the condylar facets.
5. The overhang of both condyles over the posterior surface of the tibia.
6. The articulation of the head of the fibula with the under surface of the lateral tibial condyle at the superior tibiofibular joint.

The fibrous capsule

This is essentially a sleeve of fibrous tissue enclosing the joint cavity, but its anterior part (**A**) is constituted by the broad tendon of the quadriceps femoris muscle which descends from the thigh (**329C**). Consequently, the capsule *per se* is firmly attached to the femur only on its posterior, medial and lateral sides. Anteriorly, the attachment is completed by the quadriceps muscle fibres. Study this femoral attachment of the capsule (**C, D**), noting its relationship to the margins of the condylar facets and epicondyles, and its tibial attachment (**319C, 319D, 319E**), noting the extension forwards and downwards to the tibial tuberosity.

The tendinous anterior part of the fibrous capsule contains a very large sesamoid bone, the patella. The tendinous fibres are attached to the margins of the bone and cover its superficial surface (**A**). Its deep surface (**B**) is marked by a sagittal ridge nearer its medial than its lateral margin, and is covered, except over its lowest part, by articular cartilage. This ridged deep surface of the patella glides along the grooved patellar facet on the femur (**315E, 315H**) during movement at the knee joint.

It is anatomical convention to divide the quadriceps

tendon into differently named parts according to their relationship to the patella (**312A**). The ligamentum patellae is of considerable length and it should be noted that its upper end and lower end lie appreciably above and below the joint line between the tibial and femoral condyles (**323A**).

The collateral ligaments

These strong extracapsular ligaments lie on the lateral (**C**) and medial (**D**) sides of the knee joint. Examine their bony attachments. Notice how the two ligaments differ in length, shape and inclination, and in their relationship to the underlying fibrous capsule. On the lateral side ligament and capsule are separate (**C, E**): on the medial side they are structurally continuous (**D, E**).

The intracapsular structures of the knee joint

The menisci are strips of fibrocartilage which partially separate the tibial and femoral condylar facets (**E**). Each is wedge-shaped in cross-section (**F**), diminishing in thickness from a deep peripheral surface to a thin central edge. It is the thin central parts of the menisci which are most severely compressed between the articulating bones, and these parts are consequently avascular, although the peripheral parts have an appreciable blood supply.

Observe the following differences in the two menisci.

1. The order in which their extremities or horns are attached to the anterior and posterior intercondylar areas of the tibia (**E**).
2. The difference in their shapes (**E**). The medial is semilunar and broader behind than in front, whereas the lateral is uniform in width, nearly circular, and smaller than the lateral tibial facet on which it lies.
3. The difference in their degree of attachment to the fibrous capsule (**E**). The medial meniscus is fused to the capsule throughout most of its peripheral aspect.
4. The difference in their mobility consequent on 3). The lateral meniscus has a considerable mobility whereas the medial is relatively fixed.

The anterior and posterior cruciate ligaments are attached, close to the horns of the menisci, to the anterior and posterior intercondylar areas of the tibia respectively (**G**). They extend upwards into the intercondylar fossa of the femur. The anterior ligament inclines backwards and laterally (**G**) and is attached to the lateral wall of the notch. The posterior ligament inclines forwards and medially, crosses the anterior ligament on its medial side, and becomes attached to the medial wall of the notch.

The popliteus muscle is closely associated with the knee joint both functionally and topographically. It has two origins, one tendinous and the other muscular. The tendon arises inside the fibrous capsule, from the pit below the lateral epicondyle of the femur (**H**).

KNEE JOINT: ANTERIOR ASPECT

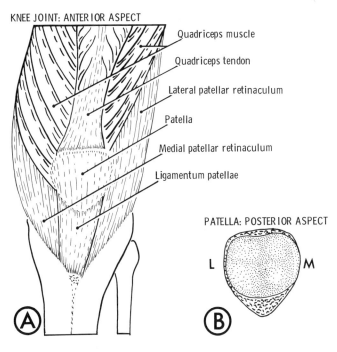

Quadriceps muscle
Quadriceps tendon
Lateral patellar retinaculum
Patella
Medial patellar retinaculum
Ligamentum patellae

PATELLA: POSTERIOR ASPECT

L   M

(B)

(A)

KNEE JOINT: LATERAL ASPECT   KNEE JOINT: MEDIAL ASPECT

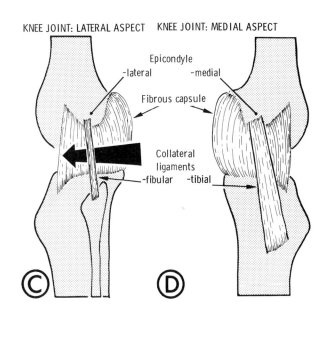

Epicondyle
-lateral   -medial
Fibrous capsule

Collateral
ligaments
-fibular   -tibial

(C)   (D)

MENISCI

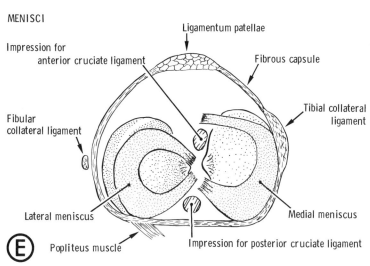

Ligamentum patellae

Impression for
anterior cruciate ligament

Fibrous capsule

Tibial collateral
ligament

Fibular
collateral ligament

Lateral meniscus

Medial meniscus

Popliteus muscle

Impression for posterior cruciate ligament

(E)

MEDIAL MENISCUS: CORONAL SECTION

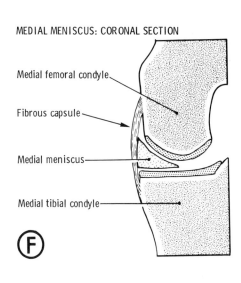

Medial femoral condyle

Fibrous capsule

Medial meniscus

Medial tibial condyle

(F)

CRUCIATE LIGAMENTS

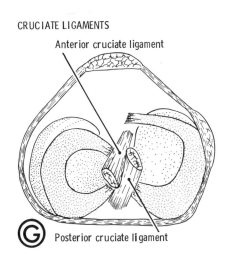

Anterior cruciate ligament

Posterior cruciate ligament

(G)

KNEE JOINT: LATERAL ASPECT

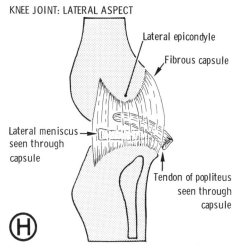

Lateral epicondyle
Fibrous capsule

Lateral meniscus
seen through
capsule

Tendon of popliteus
seen through
capsule

(H)

KNEE JOINT: POSTERIOR ASPECT

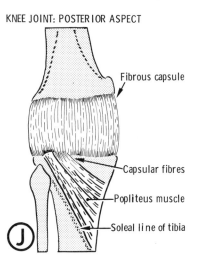

Fibrous capsule

Capsular fibres

Popliteus muscle

Soleal line of tibia

(J)

321

It extends backwards between the lateral meniscus and the capsule and, piercing the posterior part of the capsule, gives way to muscular fibres (**321J**). Other muscle fibres arise from the capsule just medial to the emerging tendon, and are indirectly attached through the capsule to the posterior margin of the lateral meniscus (**321E**). The two sets of muscle fibres blend and the single muscle belly turns downwards to be attached to the triangular area on the posterior surface of the tibia above the soleal line (**321J**).

The synovial membrane

In the knee joint the synovial membrane, essentially, lines the fibrous capsule and covers those intracapsular bone surfaces which are not covered by articular cartilage. However, this simple arrangement is modified in a number of situations.

1. Posteriorly, the membrane is invaginated forwards by the cruciate ligaments, which it consequently covers on their anterior, medial and lateral aspects (**C**).
2. On either side, the membrane is invaginated inwards by the menisci, but in adults it is recognisable only on the peripheral parts of their upper and lower surfaces (**B**). Its absence from the central parts of these surfaces is a result of the compression which they experience between the femoral and tibial condyles.
3. The wedge-shaped region between the ligamentum patellae and the anterior aspect of the tibial condyles is occupied by the infrapatellar fat (**A**). The synovial membrane runs forwards over the upper surface of this fat pad, between the anterior intercondylar area of the tibia and the lower margin of the articular surface of the patella.
4. Above and in front, where the fibrous capsule has no direct femoral attachment, the synovial membrane protrudes upwards between the quadriceps femoris muscle and tendon anteriorly, and the lower quarter of the shaft of the femur posteriorly (**A**). This is named the suprapatellar pouch, and it is very important that the presence of this part of the knee joint cavity, well above the level of the articular surfaces, should be clearly appreciated.

Bursae around the knee joint

A large number of bursae are placed in the vicinity of the knee joint, and may become enlarged as a result of repeated injury, producing tense localised swellings.

1. The prepatellar bursa lies in the superficial fascia in front, over the lower part of the patella and the upper part of the ligamentum patellae (**A**). Enlargement is known for obvious reasons as housemaid's knee.
2. The deep infrapatellar bursa lies in the lowest part of the infrapatellar pad of fat, between the ligamentum patellae and the tibia (**A**).
3. The subcutaneous infrapatellar bursa is interposed between the skin and the tibial tuberosity (**A**).

Palpation of the knee joint

Examine your own knee joint while sitting with one knee over the other.

1. The tuberosity of the tibia, the ligamentum patellae and the patella are readily palpable and the smooth, grooved patellar facet on the femur can be distinguished.
2. On the lateral side, palpate the margin of the lateral femoral condyle and identify the lateral epicondyle of the femur, the head of the fibula and the cord-like fibular collateral ligament running between these two features.
3. On the medial side, the medial femoral epicondyle, the margin of the medial condyle of the femur, the peripheral margin of the medial meniscus and the medial tibial condyle can be felt in that order from above down, but it is unusual to be able to distinguish the tibial collateral ligament, because of its flat strap-like form.

Movement and stability at the knee joint

Fundamentally, the knee is a large joint at which movement of the tibia on the femur occurs in a sagittal plane, around a transverse axis of rotation traversing the two femoral epicondyles (**C, D**). Backward movement of the tibia is flexion, and forward movement extension. The composite tibiomeniscal articular surfaces move around the curved long axes of the femoral condyles, while the patella glides along the grooved patellar facet, lying at the upper margin of the facet in extension (**A**) and close to the intercondylar notch in flexion.

The movements of flexion and extension have important effects on the state of both the cruciate and collateral ligaments. The collateral ligaments both become taut in extension (**D**) and slack in flexion (**E, F**). The effects of these movements on the cruciate ligaments are more complex. Midway between flexion and extension (**E**), both cruciate ligaments are slightly slack. This small degree of slackness can be demonstrated by firmly grasping the upper part of the leg of a colleague, who is lying supine with the knee in semiflexion, and observing that the tibia can be displaced slightly backwards and slightly forwards on the femur. Full extension of the knee joint (**D**) produces complete tightening of the anterior cruciate ligament without altering the slight laxity of the posterior ligament. In contrast, full flexion of the knee (**F**) completely tightens the posterior ligament, but does not affect the slight laxity of the anterior.

SAGITTAL SECTION OF KNEE JOINT

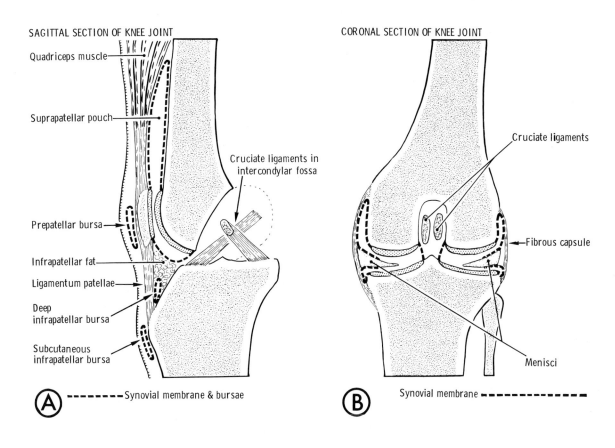

Quadriceps muscle

Suprapatellar pouch

Cruciate ligaments in intercondylar fossa

Prepatellar bursa

Infrapatellar fat

Ligamentum patellae

Deep infrapatellar bursa

Subcutaneous infrapatellar bursa

(A) - - - - Synovial membrane & bursae

CORONAL SECTION OF KNEE JOINT

Cruciate ligaments

Fibrous capsule

Menisci

(B) Synovial membrane - - - - - - -

TRANSVERSE SECTION OF KNEE JOINT

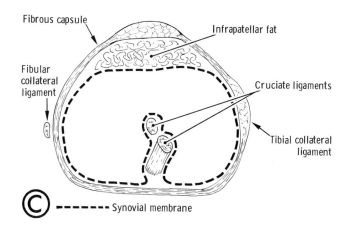

Fibrous capsule

Infrapatellar fat

Fibular collateral ligament

Cruciate ligaments

Tibial collateral ligament

(C) - - - - Synovial membrane

KNEE JOINT IN EXTENSION

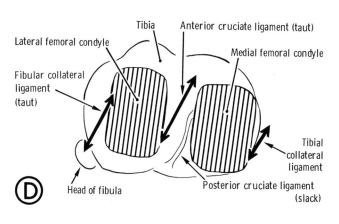

Tibia

Lateral femoral condyle

Anterior cruciate ligament (taut)

Medial femoral condyle

Fibular collateral ligament (taut)

Tibial collateral ligament

Head of fibula

Posterior cruciate ligament (slack)

(D)

KNEE JOINT: MIDWAY BETWEEN FLEXION AND EXTENSION

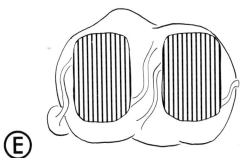

(E)

KNEE JOINT IN FLEXION

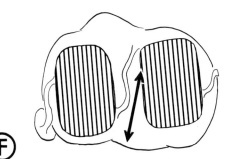

(F)

Limitation of flexion occurs only when the calf comes into contact with the thigh. The final limit of extension occurs at a sagittal angulation of about 190° between femur and tibia. This final limitation is brought about by a very complex locking mechanism which operates over the last 5° or so of the movement, and involves interaction of many joint structures. However, these terminal degrees of extension are so seldom used in the common activities of everyday life that the locking mechanism is to be regarded as being of academic rather than practical importance.

In relaxed standing, the force of body weight tends to extend the knee joint, and the quadriceps femoris is relaxed, as indicated by side to side freedom of the patella. The joint is stabilised in this position by tension in both collateral ligaments, in the anterior cruciate ligament (**323D**), in the posterior part of the fibrous capsule and in all those tissues, such as muscles, deep fascia and skin, which lie behind the capsule. But in these circumstances the joint is not fully extended. If the quadriceps muscle is strongly contracted, or if some other powerful extending force is exerted on the joint, the knee is moved even farther backwards towards its final limit. It is only in these rather unnatural circumstances that the locking mechanism becomes operative.

Rotation is the other normal movement at the joint. Description of such movement as medial or lateral rotation must always indicate which bone is being regarded as the fixed element and which the moving element. Thus medial rotation of the femur on the grounded tibia is the same movement as lateral rotation of the free tibia on the femur. Such axial rotations are only possible when the knee joint is flexed.

Sit in a chair and place one heel on another chair so that the knee joint is extended. When the raised foot is pivoted from side to side on the heel, palpation of the knee joint shows that the leg bones and the femur are rotating together. In these circumstances rotation of the limb is occurring at the hip joint. Again sit in a chair but with both knees flexed and both feet on the ground. Pivot one foot from side to side on the heel and note that now the leg bones rotate, while the patella and femur remain stationary. In other words rotation is occurring at the knee joint.

If the latter manoeuvre is repeated while the head of the fibula and the medial tibial condyle are simultaneously palpated, it will be found that during rotation of the leg, there is little backward or forward movement of the medial condyle, but pronounced displacements of the fibula. This clearly indicates that rotation at the knee joint occurs around a vertical axis traversing the medial condyles of the femur and tibia (**A, B**). In rotations of the femur on the tibia, the medial femoral condyle pivots on the medial tibiomeniscal surface, which changes little in form because of the relative fixity of the medial meniscus (**321E**). At the same time the lateral femoral condyle, accompanied by the comparatively mobile lateral meniscus, moves in an arc

backwards or forwards on the stationary lateral tibial condyle (**A, B**).

If the bony movements involved in rotation at the knee joint are considered in association with the tension changes in ligaments caused by flexion and extension, the reason why rotation occurs in the flexed but not in the extended joint becomes clear. In extension, tautness of both the anterior cruciate ligament and the fibular collateral ligament (**323D**) prevents any anteroposterior displacement of the lateral femoral condyle on the tibia. In flexion both ligaments are slack, the fibular collateral more so than the anterior cruciate, and this laxity allows the lateral femoral condyle to move freely around an arc centred on the medial condyle (**323E**).

Injuries of the knee joint

Knee joint injuries are usually associated with distension of the joint cavity by blood or by the excessive production of synovial fluid. The joint is held in a slightly flexed position in which the size of its cavity is maximal. The swelling is most obvious anteriorly, above and to either side of the patella. Because the fluid separates the patella from the femoral patellar facet, the two articular surfaces can be felt to meet, if the patella is pressed sharply backwards (patellar tap). When it is necessary to aspirate fluid from a distended knee joint for therapeutic or diagnostic purposes, the needle is inserted into the cavity above or on either side of the patella.

The patella may be fractured or dislocated. Fractures of the patella may occur in two distinct circumstances. A blow or fall on the bone may fracture it into several fragments (**C**), but these tend to be held in place by the surrounding tendon of the quadriceps femoris muscle, and do not usually interfere with active extension of the knee. Alternatively a person, often in middle life, may stumble and contract the quadriceps femoris muscle, suddenly and powerfully, in an endeavour to save himself. The patella is then fractured transversely (**D**), and the tendinous fibres over the bone, and the patellar retinacula on either side of it, are torn. The bone fragments separate and there is loss of active extension of the knee. From an anatomical point of view it is interesting that the patellar fragments can be removed and the tendon sutured, with little or no effect on the efficiency of the knee joint. Because of the obliquity of the femoral shaft from which the quadriceps muscle arises, the pull on the patella when that muscle contracts is obliquely upwards and laterally (though see **328**). It is evident that the obliquity of the pull will be increased by any valgus deformity at the knee. In some individuals the normally prominent lateral lip on the femoral patellar facet (**E**), is poorly developed and there is a tendency for contraction of the quadriceps to dislocate the patella on to the lateral side of the femur.

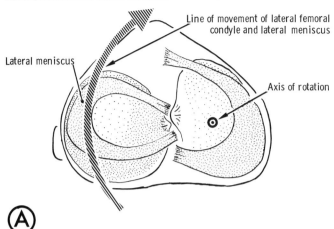

MEDIAL ROTATION OF FEMUR ON TIBIA

Line of movement of lateral femoral condyle and lateral meniscus

Lateral meniscus

Axis of rotation

(A)

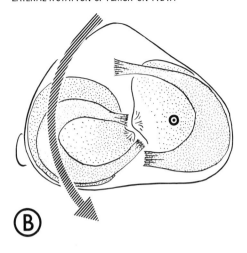

LATERAL ROTATION OF FEMUR ON TIBIA

(B)

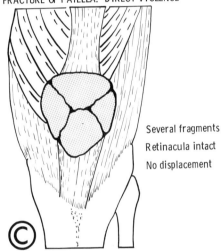

FRACTURE OF PATELLA: DIRECT VIOLENCE

Several fragments

Retinacula intact

No displacement

(C)

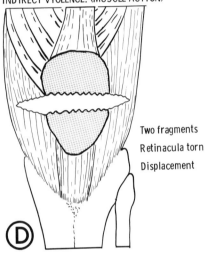

INDIRECT VIOLENCE: (MUSCLE ACTION)

Two fragments

Retinacula torn

Displacement

(D)

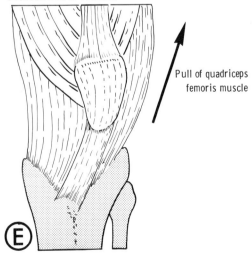

DISLOCATION OF PATELLA

Pull of quadriceps femoris muscle

(E)

The ligaments of the knee joint are frequently injured. It is a fairly easy exercise to work out the nature of the external forces which will particularly affect each ligament, and the signs which may be elicited after such injuries. It is suggested that the student should do this before reading the following paragraphs.

When a car collides with a pedestrian from one side, the car bumper often strikes the lateral side of one knee joint which is forcibly abducted. The abducted joint may then secondarily strike the medial side of the other knee which is forcibly adducted. An abducting force (**A**) causes tension medially and compression laterally, and may consequently sprain or tear the tibial collateral ligament and/or fracture the lateral tibial condyle. Similarly an adducting force (**B**) may sprain or tear the fibular collateral ligament and/or fracture the medial tibial condyle. Rupture of either ligament will allow abnormal tilting of the tibia on the femur when the surrounding muscles are relaxed.

When a car collides with a pedestrian from in front, the knee joint is forcibly hyperextended and the characteristic ligamentous injury—which may of course be associated with bony damage—is a tear or avulsion of the anterior cruciate ligament (**C**). Excessive forward mobility of the tibia on the femur can then be demonstrated.

The posterior cruciate ligament is less commonly torn, usually by a fall on the tibial tuberosity with the knee bent, so that the tibia is driven backwards in relation to the femur (**D**). Excessive backward mobility of the tibia on the femur can then be demonstrated.

Tears of the menisci are the most common internal derangements of the knee joint coming to operation. The medial meniscus is torn much more frequently than the lateral, and, typically, the injury occurs when a severe weight-bearing load is transmitted through the joint while it is semiflexed, and the femur is medially rotated on the tibia. The separated part of the meniscus frequently jams between the femoral and tibial condylar surfaces and 'locks' the joint in semi-flexion. The mechanism by which the meniscus is torn is still controversial, but there is evidence that tears occur only in menisci which have undergone some degree of degenerative change. It is of interest that when a torn medial meniscus is removed a new but more fibrous replica regenerates from the deep layers of the fibrous capsule.

THE FRONT AND MEDIAL SIDE OF THE THIGH

The adductor group of muscles

This large muscle group occupies the medial side of the thigh. The muscles arise close to one another from an area on the outer surface of the osteoligamentous pelvis below the level of the acetabulum (**E**). Except for gracilis, all are inserted into bony features on the posterior aspect of the femoral shaft (**F**).

1. The largest and most posterior muscle of the group is adductor magnus (**G**). It has a horizontal origin from the outer surface of the ischial ramus and the contiguous lower lateral region of the ischial tuberosity. It is inserted into a vertical line on the femur which runs from the adductor tubercle, along the medial supracondylar line and the linea aspera, and then upwards to the middle of the intertrochanteric crest (**F**). Consequently, the plane of the muscle twists through 90° between origin and insertion, in a direction such that the most anterior fibres of origin run horizontally and are inserted highest on the femur, while the posterior fibres of origin, from the ischial tuberosity, run vertically downwards to the adductor tubercle (**G**). In the lower third of the thigh the muscle fibres of adductor magnus give way to aponeurosis at some distance from the femur (**G**). The medial part of this aponeurosis is thick and tendon-like and is readily palpable just above the adductor tubercle into which it is inserted. The thinner lateral part of the aponeurosis is perforated by the large adductor opening which transmits the femoral vessels from the adductor canal (**331D**) to the popliteal fossa (**341C**).

2. Note the obturator externus lying above adductor magnus (**329A**). It passes laterally below and then behind the capsule of the hip joint to reach the greater trochanter.

3. The long strap-like gracilis runs downwards along the medial margin of adductor magnus (**329A**). Its tendon then crosses the medial side of the knee joint and, curving slightly forwards, inserts into the uppermost part of the medial surface of the tibial shaft.

4. Observe the relationship of adductor longus and adductor brevis. They pass in front of the upper half of the adductor magnus to reach the linea aspera.

5. Note that the lower half of adductor magnus, including the adductor opening, is not covered anteriorly by other adductor muscles.

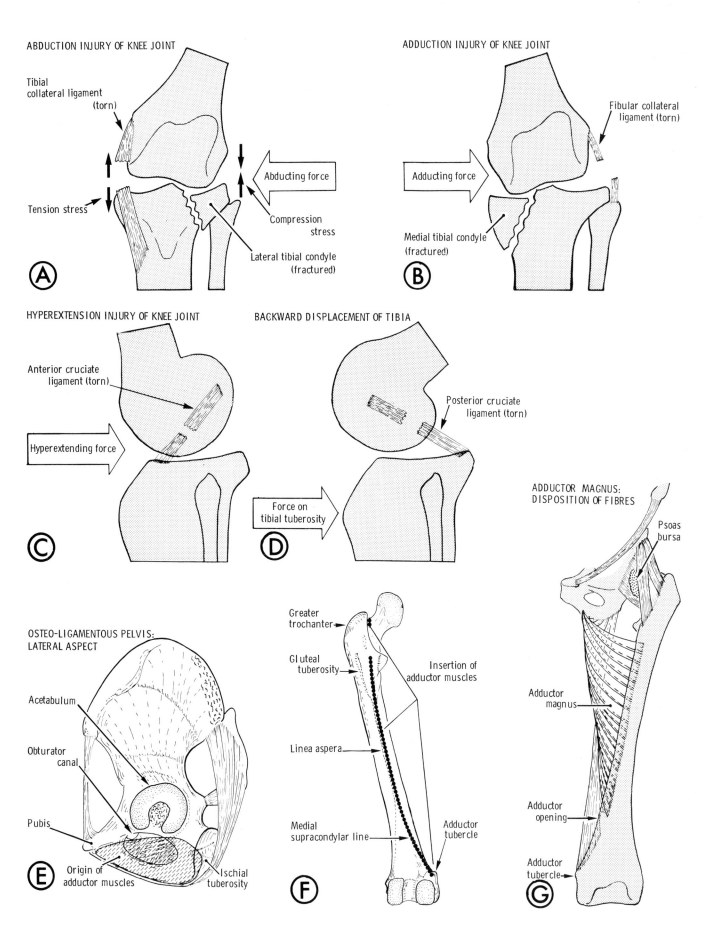

ABDUCTION INJURY OF KNEE JOINT

Tibial collateral ligament (torn)

Tension stress

Abducting force

Compression stress

Lateral tibial condyle (fractured)

(A)

ADDUCTION INJURY OF KNEE JOINT

Fibular collateral ligament (torn)

Adducting force

Medial tibial condyle (fractured)

(B)

HYPEREXTENSION INJURY OF KNEE JOINT

Anterior cruciate ligament (torn)

Hyperextending force

(C)

BACKWARD DISPLACEMENT OF TIBIA

Posterior cruciate ligament (torn)

Force on tibial tuberosity

(D)

ADDUCTOR MAGNUS: DISPOSITION OF FIBRES

Psoas bursa

Adductor magnus

Adductor opening

Adductor tubercle

(G)

OSTEO-LIGAMENTOUS PELVIS: LATERAL ASPECT

Acetabulum

Obturator canal

Pubis

Origin of adductor muscles

Ischial tuberosity

(E)

Greater trochanter

Gluteal tuberosity

Insertion of adductor muscles

Linea aspera

Medial supracondylar line

Adductor tubercle

(F)

327

The actions of the adductor muscles

All the adductor muscles except gracilis act solely on the hip joint. At this articulation they adduct and laterally rotate the thigh on the pelvis. However, neither of these movements is common in activity, and certainly neither is usually carried out with a force which would justify the great bulk of the adductor muscle group. The paradox is resolved when it is appreciated that the adductor muscles, arising from the anterior part of the pelvis, pass backwards as well as downwards and laterally, and consequently flex the hip joint (**B**), while those arising more posteriorly, pass forward as well as downwards and laterally, and consequently extend the hip. It is with flexion and extension of the hip joint that most of the activity of the adductor muscles is concerned.

Gracilis acts on the knee joint as well as on the hip. It flexes the joint and medially rotates the tibia on the femur.

The obturator nerve

This branch of the lumbar plexus is composed of fibres from the ventral rami of L2, 3 and 4. Its course in the psoas muscle and in the pelvic cavity have been considered in the appropriate sections (**205C, 269B**). The nerve enters the thigh through the obturator canal (**A**) and descends as two branches amongst the adductor muscles. It supplies all the muscles of that group except the fibres of the adductor magnus which arise from the ischial tuberosity. Those fibres are innervated by the sciatic nerve.

The quadriceps femoris muscle

This is a massive muscle which covers the anterior, medial and lateral aspects of the femoral shaft from the intertrochanteric line to the knee joint. It consists of four heads which are attached to a broad common tendon. The incorporation of this tendon into the fibrous capsule of the knee joint, its insertion into the tibia and its relationship to the patella have been considered already (**321A**) and should now be revised.

Three of the four heads, the vastus intermedius, vastus lateralis and vastus medialis, arise from the femur. Intermedius arises from the anterior and lateral aspects of the upper two-thirds of the femoral shaft and runs downwards to the knee joint. Lateralis and medialis arise from the posterior aspect of the bone on either side of the insertions of the adductor muscles (**D**), and sweep downwards and forwards to the anterior aspect of the intermedius (**C**). The fourth head is rectus femoris, a fusiform muscle belly lying in front of the vasti (**331A**). It arises by two substantial tendons (**B**). The posterior springs from the bone immediately above the acetabulum and runs forwards to join the anterior, which descends from the anterior inferior iliac spine across the capsule of the hip joint (**C**).

Note particularly the deep clefts which separate the three vasti (**331D**), the deep groove which lies between vastus medialis and the adductor muscles (**C**) and the absence of muscle attachment on the medial aspect of the femoral shaft.

All parts of the muscle are supplied by branches of the femoral nerve. Although that nerve is formed from branches of the ventral rami of L2, 3 and 4, the fibres associated with quadriceps are derived only from L3 and 4 segments of the spinal cord. The integrity of reflex activity in those segments, and the influence of higher centres upon it, can be assessed by eliciting the knee jerk. This is the reflex extension of the knee which is caused by tapping the ligamentum patellae when the knee is flexed and the quadriceps relaxed.

The actions of quadriceps femoris

Quadriceps femoris is the principal extensor of the knee joint and its rectus femoris head is a strong flexor of the hip joint. This combination of joint movements is essential in kicking, and the muscle is consequently very large in footballers.

During extension of the knee, the pull delivered by the greater part of quadriceps on the patella is upwards and laterally, owing to the inclination of the femoral shaft, so that a component of the pull tends to displace the patella laterally. This oblique pull is normally corrected by that of the lowest, almost horizontal fibres of vastus medialis, which pull medially and upwards (**E**). If the vastus medialis is weak, quadriceps contraction may dislocate the patella laterally. This is particularly so in those few individuals in whom the normally prominent lateral lip of the femoral patellar facet is poorly developed.

It is notorious that, after injuries to the knee joint, the quadriceps muscle wastes at a surprisingly rapid rate. This wasting, of itself, causes instability of the joint, and delays the correction, or may cause the recurrence, of the original joint injury. Consequently, exercises to maintain or recover the power of the quadriceps are always carried out regularly and frequently throughout any period of treatment. Thus if a supine patient raises the limb repeatedly from the bed with the knee extended, both functions of the quadriceps—flexion of the hip and extension of the knee—are exercised.

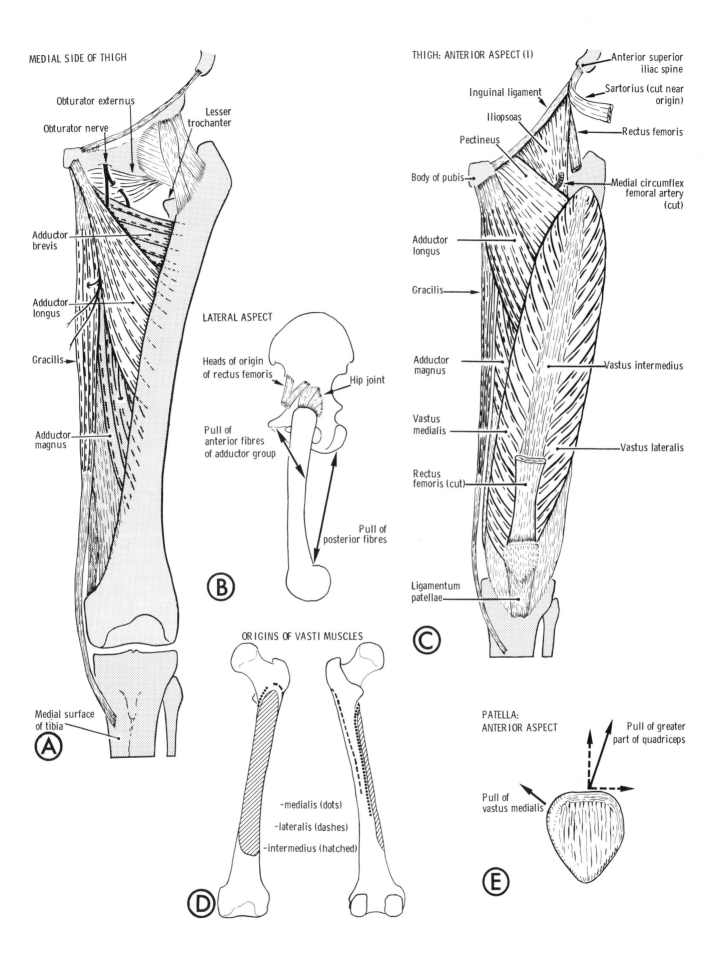

MEDIAL SIDE OF THIGH

Obturator externus

Obturator nerve

Lesser trochanter

Adductor brevis

Adductor longus

Gracilis

Adductor magnus

Medial surface of tibia

(A)

LATERAL ASPECT

Heads of origin of rectus femoris

Hip joint

Pull of anterior fibres of adductor group

Pull of posterior fibres

(B)

ORIGINS OF VASTI MUSCLES

-medialis (dots)

-lateralis (dashes)

-intermedius (hatched)

(D)

THIGH: ANTERIOR ASPECT (I)

Anterior superior iliac spine

Inguinal ligament

Sartorius (cut near origin)

Iliopsoas

Pectineus

Rectus femoris

Body of pubis

Medial circumflex femoral artery (cut)

Adductor longus

Gracilis

Adductor magnus

Vastus intermedius

Vastus medialis

Rectus femoris (cut)

Vastus lateralis

Ligamentum patellae

(C)

PATELLA: ANTERIOR ASPECT

Pull of greater part of quadriceps

Pull of vastus medialis

(E)

The flexor muscles of the hip joint

Identify the pectineus, the iliopsoas and the sartorius muscles (**A, 329C**). They and rectus femoris (**A**) are the flexors of the hip.

The pectineus arises from the pecten pubis behind the medial third of the inguinal ligament. The muscle passes downwards and laterally to reach the spiral line on the posterior aspect of the femur (**315F**). Notice that the muscle lies in front of the obturator externus (**329A, 329C**).

The psoas and iliacus heads of iliopsoas (**199E**) fuse as they pass downwards from the abdomen behind the lateral two-thirds of the inguinal ligament. The large common tendon passes in front of the capsule of the hip joint (**B**), and then turns downwards and backwards to reach the lesser trochanter on the posteromedial aspect of the femur. The tendon is separated from the hip capsule by the psoas bursa (**327G**) which in many individuals communicates with the joint cavity. Palpate on your own limb the firm rounded prominence situated a short distance below the lateral part of the inguinal ligament. This prominence is formed by the hip joint and iliopsoas tendon together.

The sartorius is a long strap-like muscle which arises from the anterior superior spine of the ilium (**195D**). Follow its sinuous, superficial course downwards across the front of the thigh to the medial side of the knee joint. There the muscle becomes tendinous. The tendon lies immediately in front of that of gracilis (**C**) and inserts into the same area on the tibia (**329A**). Notice particularly the muscles and tendons which are covered by the upper third of sartorius (**A, C**), and the relationship of the middle third of that muscle to the groove between vastus medialis and the adductor muscles (**D**).

The nerve supply of the flexors is derived from branches of the lumbar plexus. Psoas, innervated from L1, 2, and iliacus, innervated from L2, are supplied directly from the roots of the plexus within the abdomen. The other muscles receive branches from the femoral nerve (L2, 3 and 4). Pectineus and sartorius are mainly innervated from L2; rectus femoris, like the rest of quadriceps, from L3 and L4.

The femoral triangle

This is a shallow depression on the upper third of the front of the thigh. Two margins of the triangle are formed by the inguinal ligament and by the medial border of sartorius as far as the point at which the femoral artery passes deep to it. A third boundary can be constructed but is not related to any definite structure (**A**). Note the muscles which form the floor of the triangle. Its roof or anterior wall is constituted only by skin, and superficial and deep fascia. Its contents are therefore comparatively unprotected from external violence.

The adductor canal

This is an intermuscular tunnel in the middle third of the thigh which begins at the lower angle of the femoral triangle and ends at the adductor opening in adductor magnus. The canal is triangular in cross section (**D**). The posterior wall is formed by the adductor muscles (**329A**), the anterolateral wall by vastus medialis (**329C**), and the anteromedial wall by sartorius.

The femoral artery

This is the main arterial stem to the lower limb. It begins as a continuation of the external iliac artery (**C**) behind the midpoint of the inguinal ligament (**A**).

The vessel runs downwards through the femoral triangle (**A, C**) where it is covered only by skin and fascia. Because of this very superficial situation, its pulsations are readily palpable, a needle or catheter can be easily inserted into it, and it is susceptible to injury by perforating or incised wounds. Such injuries can also damage the profunda femoris branch of the artery (**C**) and the large femoral and profunda femoris veins. The massive haemorrhage which then results can be controlled, but only by very strong digital pressure applied just below the inguinal ligament.

Leaving the femoral triangle at its apex, the femoral artery traverses the length of the adductor canal (**D**) and ends by passing through the adductor opening in the adductor magnus (**C**) to become the popliteal artery (**333A**).

The femoral artery gives off numerous small branches, which supply all the tissues of the anteromedial aspect of the thigh and the superficial tissues of both the external genitalia and the lower part of the anterior abdominal wall. In addition, it gives off the much larger and more important profunda femoris artery. Observe the origin of this vessel.

The profunda femoris artery arises in the femoral triangle. Observe its position and relations in this area in **C**. Leaving the triangle it descends amongst the adductor muscles in close proximity to the linea aspera of the femur. Because of this position the artery may be torn by fractures of the femoral shaft when as much as a litre of blood may accumulate in the tissues.

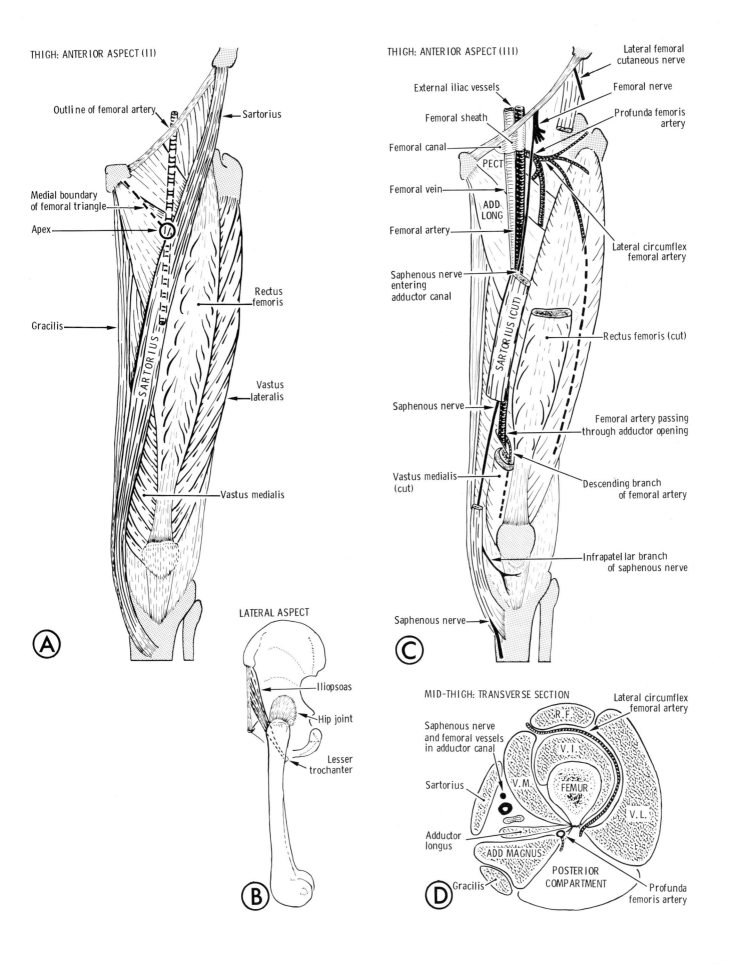

THIGH: ANTERIOR ASPECT (II)

Outline of femoral artery

Sartorius

Medial boundary of femoral triangle

Apex

Gracilis

SARTORIUS

Rectus femoris

Vastus lateralis

Vastus medialis

Ⓐ

LATERAL ASPECT

Iliopsoas

Hip joint

Lesser trochanter

Ⓑ

THIGH: ANTERIOR ASPECT (III)

Lateral femoral cutaneous nerve

External iliac vessels

Femoral nerve

Femoral sheath

Profunda femoris artery

Femoral canal

PECT

Femoral vein

ADD LONG

Femoral artery

SARTORIUS (CUT)

Lateral circumflex femoral artery

Saphenous nerve entering adductor canal

Rectus femoris (cut)

Saphenous nerve

Femoral artery passing through adductor opening

Vastus medialis (cut)

Descending branch of femoral artery

Infrapatellar branch of saphenous nerve

Saphenous nerve

Ⓒ

MID-THIGH: TRANSVERSE SECTION

Lateral circumflex femoral artery

Saphenous nerve and femoral vessels in adductor canal

R.F.

V.I.

Sartorius

V.M.

FEMUR

V.L.

Adductor longus

ADD MAGNUS

POSTERIOR COMPARTMENT

Gracilis

Profunda femoris artery

Ⓓ

331

The profunda femoris artery distributes a number of branches to the posterior aspect of the thigh and the buttock. The medial circumflex femoral branch springs from the back of the artery close to its origin (**A**) and runs backwards, amongst the muscles which lie below the femoral neck, to emerge in the buttock (**337B**). The lateral circumflex femoral branch arises from the lateral aspect of the artery at the same level (**A**), and winds, as a series of diverging divisions, round the lateral aspect of the femoral shaft to the buttock and the back of the thigh (**337B**). At a lower level the profunda femoris artery gives off four or so perforating branches which pass backwards through the adductor muscles into the posterior compartment of the thigh (**A, 337B**).

The arteries of the thigh are well shown in arteriograms of the lower limb (**B**) in which radio-opaque material has been introduced into the femoral artery just below the midpoint of the inguinal ligament.

The femoral vein

The femoral vein passes upwards on the posterior aspect of the artery through the adductor canal. In the femoral triangle, it appears at the medial margin of the artery and eventually lies completely to its medial side as it passes behind the inguinal ligament to become the external iliac vein (**C**). In the femoral triangle it receives the profunda femoris vein and the great saphenous vein (**335C**).

The femoral sheath

The external iliac vessels, with which the femoral vessels are continuous, lie in the extraperitoneal tissue inside the fascial envelope of the abdomen. As the femoral vessels pass into the femoral triangle they carry around them, behind the inguinal ligament, a conical protrusion of this envelope, which is named the femoral sheath (**C**). In the adult the sheath is about 4 cm long but in infancy and childhood it is disproportionately shorter. Observe the muscles which lie behind the sheath, and its exact relationship to the inguinal ligament (**335A**).

The sheath is divided by two rather tenuous sagittal septa into three compartments. The lateral contains the femoral artery and the femoral division of the genito-femoral nerve. The middle compartment contains the femoral vein. The conical medial compartment (**D**) is called the femoral canal, and its circular upper end is the femoral ring. The ring cannot be seen from in front because it lies behind the inguinal ligament. But it can be clearly seen from the abdominal cavity after removal of the peritoneum and extraperitoneal tissue (**C**). Identify the boundaries of the ring in this view and note the relationship of the ring to the insertion of the conjoint tendon (**207E**). The femoral canal normally contains the deep stream of lymph vessels, which have followed the femoral vein up the thigh (**331C**), and one or two deep inguinal lymph nodes. These structures are embedded in fatty areolar tissue, which is continuous through the femoral ring with the abdominal extraperitoneal tissues (**D**). In many individuals, this areolar tissue is condensed into a thin sheet of fascia in the lumen of the femoral ring: this is named the femoral septum. The femoral ring and canal are of clinical importance because they are the site of femoral herniae (**335B**).

The femoral nerve

This, which is much the largest of this group of nerves, draws its fibres from L2, 3 and 4. Recall that it descends through the iliac fossa, lying deeply in the groove between the psoas and iliacus heads of iliopsoas (**205C**). It passes behind the inguinal ligament into the femoral triangle to the lateral side of the femoral artery. It should be noted particularly that in this situation the nerve lies outside the femoral sheath, and that this is due to the fact that, within the abdomen, it lies outside the fascial envelope of that region. A centimetre or so below the inguinal ligament the nerve divides abruptly into a spray of branches (**331C**).

1. Motor branches supply pectineus (L2), sartorius (L2) and all parts of the quadriceps femoris (L3, 4).
2. Several femoral cutaneous branches run downwards and pass through the deep fascia into the superficial fascia about a handbreadth below the inguinal ligament (see below).
3. The saphenous nerve is a large cutaneous branch which draws its fibres only from L4 and innervates only skin below the knee (**373A**). In the thigh it closely follows the femoral artery through the femoral triangle and the adductor canal. At the level of the adductor opening in the adductor magnus it leaves the artery and emerges from beneath the posterior border of sartorius into the superficial fascia of the leg (**331C**).

The lateral femoral cutaneous nerve

Recall that this nerve arises from L2 and 3 and passes obliquely across iliacus to emerge into the thigh beneath the lateral end of the inguinal ligament (**205C, 331C**). Running downwards, the nerve pierces the deep fascia, usually as two branches, at about the same level as the femoral cutaneous branches (**335E**).

The femoral branch of the genitofemoral nerve

This cutaneous nerve, which contains fibres from L1 and 2, has already been seen in the lateral compartment of the femoral sheath. It passes through the anterior wall of the sheath and the overlying deep fascia into the superficial fascia (**335E**).

PROFUNDA FEMORIS ARTERY

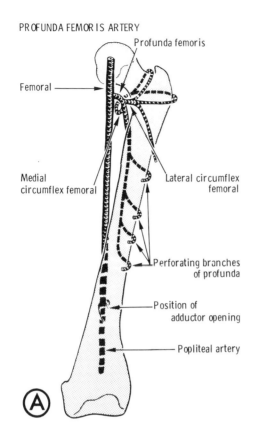

Profunda femoris
Femoral
Medial circumflex femoral
Lateral circumflex femoral
Perforating branches of profunda
Position of adductor opening
Popliteal artery

(A)

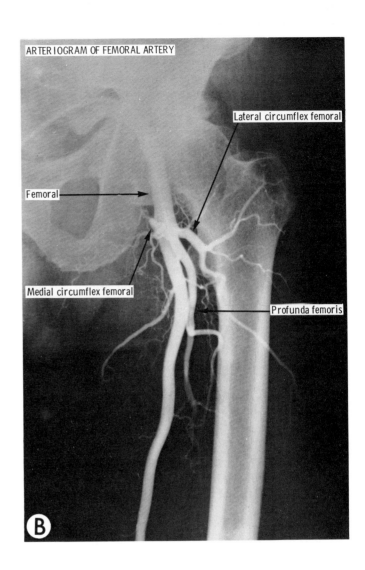

Lateral circumflex femoral
Femoral
Medial circumflex femoral
Profunda femoris

(B)

FEMORAL SHEATH: ABDOMINAL ASPECT

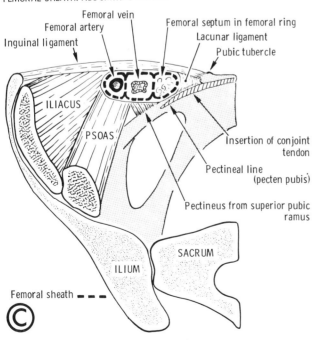

Femoral vein
Femoral artery
Inguinal ligament
Femoral septum in femoral ring
Lacunar ligament
Pubic tubercle
ILIACUS
PSOAS
Insertion of conjoint tendon
Pectineal line (pecten pubis)
Pectineus from superior pubic ramus
SACRUM
ILIUM
Femoral sheath ---

(C)

FEMORAL RING & CANAL: SAGITTAL SECTION

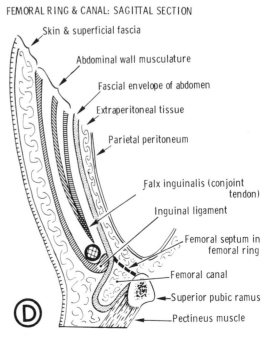

Skin & superficial fascia
Abdominal wall musculature
Fascial envelope of abdomen
Extraperitoneal tissue
Parietal peritoneum
Falx inguinalis (conjoint tendon)
Inguinal ligament
Femoral septum in femoral ring
Femoral canal
Superior pubic ramus
Pectineus muscle

(D)

333

The deep fascia of the front of the thigh

A thick layer of deep fascia forms a cylindrical investment around the muscles of the thigh and buttock. It is called the fascia lata because of its large extent. A short distance below the medial end of the inguinal ligament, the anterior part of the fascia lata splits into a superficial lateral zone and a deeper medial zone (**A**). These overlap, the superficial zone being attached above to the inguinal ligament, and the deeper zone to the pecten pubis. In this way an oblique opening, called the saphenous opening, passes through the fascia lata in a mediolateral direction. Because of the way in which it is formed, the saphenous opening has sharp upper, lateral and lower margins (**A, C**), but no definite medial margin. Despite the lack of a medial margin it is helpful to visualise the centre of the saphenous opening as being 2 cm below and lateral to the pubic tubercle.

The femoral sheath (**A**) lies in the saphenous opening between the superficial and deep layers of the fascia lata (**C**). Note the compartments of the sheath which are visible when one looks backwards through the saphenous opening.

Femoral herniae

A femoral hernia is a protrusion of a sac of parietal peritoneum through the femoral ring (**B**) into the femoral canal. The sac may be empty or, more commonly, contain parts of abdominal viscera such as the small intestine or the greater omentum. If such a hernia enlarges, because additional contents are forced into it, it tends to distend mainly the unsupported anterior wall of the femoral canal, and bulge through the saphenous opening (**B**). As enlargement continues, the hernia impinges against the sharp lower margin of the saphenous opening so that it is redirected upwards (**B**).

Note the tissues which cover the peritoneal sac of a femoral hernia, particularly the distended and thickened femoral septum. The small size of the femoral ring through which the hernial sac passes, and the rigidity of most of its boundaries (**333C, 333D**), make reduction of the hernia—that is the return of any contents to the abdominal cavity—difficult or even impossible and the procedure is seldom attempted. Moreover, the same factors frequently cause constriction of the blood vessels supplying any contents so that the hernia becomes 'strangulated'. Operative treatment is then a matter of urgency.

Surgical treatment of a femoral hernia usually involves an approach to the femoral ring from the extraperitoneal tissue of the anterior abdominal wall. Reduction of the hernial contents may require enlargement of the femoral ring, and it is evident (**333C**) that this can only be achieved by division of its anterior or medial boundaries. It will be recalled that in some individuals the obturator artery arises abnormally from the inferior epigastric and courses close to these margins of the ring. Once the hernial contents have been returned to the abdominal cavity and the hernial sac

has been removed, an attempt is made to prevent recurrence by closure of the femoral ring. This is usually achieved by stitching the back of the inguinal ligament to the ligamentous fibres on the pecten pubis (**333C**).

The superficial fascia of the front of the thigh

This fatty areolar tissue surrounds the fascia lata and is continuous above and below with similar tissue on the trunk and leg. On the front of the thigh it contains a number of structures.

1. Small arteries which arise from the deep vessels. Note that some of these spread upwards to the superficial fascia over the lower half of the abdominal wall and medially to superficial fascia of the external genitalia.
2. Larger veins which, together with veins from the superficial fasciae of the lower abdominal wall and the external genitalia, converge on the great saphenous vein, which passes through the saphenous opening and the anterior wall of the femoral sheath to join the femoral vein (**C**). As most of the course of the great saphenous vein, and many of its important connections, lie in the leg and foot, it will be considered as a whole later in this chapter (**373A**).
3. Although the lymph drainage of the lower limb as a whole is considered later in this chapter, it is convenient to describe the superficial inguinal lymph nodes here as an important content of the superficial fascia of the thigh. These nodes are arranged in horizontal and vertical groups, in the form of a T. Note the relationship of the horizontal group to the inguinal ligament, and of the vertical group to the terminal part of the great saphenous vein (**C**). Because of their superficial position, normal nodes of this group can be readily palpated in children and, indeed, in many adults. Other lymph nodes in the body are not usually palpable, unless affected by some pathological change.

It is sometimes necessary to visualise lymph nodes and their associated lymph vessels in the living patient. This can be accomplished by the injection of a radio-opaque fluid into a superficial lymph vessel, after the position of that vessel has been defined by its uptake of a subcutaneously injected dye such as Trypan Blue. A lymphangiogram prepared in this way, and showing the superficial inguinal nodes and their afferent and efferent vessels, is shown in **D**.
4. The superficial fascia contains the several cutaneous nerves indicated in **E**. Revise the source of these nerves and observe the positions and extents of the skin areas innervated by L1, the cutaneous branches of the femoral nerve, and the lateral femoral cutaneous nerve (**E**).

UPPER THIRD OF THIGH: DEEP

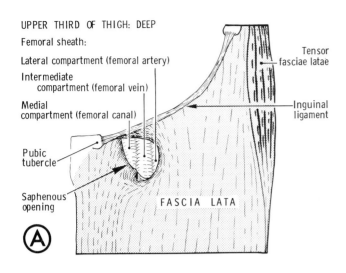

Femoral sheath:

Lateral compartment (femoral artery)

Intermediate compartment (femoral vein)

Medial compartment (femoral canal)

Pubic tubercle

Saphenous opening

FASCIA LATA

Tensor fasciae latae

Inguinal ligament

(A)

UPPER THIRD OF THIGH: SUPERFICIAL

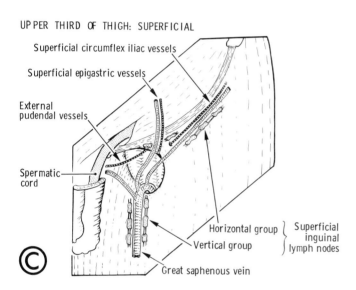

Superficial circumflex iliac vessels

Superficial epigastric vessels

External pudendal vessels

Spermatic cord

Horizontal group

Vertical group

} Superficial inguinal lymph nodes

Great saphenous vein

(C)

LYMPHANGIOGRAM

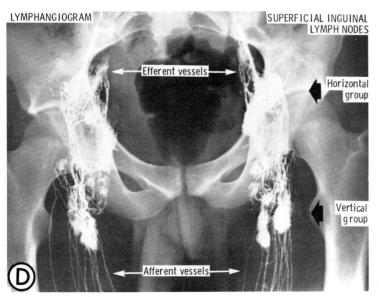

SUPERFICIAL INGUINAL LYMPH NODES

Efferent vessels

Horizontal group

Vertical group

Afferent vessels

(D)

FEMORAL HERNIA: SAGITTAL SECTION

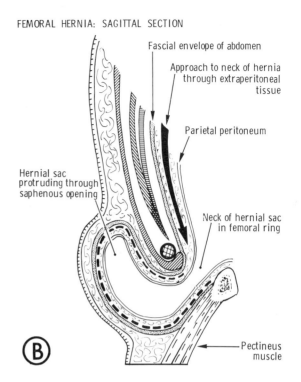

Fascial envelope of abdomen

Approach to neck of hernia through extraperitoneal tissue

Parietal peritoneum

Hernial sac protruding through saphenous opening

Neck of hernial sac in femoral ring

Pectineus muscle

(B)

CUTANEOUS INNERVATION

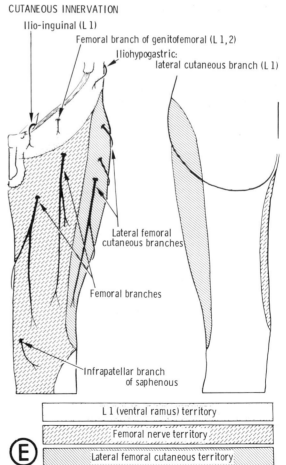

Ilio-inguinal (L 1)

Femoral branch of genitofemoral (L 1, 2)

Iliohypogastric: lateral cutaneous branch (L 1)

Lateral femoral cutaneous branches

Femoral branches

Infrapatellar branch of saphenous

L 1 (ventral ramus) territory

Femoral nerve territory

Lateral femoral cutaneous territory

(E)

335

The back of the thigh and buttock

The anterior wall of the posterior compartment of the thigh (**331D**) is formed by three muscles which have already been considered (**A**). The posterior aspect of vastus lateralis (**331A**) is separated from the posterior aspects of adductor magnus and gracilis (**329A**) by the linea aspera of the femur.

At the lower end of the linea aspera, the medial and lateral supracondylar lines diverge to outline the popliteal surface of the femur. This surface, the posterior aspect of the fibrous capsule of the knee joint and the popliteus muscle together form the floor of the popliteal fossa, which consequently lies partly in the back of the thigh and partly in the back of the leg. The fossa and its contents will be considered later.

The region above adductor magnus (**A**) constitutes the buttock. In that region identify the following features.

1. The greater and lesser trochanters of the femur joined by the intertrochanteric crest.
2. The greater and lesser sciatic foramina in the osteoligamentous pelvis. Recall that the greater foramen leads from the buttock into the pelvic cavity while the lesser foramen leads into the perineum.
3. The internal pudendal artery and the pudendal nerve as they cross the outer surface of the sacrospinous ligament. These structures are not functionally concerned with the buttock, but traverse that region for a short distance as they pass from the pelvic cavity to the perineum.

The deep muscles of the buttock

Above adductor magnus, a group of muscles pass laterally from the osteoligamentous pelvis and converge to insertions on the greater trochanter and intertrochanteric crest.

Obturator externus arises from the outer surface of the obturator membrane and passes obliquely, upwards and laterally across the back of the hip joint lying *deep* to the obturator internus. It is inserted into the medial aspect of the greater trochanter (**A**).

Obturator internus originates inside the osteoligamentous pelvis and emerges from the perineum (**B**) through the lesser sciatic foramen. It inserts into the medial aspect of the greater trochanter.

Piriformis arises inside the osteoligamentous pelvis and emerges from the pelvic cavity (**B**) through the greater sciatic foramen. It passes laterally behind the upper part of the hip joint to the summit of the greater trochanter.

Quadratus femoris passes transversely, below the obturator muscles and above adductor magnus, from the lateral margin of the ischial tuberosity to the middle of the intertrochanteric crest (**B**).

It should be recognised that this group of muscles are not of much functional significance although it is evident, from their position, that they can laterally rotate the thigh or prevent excessive medial rotation.

The gluteus minimus and the gluteus medius are of much greater fundamental importance. They lie above the hip joint (**B**), between piriformis behind and the origins of sartorius and the anterior tendon of rectus femoris (**329C**) in front. They arise respectively from the lower and upper parts of the outer surface of the ilium and are inserted into the upper lateral aspect of the greater trochanter.

These two muscles are powerful abductors of the hip joint. Abduction is not a commonly produced voluntary movement in the free limb, but, despite this fact, the two muscles are important, because, by preventing adduction of the hip, they are essential for normal walking (**369F**). Their paralysis leads inevitably to an obviously abnormal gait and considerable disability (**371A**). Gluteus minimus and medius are both innervated by the superior gluteal branch of the sacral plexus, drawing the majority of their fibres from the L5 spinal segment.

The blood vessels of the buttock and back of the thigh

The arteries in these regions arise from two sources.

The superior and inferior gluteal arteries arise in the pelvic cavity from the internal iliac artery (**269B**). They emerge into the buttock through the greater sciatic foramen, respectively above and below piriformis muscle (**B**). The superior gluteal artery ramifies between the gluteus minimus and medius muscles (**B**). The inferior gluteal divides into a spray of branches which enter and supply the bulky gluteus maximus muscle (**339C**) which overlies it.

The profunda femoris artery is a branch of the femoral artery (**333A**) but distributes most of its branches to the back of the thigh and the buttock. Identify the several perforating branches (**B**) passing backwards through the adductor magnus, the medial circumflex femoral branch (**B**), which passes backwards between the muscles below the hip joint and ramifies around the quadratus femoris muscle, and the upper terminal twigs of the lateral circumflex femoral branch, which run into the region of the greater trochanter (**B**).

The popliteal artery is the continuation of the femoral artery and enters the popliteal fossa through the adductor opening in adductor magnus (**B**).

The arteries of the buttock and thigh are associated with corresponding veins which drain eventually into the internal iliac and femoral veins.

All the arteries detailed above including the popliteal artery and its branches (**341C**) anastomose with one another to form a long anastomotic chain extending through the buttock and the back of the thigh to the popliteal fossa.

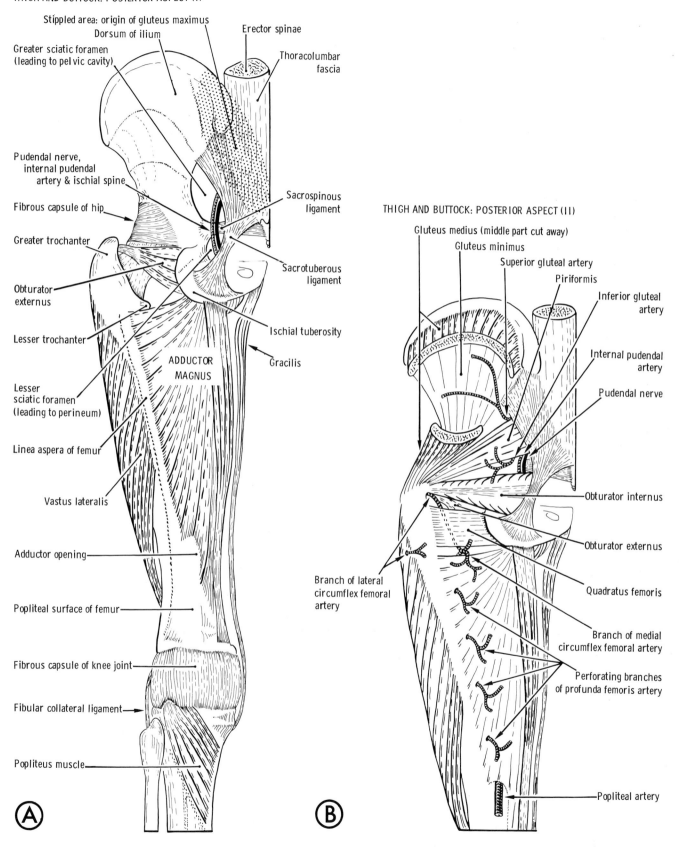

THIGH AND BUTTOCK: POSTERIOR ASPECT (I)

Stippled area: origin of gluteus maximus
Dorsum of ilium
Greater sciatic foramen (leading to pelvic cavity)
Erector spinae
Thoracolumbar fascia
Pudendal nerve, internal pudendal artery & ischial spine
Fibrous capsule of hip
Greater trochanter
Obturator externus
Lesser trochanter
Sacrospinous ligament
Sacrotuberous ligament
Ischial tuberosity
ADDUCTOR MAGNUS
Gracilis
Lesser sciatic foramen (leading to perineum)
Linea aspera of femur
Vastus lateralis
Adductor opening
Popliteal surface of femur
Fibrous capsule of knee joint
Fibular collateral ligament
Popliteus muscle

Ⓐ

THIGH AND BUTTOCK: POSTERIOR ASPECT (II)

Gluteus medius (middle part cut away)
Gluteus minimus
Superior gluteal artery
Piriformis
Inferior gluteal artery
Internal pudendal artery
Pudendal nerve
Obturator internus
Obturator externus
Quadratus femoris
Branch of lateral circumflex femoral artery
Branch of medial circumflex femoral artery
Perforating branches of profunda femoris artery
Popliteal artery

Ⓑ

In the past, the upper part of this anastomosis, between the branches of the internal iliac artery and the circumflex femoral branches of the profunda femoris artery, was of clinical importance because it provided the basis of a possible collateral circulation when the femoral artery was severed and had to be tied between the inguinal ligament and the origin of the profunda branch. Today, the severed artery would be surgically repaired so that the establishment of a collateral circulation is unnecessary.

However, the complete anastomotic chain remains of clinical importance in patients in whom the main trunk of the femoral artery below the origin of the profunda branch is gradually narrowed by obliterative disease. In these circumstances the vessels of the anastomosis are often comparatively unaffected, and the chain may become the main source of blood entering the popliteal artery and its branches in the leg and foot.

The superficial muscles of the thigh and buttock

The hamstring group of muscles descend through the posterior compartment of the thigh behind adductor magnus. It consists of the semimembranosus which has a broad aponeurosis of origin, the semitendinosus which has a long narrow tendon of insertion, and the long and short heads of biceps femoris (**A, C**). All these muscles arise from the upper half of the ischial tuberosity, except the short head of biceps. This originates instead from the lower part of the linea aspera, between adductor magnus and vastus lateralis (**A**), and joins the anterior surface of the long head.

The stout tendon of semimembranosus crosses the posteromedial aspect of the knee joint and inserts into the same aspect of the medial tibial condyle (**B**). The tendon of the semitendinosus inclines forward and comes into association with the tendon of gracilis from the medial aspect of the thigh and that of sartorius from the anterior aspect (**B**). All three tendons are inserted, one behind the other, into the upper part of the medial surface of the tibial shaft. Biceps femoris runs downwards and laterally gradually separating from the other hamstrings (**C**). Its tendon inserts into the head of the fibula.

All these muscles flex the knee and extend the hip. In addition, when the knee joint is flexed and therefore capable of rotatory movements (**325A, 325B**), the biceps laterally rotates the leg bones on the femur, whereas semimembranosus and semitendinosus produce medial rotation. The hamstring muscles are innervated by the sciatic nerve (see below) mainly from the L5 and S1 spinal segments.

The gluteus maximus and tensor fasciae latae lie superficially in the buttock and usually act in concert with one another.

Gluteus maximus is a very large, coarsely fibred rectangular muscle which covers the greater part of the buttock (**C**). Its upper border lies obliquely across the posterior part of gluteus medius. Its lower border crosses the ischial tuberosity and the upper parts of the hamstring muscles, and it is important to note that this border does not conform to the skin fold of the buttock, which is more horizontally disposed.

The muscle arises from the large area shown in **A, C**. Note the components of this area. The fibres pass laterally and somewhat downwards to two distinct insertions. The deep fibres of the lower half of the muscle are attached to the gluteal tuberosity of the femur (**A**). The other three-quarters or so are inserted with another much smaller fusiform muscle, the tensor fasciae latae (**A**), which arises near the anterior end of the iliac crest and passes downwards and somewhat backwards. Both sets of muscle fibres become tendinous and are projected into the fascia lata over the region of the greater trochanter. The thick wide strip so formed within the deep fascia is the iliotibial tract. It extends downwards and a little forwards, across the lateral aspects of thigh and knee, before inserting into the anterolateral aspect of the lateral tibial condyle (**341A**). Observe, in your own limb, that the posterior border of the lower part of the tract is readily palpable when the knee joint is semiflexed.

Consider in particular the following facts

1. The gluteus maximus and tensor fasciae latae differ both in their size and in the angle at which they join the iliotibial tract (**341A**). Acting together the two muscles tend to produce a pull in the long axis of the tract.
2. The iliotibial tract passes in front of the lateral femoral epicondyle (**341A**) which approximately coincides with the transverse axis of the knee joint (**321C, 321D**). Tension in the tract therefore extends the knee.
3. The fibres of gluteus maximus which are inserted into the femur act on the hip joint to produce extension and lateral rotation.
4. The whole of gluteus maximus and tensor fasciae latae usually operate as a single functional unit, causing simultaneous extension of hip and knee joints.
5. Surprisingly, considering 4, the two muscles have different innervations. Gluteus maximus is supplied by the inferior gluteal nerve (see below) from the S1, 2 spinal segments, whereas tensor fasciae latae is supplied, like the functionally distinct gluteus medius and minimus, by the superior gluteal nerve, predominantly from L5.
6. Gluteus maximus covers a large number of structures (**A**). Notice particularly the relationship of the sciatic nerve (see below).

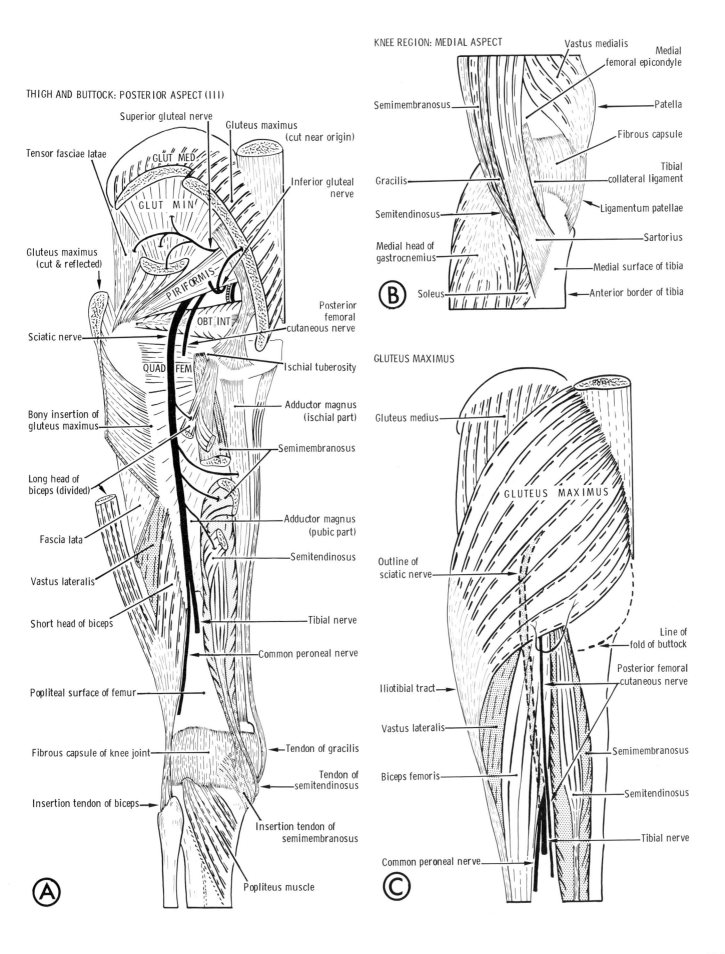

THIGH AND BUTTOCK: POSTERIOR ASPECT (III)

Superior gluteal nerve

Tensor fasciae latae

Gluteus maximus (cut near origin)

GLUT MED

GLUT MIN

Inferior gluteal nerve

Gluteus maximus (cut & reflected)

PIRIFORMIS

Sciatic nerve

OBT INT

Posterior femoral cutaneous nerve

QUAD FEM

Ischial tuberosity

Bony insertion of gluteus maximus

Adductor magnus (ischial part)

Semimembranosus

Long head of biceps (divided)

Adductor magnus (pubic part)

Fascia lata

Semitendinosus

Vastus lateralis

Tibial nerve

Short head of biceps

Common peroneal nerve

Popliteal surface of femur

Fibrous capsule of knee joint

Tendon of gracilis

Tendon of semitendinosus

Insertion tendon of biceps

Insertion tendon of semimembranosus

Popliteus muscle

Ⓐ

KNEE REGION: MEDIAL ASPECT

Vastus medialis

Medial femoral epicondyle

Semimembranosus

Patella

Fibrous capsule

Gracilis

Tibial collateral ligament

Semitendinosus

Ligamentum patellae

Medial head of gastrocnemius

Sartorius

Medial surface of tibia

Ⓑ Soleus

Anterior border of tibia

GLUTEUS MAXIMUS

Gluteus medius

GLUTEUS MAXIMUS

Outline of sciatic nerve

Line of fold of buttock

Iliotibial tract

Posterior femoral cutaneous nerve

Vastus lateralis

Semimembranosus

Biceps femoris

Semitendinosus

Tibial nerve

Common peroneal nerve

Ⓒ

339

The nerves of the buttock and back of thigh

Most of the nerves in the buttock and back of the thigh (**339A**) are branches of the sacral plexus which emerge through the greater sciatic foramen. Recall that the sacral plexus itself lies on the posterior wall of the pelvic cavity and is formed by the ventral rami of L5, S1, 2, 3, plus contributions from the ventral rami of L4 and S4 (**269A, 269B**).

Observe (**339A**) that whereas the superior gluteal nerve emerges through the upper part of the greater sciatic foramen, the pudendal, sciatic, inferior gluteal and posterior femoral cutaneous nerves emerge through the lower part of the foramen below piriformis. The pudendal nerve is not functionally associated with the buttock. It simply crosses the sacrospinous ligament and passes medially through the lesser sciatic foramen into the perineum, where its distribution has already been considered (**285D, 287B**).

The sciatic nerve (L4, 5, S1, 2, 3) is the largest nerve in the body. It appears in the buttock as a broad flattened band which runs downwards and laterally to a point somewhat nearer the ischial tuberosity than the greater trochanter, and thereafter continues vertically down the thigh. It terminates, usually at the upper angle of the popliteal fossa, by dividing into the tibial nerve medially and the common peroneal nerve laterally (**339A**). Observe the bone and muscles on which the nerve lies, and that it is covered initially by gluteus maximus and thereafter by the long head of biceps (**339C**).

Its relationship to gluteus maximus is important because intramuscular injections are often made into this muscle. To avoid the sciatic nerve, such injections are made into the upper outer quadrant of the buttock, or they may be made into the lateral aspect of the thigh, deep to the iliotibial tract.

In the thigh, the sciatic nerve supplies the hamstrings and those vertical fibres of adductor magnus which arise from the ischial tuberosity.

The posterior femoral cutaneous nerve (S2, 3) descends first deep to gluteus maximus (**339A**), then between the long head of biceps femoris and the fascia lata (**339C**), and finally through the fascia lata into the superficial fascia over the popliteal fossa and the back of the leg (**343B**).

The inferior gluteal nerve (S1) turns backwards and, breaking into a spray of branches, supplies the whole of the gluteus maximus muscle.

The superior gluteal nerve (L5) emerges through the upper part of the greater sciatic foramen above piriformis (**339A**). It turns forwards between gluteus medius and minimus and ends in tensor fasciae latae. It supplies these three muscles.

The cutaneous nerve supply of the back of thigh and buttock

The nerve supply of this area can be considered in three zones.

1. The areas supplied by the iliohypogastric, lateral femoral cutaneous, and femoral nerves, which are all derivatives of the lumbar plexus, are continuous with the areas on the front of the thigh supplied by the same nerves (**B, 335E**).
2. The posterior femoral cutaneous nerve supplies a long zone of skin which covers the lower part of the buttock, the posterior aspect of the thigh, the popliteal fossa and the upper half of the calf (**B**).
3. The skin over the upper, central and medial parts of the buttock is unique in the lower limb in being innervated by the dorsal rather than the ventral rami of spinal nerves. The four strips of skin supplied by the dorsal rami of T12, L1, 2 and 3 begin at the midline and extend downwards and laterally across the iliac crest to the region of the greater trochanter. The dorsal rami of L4 and 5 end in the erector spinae muscle (**199D**) and do not supply skin. The dorsal rami of S1, 2 and 3 supply successive skin areas over the lower medial part of the buttock (**B**). The areas supplied by the minute dorsal rami of the lowest sacral nerves and the coccygeal nerve are not visible in **B** because they lie in the natal cleft immediately behind the tip of the coccyx (**291E**).

THE POPLITEAL FOSSA

This is a diamond-shaped intermuscular space behind the knee (**C**). Observe the three components of its floor, namely the popliteal surface of the femur (**315F**), the posterior aspect of the knee joint (**321J**) and the popliteus muscle (**337A**), and identify the hamstring muscles which form its upper medial and upper lateral walls (**339C**). The adductor opening in adductor magnus lies partially deep to semimembranosus. The lower walls of the fossa are the medial and later heads of gastrocnemius, a large muscle which forms the prominence of the calf (**343A**). The two heads arise from the respective lower corners of the popliteal surface of the femur and converge rapidly as they descend. They must be artificially separated to expose the lower part of the fossa. The roof of the fossa is the thick popliteal fascia which is continuous above with the fascia lata.

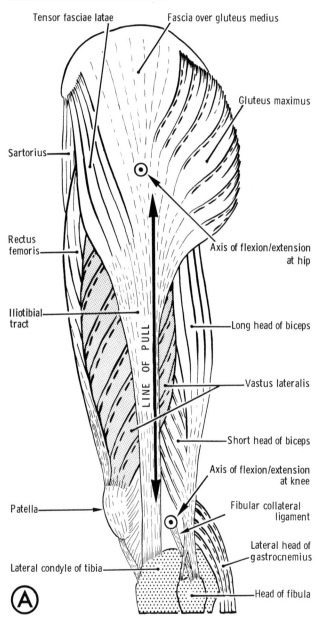

THIGH AND BUTTOCK: LATERAL ASPECT

Tensor fasciae latae

Fascia over gluteus medius

Gluteus maximus

Sartorius

Axis of flexion/extension at hip

Rectus femoris

LINE OF PULL

Iliotibial tract

Long head of biceps

Vastus lateralis

Short head of biceps

Axis of flexion/extension at knee

Patella

Fibular collateral ligament

Lateral head of gastrocnemius

Lateral condyle of tibia

Head of fibula

(A)

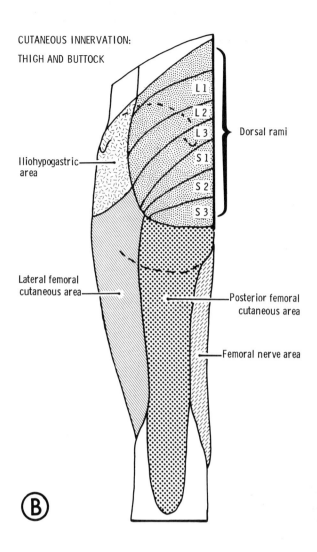

CUTANEOUS INNERVATION: THIGH AND BUTTOCK

L1
L2
L3
S1
S2
S3

Dorsal rami

Iliohypogastric area

Lateral femoral cutaneous area

Posterior femoral cutaneous area

Femoral nerve area

(B)

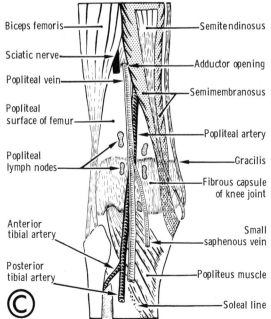

POPLITEAL FOSSA (I)

Biceps femoris

Semitendinosus

Sciatic nerve

Adductor opening

Popliteal vein

Semimembranosus

Popliteal surface of femur

Popliteal artery

Gracilis

Popliteal lymph nodes

Fibrous capsule of knee joint

Small saphenous vein

Anterior tibial artery

Popliteus muscle

Posterior tibial artery

Soleal line

(C)

341

The popliteal blood vessels

The popliteal artery is the continuation of the femoral artery at the adductor opening. From that point it passes downwards lying against the floor of the fossa to end at the lower border of popliteus by dividing into anterior and posterior tibial arteries (**241C**).

Because it is the deepest of the contents of the popliteal fossa and is covered by the thick popliteal fascia, the popliteal artery is difficult to palpate. Consequently the fossa is an unsatisfactory site to assess by palpation the efficiency of the circulation in patients in whom chronic arterial blockage is suspected.

The artery gives off a number of branches which anastomose around the knee joint with descending branches from the femoral and profunda femoris vessels (**337B**) and recurrent branches from the anterior and posterior tibial arteries in the leg. If the popliteal artery is gradually occluded by disease, or by the slow expansion of a neighbouring lesion, this genicular anastomosis can sometimes expand sufficiently to allow the establishment of some collateral circulation to the leg and foot.

The popliteal vein is formed at the lower angle of the fossa by the union of the venae comitantes of the anterior and posterior tibial arteries. It traverses the fossa lying behind the artery and becomes continuous with the femoral vein as it passes through the adductor opening. Its most important tributary is the small saphenous vein. This ascends through the superficial fascia of the calf (**273B**) and, piercing the lower part of the popliteal fascia (**241C**), ascends through the fossa to join the upper part of the popliteal vein (**A**).

In operations on varicose veins in the lower limb, the short saphenous vein may be stripped out, from the origin below to its termination. The low level at which it pierces the deep fascia, often as low as three of four fingerbreadths below the level of the knee joint, has to be remembered when the upper end of the vein is sought at operation.

The popliteal lymph nodes

About six small nodes are located along the popliteal vein (**241C**). The afferent and efferent vessels associated with them are considered later (**370**).

The nerves of the popliteal fossa

The tibial nerve (L4, 5, S1, 2, 3) is the larger and more medial terminal branch of the sciatic (**A**). It runs vertically from the upper to the lower angle of the popliteal fossa before descending into the posterior compartment of the leg (**361B**). The nerve lies superficial to (i.e. behind) the popliteal vessels and can be palpated when the knee is semiflexed. It supplies both heads of gastrocnemius (**A**) and gives off its cutaneous sural branch, which leaves the lower angle of the fossa alongside the small saphenous vein (**B**).

The common peroneal nerve (L4, 5, S1, 2) is the lateral terminal branch of the sciatic. It passes obliquely downwards and laterally and leaves the popliteal fossa by crossing the lateral head of gastrocnemius, immediately behind the biceps femoris tendon (**A**). It enters the leg round the lateral aspect of the neck of the fibula. In the popliteal fossa the nerve gives off a cutaneous branch to the upper lateral part of the leg (**B**).

THE LEG AND FOOT

The tibia and fibula and the tibiofibular joints

The tibia lies on the medial side and the fibula on the lateral (**C, D**). The tibia is a massive long bone which extends from the knee joint to the ankle joint and transmits the body weight. The slender fibula forms part of the ankle joint but not of the knee joint; it does not bear weight, but provides an extensive attachment for muscles.

The expanded proximal end of the tibia has been described already (**319**) and should now be revised. The head of the fibula is the proximal end of the bone. It is small and carries a plane articular facet which articulates with a reciprocal facet on the distal aspect of the lateral tibial condyle. This articulation is the synovial superior tibiofibular joint.

The proximal two-thirds of both tibia and fibula are triangular in cross section: observe the names of the borders and surfaces of the bones (**E**). On the posterior surface of the tibia (**D**) the rough soleal line extends obliquely from the superior tibiofibular joint to the medial border of the bone. A strong fibrous sheet, the tibiofibular interosseous membrane, joins the lateral border of the tibia to the medial border of the fibula. It is perforated above by an oval aperture which transmits the anterior tibial artery from the posterior compartment of the leg to the anterior (**341C**). This artery may be torn if the membrane is ruptured in injuries which separate the leg bones.

POPLITEAL FOSSA (II)

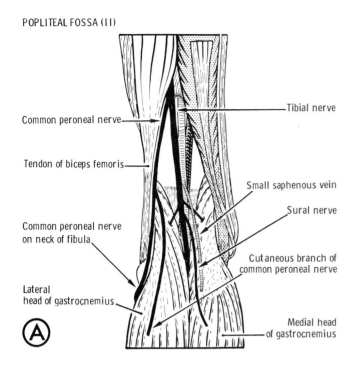

Common peroneal nerve

Tendon of biceps femoris

Common peroneal nerve on neck of fibula

Lateral head of gastrocnemius

(A)

Tibial nerve

Small saphenous vein

Sural nerve

Cutaneous branch of common peroneal nerve

Medial head of gastrocnemius

POPLITEAL FOSSA (ROOF)

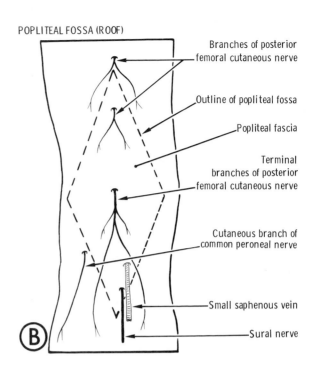

Branches of posterior femoral cutaneous nerve

Outline of popliteal fossa

Popliteal fascia

Terminal branches of posterior femoral cutaneous nerve

Cutaneous branch of common peroneal nerve

Small saphenous vein

Sural nerve

(B)

LEG BONES: ANTERIOR ASPECT

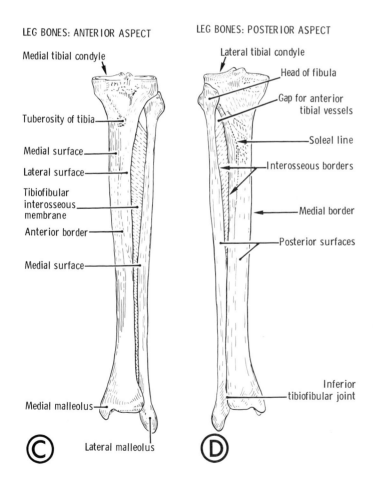

Medial tibial condyle

Tuberosity of tibia

Medial surface

Lateral surface

Tibiofibular interosseous membrane

Anterior border

Medial surface

Medial malleolus

(C)

Lateral malleolus

LEG BONES: POSTERIOR ASPECT

Lateral tibial condyle

Head of fibula

Gap for anterior tibial vessels

Soleal line

Interosseous borders

Medial border

Posterior surfaces

Inferior tibiofibular joint

(D)

LEG BONES: TRANSVERSE SECTION AT MID-LEG

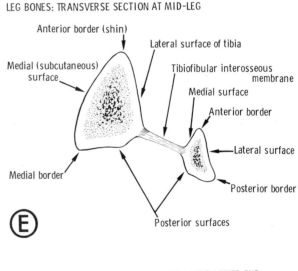

Anterior border (shin)

Medial (subcutaneous) surface

Lateral surface of tibia

Tibiofibular interosseous membrane

Medial surface

Anterior border

Lateral surface

Posterior border

Medial border

Posterior surfaces

(E)

LEG BONES: TRANSVERSE SECTION NEAR LOWER END

Tibiofibular interosseous ligament

TIBIA

FIBULA

(F)

Inferior tibiofibular joint

Traced distally, both tibia and fibula become quadrangular, while the interosseous membrane expands into the short and very strong tibiofibular interosseous ligament, which unites the two bones in a syndesmosis—the inferior tibiofibular joint (**343F**).

The superior and inferior tibiofibular joints and the interosseous membrane allow no voluntary movement between the leg bones, but some elasticity is conferred on the proximal articular surface of the ankle joint (see below).

The shaft of the tibia has two anatomical peculiarities which are of clinical significance. Examine your own leg and note that the whole of the medial surface of the bone is devoid of overlying muscles and is covered only by skin and superficial fascia. Open fractures, that is fractures in which the bone ends penetrate the overlying skin, are consequently more frequent than in most bones. When the soft tissues of the leg are considered later, it will be seen that no muscle or tendinous fibres are attached to the lower third of the tibia. Lack of such attachments is associated with a paucity of periostial and metaphysial arteries, and, because of this relatively poor blood supply, healing of fractures of the lower part of the tibia is often slow (delayed union).

From the medial aspect of the distal end of the tibial shaft, the medial malleolus projects distally as a short blunt process (**343C**). The distal end of the fibula expands and then tapers to a blunt tip, and the whole of this region of the bone is termed the lateral malleolus (**343C**). The malleoli do not end at the same level; the tip of the lateral malleolus is half an inch below, and half an inch farther back than, the medial malleolus. Check this on yourself: it is an important diagnostic point in suspected fractures of the leg bones.

The tibiofibular mortice is a complex articular surface formed by the distal ends of the tibia and fibula. It articulates with the trochlear surface of the talus (see below). The quadrangular distal surface of the tibia is coated with articular cartilage, and is concave anteroposteriorly, convex from side to side, and wider anteriorly than posteriorly. The cartilage continues without interruption on to the lateral (deep) surface of the medial malleolus. The medial aspect of the lateral malleolus carries an oval articular facet anteriorly and the deep malleolar fossa posteriorly. The fibular facet is separated from the tibial facet by a narrow cleft which contains the lowest fibres of the tibiofibular interosseous ligament (**A**).

Ossification of the patella and leg bones

The ossification of the patella occurs in cartilage, usually from a single primary centre which appears at about 4 or 5 years.

In some individuals, ossification begins at more than one centre. This may result in the adult patella consisting of two bony parts joined by the cartilage. Nearly always the smaller of two such bony segments constitutes the upper and lateral corner of the patella. This condition may be mistaken for a fracture if the patella is known to have been exposed to injury.

Ossification of the tibia and fibula involves ossification of the shaft from primary centres appearing in cartilage models about 8 weeks after conception. The proximal and distal epiphyses ossify from secondary centres which appear shortly before birth or in early childhood, as indicated in the accompanying radiographs **B, C, D, E, F**.

The only secondary centre present in either bone at birth is in the central part of the proximal tibial epiphysis (**B**). In medicolegal investigations the presence or absence of this centre may indicate if a baby died before or after the normal gestation period.

The proximal growth plate of the tibia is horizontal behind but in front turns sharply downwards to emerge at the tibial tuberosity. The resulting descending process of the proximal tibial epiphysis ossifies at about 12 years, either by extension from the main secondary centre or from a separate centre (**D**). In everyday activities the posterior part of the epiphysial plate is subject to compressive stress by body weight and the anterior part to tensile stress from the pull of the quadriceps femoris muscle through the ligamentum patellae. A sudden violent contraction of the quadriceps muscle in a young person may separate the descending epiphysial process from the diaphysis.

At the lower end of the tibia, the medial malleolus does not become bony until 7 years (**E, F**), and it too may ossify from a separate centre. The radiological appearance of separate centres in the processes of the two tibial epiphyses must be distinguished from fractures.

Rather more diaphysial growth occurs at the proximal than at the distal growth plates in the leg bones, but the growth ratio (1.3:1) is much nearer unity than it is in many other long bones, e.g. in the humerus the rate of growth at the proximal end is about four times that at the distal end.

The skeleton of the foot

At rest the foot lies approximately at right angles to the leg, and its upper and lower surfaces are usually described as dorsal and plantar respectively.

TIBIOFIBULAR MORTICE

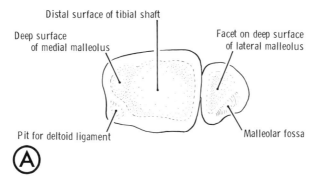

Distal surface of tibial shaft

Deep surface
of medial malleolus

Facet on deep surface
of lateral malleolus

Pit for deltoid ligament

Malleolar fossa

(A)

LEG BONES: OSSIFICATION

Anteroposterior. 2 years

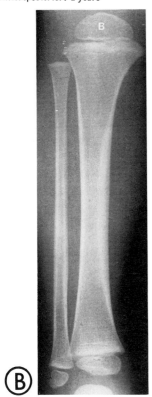

(B)

Anteroposterior. 4 years

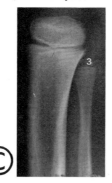

(C)

Lateral. 15 years

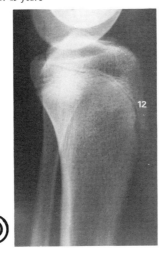

(D)

Anteroposterior. 5 years

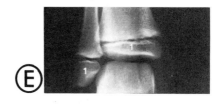

(E)

Anteroposterior. 12 years

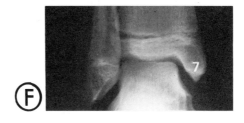

(F)

Its skeleton (**A**, **B**) consists of three groups of bones. The posterior group are several irregular tarsal bones (the tarsus). The names and positions of the individual bones should be learned at this time. Note particularly the sustentaculum tali, a thick shelf-like process from the medial side of the calcaneus, which juts medially beneath the talus. Anterior to the tarsus are five miniature long bones, called the metatarsal bones, which are numbered from medial to lateral. Another set of miniature long bones, the phalanges, lie within the toes. The great toe contains two phalanges, the proximal and the distal. The other four toes each contain three phalanges, named proximal, middle, and distal.

Functionally, another grouping of the bones of the foot is more helpful. In this the foot skeleton is divided into the talus, the foot-plate and the phalanges. The positions of talus and phalanges have been observed already. The foot-plate consists of the tarsal bones apart from the talus, the metatarsals and the numerous small joints which separate those bony elements. The region is stippled in **A**, **B**.

The talus

This very important bone is the link between the tibia and fibula and the foot-plate, and so is involved in two major joints, the ankle joint above and the subtalar joint below. Much of its surface is consequently covered with articular cartilage. Recognise the body, neck and head of the bone as they are seen from the dorsal (**C**) and plantar (**D**) aspects.

The pulley-shaped trochlear area of cartilage is associated with the body of the bone. It covers, as three continuous facets, the whole of the lateral and dorsal surfaces and the upper half of the medial surface, and fits into the tibiofibular mortice (**345A**). Thus the dorsal facet articulates with the distal surface of the tibia and is correspondingly convex sagittally, concave from side to side and wider anteriorly than posteriorly. The lateral facet is triangular (**B**) and concave from above down. It articulates with the lateral malleolus. The medial facet is comma-shaped (**A**) with the broad end anteriorly. It articulates with the medial malleolus.

On the plantar surface of the talus (**D**) the neck is crossed from side to side by a deep groove, the sulcus tali. This is narrow medially and wide laterally, and separates two articular surfaces. That behind the sulcus is concave and covers the plantar aspect of the body of the talus, while that in front is convex and covers the plantar, medial and anterior aspects of the ovoid head.

The foot-plate

This region of the foot contains the calcaneus, the navicular, the cuboid, the three cuneiform bones and the metatarsals.

Identify these bones on the dorsal aspect of the foot-plate (**E**). This aspect exhibits a group of features which, in the complete foot, are apposed to those already noted on the plantar surface of the talus (**D**). The middle third of the dorsal surface of the calcaneus carries a large convex area of cartilage which is paired with the concave facet on the plantar aspect of the body of the talus. In front of this facet the calcaneus is crossed from side to side by a groove, the sulcus calcanei, which is narrow medially and wide laterally. In the complete foot, this is apposed to the sulcus tali (**D**), and the two sulci together complete a funnel-shaped tunnel between the talus and the calcaneus called the sinus tarsi (**351B**).

In front of the sulcus calcanei lies a complex, deeply concave articular area named the calcaneonavicular socket (**E**). A cartilage facet on the sustentaculum tali usually extends on to the body of the calcaneus and forms the posterior part of the socket, while another facet on the posterior aspect of the navicular forms the anterior part. The intervening part of the socket is ligamentous. The plantar calcaneonavicular (spring) ligament is a curved structure which extends from the anterior and medial margins of the sustentaculum tali to the plantar and medial aspects of the navicular: it forms the floor and medial wall of the socket. Laterally, the bifurcated ligament extends forwards from the lateral part of the sulcus calcanei and divides, as its name implies, into two parts. The lateral band is attached to the dorsal surface of the cuboid, while the medial band reaches the lateral aspect of the navicular and completes the lateral wall of the socket. In the complete foot the calcaneonavicular socket articulates with the convex area of cartilage on the head of the talus (**D**).

Identify again the individual bones and small intervening joints which are seen on the plantar aspect of the foot-plate (**F**).

Note particularly the following features.

1. The plantar surface of the calcaneus with its three named prominences, and at a higher level the plantar aspect of the sustentaculum tali.
2. The deep groove and prominent ridge on the plantar surface of the cuboid.
3. The tuberosity of the navicular at the junction of the medial and plantar aspects of the bone.
4. The plantar calcaneonavicular (spring) ligament in the gap between the sustentaculum tali and navicular.
5. The sagittal grooves, separated by a ridge, on the plantar aspect of the articular surface on the first metatarsal head.
6. The tuberosity extending backwards and laterally from the base of the fifth metatarsal.

SKELETON OF FOOT: MEDIAL ASPECT

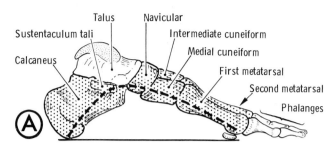

Sustentaculum tali
Calcaneus
Talus
Navicular
Intermediate cuneiform
Medial cuneiform
First metatarsal
Second metatarsal
Phalanges

Ⓐ

Medial longitudinal arch — — — — —
Bones of foot-plate - stippled ⬚⬚⬚⬚⬚
Lateral longitudinal arch ●●●●●●●●●●

SKELETON OF FOOT: LATERAL ASPECT

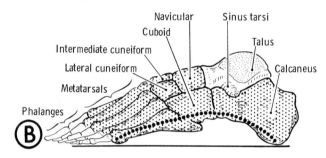

Navicular
Sinus tarsi
Cuboid
Talus
Intermediate cuneiform
Calcaneus
Lateral cuneiform
Metatarsals
Phalanges

Ⓑ

TALUS: DORSAL ASPECT

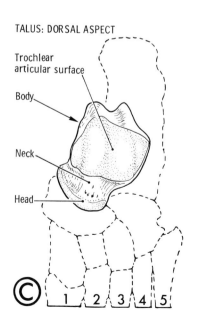

Trochlear articular surface
Body
Neck
Head

Ⓒ 1 2 3 4 5

TALUS: PLANTAR ASPECT

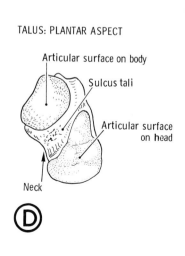

Articular surface on body
Sulcus tali
Articular surface on head
Neck

Ⓓ

FOOT-PLATE: DORSAL ASPECT

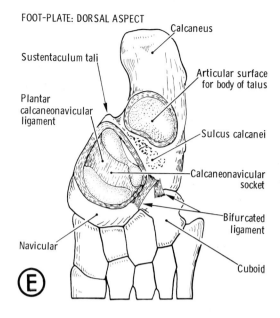

Calcaneus
Sustentaculum tali
Articular surface for body of talus
Plantar calcaneonavicular ligament
Sulcus calcanei
Calcaneonavicular socket
Bifurcated ligament
Navicular
Cuboid

Ⓔ

FOOT-PLATE: PLANTAR ASPECT

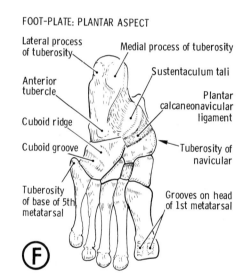

Lateral process of tuberosity
Medial process of tuberosity
Anterior tubercle
Sustentaculum tali
Plantar calcaneonavicular ligament
Cuboid ridge
Cuboid groove
Tuberosity of navicular
Tuberosity of base of 5th metatarsal
Grooves on head of 1st metatarsal

Ⓕ

FOOT-PLATE: TRANSVERSE SECTION

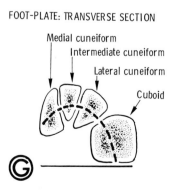

Medial cuneiform
Intermediate cuneiform
Lateral cuneiform
Cuboid

Ⓖ

The foot-plate as a whole is longitudinally arched (**347A**), so that the central part lies at a higher level than its anterior and posterior ends. The arched form adapts this part of the foot to the stresses it experiences when the heel leaves the ground in each walking step.

Because a greater proportion of body weight is transmitted to the ground through the medial metatarsal heads than through the lateral in that phase of activity, the arch is higher on the medial than on the lateral side of the foot-plate (**347A**). As a result the cuneiform and navicular bones lie above, as well as medial to, the cuboid, so that the central part of the foot-plate is sometimes described as being transversely arched (**347G**).

Ossification of the bones of the foot

At birth only the calcaneus and talus and the diaphyses of the metatarsals and phalanges are undergoing ossification from primary centres established during foetal life (**A**). Thereafter, ossification appears in the cuboid soon after birth and in the cuneiforms and navicular between 1 and 3 years.

The tarsal bones are ossified wholly from primary centres, except for the calcaneus. In the posterior part of that bone a secondary centre develops at about 7 years and produces a thin bony epiphysis which covers most of the posterior surface and extends forwards to include the tuberosity (**C**). It consequently receives the attachments of the tendo calcaneus (**361A**) and the plantar aponeurosis (**354**) and transmits a large part of the body weight to the ground in standing.

Contrary to the usual pattern of development in long bones, the metatarsals and phalanges develop bony epiphyses only at one end. The secondary centres which produce these appear at rather variable times between 3 and 6 years. Note particularly that in the phalanges and the first metatarsal the epiphyses are at the bases of the bones, whereas in the other four metatarsals they form the head (**A**, **B**).

The ankle joint

At the ankle joint the tibiofibular mortice (**345A**) articulates with the trochlear surface of the talus (**347C**). Re-examine the form of these two articular surfaces, and visualise the interrelationships of corresponding facets.

The joint cavity is enclosed by a fibrous capsule which is lined by synovial membrane and attached to bone above and below, just beyond the margins of the articular surfaces. The capsule is thin and the main bonds between the articulating bones are the strong collateral ligaments on the medial and lateral sides of the joint.

The collateral ligaments are described below, but note that some extend downwards beyond the talus to reach the foot-plate and are consequently associated, not only with the ankle joint, but also with the subtalar joint which intervenes between foot-plate and talus.

Medially, the very strong, triangular deltoid ligament (**D**) extends downwards from the medial malleolus. Its deeper and posterior fibres are attached to the medial aspect of the body of the talus and are concerned solely with the ankle joint. Many of the more superficial fibres reach the navicular and the sustentaculum tali, while others end by binding with the upper margin of the plantar calcaneonavicular (spring) ligament (**347E**).

On the lateral side of the joint there are three separate ligaments which diverge from the anterior, inferior and medial aspects of the lateral malleolus: they are described collectively as the lateral ligament of the ankle joint (**E**). The anterior band runs forwards to the lateral aspect of the neck of the talus, while the posterior, arising from the malleolar fossa (**345A**), inclines medially and somewhat backwards to the posterior aspect of the talus (**E**). Both are concerned solely with the ankle joint. On the other hand, the middle band (**E**, **F**) extends downwards and backwards to the central part of the lateral aspect of the calcaneus, and so is a ligament of both ankle and subtalar joints.

Movements of the ankle joint are restricted to the sagittal plane, both by the shape of the articular surfaces and by the disposition of the major ligaments. Unusual terms are customarily applied to these movements. Movement of the anterior part of the foot in a downward or plantar direction is called plantar flexion: movement in an upward or dorsal direction is called dorsiflexion, despite being produced by the extensor group of muscles (**357D**). Make these movements in your own limb and observe that plantar flexion is a larger movement than dorsiflexion.

These movements occur around a transverse axis of rotation. The effects of muscular and gravitational forces on the joint depend on the relationship of these forces to this axis. It traverses the tip of the lateral malleolus (**F**), but, because of the different levels of the two malleoli (**344**), it emerges on the medial side, half an inch below and behind the tip of the medial malleolus (**D**).

BONES OF FOOT:
OSSIFICATION

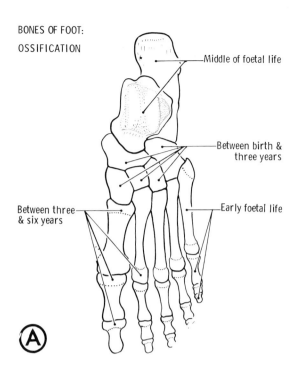

Middle of foetal life

Between birth &
three years

Between three
& six years

Early foetal life

Ⓐ

METATARSAL BONES: OSSIFICATION

Dorsoplantar. 10 years

Epiphyses of metatarsals

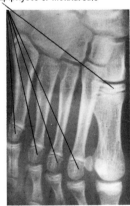

Ⓑ

CALCANEUS: OSSIFICATION

Lateral. 14 years

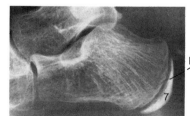

Bony epiphysis
of calcaneus

Ⓒ

ANKLE JOINT: MEDIAL ASPECT

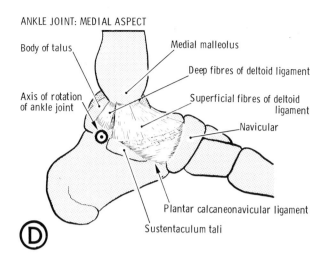

Body of talus

Medial malleolus

Deep fibres of deltoid ligament

Axis of rotation
of ankle joint

Superficial fibres of deltoid
ligament

Navicular

Plantar calcaneonavicular ligament

Sustentaculum tali

Ⓓ

ANKLE JOINT: POSTERIOR ASPECT

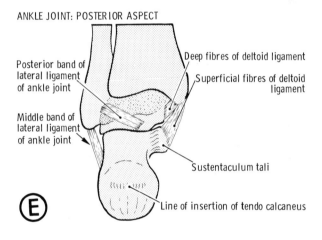

Posterior band of
lateral ligament
of ankle joint

Deep fibres of deltoid ligament

Superficial fibres of deltoid
ligament

Middle band of
lateral ligament
of ankle joint

Sustentaculum tali

Line of insertion of tendo calcaneus

Ⓔ

ANKLE JOINT: LATERAL ASPECT

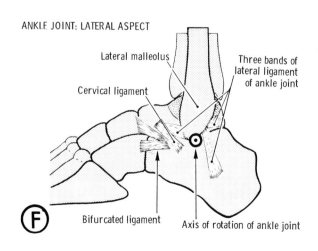

Lateral malleolus

Three bands of
lateral ligament
of ankle joint

Cervical ligament

Bifurcated ligament

Axis of rotation of ankle joint

Ⓕ

The subtalar joint

This is a complex joint between the plantar aspect of the talus (**347D**) and the dorsal aspect of the foot-plate (**347E**). It consists of two compartments, one anteromedial and the other posterolateral, which are entirely separated by the sinus tarsi (**346**). At the posterolateral or talocalcaneal compartment, the facet on the inferior surface of the body of the talus articulates with that on the middle third of the superior surface of the calcaneus, and the plane of the joint is convex upwards. At the anteromedial or talocalcaneonavicular compartment, the head of the talus articulates with the several elements of the calcaneonavicular socket and the plane of the joint is convex downwards. As a consequence of these features, movements of the foot-plate on the talus necessarily occur at both compartments, simultaneously, around a single, common axis of rotation (**A**). The axis passes upwards, forwards and medially through the calcaneus, the sinus tarsi and the head of the talus, so that it passes below the talocalcaneal compartment but above the talocalcaneonavicular (**B**).

The movements which occur at the subtalar joint are rather complex. However, in essence, the foot-plate is tilted medially or laterally beneath the talus. Because of their complexity the movements are given special names. Medial tilting of the foot-plate is called inversion, while lateral tilting is called eversion. Make these movements in your own unshod foot and observe that inversion is a considerably larger movement than eversion.

Both compartments of the subtalar joint are enclosed by tenuous fibrous capsules, and the apposed parts of these capsules complete the anterior and posterior walls of the sinus tarsi (**B**).

The ligaments of the joint lie on its medial and lateral aspects. As previously noted (**349**) the superficial part of the deltoid ligament (**C**) and the middle band of the lateral ligament of the ankle (**D**) extend over both ankle and subtalar joints. On the other hand the cervical ligament (**D**) is concerned with the subtalar joint alone. It runs downwards and laterally through the wide lateral part of the sinus tarsi, from the inferolateral aspect of the neck of the talus to the dorsal surface of the calcaneus. Inversion at the subtalar joint is limited by the cervical ligament and the middle band of the lateral ligament of the ankle joint, and eversion by the deltoid ligament.

Surface anatomy of the ankle and subtalar joints

On the medial side of the foot identify the following bony points and then draw the outline of the deltoid ligament with a skin pencil (**C**).

1. The tip of the medial malleolus.
2. The tuberosity of the navicular which projects about 4 cm below and in front of 1. Note that this separation increases when the foot is everted and decreases when it is inverted.

3. The medial aspect of the head of the talus which lies immediately behind 2. When the foot is inverted this bony feature is almost impalpable, and even in eversion it is rather indistinct because it is covered by the thick plantar calcaneonavicular ligament. The swelling caused by injury naturally obscures the feature still further, but it is still important that it should be identified, for in severe ankle injuries, it can be considerably displaced.
4. The sustentaculum tali, which is felt rather indistinctly as a blunt horizontal ridge below 3.

On the lateral side of the foot, identify the main bony features listed below, and then draw the three bands of the lateral ligament of the ankle joint, and the cervical ligament (**D**). In an injured ankle, it is the lateral side that is the more commonly affected. It will be bruised and swollen, and the bony features will be more difficult to identify than in the normal part.

1. The tip of the lateral malleolus. Compare the positions of the two malleoli and recall that the lateral normally extends to a point half an inch below and behind the medial.
2. The wide lateral end of the sinus tarsi which presents as a distinct hollow in front of 1. The bone palpable above the hollow is the neck of the talus and the bone below is the calcaneus.
3. The line of the calcaneocuboid joint, which is easily palpable when the foot is inverted.
4. The prominent tuberosity of the base of the fifth metatarsal.

Injuries of the ankle and subtalar joints

Most injuries of this region are caused by forces tending to cause excessive inversion or eversion of the foot-plate.

Inversion injuries are the more common, and often occur when a person stumbles over the edge of a pavement and the "ankle goes over". The tensile stresses which the inversion force causes on the lateral side of the foot may partially or completely tear the cervical ligament or the middle band of the lateral ligament of the ankle (**D**), or cause an oblique or a transverse avulsion fracture through the tip of the lateral malleolus (**E**).

Eversion injuries are less common. The deltoid ligament is very strong and any injury on the medial side of the foot caused by an everting force is usually transverse avulsion of the tip of the medial malleolus (**F**). In these circumstances the fibula tends to be levered laterally and may fracture transversely at any level up to the neck of the bone. Such fractures may be associated with rupture of the inferior tibiofibular ligament, and in the most severe injuries, the talus may be displaced between the long bones or out of the ankle joint.

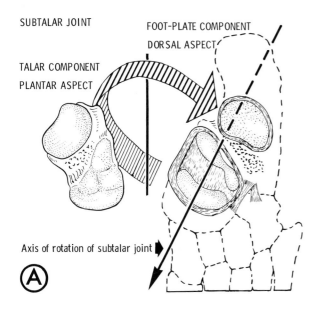

SUBTALAR JOINT

FOOT-PLATE COMPONENT
DORSAL ASPECT

TALAR COMPONENT
PLANTAR ASPECT

Axis of rotation of subtalar joint

(A)

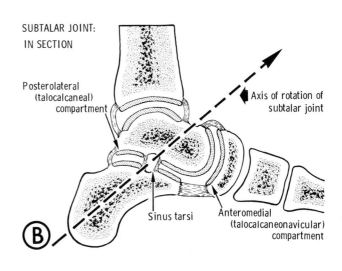

SUBTALAR JOINT:
IN SECTION

Posterolateral
(talocalcaneal)
compartment

Axis of rotation of
subtalar joint

Sinus tarsi

Anteromedial
(talocalcaneonavicular)
compartment

(B)

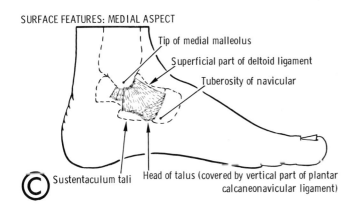

SURFACE FEATURES: MEDIAL ASPECT

Tip of medial malleolus

Superficial part of deltoid ligament

Tuberosity of navicular

Sustentaculum tali

Head of talus (covered by vertical part of plantar calcaneonavicular ligament)

(C)

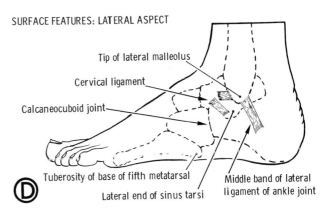

SURFACE FEATURES: LATERAL ASPECT

Tip of lateral malleolus

Cervical ligament

Calcaneocuboid joint

Tuberosity of base of fifth metatarsal

Lateral end of sinus tarsi

Middle band of lateral ligament of ankle joint

(D)

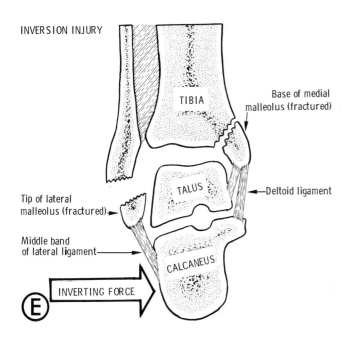

INVERSION INJURY

TIBIA

Base of medial malleolus (fractured)

TALUS

Deltoid ligament

Tip of lateral malleolus (fractured)

Middle band of lateral ligament

CALCANEUS

INVERTING FORCE

(E)

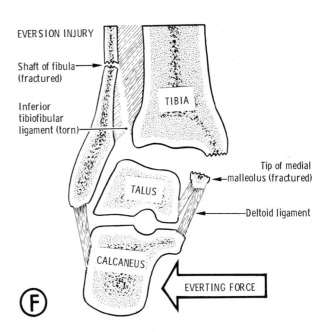

EVERSION INJURY

Shaft of fibula (fractured)

Inferior tibiofibular ligament (torn)

TIBIA

Tip of medial malleolus (fractured)

TALUS

Deltoid ligament

CALCANEUS

EVERTING FORCE

(F)

351

The joints of the foot-plate

The bones of the foot-plate are separated by numerous synovial joints which are mainly small and of the plane type. But although any one of these joints has little mobility, simultaneous movements at all the joints produce appreciable and important changes in the form of the foot-plate as a whole. Such movements do not have the freedom usually associated with synovial joints. On the contrary, they are permitted largely by slight stretching of ligaments and slight compression of joint cartilages, so that they are elastically resisted. Consequently, when a moving force ceases, the distorted foot-plate tends to spring back automatically to a neutral position. The position of the several foot-plate joints should now be revised (**347A, 347B**) but because of their small size and collective operation it is unnecessary to consider their detailed anatomy.

The ligaments of the foot-plate can be considered in three groups.

1. Several short strong ligaments which bind the apposing surfaces of adjacent bones to one another.
2. Feltworks of fibres which cover the plantar and dorsal aspects of the central part of the foot-plate, uniting the navicular, cuboid, and cuneiform bones and bases of the metatarsals.
3. This central part of the foot-plate is joined to the calcaneus by four larger ligaments. The bifurcated and plantar calcaneonavicular ligaments have been considered already (**347E**). The short plantar ligament (**A**) runs from the anterior tubercle of the calcaneus to the plantar surface of the cuboid behind the ridge. The long plantar ligament (**B**) is attached posteriorly to the plantar surface of the calcaneus. Anteriorly its deeper fibres end at the cuboid ridge, but its superficial fibres continue forwards as three bands to the bases of the second, third, and fourth metatarsals. These superficial fibres convert the groove on the cuboid into an osteoligamentous canal which is traversed by the tendon of the peroneus longus muscle.

Alterations in the shape of the foot-plate may be produced by gravitational or muscular forces and are of two broad types. First accentuation or diminution of the longitudinal curvature of the plate (**347A**) may be produced by bending or unbending forces acting in the sagittal plane. And since these movements are similar in kind and effect to those occurring at the ankle joint, bending may be termed plantar flexion of the foot-plate and unbending dorsiflexion.

The ranges of these movements vary greatly in different individuals. In most people they are small, but when a ballet dancer stands on her points, she achieves such a degree of plantar flexion, both at the ankle joint and within the foot-plate, that the metatarsals are aligned with the leg bones. On the other hand, in relaxed standing her foot-plate tends to be almost flat on the ground with very little longitudinal curvature.

In the second type of movement the foot-plate is twisted about its long axis by rotation of its anterior end in relation to its posterior end.

In the free limb, inversion of the foot resulting from muscular activity involves inversion at the subtalar joint (**350**) and, simultaneously, a longitudinal twist of the foot-plate such that the medial metatarsal heads are elevated and the lateral heads depressed (**C**). Such a twist of the foot-plate may therefore be called an inversion twist. On the other hand, eversion of the foot involves subtalar eversion (**350**) and, simultaneously, a longitudinal twist such that the medial metatarsal heads are depressed and the lateral heads elevated (**D**). Such a twist may therefore be called an eversion twist. Inversion and eversion twists of the foot-plate may also be produced by passively rotating the region of the metarsal heads in the unshod foot.

The subtalar and foot-plate joints in the weight-bearing foot

In the passive weight-bearing foot the force of body-weight produces, or tends to produce, dorsiflexion of the foot-plate and eversion of the subtalar joint, while elevation of the lateral metatarsal heads as a result of the subtalar eversion is prevented by an inversion twist of the foot-plate.

In certain circumstances it is necessary to raise the medial part of the longitudinal arch of the foot in weight-bearing, by muscle action.

The movements within the foot which the muscles produce to effect this elevation are plantar flexion of the foot-plate and inversion of the subtalar joint, while elevation of the medial metatarsal heads as a result of subtalar inversion is prevented by an eversion twist of the foot-plate. The muscles which produce these movements are noted below (**364**).

The bones and joints of the toes

The heads of the metatarsals have condyloid articular surfaces which extend over their anterior and plantar aspects, but only marginally on to their dorsal aspects (**355**). All the phalanges have gently concave facets on their bases. The heads of all proximal and middle phalanges carry trochlear (pulley-shaped) surfaces whereas the ends of the distal phalanges are non-articular.

SOLE OF FOOT: SHORT PLANTAR LIGAMENT

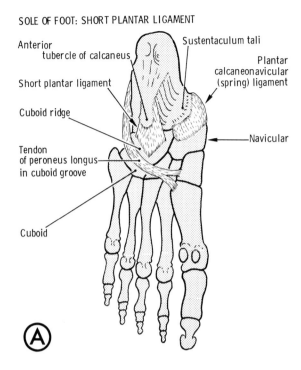

Anterior tubercle of calcaneus

Short plantar ligament

Cuboid ridge

Tendon of peroneus longus in cuboid groove

Cuboid

Sustentaculum tali

Plantar calcaneonavicular (spring) ligament

Navicular

(A)

SOLE OF FOOT: LONG PLANTAR LIGAMENT

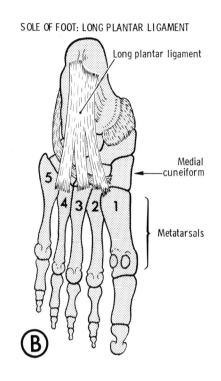

Long plantar ligament

Medial cuneiform

Metatarsals

5 4 3 2 1

(B)

FOOT-PLATE: INVERSION TWIST

Sole of foot faces downwards & medially

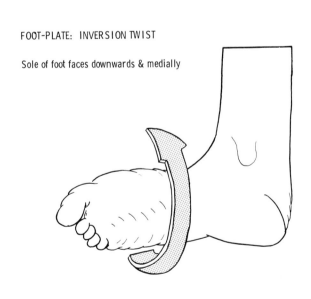

(C)

FOOT-PLATE: EVERSION TWIST

Sole of foot faces downwards & laterally

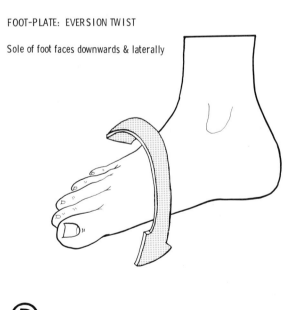

(D)

The metatarsophalangeal (MTP) and interphalangeal (IP) joints are similar. Each is enclosed by a fibrous capsule which is very considerably thickened in its plantar part (**A, B, C, D**), and is augmented medially and laterally by collateral ligaments. In the case of the MTP joints, the thickened plantar aspects of all the fibrous capsules are joined by the deep transverse metatarsal ligament (**357B**). Note that the corresponding ligament in the hand, that is the deep transverse metacarpal ligament, joins only the four medial digits and thus permits the characteristic mobility of the thumb (**545D**).

All the joints allow flexion and extension movements in the sagittal plane and, although the MTP joints can in addition be moved from side to side, at least passively, that range of mobility is seldom utilised.

The first MTP joint has special features. The plantar surface of the first metatarsal head is marked by two sagittal grooves and an intervening ridge (**347F**). The twin tendons of flexor hallucis brevis muscle (**363B**), which are inserted into the proximal phalanx of the great toe each contains a large sesamoid bone, the medial and lateral hallucial sesamoids. Both the tendons and these sesamoids are incorporated into the substance of the plantar part of the joint capsule, so that each sesamoid articulates by its deep surface with one of the grooves on the metatarsal head (**A, B**). These hallucial sesamoids are the main supporting structures at the anterior end of the foot in standing, and they may transmit very great forces when a person jumps from a height and lands on the 'ball of the foot'. Although the hallucial sesamoids usually ossify from single centres of ossification, either bone may develop from two centres which may remain separate in adult life. Radiographic examination will then suggest a fracture where none exists. Lateral angulation of the proximal phalanx of the great toe in relation to the first metatarsal is called hallux valgus (**E**). Some degree of this is present in many functionally normal feet, but in some individuals the angulation becomes excessive and pressure effects (a 'bunion') develop on the medial aspect of the MTP joint.

Movements at the MTP and IP joints can be regarded as starting from the resting, non-weight-bearing positions illustrated in the great toe in **A**, and in one of the lateral four toes in **C**. In walking, during each step, the heel is raised while the metatarsal heads and toes remain on the ground. Subsequently the toes are flexed and leave the ground, imparting a final upward and forward thrust to the body as they do so. The positions of the MTP and IP joints in the first phase of this cycle are shown in the great toe and in one of the other toes in **B, D**. Note in particular that in the lateral toes (**D**) the proximal IP joint is flexed whereas the MTP and distal IP joints are extended. This position may force the dorsum of the proximal IP joint against the uppers of the shoe and accounts for the frequency of

blisters at that site. In some people this position becomes fixed and permanent in one digit and the condition is known as hammer toe (**F**).

The deep fascia of the leg and foot

The muscles and bones of the leg are enclosed within a cylindrical sheath of deep fascia of considerable thickness and strength (**G**). In two regions, over the medial surface of the shaft and malleolus of the tibia, and over the lateral aspect of the lateral malleolus of the fibula, it is continuous with the superficial layer of the periosteum. Confirm on your own leg that these areas of bone are easily palpable. Proximally, the fascia is attached to the leg bones except posteriorly, where it is continuous with the popliteal fascia (**343A**). The space between this fascial tube and the leg bones is divided into three compartments by fibrous septa (**G**), attached to the anterior and posterior borders of the fibula. The compartments may be named according to either their position or the muscle group they contain.

This tube of deep fascia is so tough and strong that if extensive bruising occurs within it, the pressure exerted by the effused blood on the vessels of the leg may be sufficient to interfere seriously with the blood supply to the foot. The fascia then has to be widely incised to relieve the pressure.

In the ankle region, particular areas of the deep fascia of the leg become thickened, and in places firmly attached to bone, to form retinacula which hold the tendons of the three compartments of the leg in place as they change direction to pass forwards into the foot. Observe the names, positions and shapes of these retinacula (**H, J, K**). Also note carefully the relationship of the retinacula to the ligaments on the medial and lateral sides of the ankle.

The plantar aponeurosis is a greatly thickened triangular zone of deep fascia in the sole of the foot (**357A**). Over other aspects of the foot the deep fascia is thin and transparent. Observe the shape and posterior attachment of this structure. Anteriorly it divides into five digitations which are united by a band of transverse fibres. Each digitation is attached to the fibrous flexor sheath (see below) and proximal phalanx of the corresponding digit (**357A**).

Because of this anterior attachment the aponeurosis becomes taut when the metatarsophalangeal joints are extended as the heel is raised during walking (**B, D**). In those circumstances the taut aponeurosis acts as a plantar ligament which limits dorsiflexion of the foot-plate (depression of the foot arch) by body weight.

The superficial fascia in the sole of the foot is fibrous and tough. It binds the plantar aponeurosis very firmly to the overlying skin. The arrangement is similar to that in the palm of the hand, and in both cases it prevents undesirable mobility of the skin in grasping or in standing.

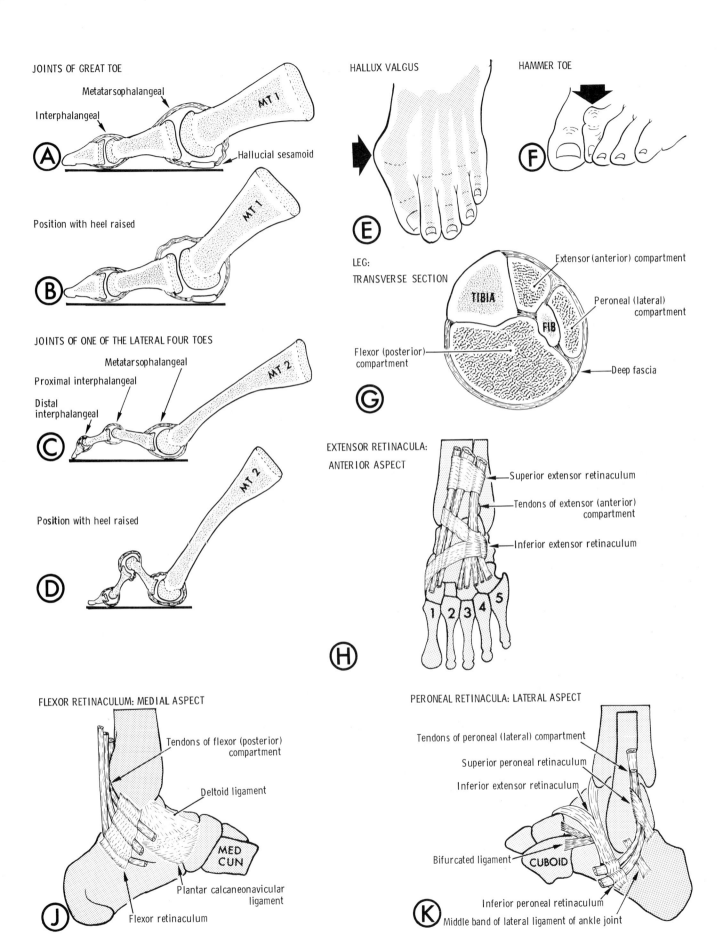

JOINTS OF GREAT TOE

A — Interphalangeal, Metatarsophalangeal, MT 1, Hallucial sesamoid

B — Position with heel raised, MT 1

JOINTS OF ONE OF THE LATERAL FOUR TOES

C — Distal interphalangeal, Proximal interphalangeal, Metatarsophalangeal, MT 2

D — Position with heel raised, MT 2

E — HALLUX VALGUS

F — HAMMER TOE

G — LEG: TRANSVERSE SECTION

Extensor (anterior) compartment
Peroneal (lateral) compartment
TIBIA
FIB
Flexor (posterior) compartment
Deep fascia

H — EXTENSOR RETINACULA: ANTERIOR ASPECT

Superior extensor retinaculum
Tendons of extensor (anterior) compartment
Inferior extensor retinaculum
1 2 3 4 5

J — FLEXOR RETINACULUM: MEDIAL ASPECT

Tendons of flexor (posterior) compartment
Deltoid ligament
MED CUN
Plantar calcaneonavicular ligament
Flexor retinaculum

K — PERONEAL RETINACULA: LATERAL ASPECT

Tendons of peroneal (lateral) compartment
Superior peroneal retinaculum
Inferior extensor retinaculum
Bifurcated ligament
CUBOID
Inferior peroneal retinaculum
Middle band of lateral ligament of ankle joint

The fibrous flexor sheaths are thick fibrous tubes associated with each toe. Each begins on the plantar aspect of the metatarsophalangeal joint and extends along the same aspect of the phalanges and interphalangeal joints to a blind end over the distal phalanx (**A**, **B**). Each contains the flexor tendons of the corresponding toe, the tube and tendons being separated by a synovial sheath (**C**).

The extensor (anterior) compartment of the leg and the dorsum of the foot

The muscles

Extensor digitorum brevis is the only muscle belly on the dorsum of the foot. Note (**E**) the origin of the muscle from the calcaneus, and its formation of four tendons which extend towards the four medial toes. The tendon to the great toe is inserted directly into the base of the proximal phalanx, while the others fuse with the corresponding tendons of extensor digitorum longus (see below). Visualise the relationship of the muscle to the fibrous structures arising from the floor of the sinus tarsi.

The muscles of the extensor compartment arise from those surfaces of the tibia, the fibula, the interosseous membrane and the deep fascia which envelop the compartment (**335G**). The largest of the group, tibialis anterior, lies medially, extensor digitorum longus laterally and extensor hallucis longus between them. The lowest muscle fibres of extensor digitorum longus differ in their insertion and function from the rest of that muscle and constitute the peroneus tertius (**D**). In the lower part of the leg the tibialis anterior, the extensor hallucis longus and the peroneus tertius muscles form single tendons, while the true extensor digitorum longus fibres form four diverging tendons. All seven tendons pass beneath the two extensor retinacula on to the dorsum of the foot (**D**). They are protected from friction against these retinacula by three synovial sheaths, one of which is common to the five tendons of extensor digitorum longus and peroneus tertius. In **D** these sheaths are indicated in stipple. Note their longitudinal extents, and particularly their relationships to the two retinacula.

On the dorsum of the foot (**D**), observe the bony insertions of the tendons of tibialis anterior, peroneus tertius and extensor hallucis longus, and the relationship of the last tendon and the four tendons of extensor digitorum longus to extensor digitorum brevis and its tendons. The tendons of extensor digitorum longus diverge towards the four lateral toes, and near the metatarsophalangeal joints all except that to the fifth toe fuse with the corresponding tendons of the short extensor. Over the proximal phalanges, the extensor tendons of the four lateral toes expand into flat sheets called dorsal digital expansions, which divide distally into three slips. The middle slip inserts near the base of the middle phalanx while the two lateral slips unite and insert near the base of the distal phalanx (**D**).

All the muscles of the extensor compartment and the dorsum of the foot are supplied by the deep peroneal nerve (see below). Tibialis anterior draws its nerve supply mainly from the L4 segment of the spinal cord, extensor hallucis longus, extensor digitorum longus and peroneus tertius from L5 and extensor digitorum brevis from S1.

Examine the relationship of each of the muscles and tendons to the axes of rotation of the ankle (**349D**, **349F**) and subtalar joints (**351A**, **351B**) to the medial and lateral borders of the foot-plate and to the joints of the toes. It is evident that, in the free foot:

1. the ankle joint is dorsiflexed by all the muscles of the extensor compartment of the leg.
2. the subtalar joint is inverted by tibialis anterior and everted by peroneus tertius.
3. an inversion twist may be imparted to the foot-plate by tibialis anterior and an eversion twist by peroneus tertius.
4. the toes are extended by extensor hallucis longus, extensor digitorum longus and extensor digitorum brevis.

The blood vessels

The anterior tibial artery arises as a terminal branch of the popliteal artery in the lowest part of the popliteal fossa (**341C**), and enters the upper part of the extensor compartment by passing through the interosseous tibio-fibular membrane (**E**). Note the similarity of this course to that of the posterior interosseous artery into the back of the forearm (**533C**). Having gained the extensor compartment, the artery gives off a few recurrent branches which contribute to the genicular anastomosis (**342**), and thereafter descends to the front of the ankle joint, lying first on the tibiofibular interosseous membrane and then on the anterior aspect of the tibia (**E**). Throughout most of its course it is deeply buried beneath the extensor group of muscles (**D**), but as these muscles narrow into their tendons in the lower part of the leg the artery becomes more superficial and lies between the tendons of tibialis anterior and extensor hallucis longus, midway between the two malleoli (**D**). Here the vessel changes its name to the dorsalis pedis artery.

The dorsalis pedis artery continues forwards, across the dorsum of the tarsus, to the proximal end of the first intermetatarsal space, where it turns downwards into the sole to take part in the formation of the plantar arterial arch. Note the relationship of the vessel to extensor hallucis longus and the extensor digitorum brevis (**D**). In clinical practice the artery is frequently palpated in patients with symptoms of arterial insufficiency in the lower limb. Absence of pulsations indicates a marked reduction of blood supply. It is important to remember the point at which the artery passes into the sole otherwise palpation may be attempted too far down the dorsum of the foot.

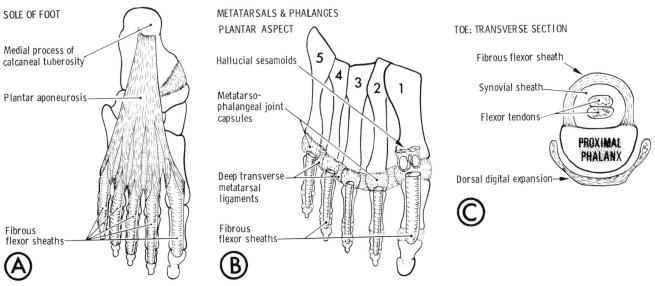

SOLE OF FOOT

Medial process of calcaneal tuberosity

Plantar aponeurosis

Fibrous flexor sheaths

Ⓐ

METATARSALS & PHALANGES PLANTAR ASPECT

Hallucial sesamoids

Metatarso-phalangeal joint capsules

Deep transverse metatarsal ligaments

Fibrous flexor sheaths

5 4 3 2 1

Ⓑ

TOE: TRANSVERSE SECTION

Fibrous flexor sheath

Synovial sheath

Flexor tendons

PROXIMAL PHALANX

Dorsal digital expansion

Ⓒ

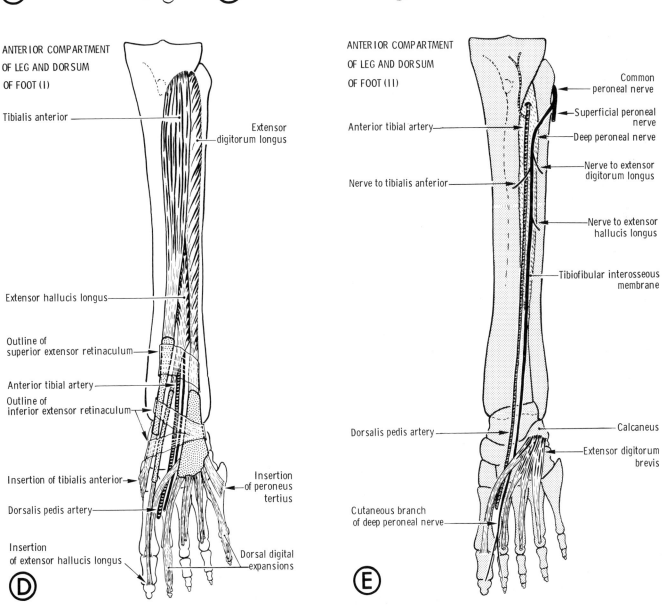

ANTERIOR COMPARTMENT OF LEG AND DORSUM OF FOOT (I)

Tibialis anterior

Extensor digitorum longus

Extensor hallucis longus

Outline of superior extensor retinaculum

Anterior tibial artery

Outline of inferior extensor retinaculum

Insertion of tibialis anterior

Dorsalis pedis artery

Insertion of extensor hallucis longus

Insertion of peroneus tertius

Dorsal digital expansions

Ⓓ

ANTERIOR COMPARTMENT OF LEG AND DORSUM OF FOOT (II)

Anterior tibial artery

Nerve to tibialis anterior

Dorsalis pedis artery

Cutaneous branch of deep peroneal nerve

Common peroneal nerve

Superficial peroneal nerve

Deep peroneal nerve

Nerve to extensor digitorum longus

Nerve to extensor hallucis longus

Tibiofibular interosseous membrane

Calcaneus

Extensor digitorum brevis

Ⓔ

357

The nerves

The deep peroneal nerve (L4, 5, S1) begins on the lateral aspect of the neck of the fibula as one of the two terminal branches of the common peroneal nerve (**A**). Curling forwards round the fibula, it enters the extensor compartment and comes into association with the anterior tibial artery (**257E**). Note that the course of this nerve into the extensor compartment differs from that followed by the anterior tibial artery, but is similar to the course of the deep branch of the radial nerve into the back of the forearm (**537A**, **537C**). The nerve follows the anterior tibial and dorsalis pedis arteries to the dorsum of the foot (**357E**), supplying all the muscles in these regions as it goes. It terminates as a small cutaneous branch supplying the adjacent halves of the dorsal skin surfaces of the great and second toes as far as the nail beds (**C**, **357E**).

The peroneal (lateral) compartment of the leg

The muscles

The peroneus longus and peroneus brevis arise, respectively, from the upper and lower parts of the lateral surface of the fibula and the related deep fascia (**A**). In the lower part of the compartment, the more superficial longus tendon and the deeper brevis tendon wind backwards on to the posterior aspect of the lateral malleolus, and hook forwards round its tip (**A**). They then run downwards and forwards across the calcaneus towards the lateral border of the foot, with the brevis tendon uppermost. Note the successive relationships of the two tendons to the superior and inferior peroneal retinacula and the lateral ligament of the ankle joint. To reduce friction against the underlying bone, the tendons are enclosed in synovial sheaths where they are directly related to the lateral malleolus and the calcaneus (**A**—stipple).

Peroneus brevis is inserted into the tuberosity of the base of the fifth metatarsal (**A**). The peroneus longus tendon turns round the lateral aspect of the cuboid into the sole and at this point contains a *sesamoid*, which articulates with a facet on the cuboid ridge (**B**, **347F**). The sesamoid is usually fibrocartilaginous and is consequently not evident in radiographs. In the sole, the tendon, protected by a second synovial sheath (**B**, **353B**), runs forwards and medially through the osteoligamentous tunnel between the cuboid groove and the superficial fibres of the long plantar ligament (**365A**). It is eventually inserted into the adjacent parts of the medial cuneiform and first metatarsal bones (**B**).

Both muscles are innervated from the S1 segment of the spinal cord through the superficial peroneal nerve (see below).

Consider the relationship of the tendons of the lateral compartment to the axes of rotation of the ankle (**349D**, **349F**) and subtalar joints (**351A**, **351B**), and also the directions of the forces which the tendons can exert on the lateral and medial borders of the foot-plate. In the free non-weight-bearing foot, both muscles plantarflex the ankle, evert the subtalar joint and produce an eversion twist of the foot-plate. Their functions in weight-bearing activities are considered later (**366**).

The nerves

The common peroneal nerve (L4, 5, S1, 2) leaves the popliteal fossa (**343A**) and enters the uppermost part of the peroneal compartment of the leg. Here it lies against the lateral aspect of the neck of the fibula in the substance of peroneus longus (**A**) where it divides into its deep and superficial peroneal branches. The deep peroneal nerve has already been traced into the extensor compartment of the leg.

The superficial peroneal nerve (L4, 5, S1) supplies the peroneus longus and brevis muscles as it descends through the peroneal compartment. Subsequently it passes through the deep fascia about halfway down the leg (**C**). In the superficial fascia its branches run downwards and supply a large skin area of the leg and foot (**C**). Note that this area does not include

1. the adjacent sides of the great and second toes.
2. the medial and lateral borders of the foot.
3. the sensitive regions of the nail beds.

Injuries to the common peroneal nerve usually occur on the lateral aspect of the neck of the fibula where the nerve is very closely related to bone. The injury may be caused by a single blow such as a kick, by prolonged pressure—sometimes caused by a plaster of Paris bandage—or by being torn by fractured bone ends.

Such injuries affect all those structures innervated by both the superficial and deep peroneal branches. The most noticeable effect is a paralysis of all the muscles capable of dorsiflexing the ankle joint and everting the subtalar joint. Consequently, in the dependent free limb, the foot hangs downwards in a plantarflexed and somewhat inverted position, the condition being known as drop-foot. In walking, instead of the anterior part of the foot being raised during each swing phase (**369A**), it is scraped forwards along the ground so that the anterior and lateral parts of the sole of the shoe quickly become worn.

Sensory loss also occurs, but the area affected is usually somewhat smaller than the total area receiving fibres from the deep and superficial peroneal nerves.

LEG: LATERAL ASPECT

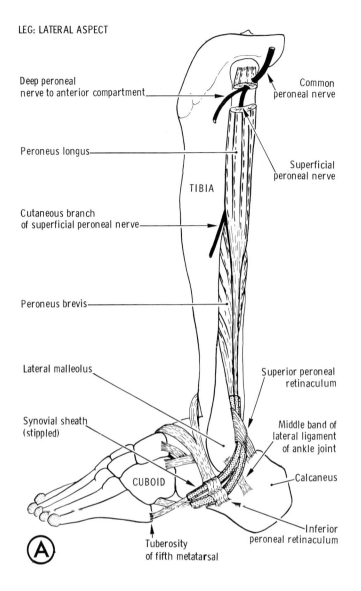

Deep peroneal nerve to anterior compartment

Common peroneal nerve

Peroneus longus

Superficial peroneal nerve

TIBIA

Cutaneous branch of superficial peroneal nerve

Peroneus brevis

Lateral malleolus

Superior peroneal retinaculum

Synovial sheath (stippled)

Middle band of lateral ligament of ankle joint

CUBOID

Calcaneus

Inferior peroneal retinaculum

Ⓐ

Tuberosity of fifth metatarsal

CUTANEOUS INNERVATION:
ANTERIOR ASPECT OF LEG AND DORSUM OF FOOT

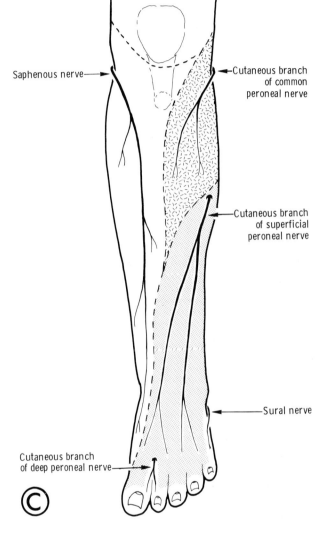

Saphenous nerve

Cutaneous branch of common peroneal nerve

Cutaneous branch of superficial peroneal nerve

Sural nerve

Cutaneous branch of deep peroneal nerve

Ⓒ

SOLE OF FOOT

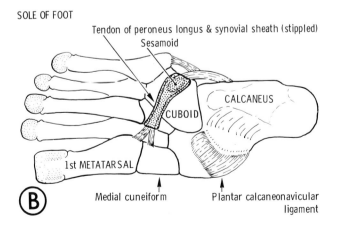

Tendon of peroneus longus & synovial sheath (stippled)
Sesamoid

CALCANEUS

CUBOID

1st METATARSAL

Ⓑ

Medial cuneiform

Plantar calcaneonavicular ligament

The flexor (posterior) compartment of the leg

The muscles

The compartment contains superficial and deep groups of muscles.

Soleus and gastrocnemius are the superficial muscles of the compartment and are inserted by a common tendon. Because gastrocnemius has two distinct bellies, the whole complex is sometimes described as the triceps surae. The common tendon of insertion, the tendo calcaneus (**A**), is very large and easily palpable in your own limb just above the heel. It extends through the lower half of the leg to be inserted into the middle part of the posterior surface of the calcaneus (**C**), and is separated from the upper part of that surface by a bursa which may become swollen and painful after unaccustomed exercise (**D**).

Examine the bony origins of soleus (**C**). The central fibres of the muscle arise from a fibrous arch running between the tibia and fibula, behind and separate from the interosseous membrane. The muscle inserts into the deep (anterior) surface of the tendo calcaneus, the lowest fibres reaching within 5 cm of the heel (**A**). The origins of the medial and lateral heads of gastrocnemius have been considered previously (**343A**). The heads remain distinct as they pass downwards, superficial to soleus, to insert into the superficial surface of the tendo calcaneus at the middle of the leg. Note the very different levels of the lowest fibres of soleus and gastrocnemius (**A**).

These superficial muscles are the chief plantarflexors of the ankle joint in the free foot and are of vital importance in weight bearing activities (**367, 369**). They are innervated through the tibial nerve (see below) from the S1, 2 segments of the spinal cord.

The deep flexor muscles should be studied in **B**. They arise from the posterior surfaces of the tibia, fibula and interosseous membrane below the origin of the soleus (**C**). Initially, their order from the medial to the lateral side is flexor digitorum longus, tibialis posterior and flexor hallucis longus (**B**). The tendons, which are formed in the lower part of the leg, incline downwards and medially and that of tibialis posterior passes in front of (deep to) flexor digitorum longus to reach its medial side (**D**). The three tendons then curve forwards below the medial malleolus, deep to the flexor retinaculum. Their positions beneath the retinaculum and their relationship to the underlying bones should be noted (**D**). Leaving the retinaculum, the tendon of tibialis posterior passes forwards across the plantar surface of the plantar calcaneonavicular ligament to insert into the tuberosity of the navicular (**D**). The other two

tendons enter the sole of the foot and continue towards the toes (see below). As the tendons turn round the medial malleolus and pass forwards beneath the retinaculum, they are enclosed and protected by individual synovial sheaths (**D**).

All three muscles are innervated by branches of the tibial nerve (see below), but the segmental origin of the fibres differs according to the function of the individual muscle. The tendon of tibialis posterior passes so close to the axis of rotation of the ankle (**D**) that the couple it produces at that joint is negligible. On the other hand, it is a powerful invertor of the subtalar joint, and consequently the motor nerve fibres it receives from the tibial nerve, like those innervating tibialis anterior from the deep peroneal nerve (**356**), are derived from L4. The tendons of the other two muscles pass farther from the axis of the ankle (**D**) and are consequently significant plantarflexors of that joint as well as flexors of the toes. In conformity with these actions their nerve supplies have a lower segmental origin than tibialis posterior, from S2.

The blood vessels

The posterior tibial artery arises at the bifurcation of the popliteal artery in the lowest part of the popliteal fossa (**B, 341C**) and immediately above the origin of soleus (**A**). Through its branches, it supplies the structures in the flexor compartment of the leg and contributes to the genicular anastomosis around the knee.

Immediately after its origin, the artery passes deep to the fibrous arch of soleus and then runs downwards and somewhat medially with the deep flexor muscles and their tendons, until it passes beneath the flexor retinaculum on the medial side of the foot. Here it divides into medial and lateral plantar arteries (**363C**).

Above, it is deeply placed beneath gastrocnemius and soleus (**A**) and is consequently impalpable, but in the lower part of its course it is covered only by skin and fascia and its pulsations can be felt clearly (**D**). Confirm this on your own leg, first at a point an inch in front of the medial edge of the tendo calcaneus, and secondly at one halfway between the medial malleolus and the medial tubercle of the calcaneal tuberosity, i.e. over the midpoint of the flexor retinaculum.

The peroneal artery arises from the posterior tibial (**B**) and descends through the flexor compartment on the lateral side of the parent stem. Like all the main arteries below the knee the posterior tibial and peroneal arteries are accompanied by venae comitantes which have important connections with the veins of the superficial fascia (**373D**).

LEG: POSTERIOR ASPECT (SUPERFICIAL)

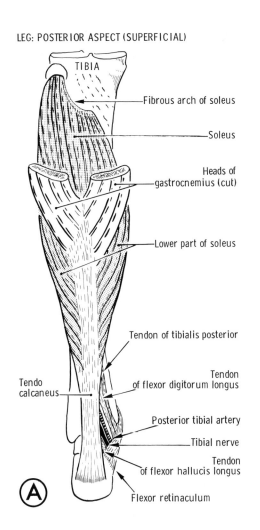

TIBIA

Fibrous arch of soleus

Soleus

Heads of gastrocnemius (cut)

Lower part of soleus

Tendon of tibialis posterior

Tendon of flexor digitorum longus

Tendo calcaneus

Posterior tibial artery

Tibial nerve

Tendon of flexor hallucis longus

Flexor retinaculum

Ⓐ

LEG: POSTERIOR ASPECT (DEEP)

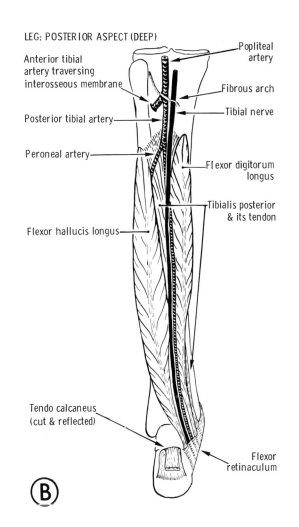

Popliteal artery

Anterior tibial artery traversing interosseous membrane

Posterior tibial artery

Peroneal artery

Flexor hallucis longus

Fibrous arch

Tibial nerve

Flexor digitorum longus

Tibialis posterior & its tendon

Tendo calcaneus (cut & reflected)

Flexor retinaculum

Ⓑ

POSTERIOR ASPECT OF LEG: MUSCLE ATTACHMENTS

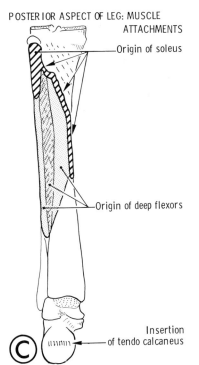

Origin of soleus

Origin of deep flexors

Insertion of tendo calcaneus

Ⓒ

LEG AND FOOT: MEDIAL ASPECT

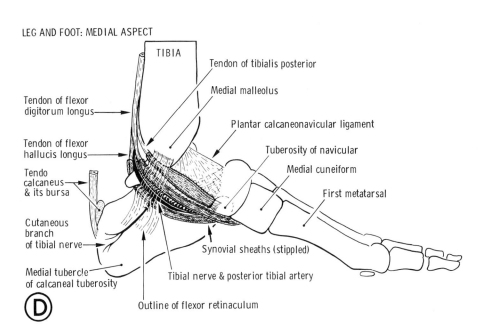

TIBIA

Tendon of tibialis posterior

Medial malleolus

Plantar calcaneonavicular ligament

Tuberosity of navicular

Medial cuneiform

First metatarsal

Tendon of flexor digitorum longus

Tendon of flexor hallucis longus

Tendo calcaneus & its bursa

Cutaneous branch of tibial nerve

Medial tubercle of calcaneal tuberosity

Synovial sheaths (stippled)

Tibial nerve & posterior tibial artery

Outline of flexor retinaculum

Ⓓ

361

The nerves

The tibial nerve (L4, 5, S1, 2, 3) in the popliteal fossa and the origins of its sural branch and its motor branches to gastrocnemius have been considered already (**343A**). It follows the posterior tibial artery beneath the fibrous arch of soleus and through the flexor compartment of the leg, to a point beneath the centre of the flexor retinaculum (**361B**). Above, it supplies the deep flexor muscles and soleus. Below, it gives cutaneous branches containing fibres from S1, which pierce the retinaculum and descend to innervate the important weight-bearing skin over the heel (**A**). Under cover of the retinaculum it divides into medial and lateral plantar nerves.

The sural nerve arises from the tibial nerve. It descends between the heads of gastrocnemius and pierces the deep fascia about halfway down the calf (**A**). In the superficial fascia it follows the short saphenous vein downwards (**373B**) and, passing behind and below the lateral malleolus, runs along the lateral border of the foot and the fifth toe. Observe the area of skin it innervates (**365C**).

The sole of the foot

The concavity of the sole of the foot contains the continuations of several tendons from the flexor and peroneal compartments of the leg, and a large number of small muscles confined to the sole and named collectively the short plantar muscles. The muscles of the latter group are similar to counterparts in the palm of the hand, but, despite this topographical similarity, the functions of palmar and plantar muscles are very different. The human hand is capable of innumerable delicately graded movements and subtle adjustments of shape, and is severely disabled by derangement or loss of any of these capabilities. The functions of the short plantar muscles are comparatively crude, and are directed simply towards the maintenance of an arched form in the weight-bearing foot, and flexion of the toes in the take-off phase of walking and running (**369**). In everyday life the muscles do no more than this. Consequently their detailed morphology is of little value in clinical practice, and only the most important will be considered individually.

In dealing with infections of the deeper tissues of the sole of the foot, these relatively crude functions allow incision and drainage of the part, without the same fears of subsequent disability which are associated with similar procedures in the palm of the hand.

Revise the fibrous structures on the plantar aspect of the foot-plate (**353A**, **353B**, **357A**) and the courses of the tendons of tibialis posterior and peroneus longus in the foot (**361D**, **359B**).

The muscles

The flexor hallucis brevis muscle (**B**) arises from the plantar surfaces of the cuboid behind the ridge, and, as it approaches the great toe, gives rise to separate medial and lateral tendons. These become incorporated into the thick plantar part of the fibrous capsule of the first MTP joint (**355A**) before being inserted into the proximal phalanx. It is these two tendons which contain the large bony hallucial sesamoids described on **354**.

The tendon of flexor hallucis longus (**C**) passes forwards in the sole of the foot dorsal to (above) that of flexor digitorum longus before the latter is joined by quadratus plantae. Thereafter, it continues on the plantar aspect of flexor hallucis brevis and passes between the two hallucial sesamoid bones into the fibrous flexor sheath of the great toe, from which it is separated by a synovial sheath. It is inserted into the base of the distal phalanx.

The tendon of flexor digitorum longus leaves the flexor retinaculum and passes towards the centre of the sole across the plantar aspect of the tendon of flexor hallucis longus (**C**). There it is joined on its lateral side by the muscle fibres of quadratus plantae, which arises as two separate heads from the medial and plantar aspects of the calcaneus (**C**). Beyond its junction with the quadratus plantae, the long flexor tendon divides into four parts. These run forwards to enter the fibrous flexor sheaths of the lateral four toes together with the tendons of flexor digitorum brevis (see below). The quadratus plantae counteracts the obliquity of the flexor digitorum longus tendon, so that a direct backward pull is applied to the toes.

The flexor digitorum brevis muscle arises from the tuberosity of the calcaneus and extensively from the deep surface of the plantar aponeurosis which covers it (**357A**). Extending forwards below the long flexor tendons, it gives rise to four tendons which enter the four lateral fibrous flexor sheaths, below the corresponding tendons of flexor digitorum longus (**357C**).

Within each of these fibrous flexor sheaths, the longus tendon runs to its insertion into the distal phalanx (**C**, **365B**), while the brevis tendon splits into two divisions, which pass dorsally on either side of the longus tendons to be inserted into the base of the middle phalanx (**D**, **365B**).

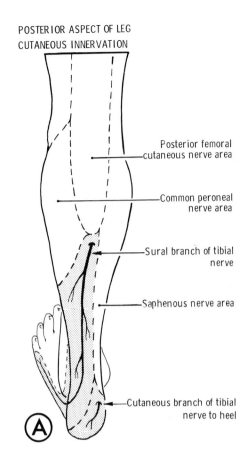

POSTERIOR ASPECT OF LEG
CUTANEOUS INNERVATION

Posterior femoral
cutaneous nerve area

Common peroneal
nerve area

Sural branch of tibial
nerve

Saphenous nerve area

Cutaneous branch of tibial
nerve to heel

(A)

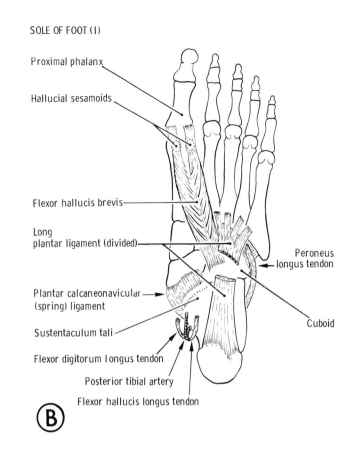

SOLE OF FOOT (I)

Proximal phalanx

Hallucial sesamoids

Flexor hallucis brevis

Long
plantar ligament (divided)

Peroneus
longus tendon

Plantar calcaneonavicular
(spring) ligament

Cuboid

Sustentaculum tali

Flexor digitorum longus tendon

Posterior tibial artery

Flexor hallucis longus tendon

(B)

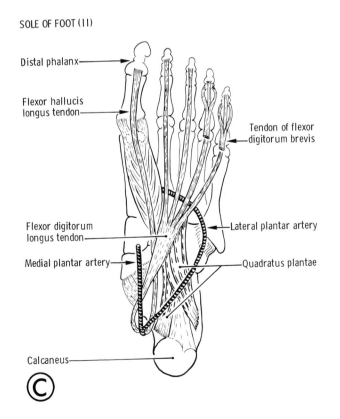

SOLE OF FOOT (II)

Distal phalanx

Flexor hallucis
longus tendon

Tendon of flexor
digitorum brevis

Flexor digitorum
longus tendon

Lateral plantar artery

Medial plantar artery

Quadratus plantae

Calcaneus

(C)

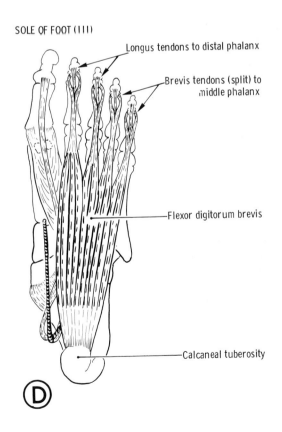

SOLE OF FOOT (III)

Longus tendons to distal phalanx

Brevis tendons (split) to
middle phalanx

Flexor digitorum brevis

Calcaneal tuberosity

(D)

A synovial sheath clothes the undivided tendon of flexor digitorum longus from beneath the flexor retinaculum to the junction of the tendon with quadratus plantae (**A**). Within each fibrous flexor sheath, the long and short tendons are enclosed in a common synovial sheath. The visceral layers surrounding the tendons are connected to the parietal layer lining the fibrous sheath by vincula which carry blood vessels to the tendons (**B**). Note that these synovial sheaths end proximally over the metatarsophalangeal joints, and that in the foot there is no sheath comparable to the ulnar bursa in the hand (**561A**).

The plantar vessels

Under cover of the flexor retinaculum, the posterior tibial artery divides into medial and lateral plantar arteries, which run forwards to supply all the tissues of the sole and the plantar aspects of the toes (**363C**). Both arteries are accompanied by venae comitantes. Note that the lateral plantar artery runs amongst the short plantar muscles towards the base of the fifth metatarsal. Then, bending sharply in a medial direction, it runs across the bases of the metatarsals above (deep to) the flexor tendons. The artery ends by joining the dorsalis pedis artery (**357D**) in the first metatarsal space and thus completes the plantar arch, which is comparable to the deep palmar arch in the hand (**563A**).

The plantar nerves

The tibial nerve (**361B**) divides into the medial and lateral plantar nerves deep to the flexor retinaculum, and the courses of these nerves within the sole are similar to those followed by the corresponding arteries.

They supply all the short plantar muscles, the motor fibres being derived from the S2, 3 spinal segments. The cutaneous branches supply the skin of the sole in front of the heel (**C**) (which is innervated directly from the tibial nerve), that of the plantar aspects of the toes, and that on the dorsal aspects of the toes round the nail beds (**D**).

Observe (**C**) the line demarcating the medial from the lateral plantar area on the skin of the sole and note its similarity to the line demarcating median and ulnar areas in the hand (**565E**). However, whereas the median and ulnar

nerves are quite frequently injured individually in the region of the wrist, individual injuries of the medial and lateral plantar nerves are rare.

Control of the arched form of the foot-plate

Refer back at this time to the arched form of the foot-plate (**346**) and the combinations of joint movements by which the arch may be relaxed or lowered (**352**).

In standing, there is no functional value in an arched foot-plate, and in individuals in whom free use of the foot has maintained free mobility of the foot-plate joints, the arch virtually disappears in that position. Such flattening of the foot-plate should not be regarded as abnormal.

Nowadays, perhaps owing to the habitual use of rather rigid footwear, few adults retain this degree of mobility. The range of movement at the joints of the foot-plate is reduced by disuse and a considerable degree of arching persists in standing. This position is maintained largely by tightening of the ligaments restricting those joint movements which would allow depression of the arch, namely the deltoid ligament (**349D**), the plantar ligaments of the foot-plate (**353A, 353B**) and the plantar aponeurosis (**357A**).

On the other hand, a highly arched form of the foot-plate suddenly becomes of functional value in that phase of the act of walking when the heel is raised and the foot-plate rests solely on the metatarsal heads (**355B, 355D**). At that time the arch is actively raised by those muscles which can produce the appropriate joint movements (**354**). Tibialis posterior inverts the subtalar joint, while the foot-plate is everted by peroneus longus and brevis, and plantar flexed by the short plantar muscles and the long flexors of the toes. It should be noted that although tibialis anterior is a strong invertor of the subtalar joint in the free toe, when the heel is raised in the weight-bearing foot the flaccidity of the palpable tendon of the muscle indicates that it is inactive. Thus in these circumstances it does not oppose the peroneus longus.

It is an inability to raise the arch in walking, rather than a flattening of the arch in standing, which constitutes the pathological condition of flat foot. This may be caused by an excessive rigidity of the foot-plate due to disease or congenital malformations of the foot-plate joints, or to a weakness of the arch-raising muscles.

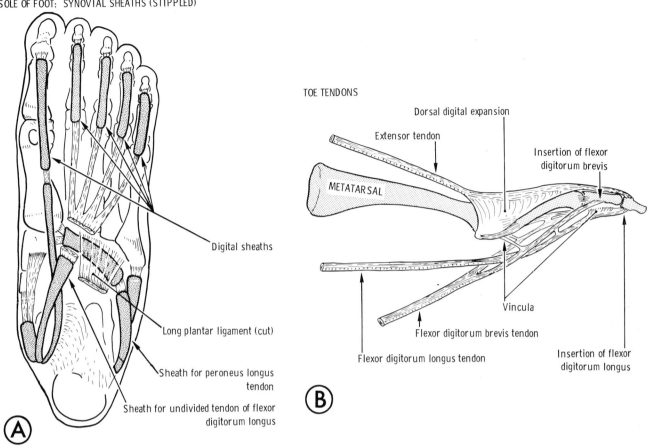

SOLE OF FOOT: SYNOVIAL SHEATHS (STIPPLED)

Digital sheaths

Long plantar ligament (cut)

Sheath for peroneus longus tendon

Sheath for undivided tendon of flexor digitorum longus

(A)

TOE TENDONS

Dorsal digital expansion

Extensor tendon

Insertion of flexor digitorum brevis

METATARSAL

Vincula

Flexor digitorum brevis tendon

Flexor digitorum longus tendon

Insertion of flexor digitorum longus

(B)

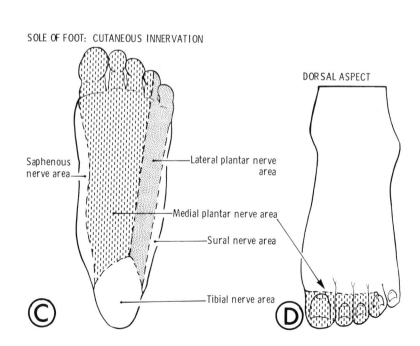

SOLE OF FOOT: CUTANEOUS INNERVATION

Saphenous nerve area

Lateral plantar nerve area

Medial plantar nerve area

Sural nerve area

Tibial nerve area

(C)

DORSAL ASPECT

(D)

WEIGHT-BEARING ACTIVITIES OF THE LOWER LIMB

Everyday life involves a wide spectrum of weight-bearing activities of the lower limb. Most of these are variations or combinations of three fundamental acts, namely, standing, walking and rising from a seated or crouched posture.

The joint movements which muscles may produce in the free lower limb have already been considered. However, in weight-bearing activities the importance of a muscle may often lie, not in its ability to produce a movement, but in its ability to restrain the opposite movement which body weight is tending to produce.

The act of standing

When people stand for any considerable length of time, they usually alternate between two rather different postures. In one of these (**A**) weight is borne equally by the two lower limbs (symmetrical standing), whereas in the other (**B**), weight is borne almost entirely by one limb, while the other is placed farther forwards and acts as a prop (asymmetrical standing).

Symmetrical standing

In this posture (**A**) the joints of the lower limbs must be stabilised against the potential effects of body-weight. The centre of gravity of the trunk lies in the lower part of the lumbar vertebral column, on a coronal plane which passes behind the flexion/extension axis of the hip joint, in front of that of the knee, and in front of the axis of the ankle. Consequently, the joint movements which body-weight tends to produce are extension of the hip, extension of the knee and dorsiflexion of the ankle. In addition, it tends to lower the arch of the foot-plate.

1. Extension at hip and knee are both limited very largely by articular mechanisms (**317F, 317G, 323D**) without the activity of flexor muscles. These articular mechanisms do not act suddenly at one position of the joint, but take the form of a rapidly increasing resistance to extension over a range of that movement. Consequently, the successful counter-action of extension by an articular mechanism does not necessarily mean that the joint cannot be farther extended. Contract one quadriceps muscle while you are standing symmetrically, and observe that the corresponding knee joint does in fact move a few degrees farther into extension.
2. In standing, the ankle joint, unlike the hip and knee, is not near one extreme of its range of movement, and cannot therefore be stabilised by an articular

mechanism. On the contrary, the dorsiflexion which body weight tends to produce has to be counteracted by activity in the plantarflexor muscles, principally soleus. However, symmetrical standing is not uncommonly an act of considerable duration, and it is important to appreciate that, in these circumstances, the ankle joint is not stabilised by continuous activity of soleus. Instead, a short burst of activity in that muscle pulls the body backwards over the foot, and this is succeeded by a period of inactivity during which body weight carries the body forwards once again. This cycle of activity and rest is repeated continuously as long as symmetrical standing persists, and it produces the slight backward and forward swaying of the body which can be readily observed if the position of a standing subject's head is compared to a fixed mark.
3. Maintenance of an arched form in the foot-plate in standing by tension in ligaments and the plantar aponeurosis has been considered already (**364**).

Asymmetrical standing

In this alternative posture (**B**) hip, knee and foot-plate in the weight-bearing limb are again stabilised by articular mechanisms, but the ankle is stabilised by the prop-like action of the other limb instead of by the intermittent activity of soleus. Asymmetrical standing is therefore the more economical of the two standing postures: indeed the great majority of individuals stand in this way most of the time.

The act of walking

In this very fundamental and complex human activity, each limb alternates between *stance phases*, when the foot contacts the ground, and shorter *swing phases*, when the limb swings forwards free of the ground (**C**). Each stance phase begins with heel contact. Towards its termination the heel is raised from the ground (*heel off*) and the phase ends when the toes leave the ground (*toe off*). The terminal part of the stance phase in one limb, overlaps the early part of the stance phase in the other limb. Consequently the act of walking, as a whole, can be regarded as an alternation between *double stance phases*, when both feet are on the ground, and *single stance phases*, when one foot is grounded while the other swings. At all times, except the middle of single stance phases, one limb (*the leading limb*) is in advance of the other (*the trailing limb*).

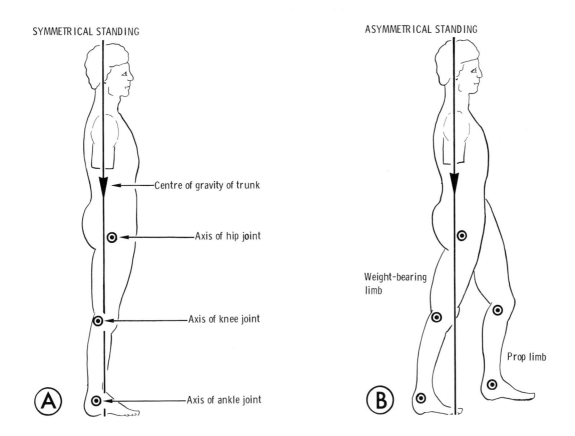

SYMMETRICAL STANDING

Centre of gravity of trunk

Axis of hip joint

Axis of knee joint

Axis of ankle joint

Ⓐ

ASYMMETRICAL STANDING

Weight-bearing limb

Prop limb

Ⓑ

PHASES OF WALKING

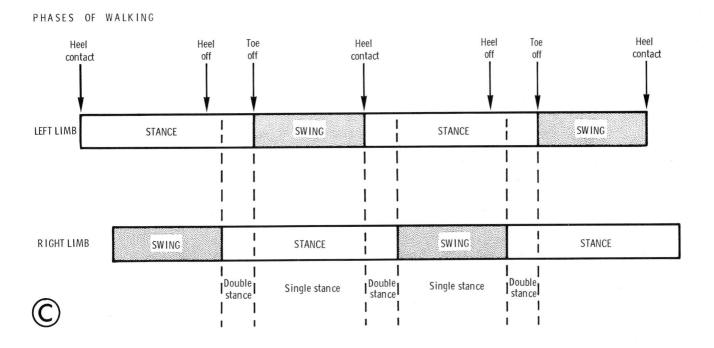

Heel contact

Heel off

Toe off

Heel contact

Heel off

Toe off

Heel contact

LEFT LIMB STANCE SWING STANCE SWING

RIGHT LIMB SWING STANCE SWING STANCE

Double stance Single stance Double stance Single stance Double stance

Ⓒ

Consider a swing phase of the left limb (**A, B, C**).

1. The limb is swung forward by flexion of the hip joint. In walking at a moderate rate this is a passive pendulum-like movement, but when the rate of walking is increased, and the limb has to be carried forward more quickly, the flexor muscles, particularly iliopsoas (**331B**), and the anterior adductors (**329A**) become involved.

2. While the limb swings forwards, the foot is raised clear of the ground through flexion of the knee by the hamstring muscles (**339A, 339C**), the dorsiflexion of the ankle by the muscles of the extensor compartment of the leg (**357D**).

3. Towards the end of the swing phase, extension of the knee by quadriceps (**329C**) to an angle of somewhat less than 180°, causes passive tightening of the hamstring muscles. This tension reverses the forward swing at the hip and plants the heel firmly on the ground.

Consider now the stance phase, again in relation to the left limb (**C, D, E**).

1. Owing to the momentum imparted to it during the previous step (see below) the trunk moves forward over the prop provided by the left limb (**C**), bringing the sole of the left foot into full contact with the ground (**D**) and thereafter passively dorsiflexing the ankle. The knee joint remains just short of 180° (see 3. above) and the tendency of body weight to increase the flexion of the joint is resisted by quadriceps.

2. At heel off (**E**) the ankle joint is forcibly plantarflexed by soleus and gastrocnemius so that an upward and forward force is applied to the body. The resultant of this force, and the downward force of body-weight, operates in a forward direction and moves the body forwards into the next step (see 1. above).

3. The forward impetus derived from plantarflexion of the ankle is augmented by flexion of the toes as the foot leaves the ground (**355B, 355D**). The movement is motivated by the long and short flexors of the hallux and other digits.

4. Between heel off (**E**) and toe off (**A**) the arch of the foot-plate is raised, so that its structure conforms to the stress pattern imposed by body-weight and the plantarflexors of the ankle. As noted previously (**364**) this change is produced by the short plantar muscles, tibialis anterior and posterior, and peroneus longus and brevis.

Throughout each single stance phase, while the body is supported only by one limb, the unbalancing effects of body weight in the coronal plane must be controlled (**F**).

1. In these circumstances, body-weight tends to depress the unsupported side of the pelvis, by adducting the supported hip joint. The displacement is prevented at each step by the activity of the gluteus medius and minimus (**337B**) on the supported side. Place your hands over these muscles in your own limbs, and confirm that right and left groups contract alternately each time the corresponding limb moves into its stance phase.

2. Once the pelvis is stabilised, the centre of gravity of the trunk must be moved over the single supporting foot. This is accomplished by slight lateral flexion of the vertebral column towards the supported side (**F**). Once equilibrium is achieved, the weight of the trunk tends to increase its own lateral flexion, and this is resisted by the vertebral muscles on the unsupported side of the body. Place your hands over the lumbar regions of your own erector spinae muscles and confirm that with each step the muscle on the unsupported side contracts.

3. When the body is balanced over one foot it is in unstable equilibrium in relation to the subtalar joint, and body weight tends to exaggerate the slightest deviation from that position. Equilibrium is maintained by balanced activities in tibialis anterior and posterior acting as invertors and the peroneal muscles acting as evertors (**F**).

The act of rising

In rising from a sitting posture, the arms are frequently used to push the trunk upwards and stabilise it over the supporting feet, but if the arms are not used, the trunk must be inclined forwards and the feet drawn back, so that the centre of gravity of the trunk lies over the feet, before rising can be accomplished (**G**). The body is straightened to a standing posture by extension of hip and knee and plantarflexion of the ankle. The hip is extended by contraction of the hamstring muscles and the femoral fibres of gluteus maximus. The contraction of these muscles can be felt in your own limbs. The knee joint is extended by quadriceps and the tibial fibres of gluteus maximus, and the activity of these muscles can be confirmed by palpating the front of the thigh and the iliotibial tract just above the lateral femoral condyle. Note that gluteus maximus is involved at both these joints, and the combined extension of hip and knee, which this muscle produces in rising, is its most important action. Plantarflexion of the ankle is caused by soleus and gastrocnemius.

Walking up steps or up a steep hill may be regarded as a combination of walking and rising, the muscle actions involved in rising being superimposed, at each step, on those characteristic of the early part of the stance phase of walking (**H**).

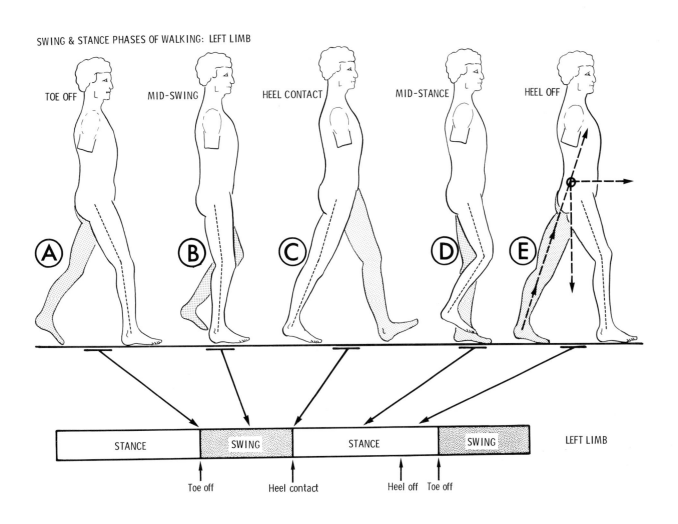

SWING & STANCE PHASES OF WALKING: LEFT LIMB

TOE OFF A

MID-SWING B

HEEL CONTACT C

MID-STANCE D

HEEL OFF E

| STANCE | SWING | STANCE | SWING | LEFT LIMB |

Toe off Heel contact Heel off Toe off

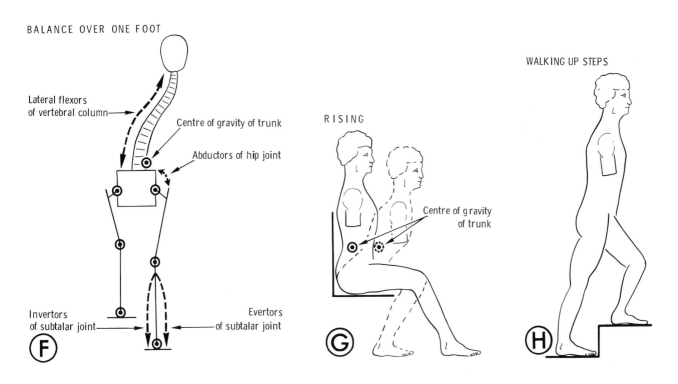

BALANCE OVER ONE FOOT

Lateral flexors of vertebral column

Centre of gravity of trunk

Abductors of hip joint

Invertors of subtalar joint

Evertors of subtalar joint

F

RISING

Centre of gravity of trunk

G

WALKING UP STEPS

H

369

Muscle paralyses in the lower limb

Paralyses of lower limb muscles or muscle groups cause loss of certain movements in the free part. They usually also have serious effects on the efficiency of weight-bearing activities, and it is these effects which are the main cause of disablement.

1. Paralysis of gluteus maximus has only a minimal effect on walking and standing. On the other hand, it will be clear that in rising from a seated or crouched posture (**369G**) the muscle is vital, and the act can only be accomplished with difficulty without it.
2. Gluteus medius and minimus are of little importance in standing or rising, but their paralysis seriously affects walking, for the pelvis can no longer be stabilised against body weight in the single stance phase (**369D**). In these circumstances, the patient learns to swing his trunk towards the paralysed side whenever the trunk is supported by the paralysed limb (**A**). This creates tension in the lateral abdominal muscles of the sound side which holds the pelvis level. But this displacement of the trunk causes a displacement of the centre of gravity in the same direction, and to maintain it over the supporting foot the pelvis is carried towards the sound side. The resulting gait is waddling and very characteristic, But it should be noted that a similar gait may be associated with congenital dislocation of the hip (**318**), because, although gluteus medius and minimus are not then paralysed, the approximation of their attachments by the dislocation prevents the muscles from exerting an abducting force at the hip joint.
3. Although paralysis of the quadriceps muscle affects both standing and rising, its most serious effect is noticed in the single stance phase of walking. Normally, throughout this phase, the muscle stabilises the supporting knee joint against body weight in a position just short of 180° (**B**). Without this muscle, the knee can only be stabilised by being locked in full extension. This is achieved by bending the trunk forwards or even by holding the knee back with one hand (**B**).
4. Paralysis of soleus and gastrocnemius is most noticeable during walking. The affected limb cannot impart a forward impetus to the body by plantarflexion of the ankle at the end of the stance phase (**C**). In consequence, the sound limb is never advanced beyond the affected limb, for no force would then be available to propel the body forwards over it. Instead, after it has delivered its force to the body at heel off (**C**), the sound limb passes through a shortened swing phase which ends when it comes level with the paralysed limb (**D**). The latter is then swung forwards by the activity of its hip flexor muscles, instead of by gravity and the trailing sound limb is ready once again to push the body forwards (**E**). This produces a staccato type of gait in which, characteristically, the paralysed limb is always leading and the sound limb always trailing.
5. Paralysis of the muscles of the extensor compartment of the leg has been considered elsewhere (**358**). It causes drop-foot, so that the foot tends to scrape against the ground during the swing phase of walking. If this is avoided by exaggerated bending of the knee, the swing phase ends with the whole foot being slapped on to the ground instead of by normal heel contact.

THE LYMPHATIC DRAINAGE OF THE LOWER LIMB

The two tissues in the lower limb which are associated with extensive lymphatic plexuses are the skin and the synovial membranes of the numerous joints. All the lymph vessels from the region eventually reach either the superficial or the deep group of inguinal nodes (**335C**), but it is important to note that both groups also receive vessels from tissues outside the lower limb.

The tributaries of the deep inguinal nodes follow the deep veins of the limb and are derived in large part from the synovial joints. This stream is joined:

1. in the popliteal fossa by lymph from the 'small saphenous area' of skin (see above) which first traverses the popliteal lymph nodes (**341C**).
2. in the upper part of the thigh by lymph from the glans penis or clitoris and, in the female, by lymph from the lateral angle of the uterus through vessels which run with the round ligament of the uterus.

The superficial inguinal nodes receive tributaries which run in the superficial fascia and come from:

1. the 'great saphenous area' of skin in the lower limb (see above).
2. the skin over the abdominal wall below the umbilicus.
3. the skin of the scrotum and penis, in the male, and the labia in the female.
4. the lining membrane of the lower half of the anal canal.

It should be noted particularly that the lymphatic vessels from the anal canal and the skin of the external genitalia to the inguinal nodes do not follow the direction of the venous drainage, as lymphatic vessels do in most regions of the body.

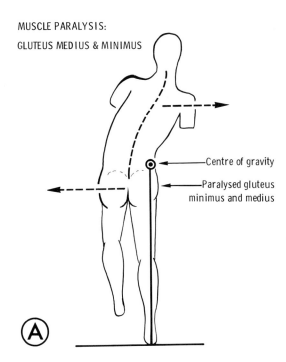

MUSCLE PARALYSIS:
GLUTEUS MEDIUS & MINIMUS

Centre of gravity

Paralysed gluteus
minimus and medius

(A)

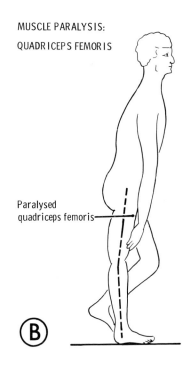

MUSCLE PARALYSIS:
QUADRICEPS FEMORIS

Paralysed
quadriceps femoris

(B)

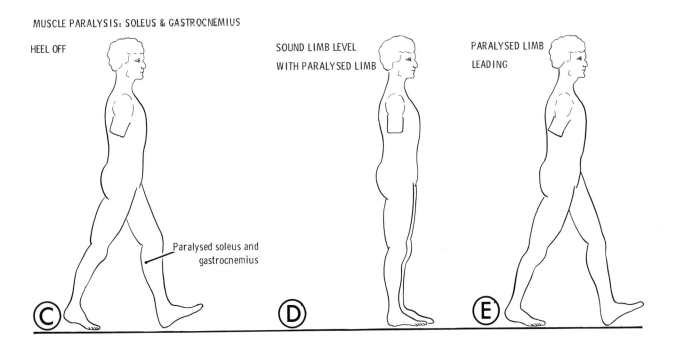

MUSCLE PARALYSIS: SOLEUS & GASTROCNEMIUS

HEEL OFF

Paralysed soleus and
gastrocnemius

(C)

SOUND LIMB LEVEL
WITH PARALYSED LIMB

(D)

PARALYSED LIMB
LEADING

(E)

371

THE SUPERFICIAL VEINS OF THE LOWER LIMB

The saphenous veins

The superficial fascia and skin of the whole lower limb are drained by two large superficial veins, the great (long) saphenous and the small (short) saphenous vein. They are equipped with numerous valves which direct the blood flow upwards. The terminations of these vessels, in the femoral and popliteal veins respectively, have been considered elsewhere (**335C, 343A**). The two veins begin at either end of a venous arch which traverses the superficial fascia on the dorsum of the foot (**A**). Observe their subsequent courses upwards through the superficial fascia (**A, B**) and note in particular the following points.

1. The relationship of the great saphenous vein to the medial border of the tibia, the medial malleolus and the saphenous nerve.
2. The relationship of the small saphenous vein to the lateral malleolus and the sural nerve.
3. The course of the great saphenous vein from the anterior aspect of the leg to the posteromedial aspect of the knee, and its return to the anterior aspect of the thigh.

The great saphenous vein is exposed throughout its length and removed when a long length of vein is required in surgery as a graft, either elsewhere in a limb or to bypass narrowed coronary arteries and so improve the blood supply to the myocardium. Although the great saphenous vein lies throughout its course in the superficial fascia, it is usually covered by a thin condensed layer of this tissue which has to be formally incised before the vein can be satisfactorily exposed.

The two saphenous veins are linked by a profuse plexus of smaller veins so that they cannot be regarded as having exact drainage areas. However, in general, the small saphenous drains from the lateral part of the foot and the posterior and lateral aspects of the leg, while the great saphenous drains the superficial fascia and skin of the rest of the lower limb. In addition it receives, near its termination (**335C**), three tributaries from the superficial tissues of the external genitalia and the anterior and lateral aspects of the abdominal wall below the level of the umbilicus. On the abdominal wall these latter tributaries are connected to the tributaries of the lateral thoracic vein which drains the superficial tissues above the umbilicus upwards to the axillary vein. These connections constitute the thoraco-epigastric venous channel (**C**). If venous drainage of the lower limb through the external iliac vein is blocked, this channel becomes dilated and varicose, and allows venous return to the heart by an alternative route. It is then readily visible through the skin.

The superficial veins of the lower limb are both connected to the deep veins by communicating vessels, often known as the perforators, which pierce the deep fascia (**D**). These connections are most numerous with the deep veins of the flexor compartment of the leg. The valves in the communicating veins are orientated so that they direct the blood flow from the superficial to the deep vessels.

In the erect posture the venous return through both the superficial and the deep vessels has to operate against a considerable hydrostatic pressure, and the origin of the force which overcomes this pressure appears to differ in the superficial and deep veins. In the deep veins it is the pressure on the vein wall caused by contraction of surrounding muscles within the rather rigid confines of osteofascial compartments (**D**), whereas in the superficial veins it is the tension created in the overlying skin by joint movements which squeezes the vessels against the underlying deep fascia or bone. In walking, both mechanisms are clearly operative but in static standing, although the intermittent contractions of the flexor muscles of the leg (**367A**) motivates flow through the deep veins, little force is exerted on the superficial vessels.

Because of the high pressures which they have to withstand, any of the veins of the lower limb may be subject to dilatation and consequent valvular incompetence (varicose veins). In this condition, the incompetency of the communicating vessels allows the blood to leak in the wrong direction from deep to superficial vessels, particularly in standing (see above). This tends to raise the pressure in the superficial veins still higher, and the resulting back pressure on the capillary plexus of the skin of the leg may interfere with the nourishment of this tissue and result in ulceration (varicose ulcer).

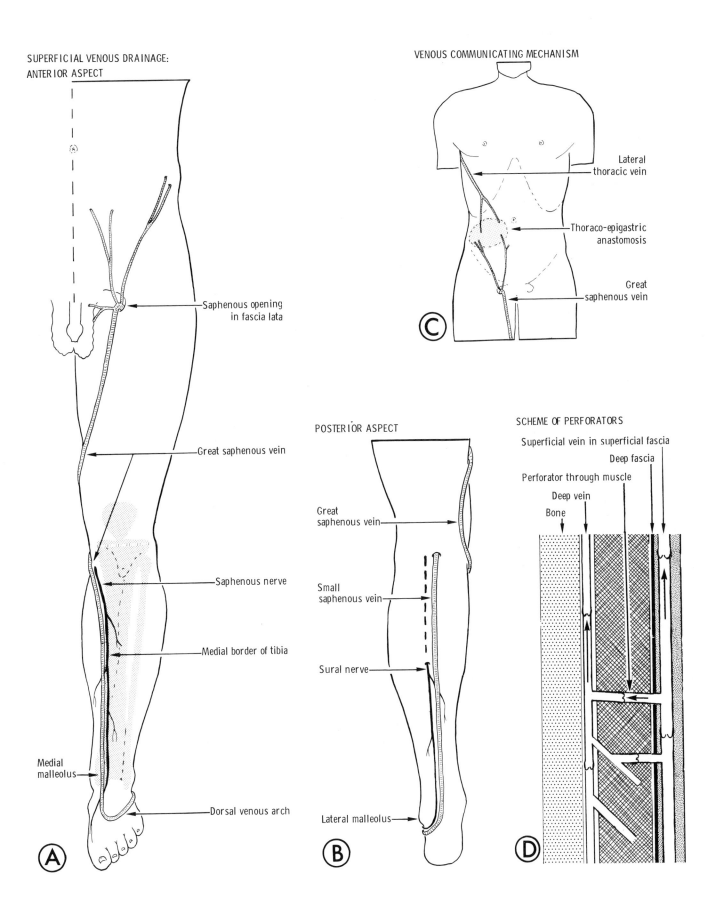

SUPERFICIAL VENOUS DRAINAGE:
ANTERIOR ASPECT

Saphenous opening
in fascia lata

Great saphenous vein

Saphenous nerve

Medial border of tibia

Medial
malleolus

Dorsal venous arch

Ⓐ

VENOUS COMMUNICATING MECHANISM

Lateral
thoracic vein

Thoraco-epigastric
anastomosis

Great
saphenous vein

Ⓒ

POSTERIOR ASPECT

Great
saphenous vein

Small
saphenous vein

Sural nerve

Lateral malleolus

Ⓑ

SCHEME OF PERFORATORS

Superficial vein in superficial fascia

Deep fascia

Perforator through muscle

Deep vein

Bone

Ⓓ

373

THE SEGMENTAL SOMATIC INNERVATION OF THE LOWER LIMB

Motor innervation

Recall certain general features of limb muscle innervation. The limb muscles are supplied by ventral rami of spinal nerves. Although most lower limb muscles receive nerve fibres from a number of spinal segments, usually the contribution from one segment predominates and those from others are of less clinical importance.

Limb muscles rarely act singly, but in groups which combine to effect specific joint movements. The joint movements which are associated with the individual spinal segments between L2 and S3, and which are seriously weakened by lesions in those segments, are shown in the following table, which is worth memorising.

L2: Flexion of the hip joint
L3: Extension of the knee joint
L4: Inversion of the subtalar joint
L5: Abduction of the hip joint
S1: Eversion of the subtalar joint
S2 and 3: Plantarflexion of the ankle joint and flexion of the toes

Cutaneous innervation

Disturbances of sensation in areas of skin in the lower limb may be due to injuries or disease processes in segments of the spinal cord, or to compression of individual spinal nerves in their intervertebral foramina, or to injury to peripheral nerves in the limb itself.

The peripheral nerves which are prone to injury are the lateral cutaneous nerve of the thigh (**332**), the saphenous nerve in the leg (**359C**) and the common peroneal nerve as it winds round the neck of the fibula (**357E**). The skin areas which these nerves supply should now be revised.

The segmental cutaneous innervation of the lower limb is illustrated in (**A**) and (**B**). Note that:

1. in broad terms the lumbar segments are associated with successive skin areas down the front of the limb and the first three sacral segments with successive areas up the back of the limb.
2. both the dorsal and plantar aspects of the foot are innervated by L4, L5 and S1 from medial to lateral side.
3. the skin areas supplied by some ventral rami are continuous with areas supplied by the numerically corresponding dorsal rami (L1, 2, S3), whereas in other cases this relationship does not exist.

It is difficult to remember the details of the complete pattern in **A** and **B** and it is perhaps more reasonable and more useful to concentrate on knowing certain localities on the skin surface which are associated with specific spinal segments. Such areas are indicated in (**A**) and (**B**) and described in the table below.

L1: Immediately below the centre of the inguinal ligament
L2: The middle of the front of the thigh
L3: Immediately above the patella
L4: The middle of the medial side of the leg
L5: The middle of the lateral side of the leg
S1: The back of the heel
S2: Over the popliteal fossa

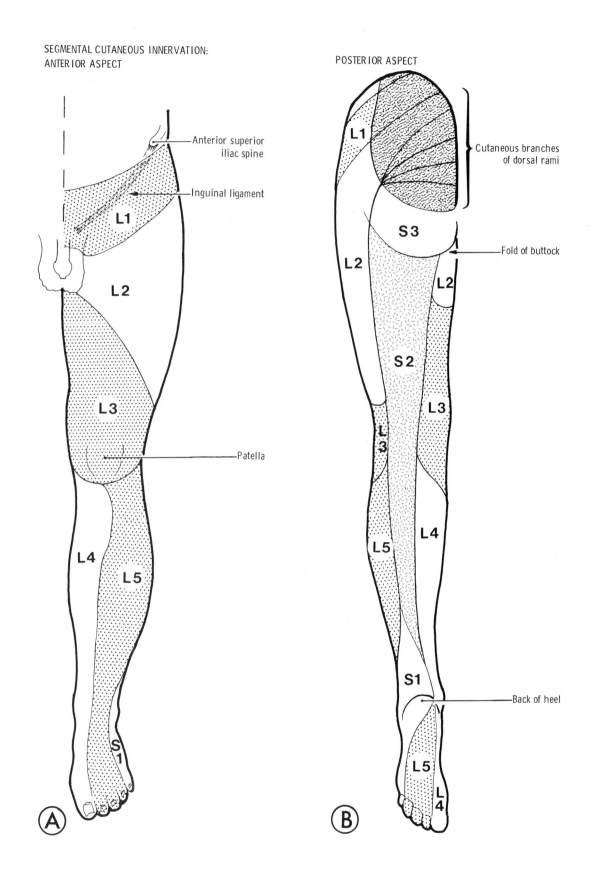

Anterior superior iliac spine

Inguinal ligament

L1

L2

L3

Patella

L4

L5

S1

(A)

POSTERIOR ASPECT

L1

Cutaneous branches of dorsal rami

S3

Fold of buttock

L2

L2

S2

L3

L3

L5

L4

S1

Back of heel

L5

L4

(B)

SYMPATHETIC INNERVATION OF THE LOWER LIMB

The autonomic supply to the lower limb consists entirely of sympathetic fibres. These control both the calibre of the blood vessels, through innervation of the plain muscle in their walls, and the degree of sweating, through innervation of the sweat glands of the skin.

The preganglionic neurons on the two-neuron sympathetic pathway have their cells in the lateral cell column of the central grey matter of the spinal cord in segments T10 to L2 inclusive, and traverse the ventral nerve roots, ventral rami and white rami communicantes to reach the corresponding ganglia on the sympathetic trunk (**A**). They then descend along the trunk to synapse with the cells of the second (postganglionic) neurons in the ganglia between L1 and S3 inclusive. Thereafter, postganglionic neurons pass through grey rami communicantes to the ventral rami of the corresponding spinal nerves and are distributed through both ventral and dorsal rami.

Every cutaneous nerve in the lower limb carries a complement of such postganglionic sympathetic fibres to the sweat glands and the superficial blood vessels in its area of distribution. Consequently division of such a nerve is associated not only with loss of sensation, but with lack of sweating and increase in the temperature of the skin in its area of distribution.

The major arteries of the lower limb are innervated by fine branches of postganglionic sympathetic fibres, which pass to them from neighbouring peripheral nerves. Thus the femoral artery and its main branches receive their supply mainly from the femoral nerve, and the anterior and posterior tibial arteries from the accompanying deep peroneal and tibial nerves.

Some clinical conditions may be alleviated by sympathetic denervation of the whole limb. Excessive sweating may be abolished, and the discomfort associated with the coldness of the skin, characteristic of degenerative arterial disease, may be greatly reduced.

From a consideration of the pathways from the spinal cord to the peripheral nerve of the lower limb (see above), it will be seen that denervation can be achieved by removal of the first three lumbar ganglia and the intervening parts of the sympathetic trunk (**B**).

SYMPATHETIC INNERVATION OF LOWER LIMB

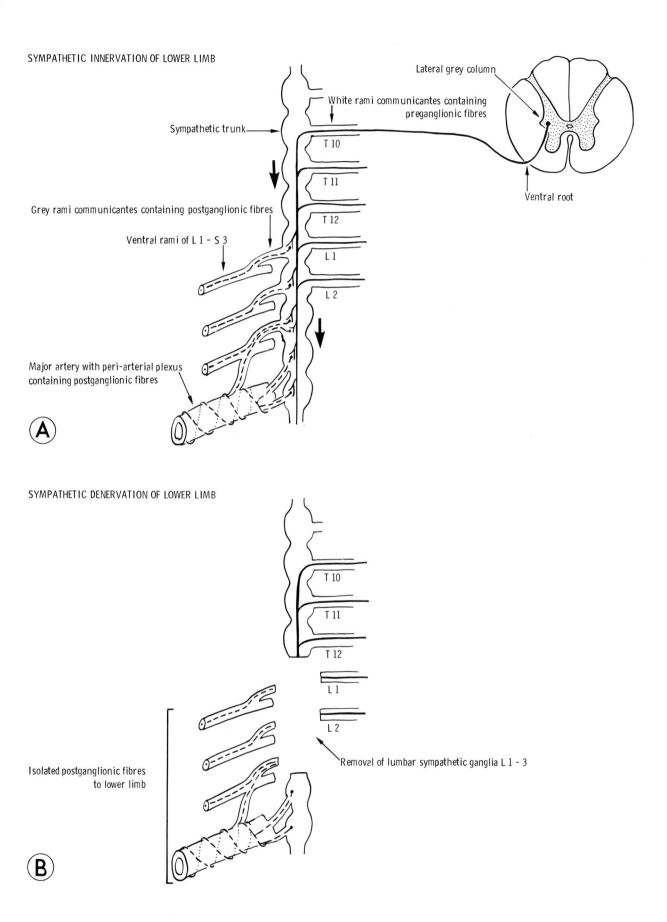

Lateral grey column

White rami communicantes containing preganglionic fibres

Sympathetic trunk

T 10

T 11

T 12

L 1

L 2

Ventral root

Grey rami communicantes containing postganglionic fibres

Ventral rami of L 1 - S 3

Major artery with peri-arterial plexus containing postganglionic fibres

A

SYMPATHETIC DENERVATION OF LOWER LIMB

T 10

T 11

T 12

L 1

L 2

Removal of lumbar sympathetic ganglia L 1 - 3

Isolated postganglionic fibres to lower limb

B

377

CHAPTER 6

The head and neck

THE SHOULDER GIRDLE AND CERVICAL VERTEBRAL MUSCLES

The cervical vertebrae and the base of the skull form the bony basis of the region of the neck. They, and the joints which separate them, have been considered previously and should now be revised (**5D, 6**). However, many of the structures in the neck are either attached to, or closely related to, the bones of the shoulder girdle by which the upper limbs are attached to the neck and thorax. It is convenient, therefore, to describe the form of the shoulder girdle here and return to its functional relationship to the upper limb in the next chapter (**494**).

The shoulder girdle

This consists of the paired clavicles (or collarbones), the paired scapulae (or shoulder blades) and the joints associated with them.

The clavicle

The clavicle lies more or less horizontally at the boundary between the neck above and the thorax and upper limbs below, and can be easily palpated throughout its length. The long axis of the shaft is S-shaped, the medial two-thirds, which is roughly cylindrical, being convex forwards and the lateral one-third, which is flattened from above down, being concave forwards (**A, B**). Observe the positions of the prominent bony features which mark the inferior aspect of the shaft (**B**). The bone has articular surfaces at its medial and lateral ends which will be described in relation to the joints with which they are associated.

Ossification begins in the clavicle earlier than in any other bone, by intramembranous ossification at the middle of a still mesenchymal model (**C**). Soon after, the remaining mesenchyme is converted to cartilage, and the original ossific centre extends towards the ends of the shaft by endochondral ossification (**D**). This process quickly reaches the lateral end of the bone, but a cartilaginous growth plate persists between the medial end of the bone and the shaft until about twenty, and it is here that all postnatal longitudinal growth of the clavicle occurs. A transitory secondary centre appears in the epiphysis at the medial end of the bone in late adolescence (**E**).

The sternoclavicular joint

The distal articular surface at this synovial joint is on the medial end of the clavicle while the proximal is formed by the clavicular notch on the manubrium sterni and upper surface of the first costal cartilage in continuity (**F**). The clavicular facet consists of dense fibrocartilage. It is convex in a downward and medial direction, particularly in its lower part, and, at rest, extends appreciably above the jugular notch of the sternum. The sternocostal facet consists of hyaline cartilage and is reciprocally curved.

The fibrous capsule is a short fibrous sleeve which is attached to the margins of the articular surfaces and is lined by synovial membrane.

An articular disc of fibrocartilage is interposed between the articular surfaces (**F**). It is most strongly attached, above, to the clavicle just beyond its articular surface and, below, to the first costochondral junction. Elsewhere its margin blends with the deep surface of the fibrous capsule so that it completely divides the joint cavity into two compartments.

The costoclavicular ligament is a strong accessory ligament lying just outside the lower part of the fibrous capsule (**F**). It is attached, below, to the first costochondral junction, close to the articular disc, and, above, to the costo-clavicular impression on the inferior aspect of the medial end of the clavicle (**B**).

The movements and stability of the joint are discussed with the mechanics of the shoulder girdle in the next chapter (**494**).

RIGHT CLAVICLE: SUPERIOR ASPECT

LATERAL   MEDIAL

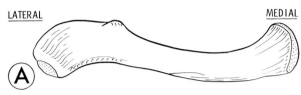

A

OSSIFICATION OF CLAVICLE:

primary ossification in mesenchymal model

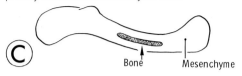

C

Bone   Mesenchyme

RIGHT CLAVICLE: INFERIOR ASPECT

Articular surfaces :stippled

LATERAL   MEDIAL

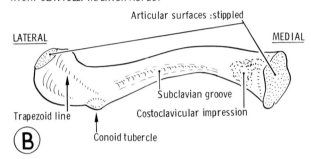

Trapezoid line

Conoid tubercle

Subclavian groove

Costoclavicular impression

B

OSSIFICATION OF CLAVICLE:

extension of ossification in cartilage model

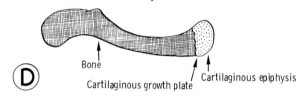

D

Bone

Cartilaginous growth plate   Cartilaginous epiphysis

OSSIFICATION OF CLAVICLE:

secondary centre in cartilaginous epiphysis

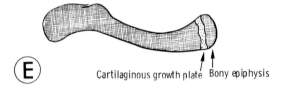

E

Cartilaginous growth plate   Bony epiphysis

RIGHT STERNOCLAVICULAR JOINT: CORONAL SECTION

Fibrous capsule

Clavicle

Fibrocartilaginous articular surface

Fibrocartilaginous articular disc

Jugular notch

Hyaline articular surface

Manubrium sterni

First rib

Costoclavicular ligament

Fibrous capsule

First costal cartilage

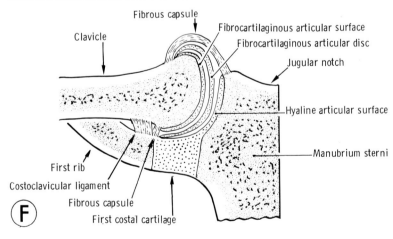

F

The scapula

The greater part of the scapula is a thin triangular plate of bone which overlies the upper part of the posterolateral aspect of the thoracic wall. It has costal and dorsal surfaces, superior, medial and lateral borders and superior, inferior and lateral angles.

Observe the following features in the isolated bone (**A**, **B**, **C**).

1. The lateral border is thick and, above, runs into the expanded lateral angle.
2. This angle carries the gently concave, oval glenoid fossa which is the proximal articular surface of the shoulder joint (**A**, **C**). The fossa is orientated at right angles to the plane of the scapula. The supraglenoid and infraglenoid tubercles lie above and below it (**C**).
3. The stout coracoid process arises from the lateral end of the superior border (**A**, **C**) and consists of two segments set at an angle, open forwards (**C**). The proximal segment is directed upwards, forwards and medially; the distal segment passes almost horizontally forwards.
4. The suprascapular notch, which marks the superior border just medial to the root of the coracoid process, is bridged by the suprascapular ligament (**B**).
5. The spine is a thick bony process which projects from the upper part of the dorsal surface (**B**). It arises along a somewhat oblique line from the junction of the upper third and lower two-thirds of the medial margin to just short of the glenoid fossa, and becomes progressively deeper from its medial to its lateral end. The posterior margin of the spine is expanded forming the crest of the spine, the junction of which with the medial border is a smooth triangular area (**B**).
6. The spine separates the smaller supraspinous fossa from the larger infraspinous fossa on the dorsal aspect of the scapula, but the two fossae communicate through the spinoglenoid notch between the lateral margin of the spine and the glenoid fossa (**B**).
7. The lateral end of the crest of the spine is continued forwards, above and behind the glenoid fossa as the flat acromion (process) which presents upper and lower surfaces and medial and lateral margins (**A**, **B**, **C**). A small articular facet (see below) lies on the anterior part of the medial margin (**A**).

8. The coraco-acromial ligament is flat and triangular (**C**), with an apical attachment to the anterior extremity of the acromion and a basal attachment to the lateral margin of the distal segment of the coracoid process. As it joins two parts of the same bone it cannot have a direct effect on any joint, but it will be seen (**498**) that it does have an indirect effect on the stability of the shoulder joint.

In the living subject, confirm that the inferior angle of the scapula, the crest of the spine and the acromion and the tip of the coracoid process are palpable.

Ossification of the greater part of the cartilaginous scapula occurs from a primary centre appearing early in intra-uterine life. Secondary centres appear in the main part of the coracoid process in the first year, and in the root of the coracoid plus the upper third of the glenoid fossa (the subcoracoid centre) at about 10 (**D**). These centres fuse with the primary bone at about 16. Other secondary centres form in the medial border, inferior angle and acromion at puberty and join the rest of the bone in the early twenties.

The acromioclavicular joint

The articular surfaces on the medial margin of the acromion and the lateral end of the clavicle are small, oval, fibrocartilaginous facets which face upwards and medially and laterally and downwards respectively (**F**).

The fibrous capsule encloses the joint and is strongest superiorly (**E**).

A wedge-shaped, fibrocartilaginous *articular disc* projects into the joint from the upper part of the fibrous capsule but does not usually separate the articular surfaces completely (**F**).

The coracoclavicular ligament is an accessory ligament of the joint and is the main factor maintaining its integrity (**E**). It consists of two usually separate parts which are named according to their shapes. The conoid part has an apical attachment to the proximal segment of the coracoid process beside the suprascapular notch, and a broader basal attachment to the conoid tubercle on the clavicle (**381B**). The trapezoid part is attached by its inferomedial margin to the upper surface of the distal segment of the coracoid process and passes upwards and laterally to the trapezoid line on the clavicle (**381B**).

The mechanics of the joint will be discussed in the following chapter (**495B**).

RIGHT SCAPULA: ANTERIOR ASPECT

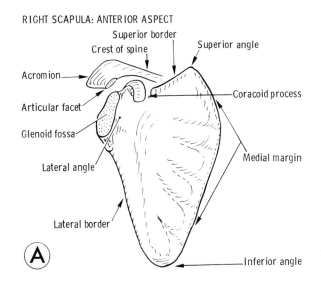

Superior border
Crest of spine
Superior angle
Acromion
Articular facet
Glenoid fossa
Coracoid process
Lateral angle
Medial margin
Lateral border
Inferior angle

(A)

RIGHT SCAPULA: POSTERIOR ASPECT

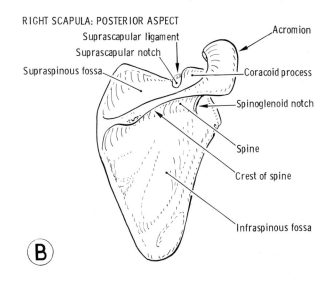

Suprascapular ligament
Suprascapular notch
Supraspinous fossa
Acromion
Coracoid process
Spinoglenoid notch
Spine
Crest of spine
Infraspinous fossa

(B)

RIGHT SCAPULA: ANTEROLATERAL ASPECT

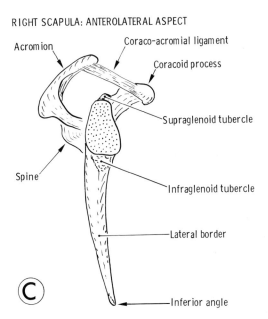

Acromion
Coraco-acromial ligament
Coracoid process
Supraglenoid tubercle
Spine
Infraglenoid tubercle
Lateral border
Inferior angle

(C)

OSSIFICATION OF SCAPULA AT 12 YEARS: ANTEROLATERAL VIEW

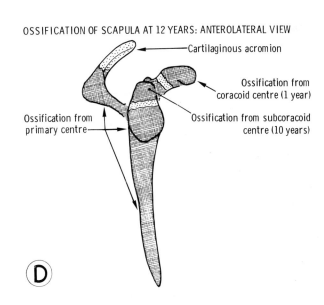

Cartilaginous acromion
Ossification from coracoid centre (1 year)
Ossification from primary centre
Ossification from subcoracoid centre (10 years)

(D)

RIGHT ACROMIOCLAVICULAR JOINT: ANTERIOR ASPECT

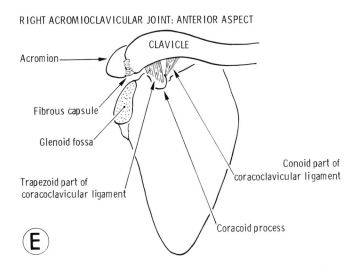

CLAVICLE
Acromion
Fibrous capsule
Glenoid fossa
Trapezoid part of coracoclavicular ligament
Conoid part of coracoclavicular ligament
Coracoid process

(E)

RIGHT ACROMIOCLAVICULAR JOINT: CORONAL SECTION

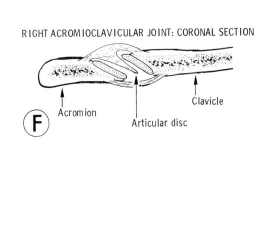

Acromion
Articular disc
Clavicle

(F)

383

The relationship of shoulder girdle, thorax, neck and upper limb

1. The medial border of the scapula lies against the posterior aspect of the chest wall, some 8 cm from the midline. At rest the superior angle is level with the spine of the second thoracic vertebra and the inferior angle with the spine of the seventh (**A**).
2. As has been noted already, at rest, the clavicle lies more or less horizontally and articulates medially at the sternoclavicular joint and laterally at the acromioclavicular joint (**B**).
3. Because of the interposition of the clavicle, the acromion and the lateral border of the scapula are held away from the chest wall (**B**). The plane of the scapula is thus oblique, passing from behind forwards and laterally so that the glenoid fossa faces in the direction of this plane and a little upwards (**B, C**). Moreover, a tissue space called the axilla (armpit) intervenes between the costal surface of the scapula and the chest wall in the uppermost part of the upper limb (**B, C**).
4. It should be recalled (**125B**) that because of the shape of the thoracic cage the shaft of the first rib, unlike the others of the series, has upper and lower surfaces and inner and outer borders. Moreover, because of the obliquity of the thoracic inlet, the neck and head of the rib lie above the level of the clavicle, whereas the anterior end of the shaft is below the level of that bone (**B**).
5. The tissues of the neck are continuous with those of the axilla through a space called the apex of the axilla. Observe that the space, which is traversed by a thick arrow in **B**, has three boundaries formed by the superior margin of the scapula, the outer border of the first rib and the posterior aspect of the clavicle.

The general arrangement of the tissues of the neck

This arrangement is most easily appreciated in a horizontal section through the neck such as that in **D**.

1. Posteriorly, the cervical part of the vertebral column is clothed by longitudinal muscles which comprise three groups called prevertebral, postvertebral and deep lateral.
2. The prevertebral and deep lateral groups are covered by the prevertebral layer of deep fascia. Above, this is attached to the base of the skull, and below, extends into both the superior mediastinum and the axilla. Posteriorly, over the postvertebral muscles, it fades out as a recognisable layer.
3. The central part of the region in front of the vertebral muscles, from the base of the skull to the thoracic inlet, is occupied by the pharynx and larynx and their downward continuations which are the cervical parts of the oesophagus and the trachea.
4. In the lower part of the neck (**D**) other viscera, the thyroid and parathyroid glands, are closely related to the anterior and lateral aspects of the digestive and respiratory passages.
5. The main neurovascular bundle of the neck, enclosed in the fascial carotid sheath, extends from the base of the skull to the root of the neck, lying in the angle between the prevertebral fascia and the midline viscera.
6. All the structures listed above are enclosed by the investing layer of deep fascia which extends as a wide tube from the skull to the shoulder girdle. On either side of the neck, the layer splits to enclose two large superficial lateral muscles called the sternocleido-mastoid (sternomastoid) and the trapezius (**D**).
7. Peripheral to this investing deep fascia are the superficial fascia and skin.

SHOULDER GIRDLE & THORACIC CAGE: POSTERIOR ASPECT

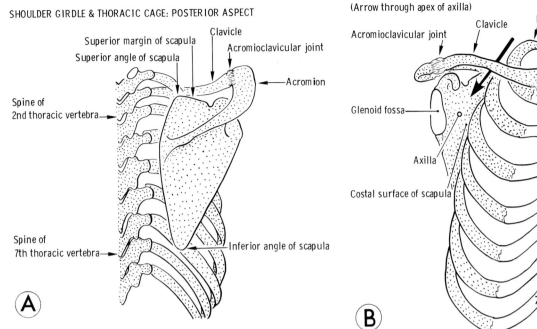

Superior margin of scapula
Superior angle of scapula
Clavicle
Acromioclavicular joint
Acromion
Spine of 2nd thoracic vertebra
Spine of 7th thoracic vertebra
Inferior angle of scapula

A

SHOULDER GIRDLE & THORACIC CAGE: ANTERIOR VIEW
(Arrow through apex of axilla)

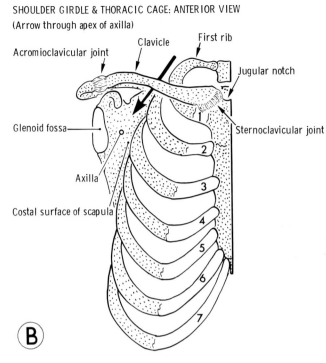

Acromioclavicular joint
Clavicle
First rib
Jugular notch
Glenoid fossa
Sternoclavicular joint
Axilla
Costal surface of scapula

B

AXILLA: HORIZONTAL SECTION (X-X scapular plane)

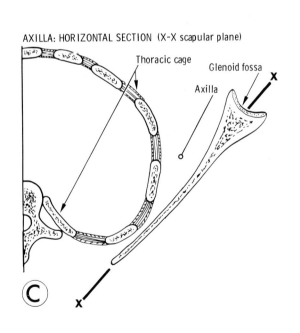

Thoracic cage
Glenoid fossa
Axilla

C

LOWER PART OF NECK: HORIZONTAL SECTION

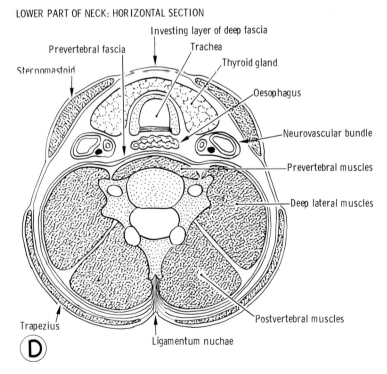

Investing layer of deep fascia
Prevertebral fascia
Trachea
Sternomastoid
Thyroid gland
Oesophagus
Neurovascular bundle
Prevertebral muscles
Deep lateral muscles
Postvertebral muscles
Trapezius
Ligamentum nuchae

D

385

The vertebral muscles

The postvertebral group

On either side of the midline a large postvertebral group of muscles, consisting of a number of separate or partially separate components, which need not be known individually, lies along the gutter formed by the cervical transverse processes, laminae and spinous processes and the ligamentum nuchae (**385D**).

Below (**A**), the group is continuous with the erector spinae muscle on the posterior thoracic wall; in the neck many of the muscle fibres are attached to the adjacent parts of the cervical vertebrae; while above many of the fibres are attached to the skull over the area between the foramen magnum and the superior nuchal line (**B**).

The group acts on the intervertebral, atlanto-axial (**6**) and atlanto-occipital (**18**) joints producing extension and rotation of the head and vertebral column.

The prevertebral group

This group also consists of a number of components, but again it is unnecessary to know these individually (**C**). The fibres are attached to the surface of the cervical and upper thoracic parts of the anterior longitudinal ligament and the anterior aspects of most of the cervical transverse processes, and many are attached to the base of the skull, anterior and lateral to the occipital condyles (**B**). The only particular feature of the group which should be noted is the lower part of its lateral border, which extends downwards and medially from the anterior aspect of the C6 transverse process to the upper thoracic vertebral bodies (**C**).

The group produces flexion of the cervical vertebral column and the head.

The deep lateral muscles

These muscles, unlike those of the previous two groups between which they lie, must be considered individually.

They arise on either side of the neck from the cervical transverse processes and incline downwards and laterally.

The levator scapulae is attached above to the posterior parts of the upper transverse processes and descends anterolateral to the postvertebral group (**A**) and behind the other deep lateral muscles (**C**). It is inserted into the medial border of the scapula above the spine (**A**). It acts primarily on the shoulder girdle (**495A**).

The scalenus posterior and medius arise from the posterior parts of most of the cervical transverse processes and pass downwards and laterally in front of levator scapulae (**C**). The small posterior muscle crosses the outer margin of the first rib and is inserted into the outer surface of the shaft of the second rib. The larger medius muscle inserts into the rough posterior third of the upper surface of the shaft of the first rib (**D**).

The scalenus anterior, unlike the other members of the deep lateral group, arises from the anterior, not the posterior parts, of most of the cervical transverse processes, in close association with the attachments of many of the prevertebral muscle fibres (see above). Inclining downwards and laterally, it is inserted by a narrow tendon into the small scalene tubercle on the first rib (**C, D**). Observe the following features of the muscle (**C**).

1. Its lowest fibres are attached, like those of the prevertebral group, to the C6 transverse process.
2. It is consequently separated from the lowest prevertebral muscle fibres by a triangular space with its apex at the C6 transverse process (**C**). The triangle is called by some the vertebral triangle because, as will be seen later, it contains part of the vertebral artery.
3. The insertion of scalenus anterior is separated from that of the scalenus medius by the subclavian groove on the first rib (**D**).

THE SPINAL NERVES OF THE NECK

These are the cervical nerves and branches of the first two thoracic nerves.

Recall (**35A**) that nerves C1–7 leave the vertebral canal above the vertebrae of corresponding number, C8 between vertebrae C7 and T1 and nerves T1 and 2 below the vertebrae of corresponding number. Revise also (**5C, 7E**) the boundaries of the typical cervical and thoracic intervertebral foramina, and the atypical forms of the apertures through which nerves C1 and 2 leave the vertebral canal.

Each nerve having emerged from the vertebral canal divides into a dorsal and a ventral ramus.

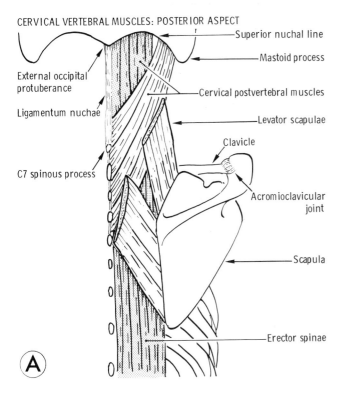

CERVICAL VERTEBRAL MUSCLES: POSTERIOR ASPECT

- Superior nuchal line
- Mastoid process
External occipital protuberance
- Cervical postvertebral muscles
Ligamentum nuchae
- Levator scapulae
Clavicle
C7 spinous process
- Acromioclavicular joint
- Scapula
- Erector spinae

(A)

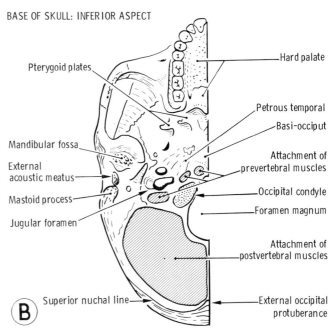

BASE OF SKULL: INFERIOR ASPECT

Pterygoid plates
- Hard palate
Mandibular fossa
- Petrous temporal
- Basi-occiput
External acoustic meatus
- Attachment of prevertebral muscles
Mastoid process
- Occipital condyle
Jugular foramen
- Foramen magnum
- Attachment of postvertebral muscles
Superior nuchal line
- External occipital protuberance

(B)

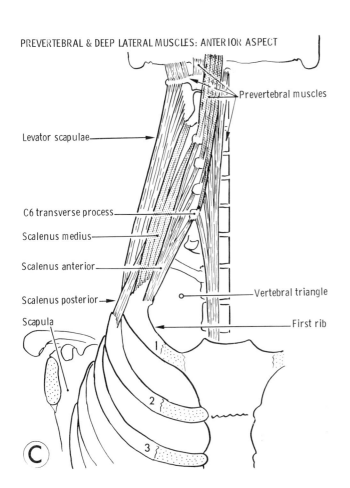

PREVERTEBRAL & DEEP LATERAL MUSCLES: ANTERIOR ASPECT

- Prevertebral muscles
Levator scapulae
C6 transverse process
Scalenus medius
Scalenus anterior
Scalenus posterior
Scapula
- Vertebral triangle
- First rib

(C)

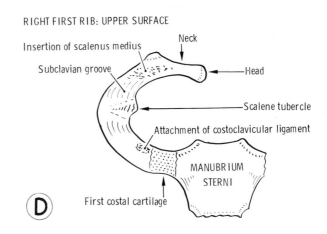

RIGHT FIRST RIB: UPPER SURFACE

Insertion of scalenus medius
Neck
Subclavian groove
- Head
- Scalene tubercle
Attachment of costoclavicular ligament
MANUBRIUM STERNI
First costal cartilage

(D)

The dorsal rami wind backwards round the posterior margin of the intervertebral foramina into the postvertebral group of muscles which they innervate (**A**). In addition, cutaneous branches arise from the dorsal rami of C2 (the greater occipital nerve), C3, 4 and 5 and T1 and 2, and supply the skin on the dorsal aspect of the body between the levels of the lambdoid suture above and the second rib below (**B**). The dorsal rami of C1, 7 and 8 are devoid of cutaneous fibres.

The ventral rami supply branches to the prevertebral and deep lateral muscles of the neck (**A**) and, passing laterally, form the roots of the cervical and brachial nerve plexuses.

The cervical plexus

The roots of this plexus are the ventral rami of the spinal nerves C1–4. The ventral ramus of C1 passes forwards above the transverse process of the atlas (**D**). The other rami run laterally over the grooved upper surfaces of the numerically corresponding transverse processes, passing in each case behind the foramen transversarium (**A, C**). As shown in **D**, the nerves emerge anterior to the levator scapulae and scalenus medius muscles, where they are joined by three loops. The branches of the plexus, which will be considered subsequently at convenient points in the text, arise from both the roots and the loops.

The brachial plexus

The constant roots of the plexus, which are considerably larger than those of the cervical plexus, are the ventral rami of C5–8 and the large ascending branch of the ventral ramus of T1. In addition, the C5 root often receives a descending branch from the ventral ramus of C4, and the T1 root an ascending branch from the ventral ramus of T2. If the communication from C4 is large, that from T2 may be absent, and the plexus is said to be prefixed. If the opposite arrangement obtains the plexus is said to be postfixed.

The plexus consists of roots, trunks, divisions, and cords. Branches arise from all these parts except the divisions. The general form of the plexus is shown diagrammatically in **C** and should be studied until it can be readily and accurately reproduced. Observe the following features.

1. The C5 and C6 roots join to form the upper trunk, the C7 root is continued unchanged as the middle trunk, while the C8 and T1 roots join to form the lower trunk.

2. Each trunk divides into anterior and posterior divisions, the posterior division of the lower trunk being small.
3. The anterior divisions of the upper and middle trunks join to form the lateral cord, the posterior divisions of the three trunks join to form the posterior cord, while the anterior division of the lower trunk becomes the medial cord.
4. Note the root sources of the fibres in the three trunks and three cords.

By reference to the diagram in **C** identify the roots, trunks and divisions of the brachial plexus in **D** and observe their relationship to neighbouring structures in the lower part of the neck. It should be noted particularly that in **D** the scalenus anterior has been removed.

The roots pass laterally from the vertebral column. Those of C5 and 6 lie on the upper surfaces of the corresponding transverse processes behind the foramina transversaria. The C7 root is in the interval between the C6 and C7 transverse processes. The C8 root is between the C7 transverse process and the neck of the first rib. The T1 root arises as a large branch of the ventral ramus of T1 between the necks of the first and second ribs, and inclines laterally and upwards over the inner border of the shaft of the first rib.

The trunks are short and converge downwards and laterally on the anterior surface of the lateral part of scalenus medius. As the lower trunk lies in front of that muscle, it is in contact with the posterior part of the subclavian groove on the upper surface of the first rib. Pressure on the nerve, resulting from this contact, will give rise to symptoms associated with the structures of the upper limb innervated by fibres in the C8 and T1 roots of the plexus.

The divisions continue downwards and laterally and converge into a closer relationship than is indicated in **D**. They then pass from the neck through the apex of the axilla into the axilla in the upper limb, where the cords are formed.

The branches may be classified as supraclavicular, arising in the neck from the roots and trunks, and infraclavicular, arising in the axilla from the cords. The individually important supraclavicular branches are the contribution to the phrenic nerve from the C5 root, and the suprascapular and long thoracic nerves which will be considered in the next chapter.

EMERGENCE OF TYPICAL SPINAL NERVE FROM VERTEBRAL CANAL

Foramen transversarium

Root of cervical or brachial plexus

Prevertebral muscle group

Deep lateral muscle group

Intervertebral foramen

Superior articular facet

Postvertebral muscle group

Dorsal ramus

Ventral ramus of typical spinal nerve

Cutaneous branches of dorsal ramus

(A)

DIAGRAMMATIC REPRESENTATION OF BRACHIAL PLEXUS

Trunks

Roots

C 5

Lateral cord (C 5, 6, 7)

Anterior divisions

Upper (C 5, 6)

C 6

Posterior cord (C 5, 6, 7, 8, T 1)

Middle (C 7)

C 7

Medial cord (C 8, T 1)

Lower (C 8, T 1)

C 8

Posterior divisions

T 1

(C)

DORSAL RAMI OF CERVICAL & UPPER THORACIC NERVES:

CUTANEOUS DISTRIBUTION (stippled area)

Area supplied by trigeminal nerve

Position of lambdoid suture

C 2

C 3

Position of superior nuchal line

C 4

Area supplied by ventral rami

C 5

Spinous processes C 7, T 1, 2, 3

T 1

T 2

(B)

CERVICAL & BRACHIAL PLEXUSES

Prevertebral muscles

Transverse process of atlas

Loops of cervical plexus

Levator scapulae

Scalenus medius

C6 transverse process

C7 transverse process

Suprascapular nerve

1

2

Scapula

Cords of brachial plexus

Subclavian groove on 1st rib

Sympathetic trunk

(D)

SOME PREVERTEBRAL STRUCTURES IN THE NECK

Excluding for the present the pharynx and larynx and the thyroid and parathyroid glands, we will now build up progressively the structures which lie in front of those shown in **389D**.

The cervical oesophagus

This muscular tube is continuous with the lower end of the pharynx at the level of the sixth cervical vertebra. Beginning in the midline it descends with a slight inclination to the left (**A**) and passes through the thoracic inlet into the superior mediastinum. It is loosely attached to the prevertebral fascia by areolar tissue. It has been noted previously that the character of the outer longitudinal and inner circular muscle coats of the oesophagus change along the length of the viscus. In the cervical region both coats consist of striated muscle.

The cervical part of the trachea

The trachea, which is continuous above with the larynx, begins at the same level as the oesophagus. Inclining very slightly to the right as it descends in front of the oesophagus it passes with that structure into the thorax (**A**). The structure of the cervical part of the trachea is the same as that of the thoracic part which has been described previously (**147C**).

The cervical pleura

As it covers the apex of the lung, the cervical pleura rises as a dome through the plane of the thoracic inlet into the root of the neck (**A**). Because of the obliquity of the first rib, the highest part of this region of pleura is level with the neck of that rib, but about 3.5 cm above the first costal cartilage. As the first rib is difficult or impossible to palpate in the living, the relationship of the cervical pleura is of much greater importance. Observe in **A** how the cervical pleura rises to a height of 2.5 cm above the medial third of the clavicle, so that a perforating injury in that region may open the pleural cavity and damage the apex of the lung.

Medially, the cervical pleura turns downwards and becomes continuous with the mediastinal pleura. In all other directions it is continuous with the costal pleura.

Note that, with the cervical pleura in position, the sympathetic trunk is now seen emerging from the thorax into the neck between the pleura and the neck of the first rib, while the ascending branch of the ventral ramus of the first thoracic nerve (the T1 root of the brachial plexus) appears, passing laterally between the pleura and the inner margin of the shaft of the first rib.

The subclavian arteries

As has been seen previously the two subclavian arteries (**A**) have asymmetrical origins. The right, with the right common carotid artery, begins at the bifurcation of the brachiocephalic artery to the right of the trachea and behind the upper border of the right sternoclavicular joint. The left, arising directly from the aortic arch, ascends through the superior mediastinum, behind and to the left of the left common carotid artery, until it is situated behind the upper part of the left sternoclavicular joint. Thereafter the courses of the two subclavian arteries are symmetrical. Each vessel curves laterally with an upward convexity across the anterior surface of the cervical pleura and continues across the subclavian groove on the upper surface of the first rib, lying immediately in front of the lower trunk of the brachial plexus. At the outer border of the first rib, which will be recalled as one of the boundaries of the apex of the axilla, the vessel becomes the axillary artery.

The relationship of the cervical pleura to the readily palpable clavicle has been stressed above. The relationship of the subclavian artery to this bone is equally important (**A**). Its curved course carries the artery above the medial half of the clavicle to a height which varies but is, on average, about 1.5 cm.

The scalenus anterior muscle

This muscle has been described already as one of the deep lateral muscles of the neck (**387C**). The left scalenus anterior is now shown in **A**. Observe that it descends to its insertion in front of the roots of the brachial plexus and in front of the subclavian artery. It is customary to describe each subclavian artery as consisting of three parts. The first part is medial to scalenus anterior, and is much shorter on the right than the left, the short second part lies behind the muscle, and the third part between the lateral border of the muscle and the outer border of the first rib.

Observe that at this stage of our build-up of the region the structures which are visible from above downwards in the vertebral triangle (**A**) are the C7 root of the brachial plexus, the C7 transverse process, the C8 root of the plexus, the neck of the first rib with the sympathetic trunk in front of it, and the cervical pleura.

DEEP STRUCTURES OF ROOT OF NECK (Right clavicle & aortic arch & its branches are indicated by interrupted lines)

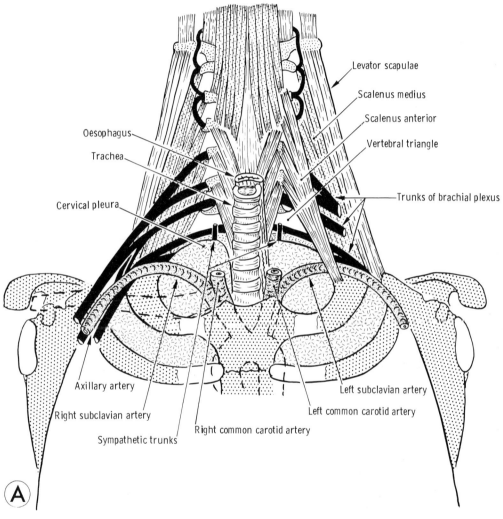

Levator scapulae

Scalenus medius

Scalenus anterior

Vertebral triangle

Trunks of brachial plexus

Oesophagus

Trachea

Cervical pleura

Axillary artery

Right subclavian artery

Sympathetic trunks

Right common carotid artery

Left common carotid artery

Left subclavian artery

(A)

As the brachial plexus and the subclavian artery emerge from between scalenus anterior and medius they carry with them a funnel-shaped extension of the prevertebral fascia. This continues as an investment of the neurovascular bundle into the axilla and is called the axillary sheath.

In **A** identify the structures which have already been illustrated on the previous page and are not labelled again.

The cervical sympathetic trunk

As it leaves the thorax between the cervical pleura and the neck of the first rib, the sympathetic trunk turns forwards and joins the inferior cervical ganglion. It will be recalled (**115C**) that frequently the inferior cervical and first thoracic ganglia are in fact continuous (a cervicothoracic or stellate ganglion).

The inferior cervical ganglion is large and lies in the vertebral triangle (**A**), on the uppermost part of the cervical pleura and in front of the C8 root of the brachial plexus.

The considerably smaller middle cervical ganglion lies on the origin of fibres of scalenus anterior and the prevertebral muscles from the anterior aspect of the C6 transverse process (**A**).

The superior cervical ganglion is fusiform in shape and is situated in front of the muscle fibres attached to the anterior aspects of the C1, 2 and 3 transverse processes (**A**).

The parts of the sympathetic trunk which join these ganglia to one another usually consist of a number of separate strands which are indicated in **B** but not in **A**.

The source of the preganglionic fibres which reach the cervical ganglia (**117B, 117C**) should be revised. In particular recall that these ganglia have no white rami communicantes. On the other hand they have a number of branches consisting mainly of postganglionic fibres.

1. Grey rami communicantes (**B**) pass from the superior ganglion to the C1, 2, 3 and 4 ventral rami and are distributed through the branches of the cervical plexus to blood vessels and skin in the head and neck region. Grey rami also pass from the middle ganglion to the C5 and 6 ventral rami, and from the inferior ganglion to the C7 and 8 ventral rami, and are thereafter distributed through the brachial plexus and its branches to the blood vessels and skin of the upper limb.
2. Vascular branches, which are mainly vasomotor in function, pass from each ganglion on to neighbouring large arteries. That from the superior ganglion forms a plexus on the wall of the internal carotid artery (**394**). Those from the middle ganglion pass onto the vertebral and inferior thyroid arteries (see below) and that from the inferior ganglion onto the wall of the subclavian artery (**390**).
3. Each cervical ganglion gives off a visceral (cardiac) branch which descends through the neck and superior mediastinum to the cardiac plexus (**B**). All the cardiac branches contain postganglionic sympathetic fibres, but in addition those from the middle and inferior ganglia contain visceral sensory fibres concerned with pain, which descend along the cervical sympathetic trunk and have their cells of origin in the spinal ganglia of the third and fourth thoracic nerves.

The cervical part of the phrenic nerve

This is formed by a large root from the C4 ventral ramus and smaller roots from C3 and 5. The roots curl downwards round the lateral border of scalenus anterior (**A**) and coalesce on its anterior surface deep to the prevertebral fascia. The nerve runs vertically downwards on the muscle and crosses the lower part of its medial border. It then immediately crosses the first part of the subclavian artery and, descending on the cervical pleura, passes into the thorax behind the first costal cartilage.

The branches of the subclavian artery

All the branches arise from the first part of the artery.

The vertebral artery is large and passes upwards from the subclavian to the C6 transverse process lying centrally in the vertebral triangle. Observe in **A** the successive posterior relations of the vessel in this part of its course. The artery then continues upwards traversing the foramen transversarium in each transverse process above that of C7. Between C6 and C2 the vessel passes in front of the ventral rami of the cervical nerves and sends a spinal branch through each intervertebral foramen into the vertebral canal (**C**). The course of the next part of the artery into the uppermost part of the vertebral canal and the cranial cavity has been considered and should now be revised (**D, 107C**).

The thyrocervical trunk passes upwards for about 1 cm along the medial margin of scalenus anterior before dividing into its branches on the anterior surface of the muscle (**A**). The most important branch is the inferior thyroid artery (**A**). It has a C-shaped course, passing first upwards on scalenus anterior medial to the phrenic nerve, then medially with a variable relationship to the middle cervical ganglion in front of the C6 transverse process, and then downwards on the prevertebral muscles to reach the thyroid gland lateral to the trachea and oesophagus (**485C**).

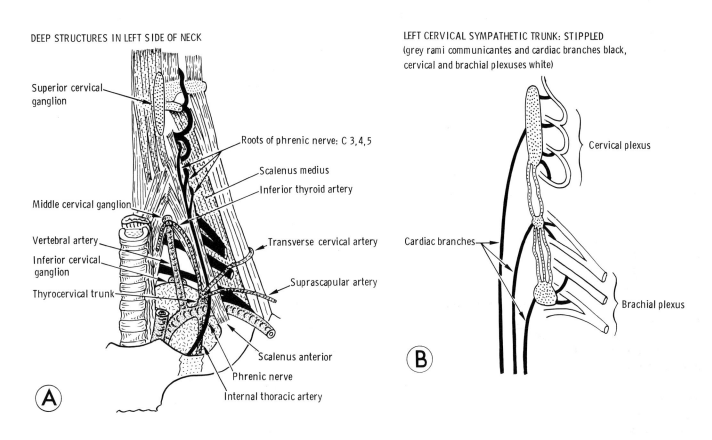

DEEP STRUCTURES IN LEFT SIDE OF NECK

Superior cervical ganglion

Roots of phrenic nerve: C 3,4,5

Scalenus medius

Inferior thyroid artery

Middle cervical ganglion

Transverse cervical artery

Vertebral artery

Inferior cervical ganglion

Suprascapular artery

Thyrocervical trunk

Scalenus anterior

Phrenic nerve

Internal thoracic artery

A

LEFT CERVICAL SYMPATHETIC TRUNK: STIPPLED
(grey rami communicantes and cardiac branches black, cervical and brachial plexuses white)

Cervical plexus

Cardiac branches

Brachial plexus

B

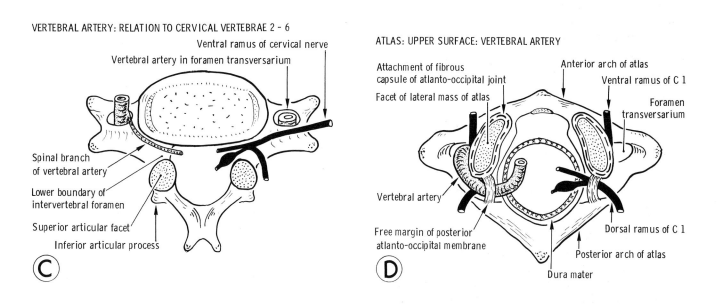

VERTEBRAL ARTERY: RELATION TO CERVICAL VERTEBRAE 2 – 6

Ventral ramus of cervical nerve

Vertebral artery in foramen transversarium

Spinal branch of vertebral artery

Lower boundary of intervertebral foramen

Superior articular facet

Inferior articular process

C

ATLAS: UPPER SURFACE: VERTEBRAL ARTERY

Attachment of fibrous capsule of atlanto-occipital joint

Facet of lateral mass of atlas

Anterior arch of atlas

Ventral ramus of C 1

Foramen transversarium

Vertebral artery

Free margin of posterior atlanto-occipital membrane

Dorsal ramus of C 1

Posterior arch of atlas

Dura mater

D

393

The transverse cervical and suprascapular branches (**393A**) run laterally across the scalenus anterior and the phrenic nerve, and continuing over or through the brachial plexus ramify in the muscles on the dorsal aspects of the neck and scapula.

The internal thoracic artery runs downwards on the anterior aspect of the cervical pleura where it is crossed from lateral to medial side by the phrenic nerve (**393A**). It then continues down the deep aspect of the anterior chest wall.

The costocervical trunk passes backwards over the cervical pleura to the neck of the first rib (**A**). Here it divides into a deep cervical branch, which runs backwards between the neck of the rib and the C7 transverse process into the postvertebral muscles, and a superior intercostal branch which descends in front of the neck of rib into the thorax and there, as has been seen (**153C**), gives off the first two posterior intercostal arteries.

The cervical part of the thoracic duct

The course of the duct in the thorax has been studied already (**147A**) and should be revised. The duct enters the neck (**B**) along the left margin of the oesophagus, lying behind the left common carotid artery, and ends in front of the first part of the left subclavian artery, where it opens into the venous system at the angle between the left subclavian and left internal jugular veins. Between these two points its course is convex upwards and reaches its highest point at the level of the C7 transverse process. Observe in **B** that it passes successively in front of the cervical pleura and the vertebral artery, and then in front of the phrenic nerve and the branches of the thyrocervical trunk as they lie on scalenus anterior.

Notice in **B** that the thoracic duct rises appreciably higher above the clavicle (4 cm) than either the cervical pleura (2.5 cm) or the subclavian artery (1.5 cm). Like these structures it is consequently prone to injury in penetrating wounds on the left side of the root of the neck.

On the right side the bronchomediastinal trunk, although much smaller than the thoracic duct, follows a similar course.

The subclavian veins

In contrast to the subclavian arteries, the subclavian veins are shorter and symmetrical on the two sides. Each begins (**B, C**) at the outer border of the first rib as a continuation of the axillary vein from the upper limb, crosses a very shallow groove on the upper surface of the rib, in front of scalenus anterior which separates it from the corresponding artery (**B**), and ends at the medial border of scalenus

anterior by joining the internal jugular vein to form the corresponding brachiocephalic vein.

The subclavian veins are thus co-extensive with the second and third parts of the arteries. And because the branches of the subclavian arteries arise from their first parts, it is not surprising that the veins corresponding to these branches drain, not into the subclavian veins, but, as will be seen later, into the brachiocephalic veins. Observe that, because of the obliquity of the first rib, the subclavian vein lies at a lower level than, as well as anterior to, the subclavian artery. Consequently, in contrast to the artery, it is very largely hidden and protected by the clavicle (**B**).

The neurovascular bundle of the neck

The neurovascular bundle extends more or less vertically from the base of the skull to the root of the neck. It rests against the lateral aspects of the pharynx, trachea and oesophagus and its long axis lies anterior to the line of cervical transverse processes. The vessels and nerves of which it is composed are enclosed in a fascial tube called the carotid sheath.

The vascular components of the bundle

The blood vessels of the bundle are shown in isolation in **C**. The internal jugular vein is continuous with the sigmoid sinus through the posterior part of the jugular foramen (**D, 101D**). The arterial stem in the lower part of the bundle is the common carotid artery, which arises on the left side from the arch of the aorta and on the right at the bifurcation of the brachiocephalic artery. The common carotid divides into internal and external carotid branches opposite the upper border of the thyroid cartilage, which can be identified in the living in the midline of the neck as the Adam's apple. The internal carotid artery continues upwards as the arterial component of the bundle. It gives off no branches in the neck and at the base of the skull enters the carotid canal through which it passes into the cranial cavity (**D, 107A**). The external carotid artery is at first anteromedial to the internal carotid and immediately leaves the neurovascular bundle in an upward and forward direction. It has numerous branches throughout its course and the presence of these facilitates its differentiation from the branchless internal carotid through a small surgical exposure.

Observe the different relationships of the arterial and venous components of the bundle at different levels (**C**).

1. Just below the base of the skull the artery is in front of the vein, in conformity to the relationship of the opening of the carotid canal to the jugular foramen (**D**).

ROOT OF NECK: SAGITTAL SECTION: COSTOCERVICAL TRUNK

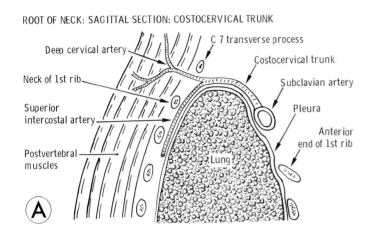

Deep cervical artery
C 7 transverse process
Costocervical trunk
Neck of 1st rib
Subclavian artery
Superior intercostal artery
Pleura
Anterior end of 1st rib
Postvertebral muscles
Lung

A

LEFT SIDE OF ROOT OF NECK: THORACIC DUCT

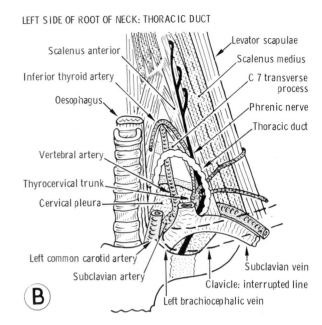

Scalenus anterior
Levator scapulae
Inferior thyroid artery
Scalenus medius
Oesophagus
C 7 transverse process
Phrenic nerve
Thoracic duct
Vertebral artery
Thyrocervical trunk
Cervical pleura
Left common carotid artery
Subclavian vein
Subclavian artery
Clavicle: interrupted line
Left brachiocephalic vein

B

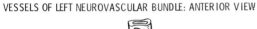
VESSELS OF LEFT NEUROVASCULAR BUNDLE: ANTERIOR VIEW

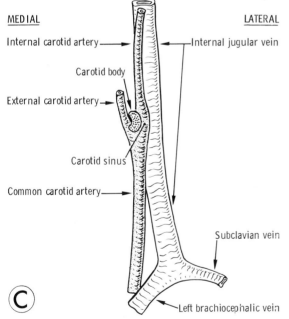

MEDIAL
LATERAL
Internal carotid artery
Internal jugular vein
Carotid body
External carotid artery
Carotid sinus
Common carotid artery
Subclavian vein
Left brachiocephalic vein

C

BASE OF SKULL (occipital bone shaded, temporal bone white)

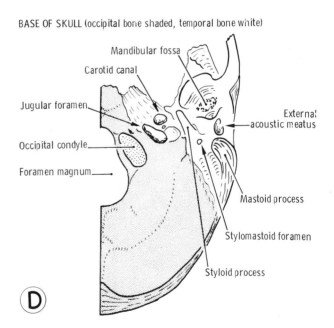

Mandibular fossa
Carotid canal
Jugular foramen
External acoustic meatus
Occipital condyle
Foramen magnum
Mastoid process
Stylomastoid foramen
Styloid process

D

395

2. Throughout the greater part of the neck the arterial stem is in contact with the medial side of the vein.

3. In the root of the neck the artery and vein become separated by a triangular interval.

The carotid sinus (**395C**) is a localised dilatation of the arterial stem which extends over the adjacent parts of the common and internal carotid arteries. It is a baroreceptor which exerts control over the blood flow to the brain.

The carotid body (**395C**) is a small cellular mass, pervaded by sinusoids, which lies in the angle between the internal and external carotid arteries and consequently in close relationship to the carotid sinus. It is a chemoreceptor which reflexly affects respiration in response to changes in the chemical composition of the blood.

Identify in **A** the deep structures of the neck which have been described already. Then consider the relationship of these structures to the vascular components of the neurovascular bundle which have been superimposed on them in **B**. Note in particular the following features:

1. The superior cervical sympathetic ganglion lies behind the internal carotid artery and, as has been seen (**392**), supplies it with a large vascular branch.

2. Several branches of the cervical plexus emerge from behind the lateral border of the upper part of the internal jugular vein.

3. All but the terminal part of the inferior thyroid artery is situated behind the neurovascular bundle.

4. The lateral half of scalenus anterior and the structures which lie on its anterior surface are visible lateral to the lower part of the internal jugular vein.

5. Where the common carotid artery and internal jugular vein separate in the root of the neck, the first part of the subclavian artery is visible through the interval.

The neural components of the bundle

The last four cranial nerves enter the upper end of the neurovascular bundle through the base of the skull. The glossopharyngeal, vagus and accessory nerves pass through the jugular foramen in front of the internal jugular vein. Observe their arrangment in that region (**C**). The glossopharyngeal, which is the most anterior of the group, exhibits superior and inferior sensory ganglia in the foramen. The larger vagus nerve, which lies between the other

two nerves, also has two sensory ganglia, the superior (or jugular) in the foramen and the inferior (or nodose) just below the foramen. The cranial and spinal parts of the accessory nerve fuse in the foramen behind the vagus. The single accessory nerve so formed divides immediately below the foramen into its original cranial and spinal parts. The cranial part then becomes incorporated into the vagus just below its inferior ganglion and is distributed subsequently through vagal branches.

The hypoglossal nerve passes downwards and laterally, through the hypoglossal canal in the occipital condyle, to join the neurovascular bundle just below the jugular foramen (**D**). In the bundle it curves round the posterior and lateral aspects of the inferior ganglion of the vagus before descending in front of that nerve. In front of the transverse process of the atlas it is joined by a branch from the upper loop of the cervical plexus which consists of fibres from the C1 ventral ramus.

For a short distance below the skull four nerves, the glossopharyngeal, the hypoglossal, now containing C1 fibres, the vagus, now containing all the cranial accessory fibres, and the spinal part of the accessory are tightly packed between the internal carotid artery in front and the internal jugular vein behind (**E**). In this region the spinal part of the accessory leaves the bundle by inclining downwards and backwards, usually across the lateral aspect of the vein, on to the tip of the transverse process of the atlas where we will leave it for the present.

As the neurovascular bundle is traced downwards the internal carotid artery inclines backwards and medially on to the medial aspect of the internal jugular vein and the three remaining nerves lie between the two vessels (**F**).

Observe in **F** that the glossopharyngeal and hypoglossal nerves both leave the neurovascular bundle in the upper half of the neck by turning forwards towards the pharynx and the tongue. In contrast, the vagus nerve continues as a component of the bundle to the root of the neck (see below). Although most of the branches of the glossopharyngeal and hypoglossal nerves will be considered later in relation to the structures they supply, it is convenient to describe here two branches which are embedded in the fascia of the carotid sheath.

The carotid branch of the glossopharyngeal (**F**) is a slender nerve which arises just below the jugular foramen and runs within the carotid sheath to the carotid body and sinus. It transmits special sensory information from these two structures.

LEFT SIDE OF NECK: DEEP STRUCTURES:

ANTERIOR VIEW

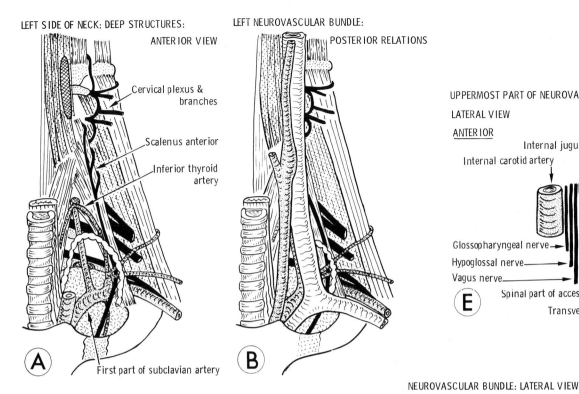

Cervical plexus & branches

Scalenus anterior

Inferior thyroid artery

First part of subclavian artery

(A)

LEFT NEUROVASCULAR BUNDLE:

POSTERIOR RELATIONS

(B)

UPPERMOST PART OF NEUROVASCULAR BUNDLE:

LATERAL VIEW

ANTERIOR   POSTERIOR

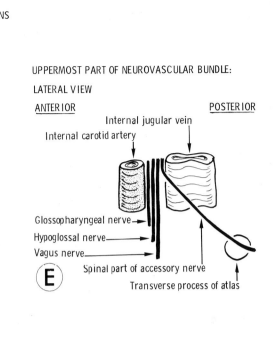

Internal jugular vein

Internal carotid artery

Glossopharyngeal nerve

Hypoglossal nerve

Vagus nerve

Spinal part of accessory nerve

Transverse process of atlas

(E)

CRANIAL NERVES IN JUGULAR FORAMEN: SAGITTAL SECTION

ANTERIOR   POSTERIOR

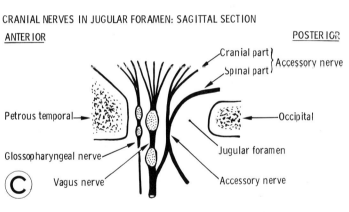

Cranial part) Accessory nerve
Spinal part)

Petrous temporal

Occipital

Glossopharyngeal nerve

Jugular foramen

Vagus nerve

Accessory nerve

(C)

HYPOGLOSSAL NERVE: CORONAL SECTION

MEDIAL   LATERAL

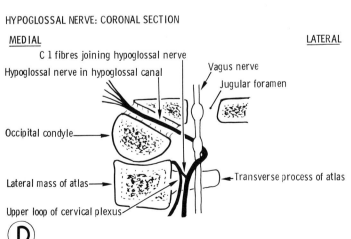

C 1 fibres joining hypoglossal nerve

Hypoglossal nerve in hypoglossal canal

Vagus nerve

Jugular foramen

Occipital condyle

Lateral mass of atlas

Transverse process of atlas

Upper loop of cervical plexus

(D)

NEUROVASCULAR BUNDLE: LATERAL VIEW

(most of internal jugular vein removed)

ANTERIOR   POSTERIOR

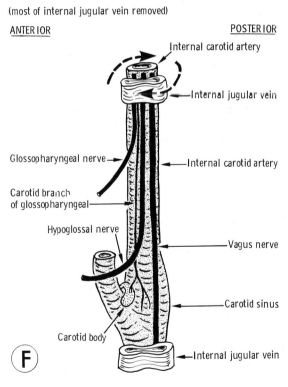

Internal carotid artery

Internal jugular vein

Glossopharyngeal nerve

Internal carotid artery

Carotid branch of glossopharyngeal

Hypoglossal nerve

Vagus nerve

Carotid sinus

Carotid body

Internal jugular vein

(F)

The ansa cervicalis is a nerve loop embedded in the anterior wall of the carotid sheath (**A**). It is formed by the junction of upper and lower roots, and gives branches to a group of muscles (the infrahyoid muscles) which lie in front of the midline viscera in the lower part of the neck (**487A, 487B**). The upper root springs from the hypoglossal nerve as it turns forwards to leave the neurovascular bundle and consists entirely of fibres which, as has been seen, join the hypoglossal nerve from the C1 ventral ramus at a higher level. The lower root is formed by the fusion of branches from the C2 and C3 ventral rami which wind downwards and forwards in the lateral wall of the carotid sheath. The ansa thus contains fibres from the ventral rami of C1, 2 and 3.

Reaching the root of the neck each vagus nerve appears in the interval created by the separation of the corresponding common carotid artery and internal jugular vein but thereafter the courses of the two nerves differ (**B**). The left vagus passes into the superior mediastinum to the left of the interval between the left common carotid and subclavian arteries, and then continues across the left side of the aortic arch. The right vagus inclines downwards and medially across the first part of the right subclavian artery and continues posterolateral to the brachiocephalic artery onto the right side of the trachea.

A recurrent laryngeal branch arises from each vagus nerve in the region shown in **B** but their origins are asymmetrical. The left arises in the superior mediastinum on the left side of the aortic arch and passes medially beneath the arch to gain its right side. It then ascends in the left tracheo-oesophageal groove. The right nerve arises in the neck, hooks round the inferior and posterior aspects of the first part of the right subclavian artery and continues upwards and medially, behind the right common carotid artery, into the right tracheo-oesophageal groove.

In **B** the two recurrent laryngeal nerves have been cut level with the upper ends of the trachea and oesophagus and their subsequent distribution to the larynx will be considered later. Meanwhile notice two features of the parts of the nerves described above.

1. The mucous membrane and muscle of the cervical parts of the trachea and oesophagus are innervated by both recurrent laryngeal nerves. On the other hand, the same structures in the superior mediastinum are innervated by the left recurrent laryngeal nerve and by direct branches from the right vagus.
2. Each recurrent laryngeal nerve comes into close but variable relationship with the corresponding inferior thyroid artery just before that vessel reaches the thyroid gland (**B**). When it is necessary to tie this artery in operations on the thyroid gland, it is usual to displace the neurovascular bundle laterally so that the tie may be applied at a safe distance lateral to the nerve.

The superficial lateral muscles of the neck

The trapezius has a long linear origin (**C**) from the medial part of the superior nuchal line, the ligamentum nuchae and the spines of all the thoracic vertebrae. The fibres converge on a continuous C-shaped insertion on the shoulder girdle (**C, D**). The upper fibres curl downwards laterally and forwards round the neck to reach the posterior surface of the lateral third of the clavicle (**D**), the middle fibres incline laterally to the acromion and the crest of the spine of the scapula (**C**), while the lower fibres converge upwards and laterally into a short aponeurosis which is inserted into the crest just beyond the smooth triangular area at its medial end (**C**). The actions of the muscle are described later (**495A**).

The sternocleidomastoid (sternomastoid) is a long bulky muscle. It has two heads of origin (**D**), a rounded tendon which quickly gives way to a muscle belly arising from the anterior surface of the manubrium sterni, and a flat muscular sheet arising from the medial third of the clavicle. Ascending, the clavicular head fuses with the deep aspect of the sternal head and the whole muscle winds round the neck to its posterolateral aspect (**C**). There it is inserted into the mastoid process and the lateral part of the superior nuchal line.

When the two muscles act together they tilt the head forwards and, if this movement is carried out against resistance, the outlines of the muscles become evident beneath the skin. When the muscle of one side acts alone, the head is tilted to that side and rotated so that it faces towards the opposite side.

Because of the obliquity of the muscle, its lower and middle parts overlie and obscure the neurovascular bundle of the neck, but lie posterior to it above. For the same reason the muscle separates two triangular regions in the neck. The anterior triangle lies between the anterior margin of the muscle and the midline, and is limited above by the lower margin of the corresponding half of the body of the mandible. The posterior triangle is bounded by the adjacent margins of sternomastoid and trapezius and the middle third of the clavicle.

The investing layer of the deep cervical fascia has already been observed in a horizontal section through the neck (**385D**). It will be recalled that it envelops both the sternomastoid and trapezius muscles, and bridges the gaps between them as a single layer.

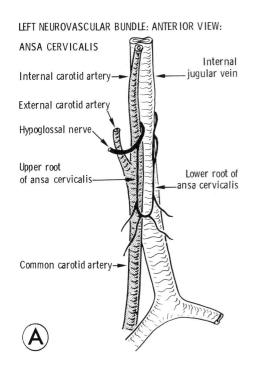

LEFT NEUROVASCULAR BUNDLE: ANTERIOR VIEW:
ANSA CERVICALIS

Internal carotid artery→

Internal jugular vein

External carotid artery→

Hypoglossal nerve→

Upper root of ansa cervicalis→

Lower root of ansa cervicalis

Common carotid artery→

(A)

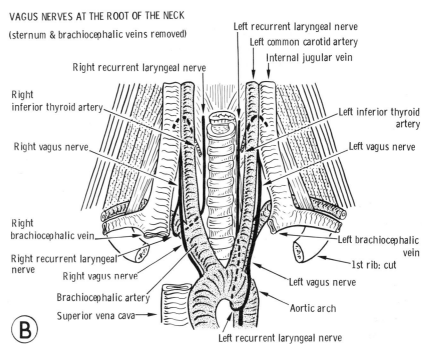

VAGUS NERVES AT THE ROOT OF THE NECK
(sternum & brachiocephalic veins removed)

Left recurrent laryngeal nerve
Left common carotid artery
Internal jugular vein

Right recurrent laryngeal nerve

Right inferior thyroid artery

Left inferior thyroid artery

Right vagus nerve

Left vagus nerve

Right brachiocephalic vein

Left brachiocephalic vein

Right recurrent laryngeal nerve

1st rib: cut

Right vagus nerve

Left vagus nerve

Brachiocephalic artery

Aortic arch

Superior vena cava→

Left recurrent laryngeal nerve

(B)

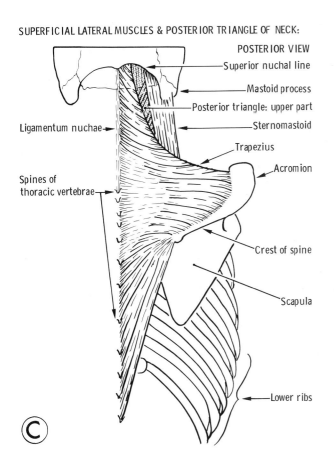

SUPERFICIAL LATERAL MUSCLES & POSTERIOR TRIANGLE OF NECK:
POSTERIOR VIEW

Superior nuchal line

Mastoid process

Posterior triangle: upper part

Ligamentum nuchae

Sternomastoid

Trapezius

Acromion

Spines of thoracic vertebrae→

Crest of spine

Scapula

Lower ribs

(C)

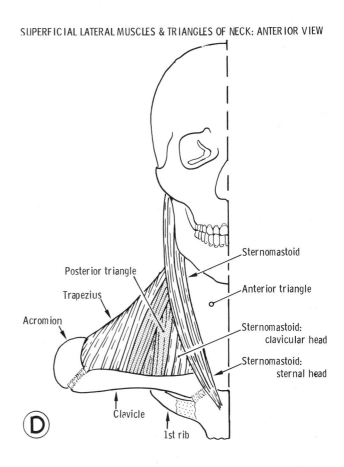

SUPERFICIAL LATERAL MUSCLES & TRIANGLES OF NECK: ANTERIOR VIEW

Sternomastoid

Posterior triangle

Anterior triangle

Trapezius

Acromion

Sternomastoid: clavicular head

Sternomastoid: sternal head

Clavicle

1st rib

(D)

399

THE POSTERIOR TRIANGLE OF THE NECK

The margins of the posterior triangle have been described (**398**) and are seen from the lateral side in **A**. Its floor is formed above by some of the postvertebral muscles of the neck but in its lower two-thirds or so by the deep lateral muscles, particularly levator scapulae and scalenus medius, covered by the prevertebral fascia. Its roof consists of the investing layer of the deep cervical fascia (see above).

A number of important structures are associated with the triangle.

1. The supraclavicular part of the brachial plexus and the third part of the subclavian artery lie in its lower part (**A**), but it should be noted that the plexus is partly obscured by the inferior belly of a digastric muscle called the omohyoid which will be considered later with the other members of the group to which it belongs (**A**, **487A**).

2. The spinal part of the accessory nerve has already been seen to leave the neurovascular bundle of the neck just below the skull, and to pass downwards and backwards, lateral to the internal jugular vein, onto the tip of the transverse process of the atlas (**397E**). This bony point can be palpated just in front of the sternomastoid and midway between the mastoid process and the angle of the mandible (**A**). Continuing downwards and backwards, the nerve pierces the investing fascia on the deep surface of sternomastoid and passes through the muscle to its posterior border slightly above its midpoint. The nerve then follows the same line across the posterior triangle to enter the trapezius through its anterior border about 5 cm above the clavicle (**A**). Thus the surface marking of the nerve in the posterior triangle can be easily constructed, and this is useful, for in this region the nerve lies in the substance of the investing fascia and consequently in a rather superficial and potentially vulnerable position.

3. *The cutaneous branches of the cervical plexus* arise from the ventral rami of C2, 3 and 4, pass laterally behind the internal jugular vein and sternomastoid, and emerge into the posterior triangle at about the middle of the posterior border of the muscle.

Piercing the investing fascia the nerves radiate upwards, forwards and downwards through the superficial fascia to supply triangular areas of skin over parts of the face, scalp and auricle, and over the whole of the neck except the area innervated by the cervical dorsal rami (**B**, **C**). Note in particular the following facts. The supraclavicular nerve divides into distinct medial, intermediate and lateral branches, and its area of distribution extends on to the anterior chest wall as far as the second rib and for about a hand's breadth beyond the acromion on the lateral aspect of the arm (**C**). The uppermost part of the cranial surface of the auricle is innervated by the lesser occipital nerve and the rest of that surface by the great auricular nerve.

4. *The external jugular vein* originates in the anterior triangle, just behind the angle of the mandible and within the superficial fascia, and crosses sternomastoid obliquely in close company with the great auricular nerve. In the lower part of the posterior triangle it pierces the investing fascia and, descending in front of omohyoid, the brachial plexus and the subclavian artery, ends by joining the subclavian vein. In its terminal part it receives the anterior jugular vein (**486**).

5. The platysma is a thin quadrilateral sheet of muscle (**D**) which lies in the superficial fascia of the neck superficial to the cutaneous nerves and the external jugular vein described above. Despite its position it is functionally a muscle of expression associated with the mouth. Its fibres arise from the deep fascia covering the superficial muscles of the anterior chest wall a short distance below the clavicle. Its borders are often visible beneath the skin in the elderly. The medial border crosses the medial end of the clavicle and ascends towards the symphysis menti. The lateral border runs from the lateral end of the clavicle over trapezius, the posterior triangle and the sternomastoid towards the angle of the mandible. The fibres insert in part into the outer surface of the body of the mandible and in part into the skin at the angle of the mouth.

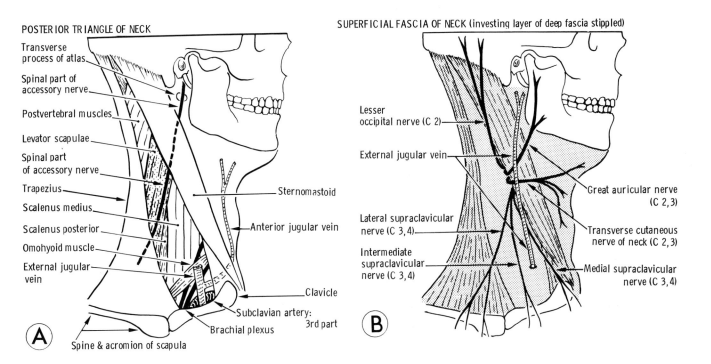

POSTERIOR TRIANGLE OF NECK

- Transverse process of atlas
- Spinal part of accessory nerve
- Postvertebral muscles
- Levator scapulae
- Spinal part of accessory nerve
- Trapezius
- Scalenus medius
- Scalenus posterior
- Omohyoid muscle
- External jugular vein
- Sternomastoid
- Anterior jugular vein
- Clavicle
- Subclavian artery: 3rd part
- Brachial plexus
- Spine & acromion of scapula

(A)

SUPERFICIAL FASCIA OF NECK (investing layer of deep fascia stippled)

- Lesser occipital nerve (C 2)
- External jugular vein
- Lateral supraclavicular nerve (C 3, 4)
- Intermediate supraclavicular nerve (C 3, 4)
- Great auricular nerve (C 2, 3)
- Transverse cutaneous nerve of neck (C 2, 3)
- Medial supraclavicular nerve (C 3, 4)

(B)

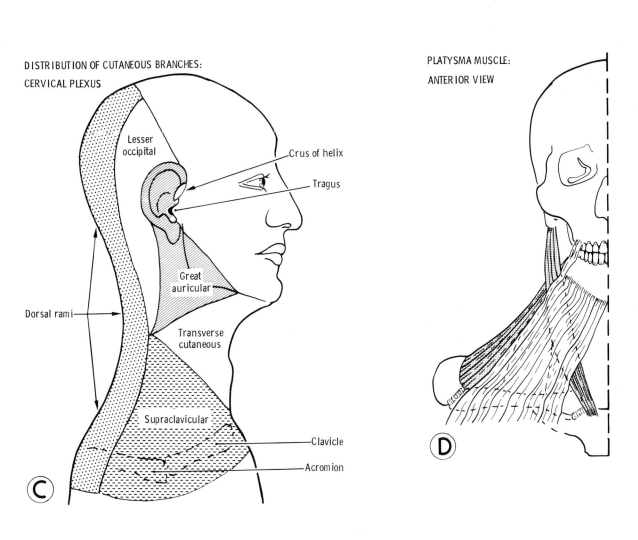

DISTRIBUTION OF CUTANEOUS BRANCHES: CERVICAL PLEXUS

- Lesser occipital
- Crus of helix
- Tragus
- Great auricular
- Dorsal rami
- Transverse cutaneous
- Supraclavicular
- Clavicle
- Acromion

(C)

PLATYSMA MUSCLE: ANTERIOR VIEW

(D)

THE EAR

The ear consists of three parts named from their relative positions as external, middle and internal.

1. The external ear is composed of a concave skin-covered plate of elastic cartilage, the auricle, which protrudes from the side of the head, and the tubular skin-lined external acoustic meatus which leads medially from the auricle into the temporal bone. It collects sound waves in the air of the external environment.
2. The middle ear is a cavity in the temporal bone which, since it communicates with the cavity of the pharynx, is lined by mucous membrane and occupied by air. Laterally, its central part is separated from the external acoustic meatus by the tympanic membrane. Sound waves travelling through the air in the meatus cause the membrane to vibrate. The middle ear cavity is crossed by an articulated chain of three small bones, the auditory ossicles, which transfer these vibrations to the internal ear.
3. The internal ear is a cavity in the temporal bone, medial to that of the middle ear. It contains a complex membranous sac surrounded by fluid. It consists of three communicating parts, named from before backwards the cochlea, the vestibule and the three semicircular canals. Movements of the auditory ossicles affect the cochlear part of the internal ear and provoke impulses in the cochlear part of the vestibulocochlear nerve. The cochlea is thus the part of the internal ear which is functionally connected to the middle and external ears and is concerned in the appreciation of sound. In contrast, the vestibule and semicircular canals are concerned with the appreciation of the position of the head and movements of the head respectively, factors which give rise to impulses in the vestibular part of the vestibulocochlear nerve.

The internal ear

In the internal ear a continuous, complex membranous sac, occupied by a fluid called endolymph, is separated by another fluid called perilymph from the serous lining of a complex cavity in the dense petrous part of the temporal bone (**A**). The membranous sac is known, because of its complex shape, as the membranous labyrinth and the bony cavity as the bony labyrinth.

The bony labyrinth

The vestibule is the central part of the labyrinth (**A**). At about the middle of its lateral wall is a reniform opening (**B**), called the fenestra vestibuli, which is occupied in the natural state by the most medial of the auditory ossicles (the stapes). On its medial wall (**C, D**) a smaller opening leads into the aqueduct of the vestibule, a tubular extension which leads downwards and backwards and opens on the posterior surface of the petrous temporal. As will be seen later it is fully occupied by a tubular extension of the membranous labyrinth (**A**). Above and in front of the orifice of the aqueduct are groups of minute foramina which communicate with the internal acoustic meatus (**C**).

The cochlea is the anterior part of the labyrinth. Its core, which is called the modiolus, is a conical region of bone lying horizontally with its apex directed forwards and laterally (**E**). The canal of the cochlea is a tubular cavity which winds in spiral fashion around the modiolus from its base to its apex where it ends blindly (**B, E**). It extends through two-and-three-quarter turns and diminishes progressively in diameter. Note that when the cochlea is viewed from base to apex the spiral formed by the cochlear canal is anticlockwise on the left side and clockwise on the right. The osseous spiral lamina is a thin bony shelf which projects from the modiolus into the cochlear canal (**E**), and is attached to the peripheral wall of that canal by a fibrous sheet called the basilar membrane (**E**). In this way the cochlear canal is divided into an apical compartment known as the scala vestibuli and a basal compartment called the scala tympani. At the apex of the cochlea the partition is deficient and the two scalae communicate through a small opening, the helicotrema.

At the beginning of the first turn of the cochlear canal, the osseous spiral lamina and the basilar membrane become continuous with the medial wall of the vestibule (**D**). This is a fundamental feature of the cochlea. As a result, the scala vestibuli opens directly into the vestibule, which explains its name. In contrast, the basal part of the scala tympani is shut off from the vestibular cavity and ends at the fenestra cochleae (**B, C, D**). This opens into the tympanic cavity and in the natural state is closed by the secondary tympanic membrane.

It can now be appreciated that, when medial displacement of the stapes through the fenestra vestibuli creates a pressure wave in the perilymph within the vestibule, that wave can pass along the scala vestibuli (**D**) and through the helicotrema, before returning along the scala tympani until its energy is absorbed by the elasticity of the secondary tympanic membrane.

In the basal wall of the scala tympani, just beyond the fenestra cochleae, is the small orifice of the aqueduct of the cochlea (**C**). This aqueduct differs from that of the vestibule (see above) in containing only perilymph (**A**).

INTERNAL EAR: SCHEMATIC REPRESENTATION

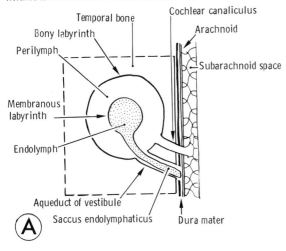

Temporal bone
Bony labyrinth
Perilymph
Cochlear canaliculus
Arachnoid
Subarachnoid space
Membranous labyrinth
Endolymph
Aqueduct of vestibule
Saccus endolymphaticus
Dura mater

A

LEFT BONY LABYRINTH: LATERAL ASPECT

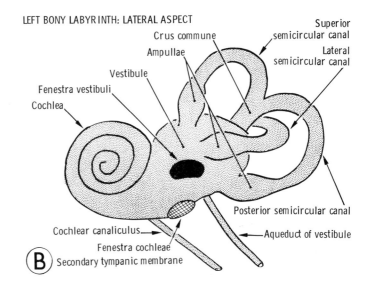

Crus commune
Ampullae
Vestibule
Fenestra vestibuli
Cochlea
Superior semicircular canal
Lateral semicircular canal
Posterior semicircular canal
Aqueduct of vestibule
Cochlear canaliculus
Fenestra cochleae
Secondary tympanic membrane

B

LEFT BONY LABYRINTH: part of lateral wall removed

Foramina leading to internal acoustic meatus

ANTERIOR

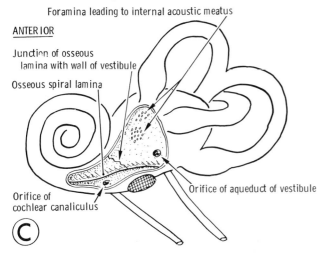

Junction of osseous lamina with wall of vestibule
Osseous spiral lamina
Orifice of cochlear canaliculus
Orifice of aqueduct of vestibule

C

LEFT BONY LABYRINTH: HORIZONTAL SECTION: bone stippled

ANTERIOR

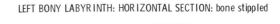
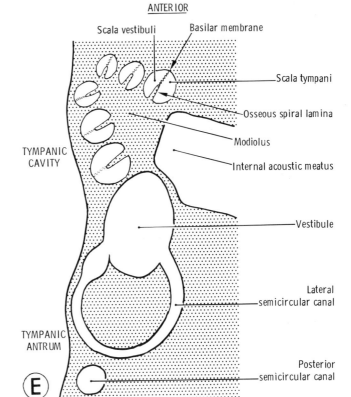

Scala vestibuli
Basilar membrane
Scala tympani
Osseous spiral lamina
Modiolus
Internal acoustic meatus
TYMPANIC CAVITY
Vestibule
Lateral semicircular canal
TYMPANIC ANTRUM
Posterior semicircular canal

E

LEFT BONY LABYRINTH: part of lateral wall removed

ANTERIOR

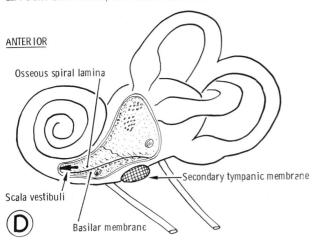

Osseous spiral lamina
Secondary tympanic membrane
Scala vestibuli
Basilar membrane

D

It opens through the dura mater and arachnoid mater into the subarachnoid space at the anterior corner of the jugular foramen, so that the perilymph of the bony labyrinth becomes continuous with the cerebrospinal fluid.

The semicircular canals (**403B**) are posterior to the vestibule and open into it. Each extends through about two-thirds of a circle and exhibits an expanded ampulla at one end. The lateral canal is convex backwards and laterally in a horizontal plane. Its lateral end is ampullated and both ends open individually into the vestibule. The superior canal is convex upwards in a vertical plane which is at right angles to the long axis of the corresponding petrous temporal (**A**). Its anterolateral end is ampullated and opens individually into the vestibule. The posterior canal is convex backwards and laterally in a vertical plane (**403B**) which is parallel to the long axis of the corresponding petrous temporal (**A**). Its inferior end is ampullated and opens individually into the vestibule. The nonampullated ends of the superior and posterior canals join to form the crus commune which opens directly into the vestibule. Thus the three semicircular canals have five, not six, openings into the vestibule.

Because the long axes of the petrous parts of the right and left temporal bones are about at right angles, it is evident that the planes of the left superior and right posterior canals are parallel, as are the planes of the right superior and left posterior canals (**A**).

The membranous labyrinth

The membranous labyrinth consists of the following interconnected parts (**B**).

The utricle and saccule are membranous sacs which lie within the posterior and anterior parts of the vestibule respectively. Their lower parts are joined by a narrow duct from which the slender saccus endolymphaticus descends through the aqueduct of the vestibule (see above) to end blindly beneath the dura mater of the posterior cranial fossa. This appears to be a mechanism which maintains constant pressure in the endolymph within the whole membranous labyrinth.

The three semicircular ducts are similar in shape to the semicircular canals in which they lie except that they are considerably narrower. They join the utricle through five openings.

The cochlear duct arises from the lower anterior part of the saccule and runs in the scala vestibuli to the apex of the cochlea where it ends blindly. It is triangular in cross section (**B, D**). Its basal wall rests on the peripheral half of the osseous spiral lamina and the basilar membrane, and its peripheral wall against the peripheral wall of the scala vestibuli. The third wall which joins the other two is the delicate vestibular membrane.

The receptor sites of the membranous labyrinth

Most of the membranous labyrinth is lined by a single layer of unremarkable squamous or cuboidal epithelial cells. However, specific sites in each section of the labyrinth are specialised as receptor areas which sense pressure waves within the adjacent endolymph. All these sites have the same basic structure. Many of the lining cells are hair cells and the numerous microvilli which project from their free surfaces are embedded in a gelatinous material which is displaced by movements of the endolymph. The deep aspects of the hair cells are intimately related to terminations of the peripheral processes of the neurons which comprise the vestibulocochlear nerve.

1. The organ of corti (**D**) extends as a continuous receptor site along the basal wall of the duct of the cochlea. The processes of its hair cells project into a gelatinous overlay called the membrana tectoria.
2. Receptor areas known as maculae are situated in the anterior wall of the saccule, and in the antero-inferior wall of the utricle, in planes at right angles to one another (**B**). The flat gelatinous masses into which the macular hair cell microvilli project contain numerous minute crystalline bodies and are called otolithic membranes.
3. In each semicircular duct hair cells are situated on an ampullary crest, which projects into the duct lumen from the peripheral wall of the ampulla (**B, C**). Gelatinous material known as a cupula projects into the endolymph from the summit of each crest.

SUPERIOR & POSTERIOR SEMICIRCULAR CANALS: VERTICAL PLANES

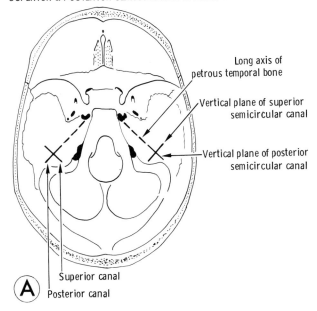

Long axis of petrous temporal bone

Vertical plane of superior semicircular canal

Vertical plane of posterior semicircular canal

Superior canal

Posterior canal

(A)

MEMBRANOUS LABYRINTH: stippled
MACULAE & AMPULLARY CRESTS: black

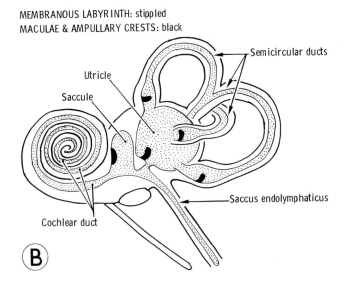

Semicircular ducts

Utricle

Saccule

Saccus endolymphaticus

Cochlear duct

(B)

SEMICIRCULAR DUCT & AMPULLARY CREST

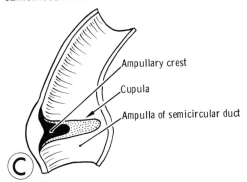

Ampullary crest

Cupula

Ampulla of semicircular duct

(C)

COCHLEAR DUCT & ORGAN OF CORTI

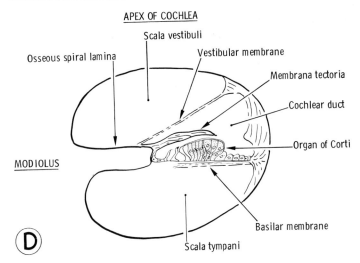

APEX OF COCHLEA

Scala vestibuli

Osseous spiral lamina

Vestibular membrane

Membrana tectoria

Cochlear duct

Organ of Corti

MODIOLUS

Basilar membrane

Scala tympani

(D)

The vestibulocochlear nerve

Traced laterally from the brain stem this nerve passes, below the two roots of the facial nerve, into the internal acoustic meatus where it divides into vestibular and cochlear parts (**A**).

The lateral end of the meatus (**B**) exhibits a posterior group of foramina which open into the vestibule of the bony labyrinth, and an antero-inferior group which open into fine canals which run longitudinally in the modiolus of the cochlea. Anterosuperiorly is the opening of the canal for the facial nerve.

Each part of the vestibulocochlear nerve has a sensory ganglion which consists, unlike those on other cranial and spinal nerves, of bipolar nerve cells. From the cells of each ganglion the central processes pass to brain stem (**51C**), while the peripheral processes pass into the internal ear, where they end in relationship to the hair cells of the receptor sites of the membranous labyrinth.

The vestibular ganglion (**A**) lies near the lateral end of the internal acoustic meatus. The peripheral processes of its cells pass as small bundles through the minute foramina in the medial wall of the vestibule and reach the maculae of the utricle and saccule and the ampullary crests of the semicircular ducts.

The cochlear ganglion (the spiral ganglion) is of very unusual shape (**A**). It occupies a spiral bony canal situated in the modiolus along the whole of the attached margin of the osseous spiral lamina. The peripheral processes of its cells radiate through fine canals in the substance of this lamina and end in relation to the hair cells of the organ of Corti in the cochlear duct. The central processes form bundles which run through narrow canals within the modiolus to its base and emerge into the internal acoustic meatus. Here they join to form the cochlear part of the vestibulocochlear nerve.

The middle ear

This consists of a continuous cavity, the greater part of which is in the temporal bone. It is divisible on functional and topographical grounds into three major parts: a central tympanic cavity, a mastoid part behind and the auditory tube in front (**C**). The latter segment opens into the upper part of the pharynx, so that the walls of the whole middle ear cavity and those structures which cross its lumen are coated by a diverticulum of pharyngeal mucous membrane and the cavity itself is occupied by air.

The tympanic cavity

This narrow cavity lies between the internal ear and the external acoustic meatus. It is obliquely orientated, extending from above downwards and medially and from behind forwards and medially. It has six walls which are described below.

1. Above (**C, D**), it is separated from the anterior surface of the petrous part of the temporal bone, and consequently from the temporal lobe of the brain in the middle cranial fossa, by a thin plate of bone called the tegmen tympani.
2. Below, the cavity is separated by another thin bony plate from the commencement of the internal jugular vein in the jugular foramen (**D**).
3. Laterally, the lower three-quarters or so of the cavity is separated from the external acoustic meatus by the tympanic membrane. The part of the tympanic cavity above the level of the membrane is called the epitympanic recess (**D**).

   The tympanic membrane (**D**), which is about 10 mm in diameter, is a trilaminar structure consisting of a central layer of connective tissue, an inner layer of mucous membrane and an outer layer of skin. It will be seen later that certain additional structures lie within the substance of the membrane between the fibrous and mucosal layers. The greater part of the margin of the membrane is firmly attached to the U-shaped medial end of the grooved upper surface of the tympanic part of the temporal bone. The corresponding part of the membrane is tense. In contrast, anterosuperiorly the fibrous lamina is attached to the squamous part of the temporal bone and is flaccid. The small flaccid part of the fibrous lamina is separated from the much larger tense part by two thickened strands called the anterior and posterior malleolar folds, which converge and meet at an obtuse angle (**D**). The membrane is convex towards the tympanic cavity and is obliquely orientated so that its concave outer surface faces laterally, downwards and forwards.
4. The lower part of the anterior wall is a thin plate of bone which separates the tympanic cavity from the vertical part of the carotid canal. Above this is the opening into the auditory tube, and above this again the opening into a smaller canal which contains the tensor tympani muscle (**D**).

VESTIBULOCOCHLEAR NERVE

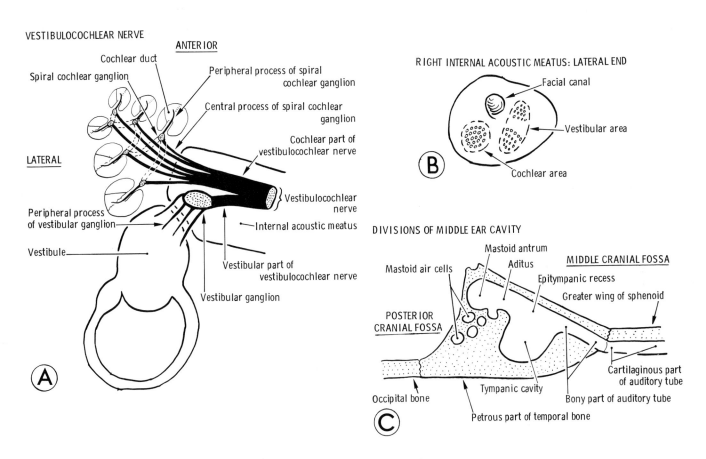

ANTERIOR

Cochlear duct

Spiral cochlear ganglion

Peripheral process of spiral cochlear ganglion

Central process of spiral cochlear ganglion

Cochlear part of vestibulocochlear nerve

LATERAL

Vestibulocochlear nerve

Peripheral process of vestibular ganglion

Internal acoustic meatus

Vestibule

Vestibular part of vestibulocochlear nerve

Vestibular ganglion

Ⓐ

RIGHT INTERNAL ACOUSTIC MEATUS: LATERAL END

Facial canal

Vestibular area

Ⓑ

Cochlear area

DIVISIONS OF MIDDLE EAR CAVITY

Mastoid antrum

Mastoid air cells

Aditus

MIDDLE CRANIAL FOSSA

Epitympanic recess

Greater wing of sphenoid

POSTERIOR CRANIAL FOSSA

Cartilaginous part of auditory tube

Occipital bone

Tympanic cavity

Bony part of auditory tube

Petrous part of temporal bone

Ⓒ

VERTICAL SECTION OF LEFT TYMPANIC CAVITY: viewed towards lateral wall

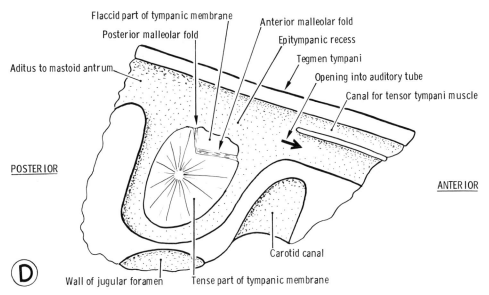

Flaccid part of tympanic membrane

Posterior malleolar fold

Anterior malleolar fold

Epitympanic recess

Tegmen tympani

Aditus to mastoid antrum

Opening into auditory tube

Canal for tensor tympani muscle

POSTERIOR

ANTERIOR

Carotid canal

Ⓓ

Wall of jugular foramen

Tense part of tympanic membrane

5. Medially, the tympanic cavity is closely related to the cochlea and vestibule of the internal ear (**A**). Antero-inferiorly, the wide initial part of the cochlear canal bulges medially producing a rounded eminence called the promontory. Above and behind this feature is a kidney-shaped aperture, the fenestra vestibuli. It leads into the vestibule, but is blocked in the undissected specimen by part of the most medial of the auditory ossicles (the stapes). Below and behind the promontory is the fenestra cochleae (**403D**), which opens upwards and forwards into the scala tympani. In the natural state it is closed by the trilaminar secondary tympanic membrane which consists of a fibrous lamina sandwiched between the lining membrane of the scala tympani and the tympanic mucosa. The two fenestrae noted above are, of course, the same as those observed earlier on the lateral aspect of the bony labyrinth (**403B**). On the medial wall of the epitympanic recess, above the features described, is a faint ridge (**A**) which marks the position of the second part of the facial canal containing part of the facial nerve (**415C**).

6. The bone which forms the lower half of the posterior boundary of the tympanic cavity contains the third part of the facial canal which passes downwards to the stylomastoid foramen (**A**). On the anterior surface of this region of bone is a forwardly directed conical projection, the pyramid (**A**). It contains a central canal which is in communication behind with the facial canal. The posterior boundary of the epitympanic recess is deficient and forms the aditus into an air space called the mastoid antrum.

The auditory ossicles

There are three minute bones forming an articulated chain which transfers the vibratory movements of the tympanic membrane to the fenestra vestibuli and so to the perilymph in the vestibule.

The malleus (**B, D**) has an expanded upper end called the head which lies in the epitympanic recess and presents an articular facet on its posteromedial surface. The short constricted neck is medial to the flaccid part of the tympanic membrane and gives rise to three processes. The slender anterior process is attached by a ligament to the bone above and in front of the tympanic membrane. The other two processes lie between the fibrous and mucosal layers of the membrane. The short, conical lateral process gives attachment to the two malleolar folds, while the longer inferior process, known as the manubrium or handle, extends downwards and somewhat backwards to the centre of the membrane, where its extremity turns sharply forwards.

The incus (**B, D**) resembles a premolar tooth in shape. The body lies in the epitympanic recess and articulates anteriorly with the facet on the head of the malleus (the incudomalleolar joint). The short process passes horizontally backwards and is fixed by a ligament to a small fossa on the lateral wall of the posterior part of the epitympanic recess. The long process extends downwards, parallel to but behind and medial to the handle of the malleus. Its lower end, which lies at the same level as the pyramid and fenestra vestibuli, turns abruptly in a medial direction to end on the small lentiform nodule which carries a convex articular facet.

The stapes (**C, D**) closely resembles a stirrup. The cup-shaped head is directly medially and articulates with the lentiform nodule of the incus (the incudostapedial joint). The short neck divides into anterior and posterior limbs, which curve medially in the same horizontal plane to join a thin vertical plate of bone called the base or footplate. The base lies within the fenestra vestibuli and is attached to its margins by the elastic anular ligament.

Movements of the ossicles

Sound waves cause vibration, that is cyclical, medial and lateral displacements of the tense part of the tympanic membrane, which are necessarily followed by the handle of the malleus. In the medial phase of each cycle the incudomalleolar joint locks because of certain conformational features of its articular surfaces, so that the malleus and incus move as a single unit around an axis which traverses the attachments of the anterior process of the malleus and the short process of the incus (interrupted line in **B**). Thus the long process of the incus moves medially with the handle of the malleus and the head of the malleus and the body of the incus are displaced laterally. The movement of the long process of the incus displaces the base of the stapes medially in relation to the margin of the fenestra vestibuli. But, because the upper part of the anular ligament is more extensible than its lower part, the movement is hinge-like in nature.

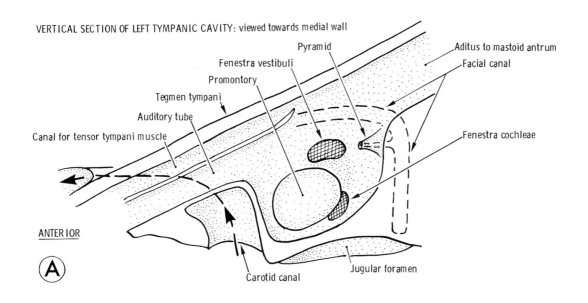

VERTICAL SECTION OF LEFT TYMPANIC CAVITY: viewed towards medial wall

Tegmen tympani
Auditory tube
Canal for tensor tympani muscle
Promontory
Fenestra vestibuli
Pyramid
Aditus to mastoid antrum
Facial canal
Fenestra cochleae

ANTERIOR

(A)

Carotid canal
Jugular foramen

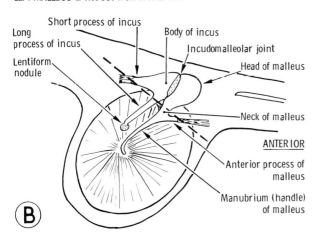

LEFT MALLEUS & INCUS: from medial side

Long process of incus
Short process of incus
Body of incus
Incudomalleolar joint
Head of malleus
Lentiform nodule
Neck of malleus

ANTERIOR

Anterior process of malleus
Manubrium (handle) of malleus

(B)

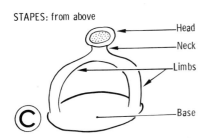

STAPES: from above

Head
Neck
Limbs
Base

(C)

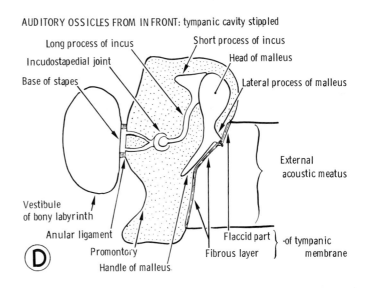

AUDITORY OSSICLES FROM IN FRONT: tympanic cavity stippled

Long process of incus
Incudostapedial joint
Base of stapes
Short process of incus
Head of malleus
Lateral process of malleus

External acoustic meatus

Vestibule of bony labyrinth
Anular ligament
Promontory
Handle of malleus.
Flaccid part
Fibrous layer
of tympanic membrane

(D)

409

In the lateral phase of the cycle, the incudomalleolar joint unlocks so that the handle and head of the malleus are able to recoil, laterally and medially respectively independently of the incus and stapes. The recoil of the latter two bones occurs rather more slowly and is motivated by the pressure of the perilymph in the bony labyrinth. Unlocking of the incudomalleolar joint prevents an excessive lateral movement of the tympanic membrane from tearing the anular ligament and pulling the base of the stapes out of the fenestra vestibuli. Excessive medial movement of the membrane cannot displace the base of the stapes into the vestibule because of the inertia of the perilymph in the bony labyrinth.

The high amplitude of the movements of the auditory ossicles, which occur in response to sounds of high intensity, are damped by two small muscles.

The stapedius muscle (**A**) arises from the walls of the central canal of the pyramid and its tendon, running forwards across the tympanic cavity, inserts into the neck of the stapes. It is innervated by the facial nerve.

The tensor tympani muscle (**A**) arises from the walls of its bony canal and from the cartilaginous part of the auditory tube (see below). Its tendon at first passes backwards but, as it emerges from its canal, turns laterally across the tympanic cavity to insert into the upper part of the handle of the malleus. The muscle is supplied by the mandibular division of the trigeminal nerve.

The nerves associated with the tympanic cavity

A tympanic branch which consists of ordinary sensory and preganglionic parasympathetic fibres arises from the inferior ganglion of the glossopharyngeal nerve (**B**). It turns upwards through the bone between the jugular foramen and the carotid canal and, entering the tympanic cavity, forms a plexus beneath the mucous membrane over the promontory. This tympanic plexus supplies sensory fibres to all parts of the mucosa of the middle ear excepting the most anterior part of the auditory tube. The parasympathetic fibres re-aggregate and, as the lesser petrosal nerve (**B**), pass forwards through the tegmen tympani into the middle cranial fossa (**C**) and thereafter downwards through the foramen ovale into the infratemporal fossa. Their subsequent distribution to the parotid salivary gland is considered later (**459C**).

The chorda tympani nerve supplies no structures in the ear but has a close and important relationship to the tympanic membrane. It is a branch of the facial nerve which arises in the descending part of the facial canal and consists of taste fibres and preganglionic parasympathetic fibres. It passes forwards to enter the tympanic cavity immediately behind the tympanic membrane (**D**). It re-enters bone immediately anterosuperior to the membrane and finally leaves it again through the lower end of the squamotympanic suture in the mandibular fossa (**413A**). Its subsequent distribution to structures in the floor of the mouth will be considered later. In the tympanic cavity it passes forwards and a little upwards, between the fibrous and mucosal layers of the tympanic membrane, and medial to the upper part of the handle of the malleus (**D**).

HORIZONTAL SECTION OF TYMPANIC CAVITY
ANTERIOR

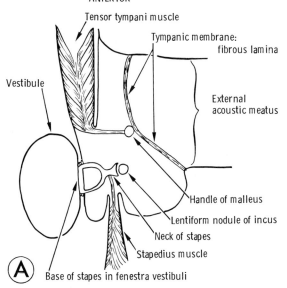

Tensor tympani muscle

Tympanic membrane:
fibrous lamina

Vestibule

External
acoustic meatus

Handle of malleus

Lentiform nodule of incus

Neck of stapes

Stapedius muscle

Base of stapes in fenestra vestibuli

(A)

MEDIAL WALL & CAVITY OF MIDDLE EAR:
TYMPANIC BRANCH OF GLOSSOPHARYNGEAL NERVE

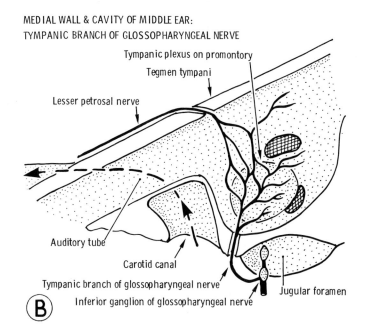

Tympanic plexus on promontory

Tegmen tympani

Lesser petrosal nerve

Auditory tube

Carotid canal

Tympanic branch of glossopharyngeal nerve

Inferior ganglion of glossopharyngeal nerve

Jugular foramen

(B)

BASE OF SKULL: INTERNAL SURFACE (Temporal bone stippled)

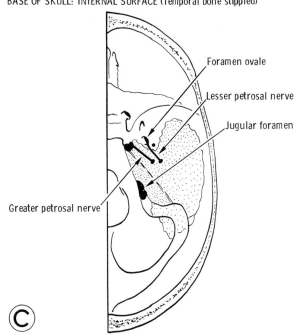

Foramen ovale

Lesser petrosal nerve

Jugular foramen

Greater petrosal nerve

(C)

LATERAL WALL OF TYMPANIC CAVITY: CHORDA TYMPANI NERVE

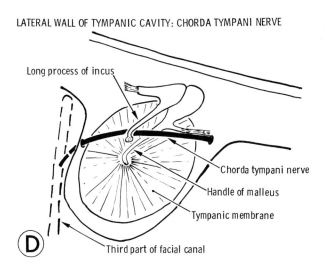

Long process of incus

Chorda tympani nerve

Handle of malleus

Tympanic membrane

Third part of facial canal

(D)

411

The mastoid antrum and air cells

The antrum is a single mucosal-lined air sinus, continuous anteriorly with the epitympanic recess through the aditus (**407C**). Its lateral wall corresponds to the suprameatal triangle on the outer surface of the skull (**A**). As the antrum is usually observed through this wall, it is important to note that whereas in the adult it is about 15 mm thick, in the infant it is only about 2 mm thick, although the antrum has reached almost its adult size. The medial wall is closely related to the semicircular canals. Above, the antrum is separated from the temporal lobe in the middle cranial fossa by the tegmen tympani (**407D**), while behind it is separated by a thin bone plate from the upper part of the sigmoid sinus and the cerebellum in the posterior cranial fossa (**B**). The floor is formed by the mastoid process and is perforated to a very variable degree by openings into the mastoid air cells (**407C**).

The mastoid air cells are a series of small intercommunicating mucosal-lined spaces, which extend progressively during infancy and adolescence from the floor of the antrum as the mastoid process enlarges downwards. Posteriorly, the air cells show a variable proximity to the sigmoid sinus and the cerebellum; anteriorly, they are closely related to the descending part of the facial canal and facial nerve.

The auditory tube

The auditory (pharyngotympanic) tube passes downwards forwards and medially from the tympanic cavity to the nasopharynx and is lined by mucous membrane (**463A**). Its patency ensures that the pressure on the inner aspect of the tympanic membrane is atmospheric. The walls of the posterior part are bony, while those of the rest consist of cartilage and fibrous tissue, the junction between the two parts being relatively constricted.

The bony part opens off the upper part of the anterior wall of the tympanic cavity and passes parallel to and below the bend of the carotid canal (**407D**). It opens on the under surface of the base of the skull in the angle between the tympanic and petrous parts of the temporal bone and the greater wing of the sphenoid (**C**).

The fibrocartilaginous part lies against the deeply grooved under surface of the suture between the petrous temporal and the greater wing of the sphenoid (**C**), and the lateral margin of its wide opening into the nasopharynx lies flush against the upper part of the posterior margin of the medial pterygoid plate. The superior and medial walls are cartilaginous and the lateral and inferior walls fibrous.

The external ear

This consists of the auricle, the convoluted concave flap which protrudes from the side of the head, and the tubular external acoustic meatus which extends from the deepest part of the auricle to the tympanic membrane.

The auricle, except for the lobule (**D**), is formed by a thin plate of elastic cartilage intimately covered by skin. The ridges and hollows which mark its lateral surface are named in **D**. The lobule is soft and occupied by loose vascular connective tissue.

The external acoustic meatus extends from the anterior part of the concha (**D**) to the tympanic membrane. Except for its posterosuperior part, which is fibrous, the wall of the lateral third of the meatus is formed by a short gutter-like extension of the auricular cartilage. In the adult the medial two-thirds of the meatus lies in the temporal bone, the grooved upper surface of the tympanic part of that bone forming its anterior, inferior and posterior walls and the squamous part its superior wall (**A**). This bony canal is related posteriorly to the mastoid process and anteriorly to the temporomandibular joint (**A**).

In infancy the length of the meatus is proportionate to its length in the adult. However, the tympanic part of the temporal bone is a simple narrow ring (**E, F**) and the wall of the segment between this and the auricular cartilage consists of fibrocartilage (**E**). As the mastoid process has yet to develop, the stylomastoid foramen is situated on the lateral aspect of the skull immediately posterior-inferior to the tympanic ring (**F**), a superficial situation which places the emerging facial nerve at risk in operations in this area.

During childhood and adolescence the tympanic ring grows laterally through the fibrocartilaginous part of the meatus (**E**). At the same time the bone of the suprameatal triangle thickens and the mastoid process bulges laterally and downwards. As a result the stylomastoid foramen becomes more deeply placed on the inferior aspect of the skull (**A**).

The skin which lines the meatus is continuous with that covering the auricle, but is characterised by ceruminous glands which secrete the ear wax.

LATERAL ASPECT OF LEFT TEMPORAL BONE

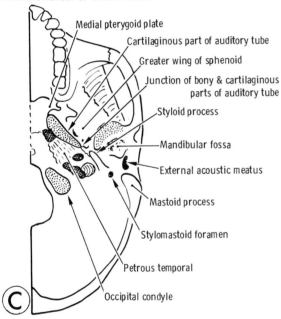

Mandibular fossa

Outline of mastoid antrum

Suprameatal triangle

Squamotympanic suture

Chorda tympani nerve

Tympanic part of temporal bone

Mastoid air cells

Stylomastoid foramen

A

INTERNAL ASPECT OF BASE OF SKULL

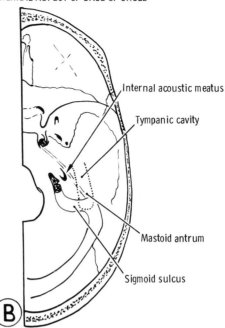

Internal acoustic meatus

Tympanic cavity

Mastoid antrum

Sigmoid sulcus

B

EXTERNAL ASPECT OF BASE OF SKULL

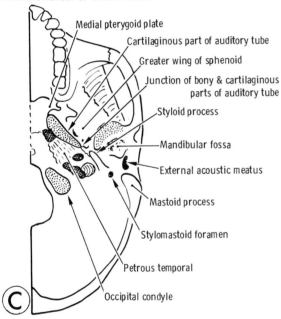

Medial pterygoid plate

Cartilaginous part of auditory tube

Greater wing of sphenoid

Junction of bony & cartilaginous parts of auditory tube

Styloid process

Mandibular fossa

External acoustic meatus

Mastoid process

Stylomastoid foramen

Petrous temporal

Occipital condyle

C

LATERAL ASPECT OF LEFT AURICLE

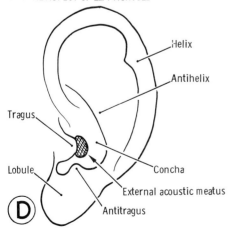

Helix

Antihelix

Tragus

Concha

Lobule

External acoustic meatus

Antitragus

D

LEFT EXTERNAL ACOUSTIC MEATUS AT BIRTH:
HORIZONTAL SECTION

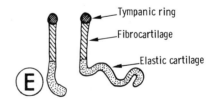

Tympanic ring

Fibrocartilage

Elastic cartilage

E

LEFT TEMPORAL BONE AT BIRTH

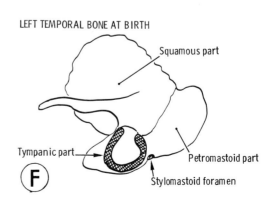

Squamous part

Tympanic part

Petromastoid part

Stylomastoid foramen

F

413

Examination of the tympanic membrane through an illuminated speculum is a common procedure and it is consequently important to appreciate certain features of the meatus.

1. Its length from the concha to the tympanic membrane is about 25 mm but, because the tympanic membrane faces downwards and forwards as well as laterally, the floor and anterior wall of the meatus are somewhat longer than the roof and posterior wall.
2. Although the main direction of the meatus is, of course, medial it is not entirely straight, inclining first anterosuperiorly, then posteriorly and finally antero-inferiorly. Consequently, passage of an auriscope through the external acoustic meatus is facilitated by pulling the auricle upwards and backwards.
3. The meatus presents two constrictions, one at the junction of the cartilaginous and osseous parts, and another within the osseous part.

On examination, the membrane is pearly grey and the malleolar folds, the flaccid and tense parts and the lateral process and handle of the malleus can be recognised (**A**). Because of the shape and orientation of the membrane, its inferior quadrant reflects the light shone down the speculum more brightly than other areas. This appearance is known as the cone of light.

The cutaneous innervation of the external ear involves a number of nerves. The distribution of cutaneous branches of the cervical plexus has been noted previously (**401C**). The auriculotemporal branch of the mandibular division of the trigeminal nerve (**B**) supplies the skin over the tragus and the anterior end of the helix, and that lining the anterior wall of the external meatus. The auricular branch of the superior ganglion of the vagus nerve passes laterally from the jugular foramen in a fine bony canal. It supplies the skin lining the posterio-inferior wall of the external meatus (**B**) and this distribution probably explains the reflex coughing, vomiting or fainting which is sometimes associated with irritation of this skin area.

The facial canal and nerve

The facial canal is closely related throughout to the internal and middle ears. It begins at the lateral end of the internal acoustic meatus, above the several foramina which transmit the fibres of the vestibulocochlear nerve to the internal ear (**407B**). The canal has three segments. The first passes laterally above the junction of vestibule and cochlea and approaches the medial wall of the epitympanic recess (**C**). The second runs backwards raising a faint ridge on this wall just above the fenestra vestibuli (**409A**). The third turns downwards, first in the bone forming the medial margin of the aditus and then in the bone forming the posterior wall of the tympanic cavity (**409A**), to reach the stylomastoid foramen (**413A, 413C**).

The facial nerve

Recall that this nerve arises from the brain stem as two parts (**39B, 51B**), a large motor root and a smaller root, known as the nervus intermedius, which is composed of taste fibres and preganglionic parasympathetic fibres. The motor root, the nervus intermedius and the vestibulocochlear nerve, in that order from above down, traverse the internal acoustic meatus within which the two parts of the facial nerve fuse (**C**). The definitive nerve then passes through the facial canal enlarging into the sensory genicular ganglion at the junction of the first and second segments (**C**). The nerve gives off three branches in the canal, and divides into a number of terminal branches once it has emerged from the stylomastoid foramen.

Two branches are composed of taste fibres, which have their cell bodies in the genicular ganglion, and preganglionic parasympathetic fibres; indeed they contain all the neurons of these types which originally formed the nervus intermedius.

1. *The greater petrosal branch* arises from the genicular ganglion and runs forwards through a canaliculus into the middle cranial fossa (**411C**).
2. *The chorda tympani nerve* arises in the third segment of the canal and its course through the temporal bone and tympanic cavity has been considered already (**411D**).

A minute branch arises in the third segment of the canal and passes forwards into the central canal of the pyramid to innervate the stapedius muscle (**409A**). This, and the terminal branch of the nerve, carry all the fibres originally situated in the motor root.

LEFT TYMPANIC MEMBRANE: SEEN THROUGH SPECULUM

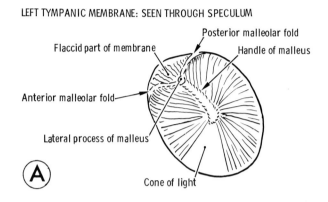

Flaccid part of membrane

Posterior malleolar fold

Handle of malleus

Anterior malleolar fold

Lateral process of malleus

Cone of light

(A)

CUTANEOUS INNERVATION: LEFT EXTERNAL ACOUSTIC MEATUS

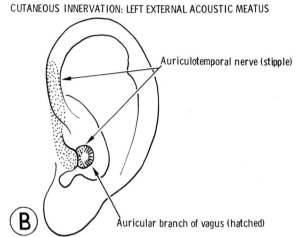

Auriculotemporal nerve (stipple)

Auricular branch of vagus (hatched)

(B)

FACIAL CANAL & NERVE: FIRST & SECOND PARTS

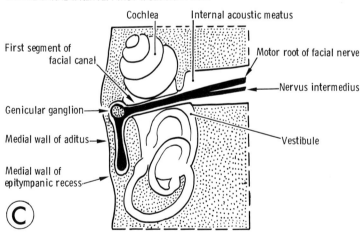

Cochlea

Internal acoustic meatus

First segment of facial canal

Motor root of facial nerve

Nervus intermedius

Genicular ganglion

Medial wall of aditus

Vestibule

Medial wall of epitympanic recess

(C)

THE ORBIT AND ITS CONTENTS

The eye

The eye, apart from a few features, is structurally symmetrical around an anteroposterior axis. Consequently, the interrelationships of the various parts of the eye are often most readily appreciated in horizontal sections through the organ, provided always that the appearance of the two-dimensional section is mentally converted to the three-dimensional structure of the actual eye.

The eye consists of three coats which are more or less concentric and enclose various transparent media.

The fibrous coat

The outer fibrous coat has two parts. About the anterior sixth is formed by the cornea and the rest by the sclera (**A**).

The sclera is white and opaque and consists of irregularly interlacing large collagen fibres. It is pierced by all the arteries and nerves which enter the eye and by the veins which leave it.

The cornea has a curvature of smaller radius than that of the sclera and is avascular and highly transparent. It is covered anteriorly by an epithelium of six to eight layers of cells, and posteriorly by a single layer of flattened cells. The substantia propria is composed of fine, collagen fibrils in an interfibrillar substance rich in proteoglycans, and the unique transparency of this connective tissue is probably related to the very regular arrangement of its fibrils and the high refractive index of the interfibrillar substance.

The corneoscleral junction

The circular junction between the two parts of the fibrous coat is bevelled so that the superficial part of the sclera overlaps the deep part of the cornea (**A**).

An anular vessel called the sinus venosus sclerae traverses the deep part of the junction (**B**). Despite its name, this vessel does not of itself contain blood though it drains into the veins of the eye. The central wall of the sinus consists of two distinct parts. The posterior part is a region of sclera, which in sections appears as a sharp forwardly directed spur (the scleral spur), but is in fact a continuous circular ridge. The anterior part is formed by the pectinate ligament which is a backward extension of the inner part of the cornea in the form of numerous anastomosing trabeculae. These trabeculae are separated by a continuous complex labyrinthine space which is lined by a continuation of the posterior endothelium of the cornea.

Although there appears to be no direct connection between this intertrabecular space and the lumen of the sinus venosus sclerae, there is no doubt that, in certain circumstances, aqueous humour (see below) escapes from the intertrabecular space into the sinus and so into the veins which drain the eye.

The vascular coat

The middle, vascular coat has three parts called from behind forwards the choroid, the ciliary body and the iris (**A**).

The choroid

The choroid lines the deep aspect of the posterior three-quarters or so of the sclera. It consists of a mesh of collagen and elastic fibres, interspersed with pigment cells and blood vessels. The outer vessels are of large calibre, while the inner ones are of capillary dimensions and constitute the choriocapillary lamina, which is concerned in the nourishment of the outer part of the retina.

The ciliary body

The ciliary body continues forwards from the choroid deep to the anterior quarter of the sclera (**C**). Its composition is similar to that of the choroid except that the choriocapillary lamina is a much less definite layer and it contains the fibres of the ciliary muscle. The posterior part of the body is called the ciliary ring and its inner surface exhibits meridionally directed ridges. Traced forwards each of these ridges divides into two or three narrower ridges, the ciliary processes (**C**), which protrude increasingly into the interior of the eye and end abruptly deep to the corneoscleral junction (**B**).

The ciliary muscle (**B, D**), which lies in the ciliary body, consists of two groups of smooth muscle fibres. The meridional fibres have a circular line of origin from the inner surface of the scleral spur and pass backwards through the outer part of the ciliary body. The circular fibres run in the anterior part of the ciliary body internal to the meriodional fibres and external to the grooves between the ciliary processes. It is innervated by the parasympathetic system (**115B**). When the ciliary muscle contracts, its two parts pull the ciliary ring and processes forwards and centrally. The important of this displacement in the process of accommodation will be considered later.

COATS OF THE EYE (X-X indicates plane of section in D)

<u>FIBROUS COAT</u>   <u>VASCULAR COAT</u>

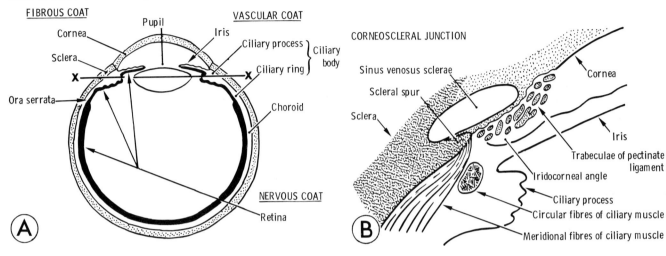

Cornea
Pupil
Iris
Sclera
Ciliary process } Ciliary body
Ciliary ring
Ora serrata
Choroid

<u>NERVOUS COAT</u>
Retina

Ⓐ

CORNEOSCLERAL JUNCTION

Sinus venosus sclerae
Scleral spur
Sclera
Cornea
Iris
Trabeculae of pectinate ligament
Iridocorneal angle
Ciliary process
Circular fibres of ciliary muscle
Meridional fibres of ciliary muscle

Ⓑ

CENTRAL ASPECT OF CILIARY BODY (Posterior half of eye removed)

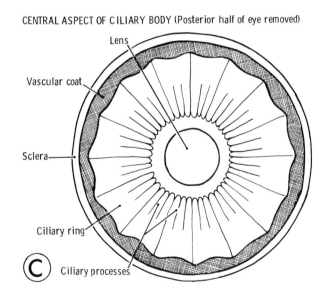

Lens
Vascular coat
Sclera
Ciliary ring
Ciliary processes

Ⓒ

CORONAL SECTION OF EYE
(Plane X-X in A)

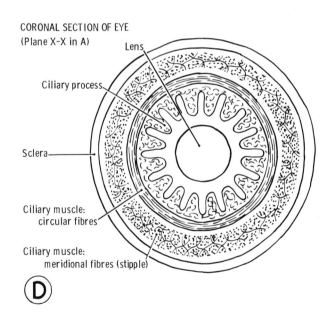

Lens
Ciliary process
Sclera
Ciliary muscle: circular fibres
Ciliary muscle: meridional fibres (stipple)

Ⓓ

417

The iris

This is a thin anular sheet of tissue which lies in or near a coronal plane in front of the lens. Its central opening is the pupil (**A**). Its peripheral margin is continuous with the anterior extremities of the ciliary processes and the pectinate ligament (**417B**).

The greater part of the iris is composed of vascular connective tissue which contains a variable number of melanocytes and circular and radial smooth muscle fibres. Its posterior surface is covered by two layers of pigmented cells which, as will be seen later, constitute the most anterior part of the retina (**A**).

Note the following features of the iris.

1. The colour of the iris depends on both the stromal melanocytes and the pigmented cells of the iridial part of the retina (**A**). When stromal melanocytes are more or less absent, as they are in the newborn, the iris is light blue, whereas when they are numerous the iris is some shade of brown.
2. The circular smooth muscle fibres which surround the margin of the pupil constitute the sphincter pupillae muscle (**B**). It is innervated by the parasympathetic system (**115B**).
3. The smooth muscle fibres which run radially from the margin of the pupil constitute the dilator pupillae muscle (**B**). It is innervated by the sympathetic system (**119A**).

The nervous coat

The retina, which is the inner nervous coat of the eye, lines the central aspects of the choroid, ciliary body and iris (**A**).

It is composed of two laminae. The outer consists, throughout, of a single layer of heavily pigmented cells. The inner varies in structure in different regions. As far forwards as the junction of the choroid and ciliary body, where its anterior limit is marked by the wavy line called the ora serrata, it is greatly thickened. The region contains all the light-sensitive elements of the retina and gives rise to the nerve fibres which form the optic nerve. The structure and features of this light-sensitive part of the retina have been described earlier and should now be revised (**81E**).

In front of the ora serrata the inner layer of the retina is reduced to a single layer of cells which are pigmented in relation to the iris but non-pigmented over the ciliary body.

The pigmentation of the outer layer of the retina prevents reflection of light within the eye once it has passed through the light sensitive part of the inner layer. The pigmentation of both layers on the posterior surface of the iris increases the opacity of that structure and ensures that only light passing through the pupil reaches the light-sensitive part of the retina.

The refractive media

As light passes through the eye to the light sensitive part of the retina, it traverses a number of transparent parts, namely the cornea which has been considered already, the aqueous humour, the lens and the vitreous body.

The aqueous humour and the chambers of the eye

The aqueous humour is a clear watery fluid which occupies both the anterior and posterior chambers of the eye. The anterior chamber is the space between the cornea and the iris, and its peripheral limit is called the iridocorneal angle (**A**). The much narrower posterior chamber separates the posterior surface of the iris from the lens and the ciliary zonule (see below) and its peripheral margin is formed by the anterior extremities of the ciliary processes (**A**). The two chambers communicate through the pupil.

The fluid is derived from capillaries in the ciliary processes, and leaves the anterior chamber by a process which is not yet understood by passing into the sinus venosus sclerae (**417B**).

The lens

The lens is a transparent biconvex body which is enclosed in a thin, highly elastic, homogeneous capsule. The radius of curvature of its anterior surface is greater than that of its posterior surface (**A**). Its essential feature is that it is elastically deformable. Thus the curvature of its surfaces can be temporarily altered, by a mechanism described below, so that an object at any distance from the observer can be focussed on the retina.

The vitreous body

This is a transparent substance of jelly-like consistency which occupies the space between the choroidal and ciliary parts of the retina and the lens (**A**).

It consists of a mesh of very fine collagen fibrils, the interstices of which are occupied by water bound to hyaluronate. A hyaloid canal, which contains only a watery fluid, extends from the optic disc to the posterior pole of the lens. It is occupied until about six weeks before birth by an artery.

HORIZONTAL SECTION OF EYE

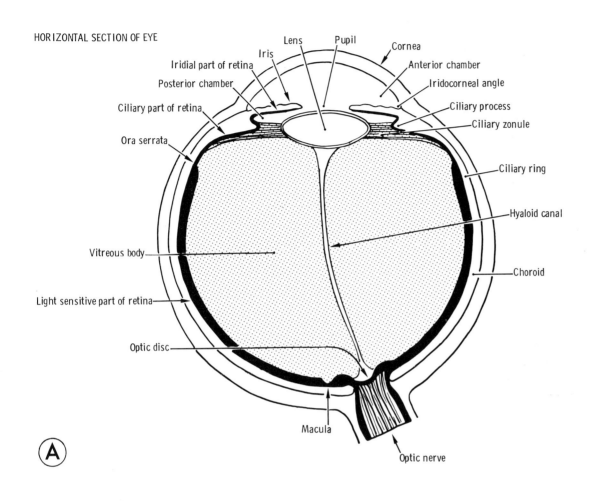

Lens
Pupil
Iris
Iridial part of retina
Cornea
Posterior chamber
Anterior chamber
Ciliary part of retina
Iridocorneal angle
Ora serrata
Ciliary process
Ciliary zonule
Ciliary ring
Hyaloid canal
Vitreous body
Choroid
Light sensitive part of retina
Optic disc
Macula
Optic nerve

Ⓐ

CORONAL SECTION OF IRIS

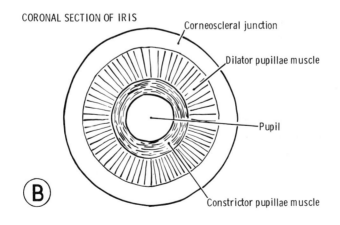

Corneoscleral junction
Dilator pupillae muscle
Pupil
Constrictor pupillae muscle

Ⓑ

The concentration of collagen fibrils in the vitreous is much greater adjacent to the ciliary processes than elsewhere (**419A**). Here the fibrils are attached to the inner lamina of cells of the ciliary part of the retina and extend centrally as an anular sheet called the ciliary zonule (**419A**).

Approaching the equator of the lens, the zonule splits into a thick anterior and a thinner posterior lamina which are attached to the corresponding aspects of the lens capsule (**419A, 419B**).

The mechanics of accommodation

The process of accommodation, by which objects at different distances from the observer are focussed on the retina, depends on alterations of the curvature of the lens surfaces. Contraction of the ciliary muscle (**A**) displaces the ciliary processes forwards and centrally, and as a result reduces the radial tension in the capsule of the lens, particularly its anterior part, which allows the anterior surface of the elastic lens to bulge forwards into a more convex shape. In these circumstances near objects are brought into focus.

When the ciliary muscle relaxes (**B**), the elasticity of the choroid slides the ciliary body backwards and peripherally thus creating tension in the ciliary zonule. This is transmitted to the lens capsule, which compresses the lens anteroposteriorly thus decreasing the convexity of its surfaces. In these circumstances distant objects are brought into focus.

Notice that the focussing of near objects is associated with active contraction of the ciliary muscle and a passive diminution in the stress within the lens, whereas the focussing of distant objects is associated with relaxation of the ciliary muscle but with an increase in the stress within the lens.

The orbit

Each orbit is a conical cavity in the facial skeleton. The anterior margin is formed by the maxillary, frontal and zygomatic bones (**C**). The orbital walls, which are not sharply demarcated from one another, converge as they are traced to the posterior end of the cavity (**C**). Observe in **C** the bones which form these walls and the several openings which pass through them.

1. Posteriorly, the optic canal traverses the root of the lesser wing of the sphenoid, while the pear-shaped superior orbital fissure separates the greater and lesser wings of the sphenoid.
2. The inferior orbital fissure extends along the angle between the lateral wall and floor and separates the greater wing of the sphenoid from the body of the maxilla.

3. From the medial part of the inferior orbital fissure the infra-orbital groove runs forwards on the upper surface of the maxilla. The groove gradually deepens into the infra-orbital canal, which continues forwards between the orbit and the air sinus within the maxilla to end at the infra-orbital foramen.
4. At the anterior end of the angle between medial wall and floor, the nasolacrimal canal opens into the orbit from the nasal cavity. Leading upwards from this opening is the lacrimal groove.

Note in the coronal section (**D**) the several important regions which are closely adjacent to the orbit.

The sagittal section through the left orbit shown in **E** illustrates the regions with which the orbit communicates through the superior and inferior orbital fissures. The superior orbital fissure leads into the middle cranial fossa in the region of the cavernous sinus (**99D**). The medial part of the inferior orbital fissure leads downwards and backwards into the pterygopalatine fossa, which in turn communicates with the middle cranial fossa through the foramen rotundum. The lateral part of the same fissure leads into the infratemporal fossa.

In the diagrammatic horizontal section (**F**) observe the planes of the medial and lateral walls of the two orbits. The medial walls are parallel, whereas the lateral walls lie at right angles to each other. Consequently, the long axes of the orbits extend obliquely forwards and laterally and it will be seen that many of the structures which pass forwards in the orbits tend towards a similarly oblique orientation. However although the eye, which lies in the anterior part of the orbit, is not fixed in its orientation, when it is focussed on infinity the visual axis which joins the anterior and posterior poles is in a sagittal plane and its equator in a coronal plane. In these circumstances the long axis of the orbit meets the posterior aspect of the eye a few millimetres medial to the posterior pole.

The fascial sheath of the eye

The eye is, of course, the essential content of the orbit and its structure has been considered already (**416**). It rests in a cup-shaped fascial sheath, the lower thicker part of which is described as the suspensory ligament. The sheath is attached to the sclera a short distance behind the corneoscleral junction. In addition it is pierced and further attached to the sclera by the tendons of all the extrinsic ocular muscles and by all the vessels and nerves which pass into the eye. Consequently, little movement is possible between the eye and its sheath and the two move within the orbit more or less as a single unit. At the sites where the sheath is pierced by the tendons of the extrinsic ocular muscles it is loosely attached to the walls of the orbit. These attachments prevent excessive movement of the eye in any direction and are called check ligaments.

MECHANICS OF ACCOMMODATION: CONTRACTION OF CILIARY MUSCLE

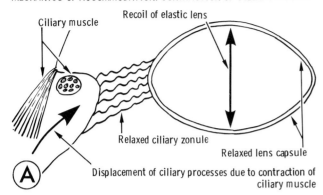

Ciliary muscle
Recoil of elastic lens
Relaxed ciliary zonule
Relaxed lens capsule
Displacement of ciliary processes due to contraction of ciliary muscle

A

MECHANICS OF ACCOMMODATION: RELAXATION OF CILIARY MUSCLE

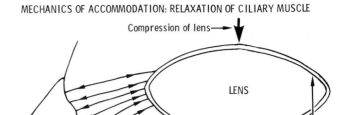

Compression of lens
LENS
Taut ciliary zonule
Taut lens capsule
Displacement of ciliary processes due to elastic pull of choroid

B

RIGHT ORBIT: ANTERIOR VIEW

Superior orbital fissure
Greater wing of sphenoid
Lesser wing of sphenoid
Orbital plate of frontal
Optic canal
Medial wall of orbit
Inferior orbital fissure
Frontal process of maxilla
Lacrimal groove
Zygomatic
Nasolacrimal canal
Maxilla
Infra-orbital foramen
Infra-orbital groove

C

CORONAL SECTION THROUGH ORBITS

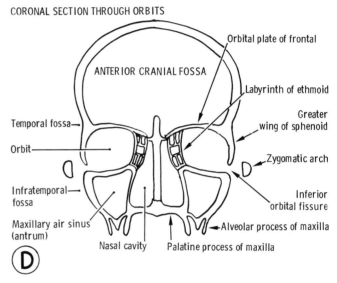

Orbital plate of frontal
ANTERIOR CRANIAL FOSSA
Labyrinth of ethmoid
Temporal fossa
Greater wing of sphenoid
Orbit
Zygomatic arch
Inferior orbital fissure
Infratemporal fossa
Maxillary air sinus (antrum)
Alveolar process of maxilla
Nasal cavity
Palatine process of maxilla

D

SAGITTAL SECTION THROUGH LEFT ORBIT:(Cut bone surfaces stippled)

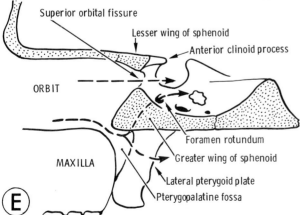

Superior orbital fissure
Lesser wing of sphenoid
Anterior clinoid process
ORBIT
Foramen rotundum
MAXILLA
Greater wing of sphenoid
Lateral pterygoid plate
Pterygopalatine fossa

E

DIAGRAM OF HORIZONTAL SECTION THROUGH ORBITS AND NASAL CAVITY

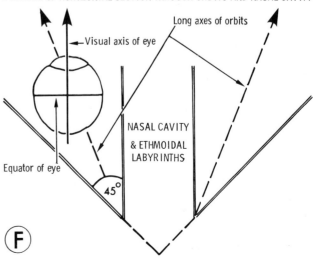

Long axes of orbits
Visual axis of eye
NASAL CAVITY & ETHMOIDAL LABYRINTHS
Equator of eye
45°

F

Orbital muscles

Six extrinsic ocular muscles, named the medial, lateral, superior and inferior recti and the superior and inferior obliques, are inserted into the scleral coat of the eye and move the eye and its fascial sheath within the orbit. The orbit also contains another muscle, which elevates the upper eyelid and is called levator palpebrae superioris.

Except for the inferior oblique, all the orbital muscles arise from a fibrous ring which is attached to the posterior wall of the orbit and encloses the openings of the optic canal and the middle part of the superior orbital fissure (**A**). Because the diameter of the fibrous ring is small in comparison to that of the eye, the muscles which arise from the ring form an expanding cone as they pass forwards to the eye (**C, D, E, F**). It will be evident (**A**) that vessels and nerves which enter the orbit through either the optic canal or the middle compartment of the superior orbital fissure, lie initially inside this cone of muscles whereas structures which enter the orbit by other routes will lie outside the cone.

Although the eye is free to rotate in any direction within the limits imposed by the check ligaments it is convenient and mechanically legitimate to resolve these movements into two components which may be visualised as occurring around vertical and transverse axes through the centre of the eye (**C, D, E, F**). The cardinal rotations of the eye may be named according to the displacements of the pupil they produce. Thus abduction, adduction, elevation and depression of the eye move the pupil laterally, medially, upwards and downwards respectively (**B**).

Examine the attachments and dispositions of the extrinsic ocular muscles (**A, C, D, E**), and note the relationships of their tendons to the vertical and transverse axes of the eye. It is these relationships which determine the actions of the muscles.

1. Both the medial and lateral rectus muscles (**A, C**) traverse the transverse axis of the eye and consequently produce no movement around it. However, the medial rectus pulls the medial aspect of the sclera backwards round the vertical axis, thus adducting the eye (**B**), whereas the lateral rectus pulls the lateral aspect of the sclera backwards round the vertical axis, thus abducting the eye (**B**).
2. The superior and inferior rectus muscles (**A, C, D**) both lie in the vertical plane which contains the long axis of the orbit. Consequently the superior rectus (**D**) pulls the anterosuperior aspect of the sclera

backwards above the transverse axis and medial to the vertical axis, and consequently both elevates and adducts the eye (**B**). Similarly the inferior rectus (**C**) pulls the antero-inferior aspect of the sclera backwards beneath the transverse axis and medial to the vertical axis and consequently both depresses and adducts the eye (**B**).

3. The superior oblique muscle (**A, D, F**) runs directly forwards along the medial wall of the orbit above the medial rectus. Its tendon passes through a cartilaginous pulley attached to the anterior part of the junction of the medial wall and roof of the orbit, and this runs backwards and laterally between the eye and the superior rectus muscle. It is inserted into the superolateral aspect of the sclera behind the equator. The muscle thus pulls this part of the sclera forwards above the transverse axis and medially behind the vertical axis and produces depression and abduction of the eye.
4. The inferior oblique muscle (**E**) differs from the other extrinsic ocular muscles in arising in the anterior part of the orbit from the maxilla just lateral to the orifice of the nasolacrimal canal. The muscle passes backwards and laterally below the eye and the inferior rectus muscle and, turning upwards, inserts into the inferolateral aspect of the sclera behind the equator. The muscle thus pulls this area of sclera forwards beneath the transverse axis and medially behind the vertical axis, so that it elevates and abducts the eye (**B**).
5. Note in **B** that, whereas abduction and adduction of the eye are each produced by a single muscle, pure elevation and depression of the eye requires the activity of two muscles acting in concert. Elevation is produced by the combined actions of inferior oblique and superior rectus, whereas depression is produced by the combined activities of superior oblique and inferior rectus.
6. The levator palpebrae superioris arises from the upper part of the fibrous ring and runs forwards and laterally against the roof of the orbit. A wide thin tendon (**F**) expands into the tissues of the upper eyelid. Its insertion will be considered later. The muscle is unusual in that it consists of two parts, an upper part which consists of voluntary muscle and a lower part which consists of smooth muscle. The significance of this will be discussed later.

FIBROUS RING ON POSTERIOR WALL OF ORBIT

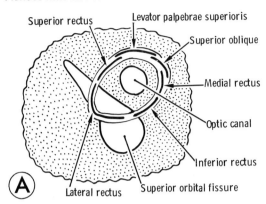

Superior rectus
Levator palpebrae superioris
Superior oblique
Medial rectus
Optic canal
Inferior rectus
Superior orbital fissure
Lateral rectus

A

DISPLACEMENT OF PUPIL BY EXTRA-OCULAR MUSCLES

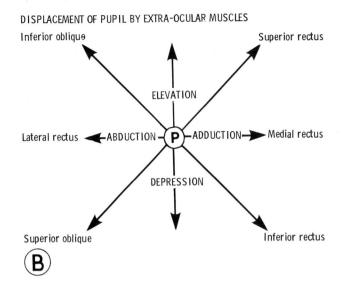

Inferior oblique
Superior rectus
ELEVATION
Lateral rectus ←ABDUCTION— P —ADDUCTION→ Medial rectus
DEPRESSION
Superior oblique
Inferior rectus

B

MUSCLES OF RIGHT ORBIT   T = transverse axis of eye   V = vertical axis of eye

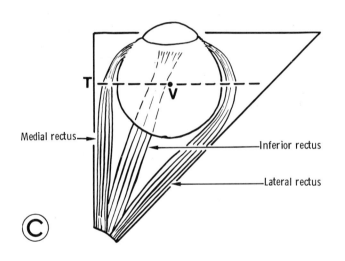

Medial rectus
Inferior rectus
Lateral rectus

C

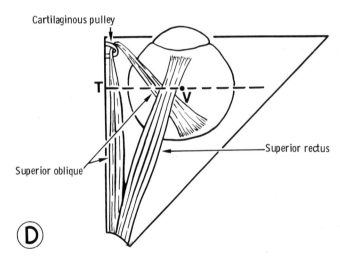

Cartilaginous pulley
Superior oblique
Superior rectus

D

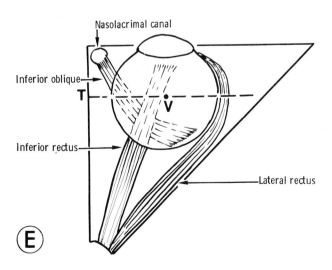

Nasolacrimal canal
Inferior oblique
Inferior rectus
Lateral rectus

E

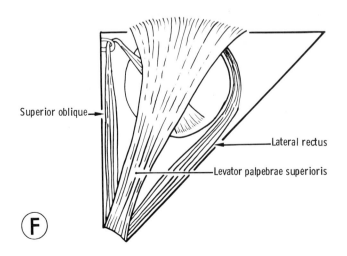

Superior oblique
Lateral rectus
Levator palpebrae superioris

F

The nerves of the orbit

All the nerves which enter the orbit approach that region in close relationship to the cavernous sinus and the internal carotid artery. Both these structures have been considered already (**99C, 99D**) and should now be revised. In particular, it may be recalled that the adventitial coat of the artery contains a profuse plexus of postganglionic sympathetic fibres derived from cell bodies in the superior cervical ganglion, and that the preganglionic neurons of this autonomic pathway have their cell bodies in the lateral grey column in the first and second thoracic segments of the spinal cord (**119A, 117B**). Branches from the internal carotid periarterial sympathetic plexus pass across the cavernous sinus and join many of the orbital nerves.

The nerves enter the orbit through the apertures already observed in the posterior part of the orbit (**421C**). Note in **A** the relationship of the nerves to these apertures and to the fibrous ring which gives origin to the cone of orbital muscles.

The optic nerve

This special sensory nerve of vision originates at the lateral end of the optic chiasma and the arrangement of its fibres in that part and in the optic tracts have been considered previously (**83C**). It passes forwards above the internal carotid artery as that vessel pierces the diaphragma sellae (**B**) and, traversing the optic canal (**A**), enters the orbit within the fibrous ring and therefore inside the cone of orbital muscles.

The nerve runs forwards and laterally along the long axis of the orbit, following a rather sinuous course which allows for movements of the eye (**D**). It reaches the eye about 3 mm medial to its posterior pole and its fibres run in bundles into the optic disc of the retina through the sclera and choroid (**C**).

In the optic canal and throughout its course in the orbit, the nerve is surrounded by concentric sheaths of pia mater, arachnoid and dura mater (**C**) which become continuous with the intracranial meninges posteriorly and fuse with the sclera anteriorly. Between the pial and arachnoid sheath is an extension of the subarachnoid space containing cerebrospinal fluid. The importance of this relationship will be discussed later (**430**).

The abducent nerve

As has been seen earlier the abducent nerve arises from the sulcus between the pons and the pyramid (**39B**) and consists of somatic motor fibres. It runs forwards and upwards in the posterior cranial fossa and, piercing the arachnoid and dura close to the inferior petrosal sinus (**B**), follows that vessel to the posterior end of the cavernous sinus. The nerve then runs longitudinally through the substance of the sinus just to the lateral side of the internal carotid artery (**E**). Leaving the anterior end of the sinus it enters to orbit within the cone of orbital muscles by passing through the middle compartment of the superior orbital fissure (**A**). Here the nerve inclines laterally to reach and supply the lateral rectus (**D**).

The oculomotor nerve

The origin of this nerve from the midbrain and the fact that it consists of somatic motor and preganglionic parasympathetic fibres have been considered earlier (**49B**). It runs forwards through the interpeduncular cistern and pierces the arachnoid and then the dura below and lateral to the posterior clinoid process (**B**). It now continues forwards immediately deep to the dura mater which forms the lateral wall of the cavernous sinus (**E**) and in this situation receives a group of postganglionic sympathetic fibres from the plexus on the wall of the neighbouring internal carotid artery. Approaching the anterior end of the sinus the nerve divides into superior and inferior divisions, the inferior division receiving all the preganglionic parasympathetic fibres. Both divisions pass through the middle compartment of the superior orbital fissure (**A**) and consequently enter the orbit inside the cone of orbital muscles. The superior division turns upwards and supplies superior rectus and levator palpebrae superioris, the smooth lower fibres of the latter muscle being innervated by the sympathetic. The inferior division turns downwards and supplies the medial and inferior recti and inferior oblique (**D**). It also gives a branch which contains all the preganglionic parasympathetic fibres of the parent nerve to the ciliary ganglion which will be considered below.

ENTRANCE OF NERVES INTO ORBIT

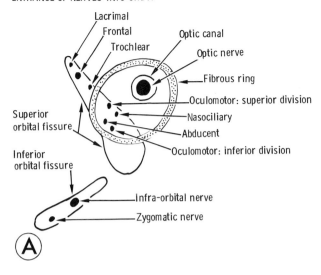

Lacrimal
Frontal
Trochlear
Optic canal
Optic nerve
Fibrous ring
Oculomotor: superior division
Nasociliary
Abducent
Oculomotor: inferior division
Superior orbital fissure
Inferior orbital fissure
Infra-orbital nerve
Zygomatic nerve

A

DURA MATER LINING BASE OF CRANIAL CAVITY

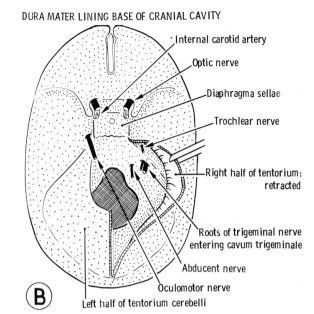

Internal carotid artery
Optic nerve
Diaphragma sellae
Trochlear nerve
Right half of tentorium: retracted
Roots of trigeminal nerve entering cavum trigeminale
Abducent nerve
Oculomotor nerve
Left half of tentorium cerebelli

B

MENINGEAL SHEATHS OF OPTIC NERVE

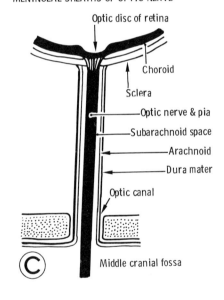

Optic disc of retina
Choroid
Sclera
Optic nerve & pia
Subarachnoid space
Arachnoid
Dura mater
Optic canal
Middle cranial fossa

C

NERVES OF LEFT ORBIT: upper orbital muscles removed

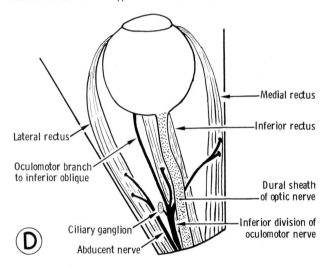

Medial rectus
Inferior rectus
Dural sheath of optic nerve
Inferior division of oculomotor nerve
Lateral rectus
Oculomotor branch to inferior oblique
Ciliary ganglion
Abducent nerve

D

CORONAL SECTION THROUGH CAVERNOUS SINUS

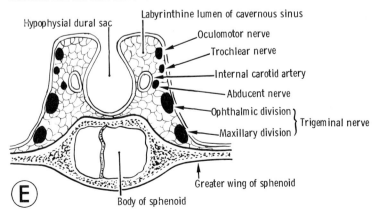

Hypophysial dural sac
Labyrinthine lumen of cavernous sinus
Oculomotor nerve
Trochlear nerve
Internal carotid artery
Abducent nerve
Ophthalmic division
Maxillary division
} Trigeminal nerve
Greater wing of sphenoid
Body of sphenoid

E

The trochlear nerve

This slender nerve consists of somatic motor fibres. Having passed forwards round the midbrain it pierces the dura on the inferior surface of the tentorium cerebelli just behind the posterior clinoid process (**425B**). It then runs forwards, deep to the dura forming the lateral wall of the cavernous sinus (**425E**), and traverses the upper compartment of the superior orbital fissure (**425A**) to enter the orbit above the cone of orbital muscles. It passes medially and forwards between the levator palpebrae superioris and the roof of the orbit (**A**) to reach and supply the superior oblique muscle.

The trigeminal nerve

This arises from the pons in the posterior cranial fossa by a small medial motor root and a large lateral sensory root (**39B**). These roots pass forwards, between the superior petrosal sinus in the attached margin of the tentorium cerebelli, and the superior border of the petrous temporal, into a dural diverticulum called the cavum trigeminale (**B**). This lies beneath the dura which lines the lateral compartment of the middle cranial fossa and against the lateral part of the foramen lacerum and the adjacent parts of the cavernous sinus and the petrous temporal (**B**).

In the trigeminal cave the sensory root enlarges into the large sensory trigeminal ganglion. The ophthalmic, maxillary and mandibular divisions, which leave the distal border of the ganglion and consist of the peripheral processes of its pseudo-unipolar cells, immediately pierce the dural cave and emerge beneath the dura which lines the lateral compartment of the middle cranial fossa (**B**). The motor root crosses below the ganglion to its lateral side, where it soon joins the mandibular division to form the mixed mandibular nerve (**B**).

The ophthalmic division of the trigeminal nerve

The ophthalmic division passes forwards from the upper medial part of the cavum trigeminale lying deep to the dura which forms the lateral wall of the cavernous sinus (**B**). Here it receives an important quota of postganglionic sympathetic fibres from the plexus on the wall of the internal carotid artery and divides into three branches called the lacrimal, frontal and nasociliary nerves (**B**). The terminal branches of these three nerves collectively innervate the ophthalmic area of skin shown in **C**.

The lacrimal nerve, which is small, enters the orbit through the uppermost part of the superior orbital fissure

(**425A**) and consequently outside the cone of orbital muscles.

It continues forwards against the lateral wall above the lateral rectus (**A**), and gives a branch to the lacrimal gland which will be discussed later. It appears at the lateral end of the supra-orbital margin (**C**).

The frontal nerve, which is considerably larger, also traverses the upper compartment of the superior orbital fissure (**425A**) and runs forwards between levator palpebrae superioris and the orbital roof (**A**). At a variable point it divides into large supra-orbital and small supratrochlear branches which appear at the middle and medial parts of the supra-orbital margin (**C**).

The nasociliary nerve enters the orbit through the central compartment of the superior orbital fissure (**425A**) within the cone of orbital muscles and lateral to the optic nerve (**D**). It then inclines medially above the optic nerve to reach the medial wall of the orbit between medial rectus and superior oblique, where it divides into an infratrochlear branch which runs forwards to appear at the medial angle of the eye (**D, C**) and a nasal branch which passes through the medial wall of the orbit into the nasal cavity. Internal nasal branches are distributed to some of the mucous membrane lining that cavity (**436**) and an external nasal branch appears at the lower margin of the bony bridge of the nose (**C**).

In the posterior part of the orbit the nasociliary nerve also gives off two or three long ciliary nerves and a communication to the ciliary ganglion (**D**). All of these consist of sensory fibres from the trigeminal ganglion and postganglionic sympathetic fibres from the plexus on the internal carotid artery.

The ciliary ganglion is one of the small isolated parasympathetic ganglia which are characteristic of the parasympathetic system in the regions of the head and neck. It lies near the back of the orbit between the optic nerve and the lateral rectus muscle (**D**). It receives fibres through two short roots and gives off numerous short ciliary branches which run forwards and pierce the sclera of the eye around the attachment of the optic nerve (**D**). One of the roots arises from the nasociliary nerve (**D**). As has been noted earlier, it is composed of ordinary sensory fibres and postganglionic sympathetic fibres, both of which continue into the short ciliary nerves without relay in the ganglion. The other root is derived from the inferior division of the oculomotor nerve (**425D**) and consists of preganglionic parasympathetic fibres. These synapse within the ganglion with postganglionic parasympathetic neurons, the axons of which pass forwards in the short ciliary nerves. The short ciliary nerves thus consist of sensory fibres and postganglionic sympathetic and parasympathetic fibres.

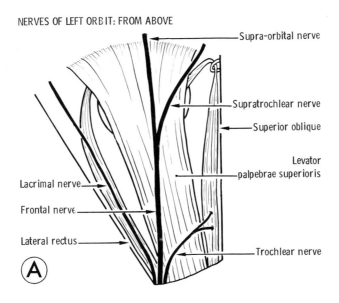

NERVES OF LEFT ORBIT: FROM ABOVE

Supra-orbital nerve

Supratrochlear nerve

Superior oblique

Levator palpebrae superioris

Lacrimal nerve

Frontal nerve

Lateral rectus

Trochlear nerve

A

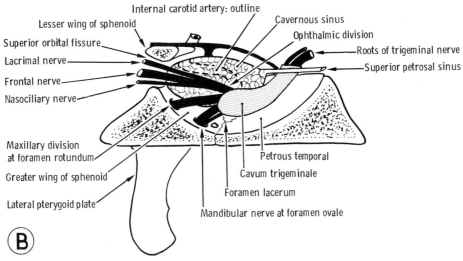

LATERAL COMPARTMENT OF MIDDLE CRANIAL FOSSA: LATERAL VIEW: lining dura removed

Internal carotid artery: outline

Lesser wing of sphenoid

Cavernous sinus

Superior orbital fissure

Ophthalmic division

Lacrimal nerve

Roots of trigeminal nerve

Frontal nerve

Superior petrosal sinus

Nasociliary nerve

Maxillary division at foramen rotundum

Greater wing of sphenoid

Petrous temporal

Lateral pterygoid plate

Cavum trigeminale

Foramen lacerum

Mandibular nerve at foramen ovale

B

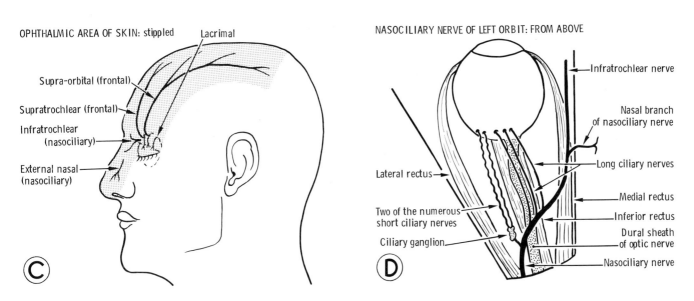

OPHTHALMIC AREA OF SKIN: stippled

Lacrimal

Supra-orbital (frontal)

Supratrochlear (frontal)

Infratrochlear (nasociliary)

External nasal (nasociliary)

C

NASOCILIARY NERVE OF LEFT ORBIT: FROM ABOVE

Infratrochlear nerve

Nasal branch of nasociliary nerve

Long ciliary nerves

Lateral rectus

Medial rectus

Two of the numerous short ciliary nerves

Inferior rectus

Dural sheath of optic nerve

Ciliary ganglion

Nasociliary nerve

D

The nerve supply to the eye reaches it entirely through the long and short ciliary nerves (see above), which pierce the sclera around the optic nerve and run forwards between the fibrous and vascular coats. The ordinary sensory fibres are distributed to the sclera, where they are stimulated by raised intra-ocular pressure, and to the cornea, where they are stimulated by surface irritation. The postganglionic parasympathetic fibres are motor to the ciliary muscle and to the constrictor pupillae muscle of the iris. The postganglionic sympathetic fibres are distributed to blood vessels, but in addition are motor to the dilator pupillae muscle of the iris.

The maxillary division of the trigeminal nerve

The maxillary division, having pierced the cavum trigeminale, runs forwards beneath the dura lining the floor of the lateral compartment of the middle cranial fossa to leave the cranial cavity through the foramen rotundum (**427B**). This foramen leads it into the upper part of the pterygopalatine fossa, where it divides into a large infra-orbital and a small zygomatic branch, both of which enter the orbit through the inferior orbital fissure (**A, C**).

The infra-orbital nerve passes along the infra-orbital groove and canal, and emerging from the infra-orbital foramen, divides abruptly into a spray of cutaneous branches (**A**). In its course it gives off three superior alveolar branches which descend in the thin bony walls of the maxillary sinus to innervate all the teeth of the upper jaw.

The zygomatic nerve runs forwards along the lower part of the lateral wall of the orbit and gives off an ascending branch, discussed below, which joins the lacrimal nerve (**A, C**). It then divides into two cutaneous branches which pass through the zygomatic bone and emerge on its anterior and lateral surfaces (**A**).

The cutaneous branches of the maxillary division described above innervate a maxillary area of skin on the face and temporal region (**B**).

The pterygopalatine ganglion is a parasympathetic ganglion which is considerably larger in size than the ciliary ganglion described above. It lies in the upper part of the pterygopalatine fossa which should be revised (**C, 17C**). The ganglion has two roots.

1. The proximal of its two connections with the maxillary division of the trigeminal nerve.
2. The greater petrosal nerve. This has already been seen to arise from the genicular ganglion of the facial nerve and pass forwards into the middle cranial fossa (**415C, 411C**). Thereafter it enters the foramen lacerum and traverses a long narrow canal through the greater wing of the sphenoid to reach the pterygopalatine fossa.

The ganglion has several branches.

1. The distal of its two connections with the maxillary division.
2. Several descending branches which leave the fossa by various routes and innervate areas of mucous membrane in the nasal cavity and the nasopharynx and on the palate.

Three functional types of nerve fibres are associated with the ganglion.

1. Ordinary sensory fibres which have their cell bodies in the trigeminal ganglion pass from the maxillary division, through its proximal connection to the ganglion and then without relay into all the descending branches.
2. Taste fibres which have their cell bodies in the genicular ganglion of the facial nerve reach the pterygopalatine ganglion in the greater petrosal nerve. Without relaying they then pass through some of the descending branches to taste buds on the palate.
3. Preganglionic parasympathetic fibres from the facial nerve also reach the pterygopalatine ganglion in the greater petrosal nerve. Here they synapse with postganglionic parasympathetic neurons whose axons follow two routes. Some pass through the descending branches to innervate glands in the areas of mucous membrane noted above. Others pass successively through the distal connection to the maxillary division, the zygomatic nerve, the communication to the lacrimal nerve and the branch of the latter nerve to the lacrimal gland to which they are secretomotor.

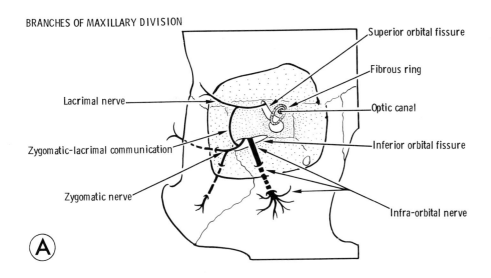

BRANCHES OF MAXILLARY DIVISION

Superior orbital fissure

Fibrous ring

Lacrimal nerve

Optic canal

Zygomatic-lacrimal communication

Inferior orbital fissure

Zygomatic nerve

Infra-orbital nerve

Ⓐ

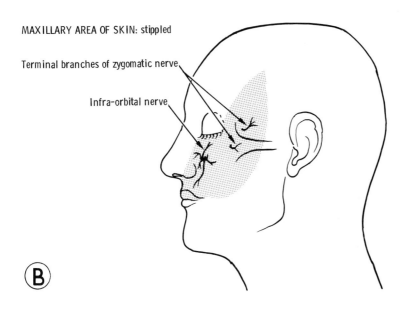

MAXILLARY AREA OF SKIN: stippled

Terminal branches of zygomatic nerve

Infra-orbital nerve

Ⓑ

PTERYGOPALATINE FOSSA & NEIGHBOURING REGIONS: DIAGRAMMATIC SAGITTAL SECTION

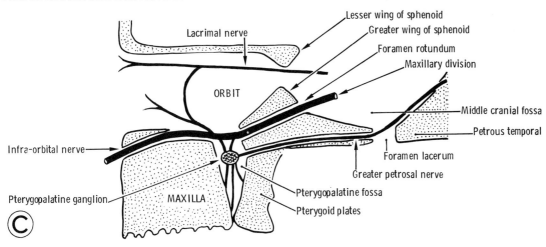

Lacrimal nerve

Lesser wing of sphenoid

Greater wing of sphenoid

Foramen rotundum

Maxillary division

ORBIT

Middle cranial fossa

Petrous temporal

Infra-orbital nerve

Foramen lacerum

Greater petrosal nerve

Pterygopalatine ganglion

MAXILLA

Pterygopalatine fossa

Pterygoid plates

Ⓒ

The arterial supply to the orbit

Almost the whole arterial supply to the contents of the orbit, including the eye, is derived from the ophthalmic artery. This arises from the internal carotid artery as soon as it has pierced the diaphragma sellae and the covering arachnoid and passes into the orbit through the optic canal (**A**). Here it is inferolateral to the optic nerve and enclosed within the same dural and arachnoid sheaths. In the orbit it leaves these sheaths and passes medially above the optic nerve to the medial wall of the orbit (**B**). It gives off a number of groups of branches.

1. The central artery of the retina, after running first within the subarachnoid space around the optic nerve, passes into the substance of the nerve and runs to the optic disc. Its branches, which are end-arteries, radiate on the inner surface of the light-sensitive part of the retina (**C**). Because of the lack of anastomoses of these arteries with adjacent vessels, occlusion causes blindness related to the corresponding area of the retina.
2. Other branches to the eye pierce the sclera either around the optic nerve (posterior ciliary) or a short distance behind its junction with the cornea (anterior ciliary). They are distributed to the choroid, ciliary body and iris and, to a lesser extent, to the sclera (**B**).
3. Branches to the extra-ocular muscles.
4. Cutaneous branches which supply the tissues of the forehead, the root of the nose and the upper and lower eyelids (**B**).

Venous drainage of the orbit

The superior and inferior ophthalmic veins pass from before backwards through the orbit. They traverse the superior orbital fissure and join the anterior end of the cavernous sinus (**D**) either singly or after union with one another. They communicate anteriorly with the facial vein around the medial angle of the eye, and with the pterygoid venous plexus in the infratemporal fossa through the inferior orbital fissure. The communication with the facial vein is important because it may allow the spread of an infective thrombophlebitis from an infective lesion on the face or forehead to the cavernous sinus.

The ophthalmic veins receive two sets of tributaries from the eye.

1. The vascular coat of the eye is drained by four veins, which, unlike the arteries supplying that area (see above), emerge through the sclera (**B**) at equally-spaced points around the equator (venae vorticosae).
2. The veins of the retina converge across its inner surface to the optic disc where they join to form the single central vein of the retina. This lies first in the centre of the optic nerve, then in the subarachnoid space around the nerve, and finally passes through the meningeal sheaths to join an ophthalmic vein (**C**).

When intracranial pressure is raised, the rise is communicated to the cerebrospinal fluid around the optic nerve and compresses the thin-walled central vein of the retina as it passes from within the optic nerve to outside its meningeal sheaths. There is little effect on the central artery because of its thicker wall and higher blood pressure.

Such compression of the central vein of the retina causes engorgement of the retinal veins, and oedema (swelling) of the optic disc. The appearance is known as papilloedema.

The eyelids and lacrimal apparatus

The eyelids or palpebrae are two mobile folds of tissue which lie in front of and protect the eye (**E**). When the eye is open the lid margins are separated by the palpebral fissure (**E**). The lateral extremity of the fissure, or the lateral angle of the eye, overlies the sclera, whereas the medial extremity or medial angle is situated some 6 mm medial to the sclera (**F**).

The space between the eye and the eyelids is lined by a transparent mucous membrane called the conjunctiva and is known as the conjunctival sac. Its upper and lower limits are the conjunctival fornices (**E**). The palpebral conjunctiva is highly vascular and is innervated by the same nerves as the palpebral skin (**427C, 429B**). The ocular conjunctiva is thin and contains few blood vessels over the sclera and centrally becomes continuous with the anterior epithelium of the cornea (**E**). Its sensory innervation is derived from the nasociliary nerve through the long and short ciliary nerves (**427D**). Conjunctiva also covers the lid margins and the small triangular area between the sclera and the medial angle of the eye which is called the lacus lacrimalis (**F**).

OPHTHALMIC ARTERY

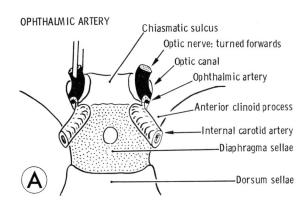

Chiasmatic sulcus
Optic nerve: turned forwards
Optic canal
Ophthalmic artery
Anterior clinoid process
Internal carotid artery
Diaphragma sellae
Dorsum sellae

A

OPHTHALMIC ARTERY: ARTERIES & VEINS OF EYE

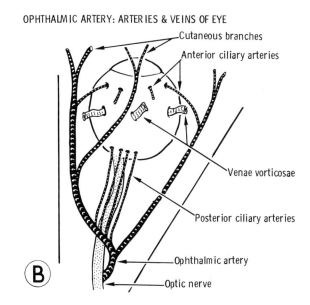

Cutaneous branches
Anterior ciliary arteries
Venae vorticosae
Posterior ciliary arteries
Ophthalmic artery
Optic nerve

B

CENTRAL VESSELS OF RETINA

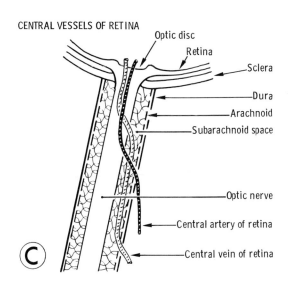

Optic disc
Retina
Sclera
Dura
Arachnoid
Subarachnoid space
Optic nerve
Central artery of retina
Central vein of retina

C

OPHTHALMIC VEINS

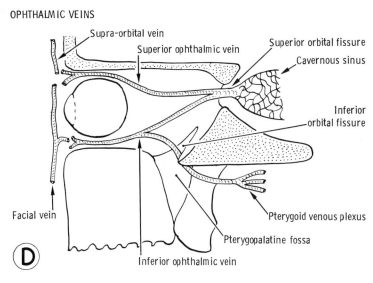

Supra-orbital vein
Superior ophthalmic vein
Superior orbital fissure
Cavernous sinus
Inferior orbital fissure
Facial vein
Pterygoid venous plexus
Pterygopalatine fossa
Inferior ophthalmic vein

D

EYELIDS & CONJUNCTIVAL SAC: SAGITTAL SECTION

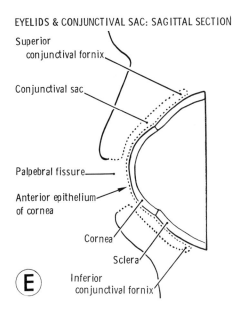

Superior conjunctival fornix
Conjunctival sac
Palpebral fissure
Anterior epithelium of cornea
Cornea
Sclera
Inferior conjunctival fornix

E

PALPEBRAL FISSURE: RIGHT EYE

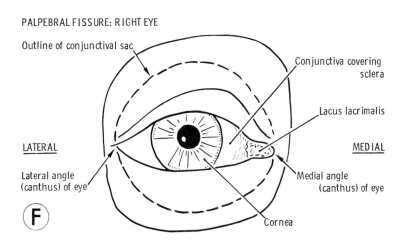

Outline of conjunctival sac
Conjunctiva covering sclera
Lacus lacrimalis

LATERAL

MEDIAL

Lateral angle (canthus) of eye
Medial angle (canthus) of eye
Cornea

F

The lacrimal gland

The conjunctival sac is constantly occupied by tears which are continually produced, albeit at varying rates, by the lacrimal gland. The gland lies in a fossa immediately behind the superolateral part of the orbital margin. However, it is partially divided into two parts by the sharp lateral edge of the tendon of levator palpebrae superioris as it expands into the upper eyelid, so that a small part of the gland lies below and behind that tendon in close relationship to the lateral part of the superior conjunctival fornix (**A**). It is from this part of the gland that multiple short ducts deliver the tears into the conjunctival sac.

The complex route of the parasympathetic secretomotor supply to the gland has been considered already (**428**)

Escape of tears from the conjunctival sac

Some of the tears are lost from the conjunctival sac by evaporation. The rest escapes through a system of passages into the nasal cavity (**A**).

Opposite the dividing line between the lacus lacrimalis and the medial part of the sclera, each lid margin exhibits a small backwardly-directed lacrimal papilla on the summit of which is a small opening named the lacrimal punctum. From each punctum the excess of tears passes through a narrow lacrimal canaliculus. The superior and inferior canaliculi pass initially upwards and downwards respectively into the corresponding lids and then, turning at right angles, each courses medially to reach the lacrimal sac.

The sac lies in the lacrimal groove on the lower anterior part of the medial wall of the orbit, where it is situated medial to the lacus lacrimalis and the medial angle of the eye. Above, it ends blindly, while below it becomes continuous with the nasolacrimal duct.

The duct, which is about 1 cm long, runs downwards through the bony nasolacrimal canal to open on the lateral wall of the lower part of the nasal cavity.

The structure of the eyelids

Between the palpebral conjunctiva and the skin the eyelids contain the following structures.

1. The curved form of the lids is maintained by correspondingly curved plates of tough fibrous tissue called the tarsi (**C, D**). Observe that the superior and inferior tarsi differ in size, and that their narrow extremities unite beyond the corresponding angles of the eye to form the palpebral ligaments. The lateral ligament is attached to bone just within the lateral orbital margin, while the medial ligament passes in front of the lacrimal sac to be attached to the anterior edge of the lacrimal groove.

2. In both eyelids, except in the regions medial to the lacrimal papillae, 20 or so straight parallel tarsal glands (**B**) pass towards the lid margins on which their ducts open, close to the posterior edge (**D**). The glands lie between the conjunctiva and the tarsi in which they are partially embedded (**D**). Consequently, if a cyst forms as a result of blockage of one of the ducts, it bulges posteriorly. The tarsal glands are modified sebaceous glands. The material they secrete has a high surface tension and thus tends to prevent tears spilling over the lid margins except when the lacrimal gland is hyperactive, as in weeping.

3. The eyelashes are two or three rows of short thick hairs which protrude with a forward inclination from the lid margins anterior to the orifices of the tarsal glands (**D**). They are absent from those parts of the lid margins bordering the lacus lacrimalis.

4. The levator palpebrae superioris muscle has been observed already in the orbit. Its tendon widens as it passes forwards and downwards into the upper eyelid. The relationship of the tendon to the lacrimal gland has been noted (**A**). Its deeper fibres, which are continuous with the involuntary part of the muscle, are attached to the upper margin of the superior tarsal plate (**C, D**), while the superficial fibres, which are continuous with the voluntary part of the muscle, spray downwards and forwards through the orbicularis oculi muscle (see below) to reach the overlying skin (**D**). The lateral and medial margins of the tendon are attached to the corresponding palpebral ligaments (**C**) and prevent excessive elevation of the eyelid. No corresponding muscle is associated with the lower eyelid.

5. The fibres of the orbicularis oculi muscle (**E**) arise from the medial palpebral ligament and from the bone above and below its attachment. The palpebral fibres extend laterally beneath the skin of both eyelids and end by interlacing superficial to the lateral palpebral ligament. They close the palpebral fissure in the involuntary blinking which smears the tears over the surface of the eye at frequent intervals. Because the fibres lack a lateral bony attachment they move the lids medially as well as towards each other and thus tend to sweep the tears from the lateral part of the conjunctival sac towards the lacrimal canaliculi. The orbital fibres describe continuous circles around the orbital margin and are inserted into the skin of the forehead and eyebrow, the temporal region and the cheek. They contract when some external violence threatens the eye and draw the skin surrounding the orbital margin over the eye as a thick protective pad. The whole of the orbicularis oculi is innervated by the facial nerve (see below).

LACRIMAL APPARATUS

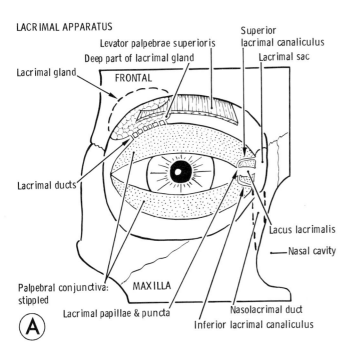

Levator palpebrae superioris
Deep part of lacrimal gland
Superior lacrimal canaliculus
Lacrimal gland
FRONTAL
Lacrimal sac
Lacrimal ducts
Lacus lacrimalis
Nasal cavity
Palpebral conjunctiva: stippled
MAXILLA
Lacrimal papillae & puncta
Nasolacrimal duct
Inferior lacrimal canaliculus

(A)

TARSAL GLANDS

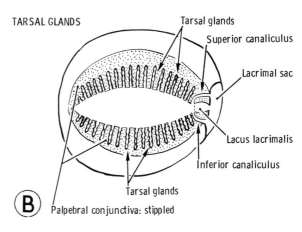

Tarsal glands
Superior canaliculus
Lacrimal sac
Lacus lacrimalis
Inferior canaliculus
Tarsal glands
Palpebral conjunctiva: stippled

(B)

THE TARSI

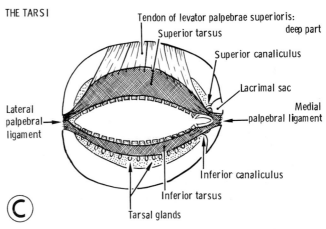

Tendon of levator palpebrae superioris: deep part
Superior tarsus
Superior canaliculus
Lacrimal sac
Lateral palpebral ligament
Medial palpebral ligament
Inferior canaliculus
Inferior tarsus
Tarsal glands

(C)

EYELIDS: SAGITTAL SECTION (thickness of eyelids exaggerated)

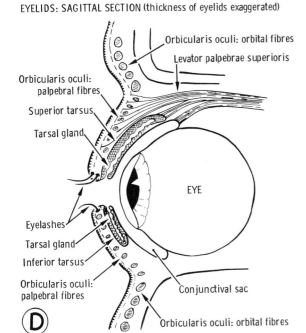

Orbicularis oculi: orbital fibres
Levator palpebrae superioris
Orbicularis oculi: palpebral fibres
Superior tarsus
Tarsal gland
EYE
Eyelashes
Tarsal gland
Inferior tarsus
Orbicularis oculi: palpebral fibres
Conjunctival sac
Orbicularis oculi: orbital fibres

(D)

ORBICULARIS OCULI

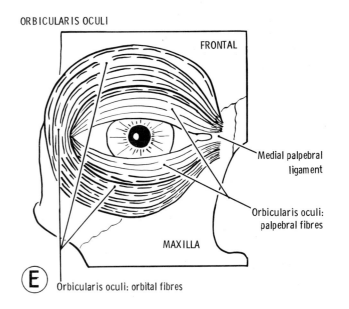

FRONTAL
Medial palpebral ligament
Orbicularis oculi: palpebral fibres
MAXILLA
Orbicularis oculi: orbital fibres

(E)

THE NOSE

The nasal cavity consists of a bony part, which is situated centrally in the facial skeleton, and a smaller cartilaginous part which protrudes as a conical eminence beyond the plane of the rest of the face. It is divided into right and left halves by a septum which, not uncommonly, deviates from the median plane. Both halves open to the exterior through the pear-shaped nostrils or nares on the inferior aspect of the cartilaginous part. The lateral boundaries of the nostrils are called the alae. Posteriorly, the two halves open into the uppermost part of the pharynx (the nasopharynx) through the posterior nasal apertures.

The cartilaginous part

In this region the two halves of the nasal cavity are separated by the septal cartilage, which is a flat quadrilateral plate of hyaline cartilage (**A**). Its posterior angle extends backwards between the two bony elements of the septum and its inferior margin lies between the nostrils (**A**).

The lateral walls of this part are formed by the several cartilage plates shown in **B** and the zones of fibrous tissue between them. Observe that the anterosuperior margin of the lateral cartilage is continuous with the corresponding margin of the septal cartilage (**A**) and that the anterior end of the greater alar cartilage has a narrow septal process. This is attached by fibrous tissue to the inferior margin of the septal cartilage (**A**, **B**).

The bony part

In **C** and **D** the ethmoid and palatine bones are shown as simple geometric shapes. Recall the basic parts of the ethmoid (**15B**) and note that the palatine bone consists essentially of thin sagittal (perpendicular) and horizontal plates joined at right angles.

As seen in the coronal section (**E**) the bony part has a narrow roof, and a comparatively wide floor.

From each lateral wall three curled bony plates, called the conchae, protrude medially and then downwards into the corresponding half of the nasal cavity (**E**) partially dividing it into compartments, the names of which should be noted.

The bony part of the nasal septum contains two thin flat bony elements (**A**). Above is the perpendicular plate of the ethmoid, which descends from the junction of the cribriform plates and articulates with the anterior and posterior parts of the roof of the nasal cavity. Below is the unpaired vomer bone. Note its articulations and its free posterior margin which separates the posterior nasal apertures.

The floor is the hard palate which separates it from the cavity of the mouth. Its anterior two-thirds is formed by the palatine processes of the maxillary bones and its posterior third by the horizontal processes of the palatine bones (**F**).

The roof consists of three parts (**F**). The anterior part slopes downwards and forwards and consists of the nasal bones and the nasal process of the frontal bone. The outer aspect of these elements form the bridge of the nose. The posterior part of the roof inclines first downwards and then backwards and is formed by the body of the sphenoid. The middle and highest part of the roof is horizontal. It consists of the cribriform plates of the ethmoid which separate the nasal cavity from the anterior cranial fossa.

The lateral wall is composed of a number of bones. The general positions of these, though not the details of their shapes, are shown in **F**. Observe the following features.

1. The ethmoidal labyrinth which separates the nasal cavity from the orbit, exhibits a round eminence, the bulla ethmoidalis on the lower part of its nasal surface.
2. The thin lacrimal bone lies between the same two regions. The anterior and posterior edges of its lower part articulate with the margins of a vertical groove on the medial surface of the maxilla. The short bony channel so formed is the nasolacrimal canal.
3. The narrow medial pterygoid plate marks the lateral margin of the posterior nasal aperture.
4. The posterior part of the vertical plate of the palatine (stippled) separates the nasal cavity from the pterygopalatine fossa.

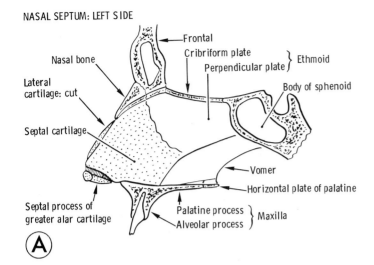

NASAL SEPTUM: LEFT SIDE

Frontal
Cribriform plate
Perpendicular plate } Ethmoid
Nasal bone
Body of sphenoid
Lateral cartilage: cut
Septal cartilage
Vomer
Horizontal plate of palatine
Septal process of greater alar cartilage
Palatine process
Alveolar process } Maxilla

A

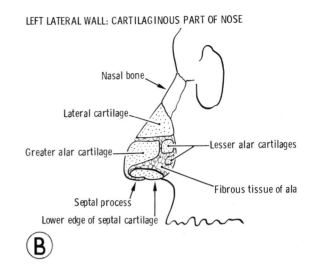

LEFT LATERAL WALL: CARTILAGINOUS PART OF NOSE

Nasal bone
Lateral cartilage
Greater alar cartilage
Lesser alar cartilages
Fibrous tissue of ala
Septal process
Lower edge of septal cartilage

B

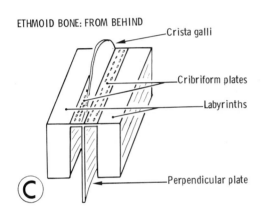

ETHMOID BONE: FROM BEHIND

Crista galli
Cribriform plates
Labyrinths
Perpendicular plate

C

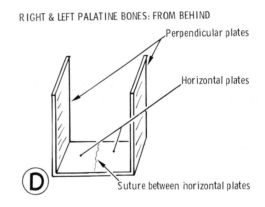

RIGHT & LEFT PALATINE BONES: FROM BEHIND

Perpendicular plates
Horizontal plates
Suture between horizontal plates

D

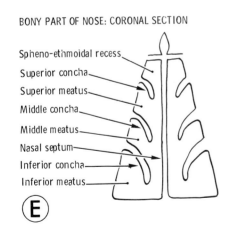

BONY PART OF NOSE: CORONAL SECTION

Spheno-ethmoidal recess
Superior concha
Superior meatus
Middle concha
Middle meatus
Nasal septum
Inferior concha
Inferior meatus

E

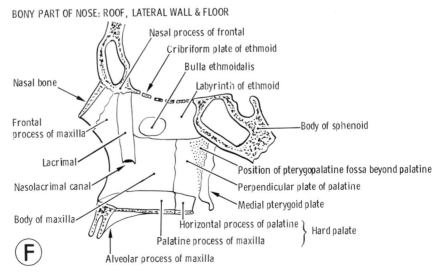

BONY PART OF NOSE: ROOF, LATERAL WALL & FLOOR

Nasal process of frontal
Cribriform plate of ethmoid
Bulla ethmoidalis
Labyrinth of ethmoid
Nasal bone
Frontal process of maxilla
Body of sphenoid
Lacrimal
Position of pterygopalatine fossa beyond palatine
Perpendicular plate of palatine
Nasolacrimal canal
Medial pterygoid plate
Body of maxilla
Horizontal process of palatine } Hard palate
Palatine process of maxilla
Alveolar process of maxilla

F

435

5. The appearance of the nasal conchae from within the nasal cavity is shown in **A**, and the lines of their attachments to the lateral wall in **B**. The superior and middle conchae, which are continuous anteriorly, are both processes arising from the nasal surface of the ethmoidal labyrinth above the bulla ethmoidalis. In contrast, the inferior concha is a separate bone which articulates by its upper margin with a number of the bones in the lateral wall of the nasal cavity.

6. On the lateral walls of the nasal meatuses, note the positions of the bulla ethmoidalis, the sickle-shaped depression named the hiatus semilunaris and the orifice of the nasolacrimal duct. The several other orifices are the openings of the paranasal air sinuses which are described below.

The lining membrane of the nose

The vestibule is the somewhat dilated anterior part of the nasal cavity corresponding in extent to the greater and lesser alar cartilages (**A**). It is lined by skin which is associated with coarse hairs and sebaceous and sweat glands. The rest of the cavity may be divided into two functionally distinct regions which are lined by different types of mucous membrane.

The olfactory region extends over the roof and the walls of the spheno-ethmoidal recess. Here the epithelium of the mucous membrane contains the bipolar olfactory receptor cells whose central processes pass upwards in bundles through the apertures in the cribriform plate of the ethmoid (**87A**).

The respiratory region, which is the rest of the nasal cavity, has a mucous membrane covered by ciliated columnar epithelium.

The blood and nerve supply of the lining membrane of the nose are both derived from several sources.

1. The upper anterior part of the cavity receives branches from the ophthalmic artery and the nasociliary nerve which pass into the nasal cavity from the orbit.
2. The posterior and lower parts receive branches from the maxillary artery and the pterygopalatine ganglion (**429C**) which pass into the nasal cavity from the pterygopalatine fossa.
3. The skin of the vestibule is supplied by branches of the facial artery and the infra-orbital nerve.

The paranasal sinuses

Most of the bones which contribute to the walls of the nasal cavity contain air-filled spaces of various sizes and shapes, which communicate through apertures with the cavity of the nose. They are lined by a respiratory type of mucous membrane containing mucous glands, and inflammation frequently spreads into them from the nose.

They are absent or very small at birth but appear during childhood and grow most rapidly at puberty.

The paired maxillary sinuses are large conical cavities which occupy the bodies of the maxillary bones (**C**). The base of each sinus is formed by the lower half of the lateral wall of the bony part of the nose and its apex is directed upwards and laterally into the zygomatic process of the maxilla. Above is the floor of the orbit, while below the inferior margin of the sinus protrudes into the alveolar process of the maxilla, where it is closely related to the roots of the upper teeth particularly those of the first and second molars.

On either side the maxillary sinus opens into the posterior part of the hiatus semilunaris (**B**). The aperture lies near the uppermost part of the base (**C**) and consequently does not favour efficient drainage when the sinus is infected.

Two sphenoidal sinuses are situated side by side in the body of the sphenoid. They frequently differ in size and, although they are often restricted to the anterior part of the sphenoid, one or both may extend further backwards. It is important to observe in **B** the close relationships of the sinuses to the hypophysial fossa and the cavernous dural venous sinuses. Each sinus opens into the spheno-ethmoidal recess of the nose through an orifice which is situated high on its anterior wall and is consequently ill-placed for efficient drainage (**B**).

Each of the two ethmoidal sinuses takes the form of a variable number of intercommunicating, bubble-like cavities of air cells which occupy the corresponding ethmoidal labyrinth (**C**). Although the anterior, middle and posterior groups of air cells communicate, they usually open into the nasal cavity through separate apertures (**B**). Thus the anterior group open at the anterior end of the hiatus semilunaris, the middle group on the bulla ethmoidalis and the posterior group on the lateral wall of the superior meatus.

Two frontal sinuses separated by a septum lie in the lower central part of the frontal bone, above and medial to the orbital margin (**D**). They usually have scalloped upper margins and are often markedly unequal in size. Below, each narrows into a canal called the infundibulum (**B, D**), which descends through the corresponding anterior group of ethmoidal air cells to a common aperture at the anterior end of the hiatus semilunaris (**B**).

LATERAL WALL OF NASAL CAVITY

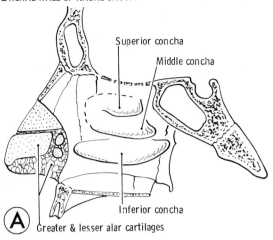

Superior concha
Middle concha
Inferior concha
Greater & lesser alar cartilages

(A)

LATERAL WALL OF NASAL CAVITY: CONCHAE REMOVED

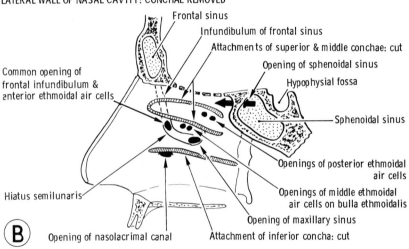

Frontal sinus
Infundibulum of frontal sinus
Attachments of superior & middle conchae: cut
Opening of sphenoidal sinus
Hypophysial fossa
Common opening of frontal infundibulum & anterior ethmoidal air cells
Sphenoidal sinus
Openings of posterior ethmoidal air cells
Openings of middle ethmoidal air cells on bulla ethmoidalis
Opening of maxillary sinus
Hiatus semilunaris
Opening of nasolacrimal canal
Attachment of inferior concha: cut

(B)

CORONAL SECTION OF SKULL

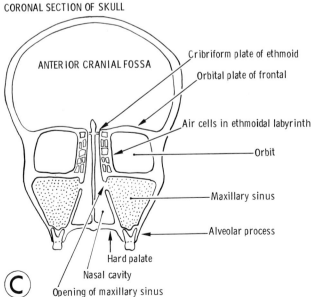

ANTERIOR CRANIAL FOSSA
Cribriform plate of ethmoid
Orbital plate of frontal
Air cells in ethmoidal labyrinth
Orbit
Maxillary sinus
Alveolar process
Hard palate
Nasal cavity
Opening of maxillary sinus

(C)

FRONTAL SINUSES: ANTERIOR WALLS REMOVED

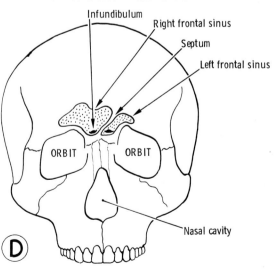

Infundibulum
Right frontal sinus
Septum
Left frontal sinus
ORBIT   ORBIT
Nasal cavity

(D)

THE REGION OF THE MOUTH

The bones

Consider the bones which are involved in the anatomy of this region.

The inferior aspect of the facial skeleton

1. Observe the hard palate and its constituent parts which are demarcated by a cruciform suture (**A**).
2. Note that the alveolar processes of the maxillae, marked by the sockets of the upper teeth articulate anteriorly to form the alveolar arch and extend back beyond the palatine processes of the maxillae on the lateral aspects of the palatine bones (**A**).
3. Each greater palatine foramen opens above into the corresponding pterygopalatine fossa. The single incisive fossa opens above through two incisive canals into the two halves of the nasal cavity.
4. On both sides the lower parts of the medial and lateral pterygoid plates are situated behind the posterior ends of the alveolar arch (**A**).

The mandible

After the first year of life this is a single bone consisting of a horizontal U-shaped body and two thin quadrilateral rami (**B**). The rami end above in a coronoid process and a condylar process which consists of a neck and a head. The narrow upper part of the body contains the sockets for the roots of the lower teeth and is called the alveolar arch.

Observe the features on the deep (**C**) and superficial (**B**) aspects of the mandible.

1. The mental foramen is on the outer surface of the body (**B**) about midway between its upper and lower margins and below the interval between the two premolar teeth.
2. The mylohyoid line extends across the deep surface of the body from the lower margin in the midline to just below the third molar tooth (**C**). The sublingual and submandibular fossae which it separates are shallow.

3. The mandibular foramen is at about the centre of the deep surface of the ramus (**C**) and is partially overlapped from below by a thin bony process called the lingula.
4. The mandibular canal runs from the mandibular foramen through the ramus and the alveolar part of the body (**C**). It gives off narrow branch canals to the tooth sockets and, near its anterior end, the mental canal which opens at the mental foramen (**B**).

The hyoid bone

The hyoid bone (**D**) can be readily palpated lying across the midline of the neck below and behind the body of the mandible. The body is a transverse bar of bone from both ends of which two processes arise. The slender greater horns project backwards. The lesser horns are short and conical and project upwards, backwards and laterally.

The teeth

A tooth (**E**) consists of a crown which protrudes from the alveolar process and one, two, or three roots, each of which is fixed in an individual socket. Loose connective tissue called the pulp occupies the centre of each root and extends for some distance into the crown. The pulp cavity is surrounded by dentine, an avascular highly mineralised connective tissue which is very sensitive to both touch and temperature. In the root the dentine is enveloped by a thin layer of cementum, which closely resembles bone and is attached to the walls of the root socket by bundles of collagen fibres which constitute the periodontal ligament (membrane). At the extremity of each root the dentine and cementum are deficient at the apical foramen, which allows the entrance of nerves and vessels into the pulp cavity.

In the crown the dentine is covered by enamel, an extremely hard, avascular and insensitive substance which consists of mineral crystals held together by a small amount of organic materal.

The teeth erupt as two successive dentitions, the deciduous or milk teeth and the permanent teeth.

FACIAL SKELETON: INFERIOR ASPECT

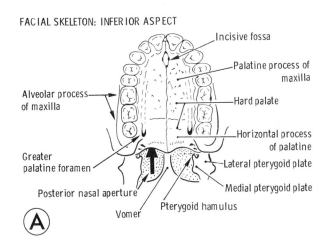

Incisive fossa

Palatine process of maxilla

Alveolar process of maxilla

Hard palate

Horizontal process of palatine

Greater palatine foramen

Lateral pterygoid plate

Medial pterygoid plate

Posterior nasal aperture

Pterygoid hamulus

Vomer

A

MANDIBLE: FROM LEFT SIDE

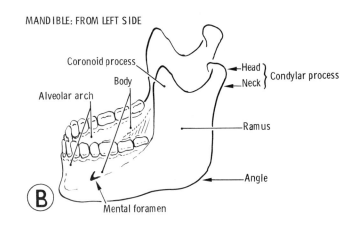

Coronoid process

Body

Head

Condylar process

Neck

Alveolar arch

Ramus

Angle

Mental foramen

B

RIGHT HALF OF MANDIBLE: DEEP SURFACE

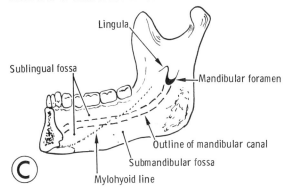

Lingula

Sublingual fossa

Mandibular foramen

Outline of mandibular canal

Submandibular fossa

Mylohyoid line

C

HYOID BONE: FROM ABOVE

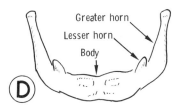

Greater horn

Lesser horn

Body

D

LONGITUDINAL SECTION OF TOOTH

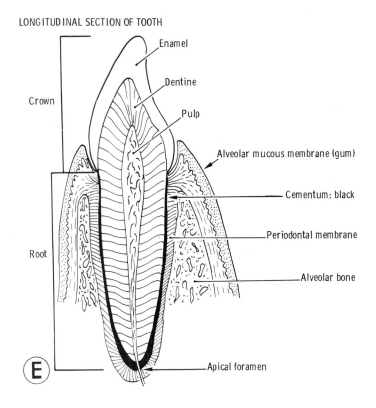

Enamel

Dentine

Pulp

Crown

Alveolar mucous membrane (gum)

Cementum: black

Periodontal membrane

Alveolar bone

Root

Apical foramen

E

439

The deciduous dentition

This comprises 20 teeth. Each half of each alveolar arch carries, from before backwards, a central incisor (6–8 months), a lateral incisor (8–10 months), a canine (16–20 months), a first molar (12–16 months) and a second molar (20–30 months). The ages in brackets are the average ages of eruption of the teeth, and it may be noted that, although in general the age of eruption increases from before backwards, the first molar erupts before the canine. Note also that there are no premolar teeth in the deciduous dentition.

The permanent dentition consists of 32 teeth.

Each half of each alveolar arch carries, from before backwards, a central incisor (6–8 years), a lateral incisor (7–9 years), a canine (9–12 years), first and second premolars (10–12 years), a first molar (6–7 years), a second molar (11–13 years) and a third molar (17–21 years). Note that in this dentition also the eruption of one tooth, the first molar, does not conform to the general anteroposterior order.

Examine the features of the right permanent teeth as seen from their outer (labial and buccal) aspect (**A**). The incisors, which are the cutting teeth, have sharp chisel-like crowns and single roots. The canines, which are adapted to securing and holding food, have conical crowns and long single roots. The premolar and molar teeth, which are adapted to grinding food, all have a number of elevations or cusps on their broad crowns. The premolars have single roots and two cusps on their crowns. The upper molars have three roots and their crowns four cusps. The lower molars have two roots and their crowns five cusps.

Loss of permanent teeth is always followed by absorption of the corresponding parts of the alveolar processes. If all the lower teeth are lost the mandibular canal and the mental foramen come to lie close to the upper margin of the body of the mandible.

The muscles

The buccinator muscle lies between the skin and mucous membrane of the cheek (**443A**). Each has a C-shaped origin (**B**). Its upper fibres arise from the outer surface of the alveolar process of the maxilla above the molar teeth, and its lower fibres from the same extent of the outer surface of the alveolar part of the body of the mandible. Its middle fibres spring from the inferior margin and hamulus of the medial pterygoid plate, and from the pterygomandibular raphe, which is a zone of fibrous tissue joining the hamulus to the alveolar part of the mandible behind the third molar tooth. The muscle is directed forwards towards the oral fissure (**C**) where its fibres diverge into the upper and lower lips (**D**). Note in **C** that the posterior part of the origin of buccinator is hidden deep to the masseter muscle, one of the muscles of mastication which move the mandible on the skull.

The orbicularis oris muscle (**D**) consists of an ellipse of fibres lying in the substance of the lips around the oral fissure. These fibres intermingle with those of numerous muscles, including buccinator, which approach the oral fissure radially and are inserted into the skin and mucous membrane of the lips.

The paired radial muscles around the oral fissure (**D**) include the buccinator and the posterior fibres of the platysma muscle which has been considered earlier. The other radial muscles are small and not of individual importance.

The mylohyoid muscle (**E**) consists of two symmetrical halves. The fibres arise from both sides of the whole length of the median fibrous raphe which joins the centre of the body of the hyoid bone to the centre of the lower margin of the body of the mandible. They extend upwards, laterally and backwards into the whole lengths of the corresponding mylohyoid lines on the mandible. The course of the fibres is somewhat curved so that the whole muscle forms a diaphragm, concave upwards, across the concavity of the body of the mandible.

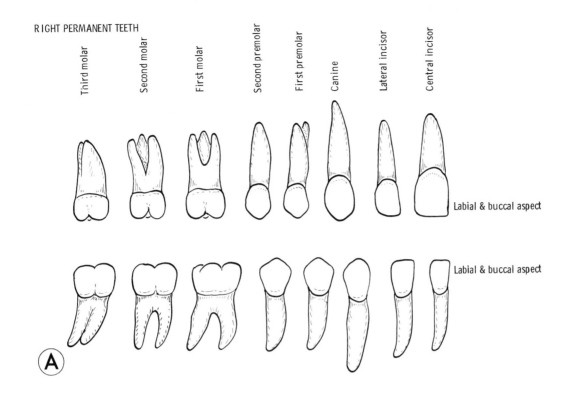

RIGHT PERMANENT TEETH

Third molar   Second molar   First molar   Second premolar   First premolar   Canine   Lateral incisor   Central incisor

Labial & buccal aspect

Labial & buccal aspect

(A)

ORIGIN OF BUCCINATOR MUSCLE
(lateral pterygoid plate & ramus of mandible removed)

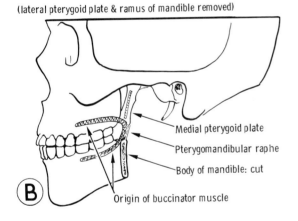

Medial pterygoid plate

Pterygomandibular raphe

Body of mandible: cut

Origin of buccinator muscle

(B)

BUCCINATOR MUSCLE

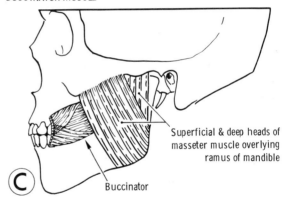

Superficial & deep heads of masseter muscle overlying ramus of mandible

Buccinator

(C)

CIRCULAR & RADIAL MUSCLES OF LIPS

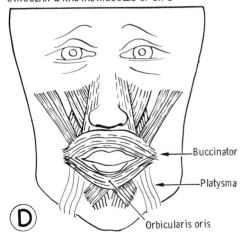

Buccinator

Platysma

Orbicularis oris

(D)

LEFT HALF OF MYLOHYOID MUSCLE

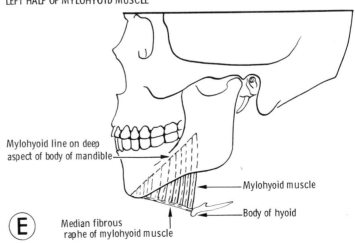

Mylohyoid line on deep aspect of body of mandible

Mylohyoid muscle

Body of hyoid

Median fibrous raphe of mylohyoid muscle

(E)

The cavity of the mouth

Examine the boundaries of the cavity of the mouth (oral cavity) in a coronal section (**A**) and a median section (**B**).

The vestibule is a narrow space lined externally by the buccinator and orbicularis oris muscles in the cheeks and lips and internally by the alveolar arches and teeth of the maxillae and mandible. It communicates with the exterior through the oral fissure between the lips.

The oral cavity proper is bounded anteriorly and laterally by the alveolar arch and teeth of the maxillae and by the lower teeth and upper part of the body of the mandible. Its roof is the hard palate and its floor the diaphragm formed by the mylohyoid muscle. The cavity communicates pos-teriorly with the oral part of the pharynx through the oropharyngeal isthmus, the position and boundaries of which will be discussed later (**446, 464**).

The contents of the oral cavity proper, which include the muscular substance of the tongue and certain salivary glands, lie close to the floor above the mylohyoid muscle. They will be considered later.

The mucous membrane is covered by non-keratinising stratified squamous epithelium and is associated with numerous small mucous glands. It covers the lips and cheeks, the hard palate and the alveolar processes (the gums). On the other hand, it is separated from the mylo-hyoid muscle by the contents of the cavity mentioned above.

THE REGIONS OF THE FACE AND SCALP

The scalp

The scalp covers the vault of the skull and is considered here as it contains a muscle which affects the disposition of the skin around the orbit. It consists of a number of layers of soft tissue (**C**).

1. An outer periosteum (the pericranium) is loosely attached to the intervening sutures.
2. The occipitofrontalis muscle has two short, separate occipital bellies attached to the superior nuchal line (**D**) and two larger frontal bellies which blend in the midline and, mingling with the orbital fibres of orbicularis oculi, are inserted into the skin of the eyebrows (**E**). Between the two pairs of bellies is the epicranial aponeurosis (the galea aponeurotica).
3. The aponeurosis is attached to the pericranium by a very loose connective tissue which allows considerable movement between the two layers.
4. The aponeurosis is very firmly bound to the overlying skin by a tough, fibrous superficial fascia resembling that of the palm of the hand and the sole of the foot.

Contraction of occipitofrontalis thus displaces the skin of the scalp backwards in relation to the bones of the cranial vault and elevates the skin of the eyebrow as in the expressions of surprise and doubt.

Both the occipital and frontal bellies of occipitofrontalis are innervated by the facial nerve (see below).

The arteries of the scalp enter the region around its periphery and run centripetally in the superficial fascia anastomosing freely (**F**).

Partial avulsion of the scalp is a not uncommon injury in road traffic accidents and also in industry, when the hair may be caught in moving machinery. Because of the toughness of the superficial fascia, avulsion occurs through the loose layer of connective tissue between the epicranial aponeurosis and the pericranium. Furthermore, because of the orientation of the arteries and their free anastomosis, the avulsed part of the scalp usually survives and can be stitched back in position.

CORONAL SECTION OF MOUTH

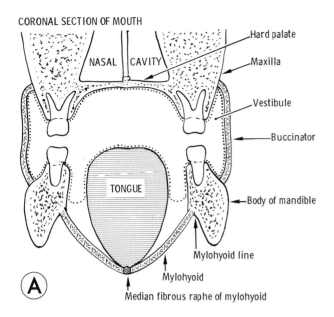

- Hard palate
- Maxilla
- Vestibule
- Buccinator
- Body of mandible
- Mylohyoid line
- Mylohyoid
- Median fibrous raphe of mylohyoid

NASAL CAVITY

TONGUE

A

MEDIAN SECTION OF MOUTH

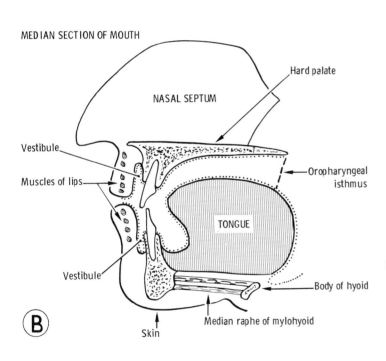

- Hard palate
- Vestibule
- Muscles of lips
- Vestibule
- Oropharyngeal isthmus
- Body of hyoid
- Skin
- Median raphe of mylohyoid

NASAL SEPTUM

TONGUE

B

LAYERS OF SCALP

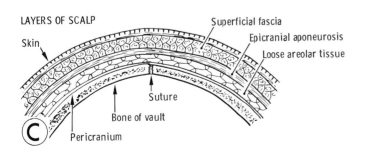

- Skin
- Superficial fascia
- Epicranial aponeurosis
- Loose areolar tissue
- Suture
- Bone of vault
- Pericranium

C

OCCIPITOFRONTALIS MUSCLE: POSTERIOR VIEW

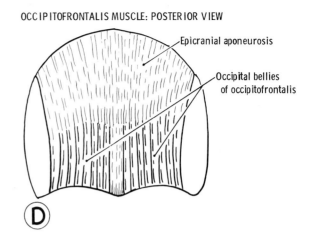

- Epicranial aponeurosis
- Occipital bellies of occipitofrontalis

D

OCCIPITOFRONTALIS MUSCLE: ANTERIOR VIEW

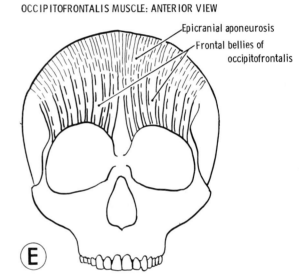

- Epicranial aponeurosis
- Frontal bellies of occipitofrontalis

E

ARTERIES OF SCALP

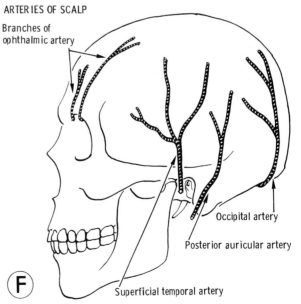

- Branches of ophthalmic artery
- Occipital artery
- Posterior auricular artery
- Superficial temporal artery

F

443

The muscles of expression

In the preceding sections a number of muscles in the face, scalp and neck have been described which are grouped around the palpebral fissure, the oral fissure and the nostrils. Their function is to move the skin and mucous membranes surrounding these openings and thereby, amongst other things, alter the expression of the face.

Around the two palpebral fissures are the orbicularis oculi muscles, the levator palpebrae superioris muscles and the occipitofrontalis muscle. Their actions have been discussed already (**422, 432, 442**).

Around the single oral fissure (**440**) is the elliptical part of the orbicularis oris muscle which closes the fissure. The buccinator muscles, acting together, assist in closure of the fissure and compress the vestibule of the mouth. Acting singly, each muscle displaces the oral fissure towards the corresponding side. The radial muscles, according to their positions, elevate the upper lip, depress the lower lip or displace the fissure towards the corresponding side. One of the radial elevators of the upper lip gives off a small slip which is attached to the greater alar cartilage of the nose and dilates the nostril.

The motor innervation of the muscles of expression.

With the exception of the levator palpebrae superioris which, it will be recalled, is innervated by the oculomotor nerve, all the muscles of expression receive their motor nerve supply through branches arising from the facial nerve after it has emerged from the stylomastoid foramen (**A**). One branch runs upwards and backwards behind the external ear to supply the occipital belly of occipitofrontalis. The nerve then turns forwards into the parotid salivary gland and divides into a number of branches which radiate forwards through its substance. The majority of these branches leave the anterior margin of the gland and diverge forwards across the face and forehead to supply the frontal belly of occipitofrontalis and the muscles of expression in the face. The lowest branch emerges from the lower pole of the gland and passes into the neck (the cervical branch). There it runs downwards about 1 cm behind the angle of the jaw lying deep to the platysma which it supplies.

It should be noted that there are numerous connections on the face and scalp between the motor branches of the facial nerve and the cutaneous nerves in the same areas (**427C, 429B, 459D**) which allow transfer of proprioceptive impulses from the muscles of expression.

Paralysis of the muscles of expression

There are two common causes of paralysis of the muscles supplied by the facial nerve.

1. Inflammation of the facial nerve in the region of the stylomastoid foramen causes unilateral paralysis of the muscles of the same side (Bell's palsy).

   Tears tend to spill from the conjunctival sac because the orbicularis oculi fails to hold the lacrimal puncta against the eye. The mouth is displaced towards the normal side and saliva tends to dribble through the oral fissure on the paralysed side. Food tends to accumulate in the vestibule of the mouth on the paralysed side because buccinator fails to hold the cheek against the teeth.
2. In the case of a cerebral vascular accident affecting the upper motor neurons associated with these muscles, the muscles around the orbit are less affected than those around the mouth, because the corresponding parts of the facial motor nuclei receive corticonuclear fibres from both cerebral hemispheres. Also, for reasons which are not clear, deliberate voluntary movements of the muscles are more severely affected than those which express emotions.

The facial vessels

The facial artery arises from the external carotid artery in the neck and enters the face deep to platysma by curling round the lower margin of the body of the mandible immediately in front of the masseter muscle (**B**). The pulse can be readily felt in this situation by gentle compression of the artery against the bone. In the face, the vessel runs upwards and medially to the medial angle of the eye, lying amongst the muscles of expression. Its course is very tortuous to allow for opening and closing of the mouth.

The facial vein in the face (**B**) lies posterior to the artery and follows a straighter course. It receives numerous tributaries and establishes two connections of clinical importance. At the medial angle of the eye it communicates with the superior ophthalmic vein of the orbit and through that vessel is connected to the cavernous sinus (**431D**). The deep facial vein passes into the infratemporal fossa between the buccinator and masseter muscles and there joins the pterygoid venous plexus (**431D**). The termination of the facial vein is described later (**461D**).

BRANCHES OF FACIAL NERVE TO MUSCLES OF FACIAL EXPRESSION

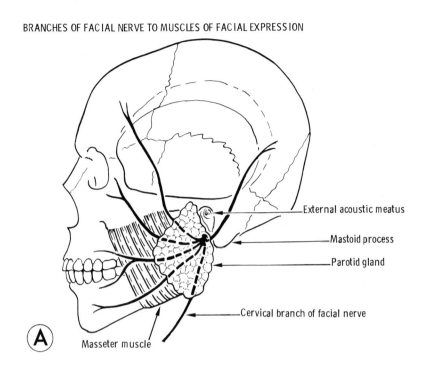

External acoustic meatus

Mastoid process

Parotid gland

Cervical branch of facial nerve

Masseter muscle

(A)

FACIAL ARTERY & VEIN

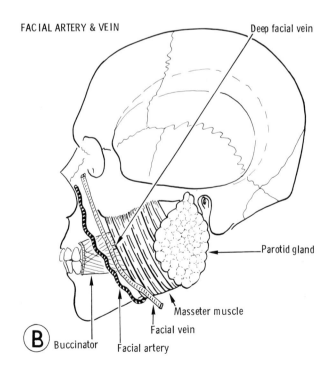

Deep facial vein

Parotid gland

Masseter muscle

Facial vein

(B) Buccinator   Facial artery

THE PHARYNX

The pharynx is a tubular structure which lies in the midline of the neck from the base of the skull to its junction with the cervical oesophagus at the level of the sixth cervical vertebra (**A**). Posteriorly, it is separated from the pre-vertebral muscles and fascia by loose areolar tissue which provides little obstruction to the spread of fluids. Anteriorly, the nasopharynx opens into the nasal cavity through the posterior nasal apertures. At a lower level the oropharynx opens into the cavity of the mouth through the oropharyngeal isthmus. The lowest part of the pharynx is called the laryngeal part. It opens forwards and downwards into the cavity of the larynx and encroaches forwards on either side of the wall of the larynx so that its lumen is crescentic in shape (**B**).

The anterior wall of the lower part

Observe the structures which contribute to this wall.

The hyoid bone which has been considered earlier (**439D**) is shown from the left side in **E**. Note how it is suspended from the mandible by the mylohyoid muscle and its raphe, and from the styloid processes by the stylohyoid ligaments.

The thyroid cartilage protrudes forwards as the Adam's apple a short distance below the hyoid bone (**C**, **E**). It consists in large part of two quadrilateral laminae set at an angle which is open backwards. The lower two-thirds of their anterior margins are continuous in the midline while their upper parts are separated by a notch. Their posterior margins are widely separated and each is continued up-wards and downwards as superior and inferior horns (cornua). The slender superior horns end a short distance below the greater horns of the hyoid. The inferior horns are shorter and thicker and incline medially. The inferior margin of each lamina is marked by an inferior tubercle from which an oblique line extends upwards and back-wards towards the root of the superior horn.

The thyrohyoid membrane, the left half of which is shown in **E**, is a gutter-shaped sheet of fibro-elastic tissue which occupies the interval between the U-shaped hyoid bone and the V-shaped thyroid cartilage.

The paired thyrohyoid muscles are attached on each side to the oblique line of the thyroid lamina and the greater horn of the hyoid bone. The left muscle is shown in outline in **E**. Note the parts of the thyroid lamina and the thyrohyoid membrane which it covers.

The cricoid cartilage (**D**, **E**) is shaped like a signet ring. The broad posterior part, called the lamina, is marked on its posterior surface by a median vertical ridge and on its upper surface by paired articular facets. The rest of the cartilage, which is called the arch, becomes progressively narrower as it is traced forwards. Its lateral aspects arti-culate with the inferior horns of the thyroid cartilage at the small cricothyroid joints, while its median part, which is readily palpable, lies a short distance below the thyroid laminae. The inferior margin of the whole cricoid cartilage is horizontal and is joined to the first tracheal ring by the cricotracheal ligament (**E**).

The paired cricothyroid muscles (**E**) arise on each side from a C-shaped origin on the thyroid cartilage between the inferior tubercle and the cricothyroid joint. The fibres converge downwards and forwards to be inserted into the lateral aspect of the cricoid arch. A fibrous arch passes across the muscle from the inferior thyroid tubercle to the cricoid arch.

The lateral and posterior walls

The constrictor muscles

These are three symmetrical pairs of thin muscles named the superior, middle and inferior constrictor muscles. They arise anteriorly (see below) and curve backwards and medially into a posterior median raphe which runs down the posterior pharyngeal wall from the pharyngeal tubercle on the basi-occiput.

DIAGRAM OF MEDIAN SECTION OF PHARYNX

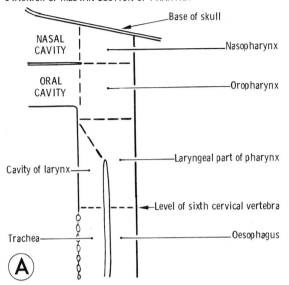

Base of skull

NASAL CAVITY — Nasopharynx

ORAL CAVITY — Oropharynx

Cavity of larynx — Laryngeal part of pharynx

— Level of sixth cervical vertebra

Trachea — Oesophagus

Ⓐ

DIAGRAM OF TRANSVERSE SECTION OF LARYNGEAL PART OF PHARYNX

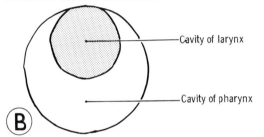

— Cavity of larynx

— Cavity of pharynx

Ⓑ

THYROID CARTILAGE: ANTERIOR ASPECT

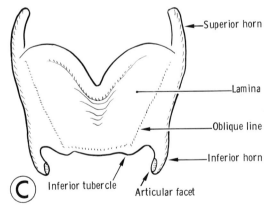

— Superior horn

— Lamina

— Oblique line

— Inferior horn

Ⓒ   Inferior tubercle   Articular facet

CRICOID CARTILAGE: LEFT ASPECT

ANTERIOR

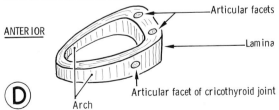

— Articular facets

— Lamina

Ⓓ   Arch   Articular facet of cricothyroid joint

STRUCTURES INVOLVED IN ANTERIOR WALL OF PHARYNX: LEFT ASPECT

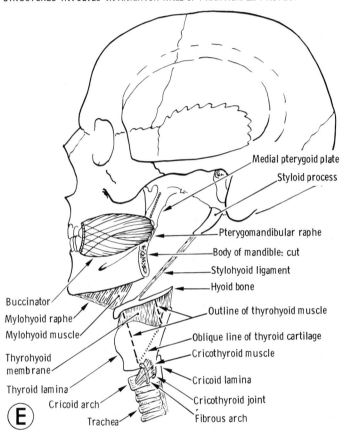

Medial pterygoid plate

Styloid process

Pterygomandibular raphe

Body of mandible: cut

Stylohyoid ligament

Hyoid bone

Outline of thyrohyoid muscle

Oblique line of thyroid cartilage

Cricothyroid muscle

Cricoid lamina

Cricothyroid joint

Fibrous arch

Buccinator

Mylohyoid raphe

Mylohyoid muscle

Thyrohyoid membrane

Thyroid lamina

Cricoid arch

Trachea

Ⓔ

As the constrictor muscles sweep backwards, their upper margins also ascend, so that those of the superior constrictors reach the pharyngeal tubercle and those of the middle and inferior constrictors overlap the superior and middle constrictors respectively (**A**). The inferior margins of the superior and middle constrictors descend, but those of the inferior constrictors are horizontal and merge with the circular muscle of the cervical part of the oesophagus.

Each superior constrictor (**A**) has a continuous linear origin from the lower half of the posterior margin of the medial pterygoid plate, the pterygoid hamulus, the pterygomandibular raphe (which separates the muscle from the buccinator) and from the alveolar part of the mandible behind the third molar tooth. It will be shown later (**482**) that the middle fibres of the muscle, which arise from the pterygoid hamulus, constitute a thickened horizontal band which is often called the palatopharyngeal sphincter and is important in the mechanism of swallowing.

Each middle constrictor (**A**) has a continuous C-shaped origin from the lower part of the stylohyoid ligament and from the lesser and greater horns of the hyoid bone.

Each inferior constrictor (**A**) has a continuous origin from the oblique line of the thyroid lamina and from the whole of the fibrous arch which crosses the cricothyroid muscle, including the attachment to the cricoid. Observe by comparison of **A** and **447E** that, as the muscle passes backwards, it passes superficial to a number of structures. These are the posterior part of the lamina and the inferior horn of the thyroid cartilage, the cricothyroid joint and the posterior part of the cricothyroid muscle, and the cricoid lamina. The lowest part of the muscle which arises from the cricoid arch is thicker than the rest and is often called the cricopharyngeal sphincter.

The triangular gaps

Although the constrictor muscles form a complete posterior pharyngeal wall, three triangular gaps are present in each lateral wall (**A**). They are occupied by loose connective tissue and provide routes through which structures arising outside the pharynx can pass into the pharyngeal and oral cavities. Observe the positions and boundaries of these gaps.

1. Each superior gap is bounded by the upper margin of the superior constrictor, the upper half of the posterior margin of the medial pterygoid plate, and the base of the skull. It opens into the nasopharynx.
2. Each middle gap is bounded by the posterior margin of the mylohyoid and the adjacent margins of the superior and middle constrictors. Structures pass through it into the oropharynx and the mouth.
3. Each inferior triangular gap lies between the posterior margin of the thyrohyoid muscle and the adjacent margins of the middle and inferior constrictors. It opens into the laryngeal part of the pharynx.

The roof

This consists of the approximately quadrangular area on the base of the skull indicated in **B**. It extends from the pharyngeal tubercle to a line joining the roots of the medial pterygoid plates. The lateral boundary can be regarded as the lines of attachment to the skull of the connective tissue which occupies the superior triangular gaps in the pharyngeal wall. Note that the roof includes parts of the body of the sphenoid, the basi-occiput and the petrous part of the temporal bone, together with the fibrocartilaginous plug which occupies the lower half of the foramen lacerum. Lateral to it is the roof of the infratemporal fossa containing the jugular foramen, the opening of the carotid canal, the foramen spinosum and the foramen ovale.

Structures related to lateral wall of pharynx

The cartilaginous part of the auditory tube

The form and structure of this part has been considered earlier in connection with the middle ear (**412**) and it will be recalled that its lateral and inferior walls consist of fibrous tissue. It joins the bony part deep to the spine of the sphenoid and runs downwards, forwards and medially on the grooved suture between the petrous temporal and the greater wing of the sphenoid, to end immediately deep to the upper part of the posterior margin of the medial pterygoid plate (**A**, **B**). Thus, as is evident in **B**, it begins lateral to the pharynx and ends within its cavity, passing obliquely through the superior triangular gap (**A**).

CONSTRICTOR MUSCLES OF PHARYNX

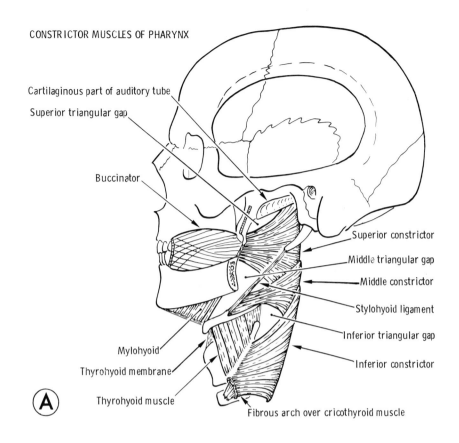

Cartilaginous part of auditory tube
Superior triangular gap
Buccinator
Superior constrictor
Middle triangular gap
Middle constrictor
Stylohyoid ligament
Inferior triangular gap
Inferior constrictor
Mylohyoid
Thyrohyoid membrane
Thyrohyoid muscle
Fibrous arch over cricothyroid muscle

(A)

ROOF OF PHARYNX

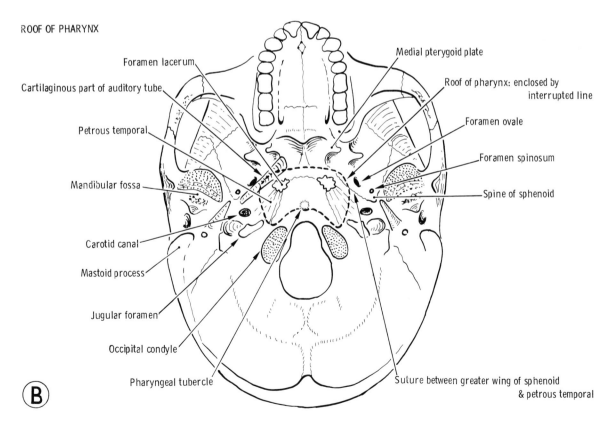

Foramen lacerum
Cartilaginous part of auditory tube
Petrous temporal
Mandibular fossa
Carotid canal
Mastoid process
Jugular foramen
Occipital condyle
Pharyngeal tubercle
Medial pterygoid plate
Roof of pharynx: enclosed by interrupted line
Foramen ovale
Foramen spinosum
Spine of sphenoid
Suture between greater wing of sphenoid & petrous temporal

(B)

The tensor palati muscle

This is a small triangular muscle. Its deep fibres arise from the fibrous lateral wall of the cartilaginous auditory tube. Its superficial fibres have a linear origin from the greater wing of the sphenoid between the root of the medial pterygoid plate and the spine of the sphenoid, lateral to the cartilaginous part of the auditory tube, and medial to the foramen ovale and the foramen spinosum (**449B**). This last relationship is important because it means that the structures which traverse these two foramina lie on tensor palati immediately below the base of the skull.

The muscle fibres converge downwards and forwards to a slender tendon which lies on the lateral side of the medial pterygoid plate. Below, the tendon turns abruptly medially through the origin of buccinator just in front of the pterygoid hamulus to enter the soft palate (**A**). Its termination in that structure will be considered later (**483E**).

The hyoglossus muscle

This is a small quadrilateral muscle which arises from the greater horn of the hyoid bone. It passes upwards and forwards, superficial to the fibres of origin of the middle constrictor, and enters the cavity of the mouth by passing obliquely through the lower angle of the middle triangular gap in the pharyngeal wall (**A**). As will be seen later (**466**) it is then incorporated into the substance of the tongue.

THE NEUROVASCULAR BUNDLE OF THE NECK

The neurovascular bundle has already been described in relation to the prevertebral muscles. It can now be appreciated that the greater part of the bundle runs longitudinally along the posterolateral aspect of the pharynx (**A**). Note that, in that diagram, the greater part of the internal jugular vein has been removed to expose the internal carotid artery. The uppermost part of the bundle, which is enclosed in a very dense part of the carotid sheath, is crossed downwards and forwards by the styloid process. Observe two of the fusiform muscles which arise from the styloid process.

The stylopharyngeus (**A**) arises near the base of the styloid process and, passing downwards and somewhat forwards across the neurovascular bundle, enters the pharyngeal cavity through the posterior angle of the middle triangular gap.

The styloglossus muscle arises near the tip of the styloid process and passes more horizontally forwards through the superior corner of the middle triangular gap into the cavity of the mouth, where it is incorporated into the tongue (**A**).

Glossopharyngeal nerve

The entrance of the glossopharyngeal nerve into the neurovascular bundle, and its tympanic and carotid branches, have been considered earlier (**396**). The nerve leaves the bundle just below the styloid process by passing forwards between the internal carotid artery and the internal jugular vein. It crosses the lateral aspect of the stylopharyngeus muscle and thereafter enters the pharynx through the middle triangular gap a little below the styloglossus muscle (**A**). It supplies the following branches.

1. A motor branch to stylopharyngeus, which is the only muscle it supplies.
2. Sensory branches which pierce the middle constrictor

muscle and innervate the greater part of the mucous membrane of the pharynx.
3. Terminal sensory branches which innervate the mucous membrane of the tonsil (palatine tonsil) and the posterior (pharyngeal) third of the tongue.

Branches of the vagus nerve

The course of the vagus nerve as a component of the neurovascular bundle in the neck and its auricular (**414**), cardiac (**185D**) and recurrent laryngeal branches (**339B**) have been considered earlier.

The pharyngeal branch, which is not shown in **A**, arises from the inferior ganglion of the vagus and is said to consist mainly or wholly of fibres which have joined the vagus from the cranial part of the accessory nerve. It passes forwards from between the internal carotid artery and the internal jugular vein and divides on the middle constrictor into numerous fine branches which supply all the muscles of the pharynx except tensor palati and stylopharyngeus.

The superior laryngeal branch, which is larger than the pharyngeal, also arises from the inferior ganglion of the vagus. Passing medial to the internal carotid artery on the surface of the superior constrictor, it divides into two unequal parts (**A**).

1. The internal laryngeal nerve runs downwards and forwards on the middle constrictor and turns forwards through the inferior triangular gap into the interval between the thyrohyoid muscle and thyrohyoid membrane. It enters the pharynx by piercing that membrane, and its subsequent distribution to the pharynx and larynx will be described later.
2. The finer external laryngeal nerve passes more steeply downwards across the middle and inferior

PHARYNX: LATERAL ASPECT

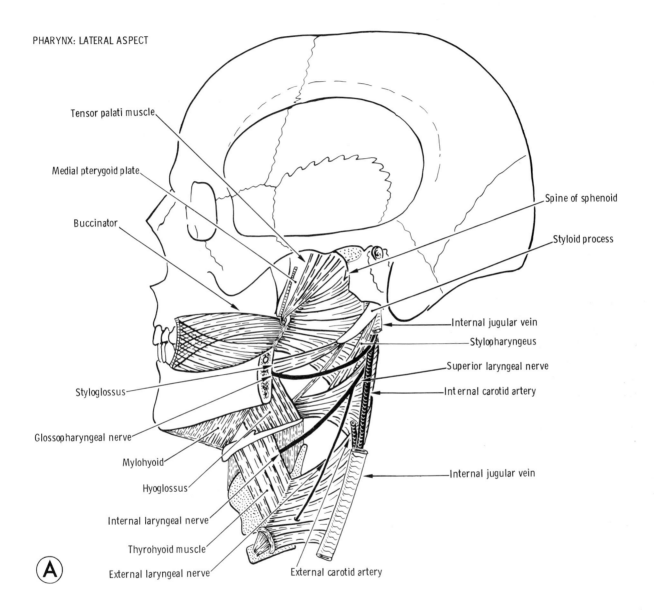

Tensor palati muscle

Medial pterygoid plate

Buccinator

Spine of sphenoid

Styloid process

Internal jugular vein

Stylopharyngeus

Styloglossus

Superior laryngeal nerve

Internal carotid artery

Glossopharyngeal nerve

Mylohyoid

Hyoglossus

Internal jugular vein

Internal laryngeal nerve

Thyrohyoid muscle

External laryngeal nerve

External carotid artery

(A)

451

constrictors. It pierces and supplies the lower part of the inferior constrictor and ends by supplying the cricothyroid muscle.

The external carotid artery

It will be recalled that this large vessel is formed by the bifurcation of the common carotid artery at the level of the upper border of the thyroid lamina. At first it passes upwards and somewhat forwards, anterior to the internal carotid artery and the internal jugular vein (**A**), and lying against the inferior and middle constrictor muscles and the superior laryngeal nerve. Later it inclines backwards and laterally so that it comes to lie superficial to the styloid process and the origins of the stylopharyngeus and styloglossus muscles, which separate it from the great vessels of the neurovascular bundle (**A**). The vessel has been cut off at this point in **A** and its subsequent course will be considered later (**461A**). This part of the artery gives off numerous branches, the more important of which are described below.

The superior thyroid artery arises anteriorly, just below the greater horn of the hyoid bone, and runs downwards on the inferior constrictor in close association with the external laryngeal nerve. Below, it reaches and helps to supply the thyroid gland (**484**).

The lingual artery arises anteriorly at the level of the hyoid bone and describes a characteristic loop, convex upwards, on the surface of the middle constrictor. It then enters the cavity of the mouth by passing forwards deep to the lowest part of the hyoglossus muscle (**A**).

The facial artery arises anteriorly, a short distance above the lingual. It first passes upwards and forwards, over the middle constrictor and styloglossus, to the inferior margin of the superior constrictor. Here it turns downwards and forwards deep to the angle of the mandible. It then enters the face, where its course has been described earlier (**444**), by turning round the posterior end of the inferior margin of the body of the mandible (**A**).

The occipital artery (**A**) arises posteriorly, at the same level as the origin of the facial artery, and passes upwards and backwards lateral to the neurovascular bundle, the spinal part of the accessory nerve, and the tip of the transverse process of the atlas. It continues backwards, medial to the mastoid process, amongst the cervial postvertebral muscles and turns upwards into the superficial fascia of the scalp between sternomastoid and trapezius. In its sinuous course in the scalp it is accompanied by the greater occipital nerve.

The hypoglossal nerve

The entry of the hypoglossal nerve into the upper part of the neurovascular bundle, and its acquisition of fibres from the ventral ramus of the first cervical nerve, have been described earlier (**397D**). The nerve leaves the bundle by curving forwards just below the origins of the occipital and facial arteries. It then continues forwards across the loop of the lingual artery and enters the cavity of the mouth between the hyoglossus and mylohyoid muscles. Note that hyoglossus separates the lingual artery and the hypoglossal nerve. The nerve gives off the following branches.

1. The superior root of the ansa cervicalis which consists solely of C1 fibres and has been considered earlier (**399A**).
2. A branch which arises from the nerve as it crosses the loop of the lingual artery and passes downwards to supply the thyrohyoid muscle. It also consists of C1 fibres.
3. The terminal branches, consisting of fibres derived from the hypoglossal nucleus, innervate the muscles of the tongue, except palatoglossus which is innervated like a pharyngeal muscle by the vagus.

The stylohyoid and digastric muscles

Observe these two muscles in (**B**).

The stylohyoid is a slender muscle which arises from the base of the styloid process and runs downwards and forwards to be inserted by a bifid tendon into the junction of the body and greater horn of the hyoid bone. The digastric muscle consists of anterior and posterior muscle bellies joined by an intermediate tendon. The longer posterior belly is attached to a groove on the base of the skull medial to the mastoid process, and runs downwards and forwards parallel to, and below, the stylohyoid. The anterior belly is attached to the inferior margin of the body of the mandible close to the midline and runs downwards, backwards and laterally. The intermediate tendon passes between the two parts of the stylohyoid tendon and is held to the hyoid bone by a fascial loop.

The deep relations of the two muscles may be studied by comparison of **A** and **B**. Note in particular that, where the external carotid artery is cut off in **B**, it is emerging from between two pairs of small muscles, the stylopharyngeus and styloglossus being deep to it, and the stylohyoid and the posterior belly of the digastric superficial.

The facial nerve

Observe in **B** the facial nerve emerging from the stylomastoid foramen and turning forwards onto the lateral side of the styloid process, where it will enter the parotid salivary gland. Before entering the gland it gives branches to stylohyoid and the posterior belly of digastric. It will be noted later that the anterior belly of digastric has a different nerve supply.

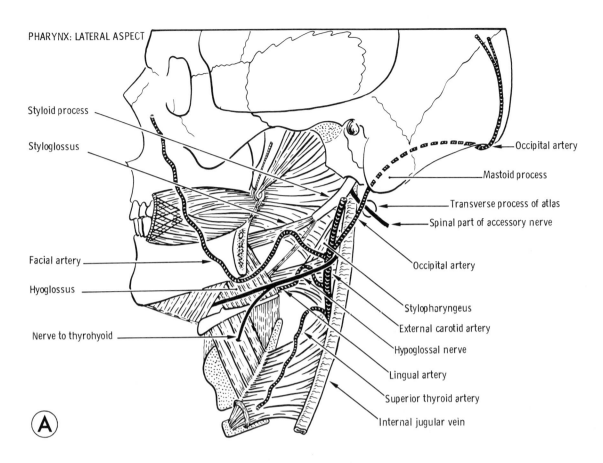

Styloid process
Styloglossus
Facial artery
Hyoglossus
Nerve to thyrohyoid

Occipital artery
Mastoid process
Transverse process of atlas
Spinal part of accessory nerve
Occipital artery
Stylopharyngeus
External carotid artery
Hypoglossal nerve
Lingual artery
Superior thyroid artery
Internal jugular vein

Ⓐ

External carotid artery
Facial nerve

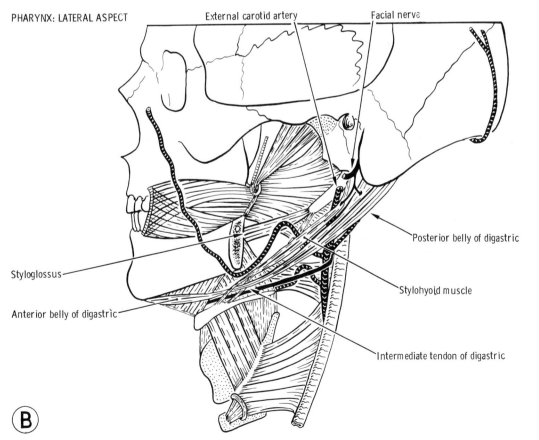

Posterior belly of digastric
Styloglossus
Stylohyoid muscle
Anterior belly of digastric
Intermediate tendon of digastric

Ⓑ

THE INFRATEMPORAL FOSSA

It will be recalled that this is the region between the lateral wall of the upper part of the pharynx and the ramus of the mandible. It is linked above by that part of the base of the skull formed by the temporal and sphenoid bones.

The temporomandibular joint

This is a synovial joint between the head of the mandible and the base of the skull.

The articular surfaces

Revise the appearance of the inferior aspect of the temporal bone in **A**. Immediately in front of the external acoustic meatus is the mandibular fossa, which consists of a posterior tympanic part and an anterior squamous part, separated by the squamotympanic suture. The fossa is limited anteriorly by a rounded transverse ridge called the articular tubercle, which is part of the root of the zygomatic process.

The proximal articular surface extends from the squamotympanic suture over the anterior part of the mandibular fossa and the articular tubercle (**A**). It is thus concavoconvex from behind forwards and gently concave from side to side.

The distal surface is situated on the elliptical head of the mandible so that it is wide and gently convex transversely and narrower and more acutely convex sagitally.

The ligaments

The fibrous capsule is a sleeve of fibrous tissue which extends between the margins of the two articular surfaces (**B**). It should be noted (**B**) that the tympanic part of the temporal bone is not involved in the joint, and that its anterior surface is separated from the posterior aspect of the fibrous capsule by a wedge-shaped recess.

An articular disc of fibrocartilage intervenes between the two articular surfaces and is attached peripherally to the deep surface of the fibrous capsule. It thus divides the joint cavity into two parts (**C**). Synovial membrane lines the free parts of the capsule. The lower surface of the disc conforms in shape to the distal articular surface (**C**), while its upper surface conforms in shape to the proximal articular surface but is somewhat shorter in the sagittal plane.

The sphenomandibular ligament (**D**) is attached above to the spine of the sphenoid which projects from the greater wing of that bone just medial to the medial end of the squamotympanic suture (**A, D**). It runs downwards, forwards and laterally to the lingula on the deep surface of the ramus of the mandible (**D**). As will be seen below, the ligament has an important influence on temporomandibular movements.

The stylomandibular ligament extends between the styloid process and the angle of the mandible. The ligament is a thickened part of the investing layer of the deep cervical fascia and, as it only becomes taut when the upper and lower teeth come into contact, it has no mechanical influence on temporomandibular movements.

Movements

The terms protraction and retraction refer to movements in which the head of the mandible moves forwards and backwards respectively on the base of the skull without undergoing any simultaneous rotation. In both cases the joint movement occurs solely at the upper compartment of the joint between the articular disc and the proximal articular surface (**C**).

Although like movements can be carried out simultaneously at both temporomandibular joints, this is uncommon as the resulting displacements of the mandible are of little functional value. Usually protraction at one temporomandibular joint is accompanied by retraction at the other, so that the mandible is moved from side to side as in the grinding component of chewing.

The terms elevation and depression of the mandible are self-explanatory. Both involve simultaneous like movements at the two temporomandibular joints, around a transverse axis which is fixed by the sphenomandibular ligament and consequently passes through the mandibular foramina.

In depression the heads of the mandible rotate against the concave under surfaces of the articular discs and simultaneously the discs slide forwards on, and become incongruent with, the proximal articular surfaces of the temporomandibular joints (**C**). If the amplitude of depression is excessive, as it may be in yawning, the convexity of the articular disc may move on to the anterior slope of the articular tubercle and become locked in that position by muscular spasm.

In elevation of the mandible, rotation of the mandibular heads against the under surface of the articular disc is associated with backward displacement of the disc on the proximal articular surface until congruence is reestablished (**C**).

LEFT TEMPORAL BONE: INFERIOR ASPECT
(Interrupted line surrounds mandibular fossa. Stipple indicates articular surface of temporomandibular joint.)

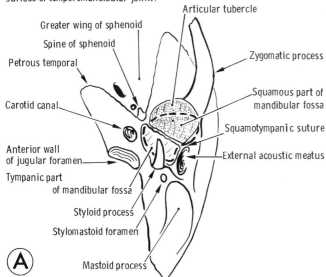

Greater wing of sphenoid
Spine of sphenoid
Petrous temporal
Carotid canal
Anterior wall of jugular foramen
Tympanic part of mandibular fossa
Styloid process
Stylomastoid foramen
Mastoid process
Articular tubercle
Zygomatic process
Squamous part of mandibular fossa
Squamotympanic suture
External acoustic meatus

(A)

LEFT TEMPOROMANDIBULAR JOINT

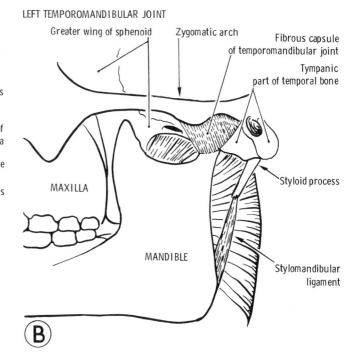

Greater wing of sphenoid
Zygomatic arch
Fibrous capsule of temporomandibular joint
Tympanic part of temporal bone
Styloid process
MAXILLA
MANDIBLE
Stylomandibular ligament

(B)

TEMPOROMANDIBULAR JOINT: SAGITTAL SECTIONS

ANTERIOR   POSTERIOR

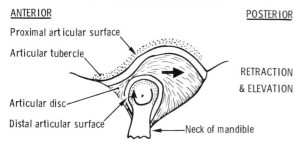

Proximal articular surface
Articular tubercle
Articular disc
Distal articular surface
Neck of mandible
RETRACTION & ELEVATION

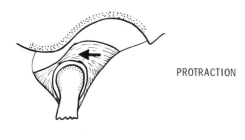

PROTRACTION

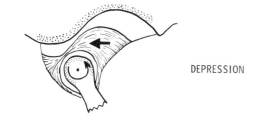

DEPRESSION

(C)

LEFT INFRATEMPORAL FOSSA : upper half of mandibular ramus removed

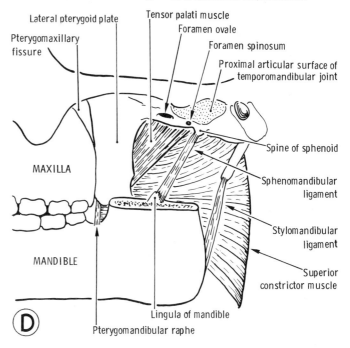

Lateral pterygoid plate
Pterygomaxillary fissure
Tensor palati muscle
Foramen ovale
Foramen spinosum
Proximal articular surface of temporomandibular joint
MAXILLA
MANDIBLE
Spine of sphenoid
Sphenomandibular ligament
Stylomandibular ligament
Superior constrictor muscle
Lingula of mandible
Pterygomandibular raphe

(D)

The muscles of mastication

These are the four muscles which act solely at the temporomandibular joint. They have a common nerve supply from the mandibular nerve (see below).

The medial pterygoid muscle arises from the medial surface of the lateral pterygoid plate (**A**) and passes downwards, backwards and laterally to be inserted into the postero-inferior quadrant of the deep surface of the ramus of the mandible. In **A** and **C** the muscle is cut through at its insertion and the ramus of the mandible has been removed.

The lateral pterygoid muscle consists of upper and lower heads (**B**). The upper head arises from that part of the infratemporal surface of the greater wing of the sphenoid which is lateral to the foramen ovale and the foramen spinosum (**449B**). If the origin of tensor palati is recalled (**450**) it will be evident that all the structures which traverse these two foramina must lie between tensor palati and the upper head of lateral pterygoid.

The larger, lower head of the muscle arises from the lateral surface of the lateral pterygoid plate and passes upwards and backwards across the lateral aspect of the medial pterygoid.

The two heads of the muscle join a single tendon which is inserted into both the anterior aspect of the neck of the mandible and, through the fibrous capsule, into the anterior aspect of the articular disc of the temporomandibular joint.

The temporalis muscle arises from the floor of the temporal fossa (**459A**) and from the deep aspect of the thick temporal fascia which covers it. The muscle fibres converge on a strong tendon, the anterior fibres being almost vertical and the posterior almost horizontal (**459A**). The tendon passes deep to the zygomatic arch and is inserted into the ramus of the mandible over the medial aspect of the coronoid process and along the whole length of the anterior border.

The masseter muscle (**459B**) consists of two parts. The deep fibres arise from the deep surface of the posterior part of the zygomatic arch and pass vertically downwards in front of the temporomandibular joint to insert into the superficial surface of the anterosuperior quadrant of the mandibular ramus. The superficial fibres arise from the zygomatic process of the maxilla and the anterior part of the zygomatic arch and pass downwards and backwards, partially covering the deep fibres, and are inserted into the lower half of the superficial surface of the mandibular ramus.

The actions of the muscles of mastication

The effects of these muscles on the temporomandibular joint depend, on the one hand, on their directions in relation to the mandible, and on the other, on their positions in relation to the axis of rotation of the joint which, it will be recalled, traverses the mandibular foramina.

1. The medial pterygoid passes backwards into the mandible below and in front of the axis of rotation and consequently protracts and elevates the mandible.
2. The lateral pterygoid passes backwards into the mandible above the axis of rotation and thus protracts and depresses the mandible. The insertion of the muscle into both the neck of the mandible and the articular disc results in both these structures moving forwards during the latter movement.
3. The posterior fibres of temporalis pass forwards into the mandible (**459A**) and consequently retract the bone. The tendon of the whole muscle passes downwards in front of the axis of rotation so that it elevates the mandible.
4. All the fibres of masseter pass downwards in front of the axis of rotation and therefore elevate the mandible. Because of their backward obliquity the superficial fibres of the muscle also protract the bone.
5. Note that elevation of the mandible is produced by medial pterygoid, temporalis and masseter and is consequently a much more powerful movement than depression, which is produced by lateral pterygoid, with some assistance from mylohyoid.

The middle meningeal artery

This important vessel arises from the maxillary artery (**461A**) at the lower border of the lateral pterygoid muscle and ascends between that muscle and tensor palati to the foramen spinosum (**A**). Through this foramen it enters the cranial cavity in which its course has been considered previously (**103A**).

The chorda tympani nerve

It has been seen already (**411D**) that this nerve is a branch of the facial nerve, consisting of taste fibres which are the processes of cells in the genicular ganglion, and preganglionic parasympathetic fibres which arise from the cells of superior salivatory nucleus in the brain stem (**51B**). It emerges into the infratemporal fossa through the lower part of the squamotympanic suture, and passes forwards across the deep aspect of the spine of the sphenoid (**455A**). The nerve then passes forwards and downwards between tensor palati and the upper head of lateral pterygoid, and deep to the middle meningeal artery (**A**) to join the lingual nerve (see below) through which its fibres are subsequently distributed.

LEFT INFRATEMPORAL FOSSA: ramus & angle of mandible removed

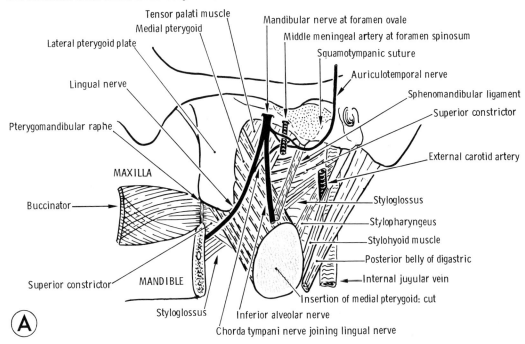

Tensor palati muscle
Medial pterygoid
Lateral pterygoid plate
Lingual nerve
Pterygomandibular raphe
MAXILLA
Buccinator
Superior constrictor
MANDIBLE
Styloglossus
Mandibular nerve at foramen ovale
Middle meningeal artery at foramen spinosum
Squamotympanic suture
Auriculotemporal nerve
Sphenomandibular ligament
Superior constrictor
External carotid artery
Styloglossus
Stylopharyngeus
Stylohyoid muscle
Posterior belly of digastric
Internal jugular vein
Insertion of medial pterygoid: cut
Inferior alveolar nerve
Chorda tympani nerve joining lingual nerve

(A)

LEFT INFRATEMPORAL FOSSA:

upper part of mandibular ramus removed, head & neck of mandible retained

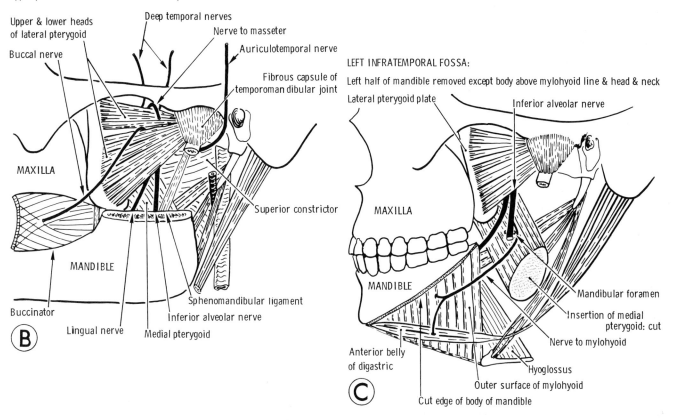

Upper & lower heads of lateral pterygoid
Buccal nerve
MAXILLA
MANDIBLE
Buccinator
Lingual nerve
Deep temporal nerves
Nerve to masseter
Auriculotemporal nerve
Fibrous capsule of temporomandibular joint
Superior constrictor
Sphenomandibular ligament
Inferior alveolar nerve
Medial pterygoid

(B)

LEFT INFRATEMPORAL FOSSA:

Left half of mandible removed except body above mylohyoid line & head & neck

Lateral pterygoid plate
Inferior alveolar nerve
MAXILLA
MANDIBLE
Anterior belly of digastric
Cut edge of body of mandible
Outer surface of mylohyoid
Hyoglossus
Nerve to mylohyoid
Insertion of medial pterygoid: cut
Mandibular foramen

(C)

457

The mandibular nerve

The longest division of the trigeminal nerve, this is a mixed nerve formed by the fusion of a large somatic sensory root from the trigeminal ganglion and a small branchial motor root from the pons (**49D**). The nerve emerges from the cranial cavity through the foramen ovale into the interval between tensor palati and the upper head of lateral pterygoid (**457A**) where it divides into its branches (see below).

All these branches originate deep to the lateral pterygoid and the different routes by which they escape from beneath that muscle should be observed in **457B**.

The lingual nerve

At its origin the lingual nerve consists solely of somatic sensory fibres. It descends between tensor palati and the lateral pterygoid muscles and is joined from behind by the chorda tympani (**457A**). Beyond this point the lingual nerve contains three functional types of fibres, somatic sensory fibres, taste fibres and preganglionic parasympathetic fibres.

The nerve emerges from beneath the lower border of lateral pterygoid (**457B**) and passes downwards and forwards in the interval between the mandibular ramus and medial pterygoid. It then runs across the lowest fibres of the superior constrictor (**457A**) and enters the cavity of the mouth, in close association with styloglossus, by passing deep to the posterior border of mylohyoid (**457C**). Its subsequent course and distribution in the mouth is described later (**471B**).

The inferior alveolar nerve

This mixed nerve runs a short distance behind the lingual nerve in the infratemporal fossa (**457A**) to reach the mandibular foramen. Here it gives off the nerve to mylohyoid, which sweeps downwards and forwards on the outer surface of that muscle, supplying it, and ends by supplying the anterior belly of the digastric muscle (**457C**).

The alveolar nerve itself continues through the mandibular canal supplying branches to the teeth and gums of the lower jaw. In the anterior part of its course it gives off a mental branch (**A**) which emerges through the mental foramen (**B**) and innervates the skin of the chin and the skin and mucous membrane of the lower lip (**D**).

The buccal nerve

This nerve passes between the two heads of the lateral pterygoid (**457B**) and passes downwards and forwards deep to the mandibular ramus, the tendon of insertion of temporalis and the superficial fibres of masseter into the superficial fascia over the buccinator muscle (**457B**). It supplies the skin and mucous membrane of the cheek (**D**).

The auriculotemporal nerve

This sensory branch arises by two roots which encircle the middle meningeal artery (**C, 457A**). It passes backwards between tensor palati and the upper head of lateral pterygoid, and then between the sphenomandibular ligament and the neck of the mandible (**457A**). Thereafter, it turns upwards in front of the auricle into the superficial fascia (**B**). It supplies the skin over the central part of the temporal region, the tragus and the adjoining part of the helix of the auricle, and the anterior wall of the external acoustic meatus (**D**).

The motor branches

1. Branches which supply the medial and lateral pterygoid muscles run directly into the deep surfaces of those muscles.
2. Two branches pass between the upper head of lateral pterygoid and the skull (**457B**) and subsequently enter and supply temporalis.
3. The nerve to the masseter muscle also appears between the upper head of lateral pterygoid and the skull (**457B**). It then turns laterally through the mandibular notch between the temporomandibular joint and the tendon of temporalis (**A**) and enters masseter.
4. The motor fibres which supply the tensor tympani (**411A**) and tensor palati muscles pass without relay through the otic ganglion (see below).

The otic ganglion

This small parasympathetic ganglion lies between tensor palati and the mandibular nerve immediately below the foramen ovale (**C**). It receives preganglionic parasympathetic fibres which arise from the cells of the inferior salivary nucleus in the brain stem (**53A**) and pass successively through the glossopharyngeal nerve, its tympanic branch, the tympanic plexus on the medial wall of the middle ear (**411B**) and the lesser petrosal nerve (**411C**). Postganglionic fibres, originating from the cells of the otic ganglion, pass through a communicating branch to the auriculotemporal nerve. They leave that nerve as it traverses the upper part of the parotid salivary gland (see below) and form its secretomotor supply.

Like most parasympathetic ganglia, the otic is traversed without relay by other fibres. The motor fibres have been noted already. In addition some of the taste fibres in the chorda tympani (**456**) pass through the ganglion, the lesser petrosal nerve, the tympanic plexus, and then through a communication to the genicular ganglion of the facial nerve where their cells of origin are situated.

MUSCLES OF MASTICATION

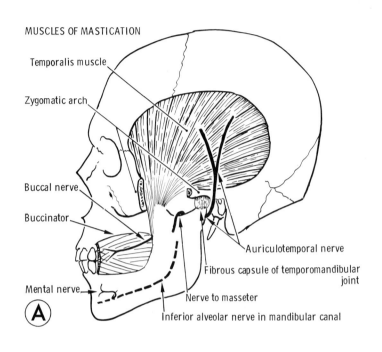

Temporalis muscle

Zygomatic arch

Buccal nerve

Buccinator

Mental nerve

Auriculotemporal nerve

Fibrous capsule of temporomandibular joint

Nerve to masseter

Inferior alveolar nerve in mandibular canal

(A)

MUSCLES OF MASTICATION

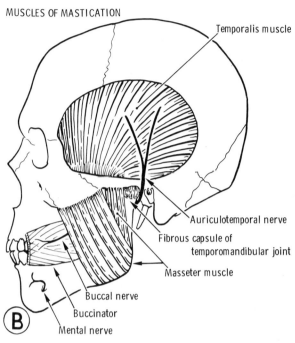

Temporalis muscle

Auriculotemporal nerve

Fibrous capsule of temporomandibular joint

Masseter muscle

Buccal nerve

Buccinator

Mental nerve

(B)

OTIC GANGLION

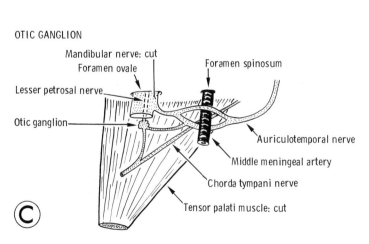

Mandibular nerve: cut

Foramen ovale

Foramen spinosum

Lesser petrosal nerve

Otic ganglion

Auriculotemporal nerve

Middle meningeal artery

Chorda tympani nerve

Tensor palati muscle: cut

(C)

MANDIBULAR AREA OF SKIN OF FACE

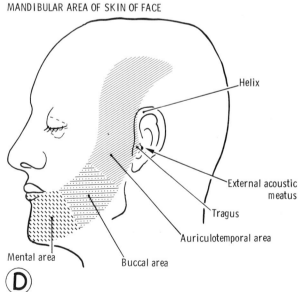

Helix

External acoustic meatus

Tragus

Auriculotemporal area

Mental area

Buccal area

(D)

The terminal branches of the external carotid artery

Soon after the external carotid artery has passed upwards into the infratemporal fossa, superficial to styloglossus and stylopharyngeus, and deep to stylohyoid and the posterior belly of digastric, it divides into two terminal branches (**A**).

The superficial temporal artery

This ascends behind the temporomandibular joint and over the posterior end of the zygomatic arch, immediately in front of the auriculotemporal nerve (**A**). It continues through the superficial fascia of the temporal region and makes a large contribution to the centripetal blood supply of the scalp (**443F**).

The maxillary artery

The larger of the terminal branches of the external carotid, the maxillary artery runs forwards through the infratemporal fossa to the pterygopalatine fossa (**A**). It passes between the neck of the mandible and the sphenomandibular ligament, and either superficial or deep to the lower head of lateral pterygoid.

The vessel gives off a large number of branches. Of those which arise in the infratemporal fossa note the middle meningeal artery which has been considered already (**457A**) and the inferior alveolar artery which accompanies the corresponding nerve throughout its course (**458**).

The branches which arise in the pterygopalatine fossa accompany the branches of the maxillary nerve and the pterygopalatine ganglion (**429C**).

The pterygoid venous plexus

The areolar tissue in the infratemporal fossa is pervaded by a plexus of small veins. This receives tributaries corresponding to the branches of the maxillary artery and communicates with the facial vein through the deep facial vein (**455B**) and with the cavernous venous sinus through an emissary vein passing through the foramen ovale (**99D**). Posteriorly, it drains into the short maxillary vein which accompanies the initial part of the maxillary artery.

The parotid gland

The parotid is the largest of the salivary glands. Its shape and contents are shown diagrammatically in **B** and it can be seen to approximate to an inverted three-sided pyramid.

The gland is closely invested by the investing layer of the deep cervical fascia so that swelling, usually from inflammation of the gland, causes considerable pain.

The superior surface is moulded against the mastoid process and the floor of the external acoustic meatus and extends into the posterior, nonarticular part of the mandibular fossa behind the temporomandibular joint (**C**).

The posteromedial surface is more or less flat and is opposed to structures which collectively form an oblique plane extending from behind, forwards and medially (**C**). Posteriorly is the anterior margin of sternomastoid. More anteriorly, the posterior belly of digastric, the styloid process and its muscles separate the gland from the neurovascular bundle. Further forwards still is the superior constrictor muscle forming the lateral wall of the pharynx.

The anteromedial surface is wrapped round the posterior margin of the ramus of the mandible so that it is deeply grooved from above down (**B**). Its deep part extends on to the deep surface of medial pterygoid and its superficial part on to the superficial surfaces of masseter and the temporomandibular joint (**D**).

The mandibular superficial surface (**D**) is subcutaneous. *The apex* of the gland overlaps the posterior belly of digastric in the interval between the angle of the mandible and sternomastoid (**D**).

The contents of the gland

The gland is traversed by a number of important structures and this naturally complicates surgical procedures in the region.

1. The external carotid artery enters the lower part of the posteromedial surface of the gland (**B**) as soon as it has passed between the styloid muscles (**C**). Passing upwards until it lies behind the neck of the mandible (**A**), it divides into maxillary and superficial temporal branches. The former leaves the anteromedial surface of the gland and, as has been seen, passes forwards through the infratemporal fossa. The latter leaves the superior surface and, as has been seen, passes into the temporal region.
2. The superficial temporal and maxillary veins enter the superior and anteromedial surfaces of the gland respectively and join, lateral to the bifurcation of the external carotid artery, to form the retromandibular vein (**B**). This vessel descends to the lower part of the gland and divides into anterior and posterior divisions which emerge on either side of the apex (**D**). The anterior division joins the facial vein below the angle of the mandible while the posterior division joins the posterior auricular vein on sternomastoid to form the external jugular vein.

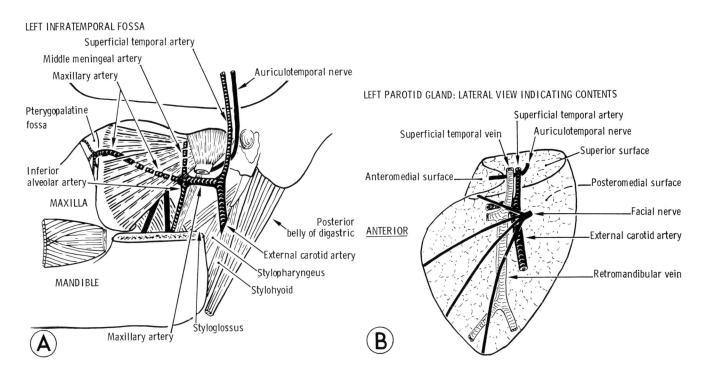

LEFT INFRATEMPORAL FOSSA

Superficial temporal artery
Middle meningeal artery
Maxillary artery
Auriculotemporal nerve
Pterygopalatine fossa
Inferior alveolar artery
MAXILLA
Posterior belly of digastric
External carotid artery
Stylopharyngeus
Stylohyoid
MANDIBLE
Maxillary artery
Styloglossus

(A)

LEFT PAROTID GLAND: LATERAL VIEW INDICATING CONTENTS

Superficial temporal vein
Superficial temporal artery
Auriculotemporal nerve
Superior surface
Anteromedial surface
Posteromedial surface
ANTERIOR
Facial nerve
External carotid artery
Retromandibular vein

(B)

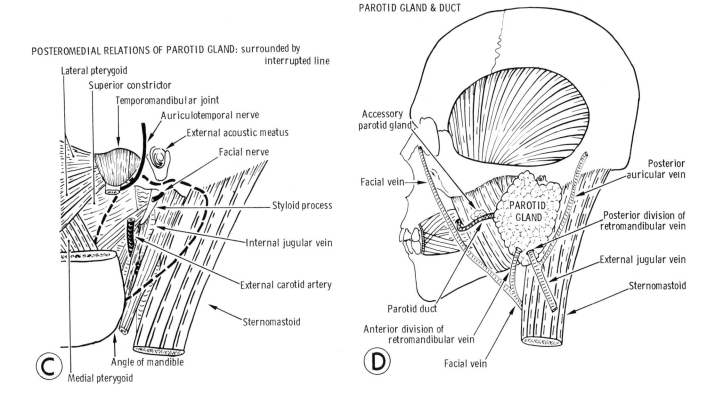

POSTEROMEDIAL RELATIONS OF PAROTID GLAND: surrounded by interrupted line

Lateral pterygoid
Superior constrictor
Temporomandibular joint
Auriculotemporal nerve
External acoustic meatus
Facial nerve
Styloid process
Internal jugular vein
External carotid artery
Sternomastoid
Angle of mandible
Medial pterygoid

(C)

PAROTID GLAND & DUCT

Accessory parotid gland
Facial vein
Posterior auricular vein
PAROTID GLAND
Posterior division of retromandibular vein
External jugular vein
Sternomastoid
Parotid duct
Anterior division of retromandibular vein
Facial vein

(D)

461

3. After passing backwards between the neck of the mandible and the sphenomandibular ligament, the auriculotemporal nerve (**458**) enters the gland through the uppermost part of its anteromedial surface (**461B**) and, after a short intraglandular course, leaves the superior surface for the temporal region. In the gland the nerve gives off secretomotor branches which carry all the postganglionic parasympathetic fibres originating in the otic ganglion (**459C**).

4. As the facial nerve emerges from the stylomastoid foramen it gives motor branches to the stylohyoid, the posterior belly of digastric (**453B**), and the occipital belly of occipitofrontalis (**445A**). It then turns forwards on the lateral aspect of the styloid process and enters the upper part of the posteromedial surface of the parotid gland. Here it divides into branches which radiate through the gland superficial to the retromandibular vein and external carotid artery (**461B**). As has been seen (**445A**) they leave the anterior border and lower pole of the gland to supply muscles of expression in the face and neck.

The parotid duct

The single duct arises from the anterior margin of the gland and passes forwards across masseter where it is palpable about 2 cm below the zygomatic arch (**461D**). It then turns medially round the anterior border of masseter and, piercing buccinator, opens into the mouth on a papilla of the mucous membrane of the cheek opposite the crown of the second upper molar tooth.

A small accessory parotid gland usually lies above the duct as it crosses masseter.

THE INTERIOR OF THE NASOPHARYNX AND OROPHARYNX

Recall the regions into which the upper parts of the digestive and respiratory tracts are divided (**447A**, **447B**) and correlate the regions shown in those diagrams with the regions seen in the median section in **A**.

To reduce the amount of detail in **A** the lateral wall of the nasal cavity is not illustrated as its features have been studied already (**437A**).

Below the hard palate in **A** is the oral cavity. Revise the form of this cavity in (**443A**, **443B**) and the form and attachments of the buccinator and mylohyoid muscles (**441B**, **441C**, **441E**). Although the tongue will be considered fully later, it is convenient to note some of its features at this time. It is a muscular organ, divided into symmetrical halves by a median fibrous septum (**465A**), which rests on the central part of mylohyoid (**443A**). Its dorsum is covered by mucous membrane and this is demarcated by a V-shaped groove (the sulcus terminalis) and a pit (the foramen caecum) into an anterior two-thirds which faces the hard palate and a posterior third which faces backwards towards the pharynx (**C**).

Behind the nasal cavity and the oral cavity respectively lie the nasopharynx and the oropharynx (**A**). In the lateral and posterior walls of these parts recognise the superior and middle constrictor muscles and the upper and middle triangular gaps which have been seen previously from the lateral side (**449A**), and revise the area on the base of the skull which forms the roof of the nasopharynx (**449B**).

The region in **A** below the level of the oral cavity is that common tube which we will later divide into the larynx and the laryngeal part of the pharynx (**447A**, **447B**).

The cartilaginous part of the auditory tube

The structure of this tube (**412**), its relationship to the base of the skull (**449B**), and its oblique passage through the upper triangular gap (**449A**), have been considered already. Its pharyngeal opening (**A**) is immediately behind the upper part of the medial pterygoid plate, a short distance behind the inferior nasal concha (**437A**), and its medial lip forms a prominence on the lateral wall of the nasopharynx called the tubal elevation.

The salpingopharyngeus muscle (**A**, **B**) is a slender fasciculus which arises from the tubal elevation and descends across the inner aspects of the three constrictor muscles. Below, it blends with other longitudinal pharyngeal muscles.

The soft palate

The soft palate (**A**, **B**, **C**) is a shelf of soft tissue which lies between the nasopharynx and the oropharynx. It is attached in front to the posterior margin of the hard palate and on either side to the deep surface of the superior constrictor muscles. Its posterior margin is free, and from its central part a conical process, called the uvula, hangs downwards (**B**, **C**). When its muscles (see below) are relaxed, the soft palate inclines downwards and backwards and is concave downwards in both coronal and sagittal planes (**A**, **B**).

The palate contains a thin plate of dense fibrous tissue called the palatine aponeurosis, which gives attachment to its muscles.

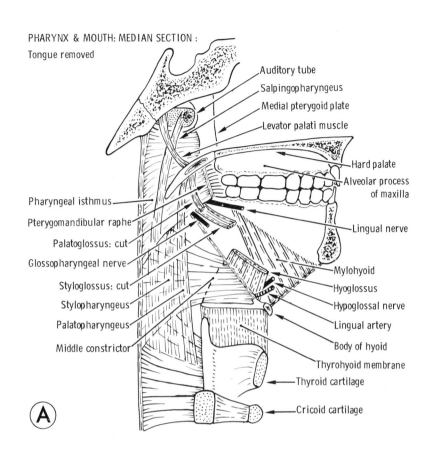

PHARYNX & MOUTH: MEDIAN SECTION :
Tongue removed

Auditory tube
Salpingopharyngeus
Medial pterygoid plate
Levator palati muscle
Hard palate
Alveolar process of maxilla
Lingual nerve
Mylohyoid
Hyoglossus
Hypoglossal nerve
Lingual artery
Body of hyoid
Thyrohyoid membrane
Thyroid cartilage
Cricoid cartilage

Pharyngeal isthmus
Pterygomandibular raphe
Palatoglossus: cut
Glossopharyngeal nerve
Styloglossus: cut
Stylopharyngeus
Palatopharyngeus
Middle constrictor

A

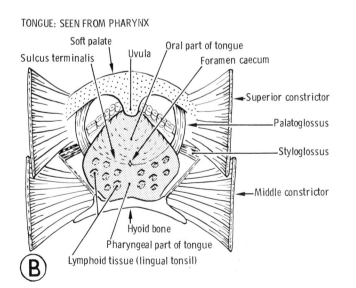

TONGUE: SEEN FROM PHARYNX

Soft palate
Sulcus terminalis
Uvula
Oral part of tongue
Foramen caecum
Superior constrictor
Palatoglossus
Styloglossus
Middle constrictor
Hyoid bone
Pharyngeal part of tongue
Lymphoid tissue (lingual tonsil)

B

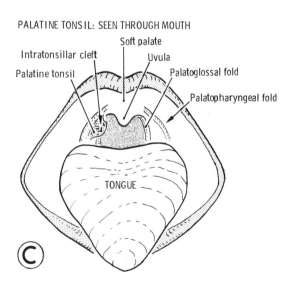

PALATINE TONSIL: SEEN THROUGH MOUTH

Intratonsillar cleft
Palatine tonsil
Soft palate
Uvula
Palatoglossal fold
Palatopharyngeal fold
TONGUE

C

The tensor palati muscle has a triangular muscle belly (**451A**) which lies lateral to the cartilaginous part of the auditory tube and the upper part of the superior constrictor, and is consequently not visible in **463A**. Its slender tendon turns at right angles below the medial pterygoid plate and passes medially through buccinator into the palatine aponeurosis.

The levator palati muscle (**463A**) arises from the medial aspect of the cartilaginous auditory tube and from the adjacent inferior aspect of the petrous part of the temporal bone (**449B**). Passing downwards and forwards, internal to the superior constrictor and salpingopharyngeus (**463A**), it enters the soft palate and inserts into the palatine aponeurosis.

The palatopharyngeus muscle passes laterally in the soft palate from the palatine aponeurosis. It then turns downwards over the internal aspects of the constrictor muscles in close association with salpingopharyngeus (**463A**). It raises the overlying mucous membrane into a ridge called the palatopharyngeal fold (**B, 463A, 463C**).

The palatoglossus muscle also passes laterally from the palatine aponeurosis and then turns downwards on the internal aspect of superior constrictor (**463A**). Thereafter it bends medially into the tongue (**463A, 463B**), which it enters at the lateral end of the sulcus terminalis (**463B**), so that the whole muscle is C-shaped.

The muscle is covered by a palatoglossal fold of mucous membrane. This lies further from the median plane than the palatopharyngeal fold so that both can be seen through the oral cavity (**463A, 463C**).

The uvular muscles arise from the posterior margin of the hard palate and pass backwards in the soft palate to be inserted into the mucous membrane of the uvula.

The isthmuses

1. The space between the posterior margin of the soft palate and the posterior pharyngeal wall is the pharyngeal isthmus through which except during swallowing (**482**) nasopharynx and oropharynx are in communication.
2. The space surrounded by the soft palate, the palatoglossal folds and the sulcus terminalis is the oropharyngeal isthmus through which the oral cavity communicates with that of the oropharynx. It is evident therefore that the anterior two-thirds of the dorsum of the tongue which lies in front of the sulcus terminalis may alternatively be called the oral part, whereas the posterior one-third may be called the pharyngeal part (**463B**).

The longitudinal pharyngeal muscles

The salpingopharyngeus and palatopharyngeus muscles have been considered above. Note in (**463A**) that these blend on the deep aspect of the middle constrictor with the stylopharyngeus muscle (**451A**) which enters the pharynx through the posterior corner of the middle triangular gap. Of the fibres in this composite bundle, many are attached to the posterior margin of the lamina of the thyroid cartilage, while others fade out on the inner aspect of the inferior constrictor muscle.

The nerve supply of the pharyngeal muscles

The constrictor muscles, the longitudinal pharyngeal muscles and the muscles of the soft palate are all innervated by the pharyngeal branch of the vagus nerve (**450**), except the tensor palati which is supplied by the mandibular nerve (**458**), and the stylopharyngeus which is supplied by the glossopharyngeal nerve (**450**).

The pharyngeal mucous membrane

The mucous membrane of the nasopharynx has a ciliated columnar epithelium and is associated with numerous mucous glands. That of the oropharynx has a non-keratinising stratified squamous epithelium which contains taste buds over the under surface of the soft palate, the palatoglossal fold and the pharyngeal part of the tongue.

The palatine and pharyngeal branches of the pterygopalatine ganglion (**428**) transmit ordinary sensations from the anterior part of the nasopharynx, and both ordinary sensations and that of taste from the under surface of the soft palate. The pharyngeal and lingual branches of the glossopharyngeal nerve (**450**) transmit ordinary sensations from the oropharynx except the soft palate and the sensation of taste from the pharyngeal part of the tongue (**450**). The mucosa of the laryngeal part of the pharynx will be considered later (**476**).

The lymphoid tissue of the pharynx

Masses of lymphoid tissue lie deep to the epithelium of the mucous membrane in certain situations in the pharynx. These are usually large in early life but atrophy with age and are not usually evident in dissecting room cadavers.

The two palatine tonsils lie in triangular depressions on the lateral walls of the oropharynx. The borders of this depression or tonsillar bed are the palatoglossal and palatopharyngeal muscles, the soft palate and the pharyngeal part of the tongue (**B, 463A, 463C**), and into each of these the lymphoid tissue tends to encroach to some extent. The lateral aspect of the palatine tonsil is firmly adherent to a layer of connective tissue (**A**), which separates it from the lower part of the superior constrictor and styloglossus (**463A**).

PHARYNX & MOUTH: MEDIAN SECTION: Compare with 463 A

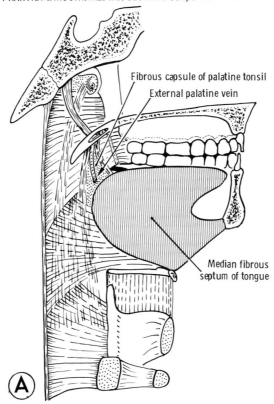

Fibrous capsule of palatine tonsil

External palatine vein

Median fibrous septum of tongue

(A)

PHARYNX: MEDIAN SECTION: Lymphoid tissue

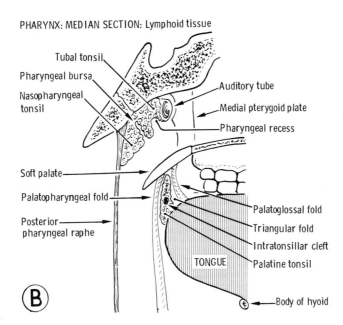

Tubal tonsil

Pharyngeal bursa

Nasopharyngeal tonsil

Auditory tube

Medial pterygoid plate

Pharyngeal recess

Soft palate

Palatopharyngeal fold

Posterior pharyngeal raphe

Palatoglossal fold

Triangular fold

Intratonsillar cleft

Palatine tonsil

TONGUE

Body of hyoid

(B)

Through the connective tissue layer an external palatine vein descends from the soft palate (**465A**). It may be the source of haemorrhage during surgical removal of the tonsil. The medial surface is covered by stratified squamous epithelium and bulges to a variable degree towards the midline (**463C**). The epithelium lines some 15 blind tonsillar crypts which penetrate into the lymphoid tissue, and also lines a larger intratonsillar cleft which runs into the upper part of the tonsil (**465B**). Especially in the young, a triangular fold of mucous membrane arising from the palatoglossal fold may obscure the anterior part of the tonsil.

The main blood supply to the tonsil comes from a tonsillar branch which arises from the apex of the loop of the facial artery (**453A**) and pierces the muscular tonsillar bed.

The pharyngeal tonsil (adenoid) is a single subepithelial mass of lymphoid tissue which lies against the roof and posterior wall of the nasopharynx (**465A**). Its free surface is thrown into a number of folds which radiate from the orifice of a blind recess called the pharyngeal bursa. This tonsil is separated from a smaller collection of lymphoid tissue over the tubal elevation (the tubal tonsil) by the part of the nasopharyngeal lumen called the pharyngeal recess.

The lingual tonsil consists of a considerable number of small masses of lymphoid tissue beneath the epithelium on the pharyngeal part of the tongue. The masses are seen as a number of low smooth elevations.

THE TONGUE AND THE FLOOR OF THE MOUTH

The tongue consists of a compact mass of voluntary muscles, divided into symmetrical halves by a median fibrous septum. Recall its general position and shape (**442**). Its inferior part or root is attached to the lower central part of the body of the mandible and to the hyoid bone (**443B**), and between these attachments rests on the upper surface of the central part of the mylohyoid (**443A**). Its posterior and superior surfaces are smoothly continuous and are known collectively as the dorsum (**443B**).

The tongue may be divided into pharyngeal and oral parts; the demarcation being marked on the dorsum by the sulcus terminalis and the foramen caecum. The narrow anterior region of the oral part protrudes forwards from the rest of the tongue as the conical tip, which has a free inferior surface (**C**).

The muscles of the tongue

Intrinsic muscle fibres pass between different areas of the tongue as longitudinal, vertical and transverse bundles, which interlace with a number of paired extrinsic muscles.

The geniohyoid muscles do not develop with the other extrinsic muscles of the tongue and consequently have a different nerve supply. But, since functionally they act in concert with the extrinsic tongue muscles, they are described here as belonging to that group. The paired fusiform muscles arise from the lower central part of the body of the mandible and pass backwards on either side of the midline to the body of the hyoid bone (**A**).

The genioglossus muscles arise from the mandible immediately above the corresponding geniohyoid. The fibres fan out through the tongue on either side of the median septum as shown in **A**, and reach the body of the hyoid bone and the mucous membrane covering the dorsum of the tongue as far as the tip.

The hyoglossus muscles arise from the corresponding greater horns of the hyoid bone (**451A**). After passing superficial to the middle constrictor muscle, each inclines upwards, forwards and medially through the middle triangular gap (**449A**, **451A**) on to the lateral aspect of genioglossus, with which it interlaces (**A**).

The styloglossus muscles arise from the styloid processes and pass forwards and downwards on the superior constrictor muscles (**451A**). Each then inclines forwards and medially through the middle triangular gap (**453A**) on to the lateral aspect of the tongue, where it interlaces with hyoglossus and genioglossus (**A**).

The palatoglossus muscle has been considered above (**464**). Its relationship to the other extrinsic muscles of the tongue is shown in **A**.

The mucous membrane of the tongue and the floor of the mouth

The mucous membrane of the tongue, like that throughout the oral cavity, has a stratified squamous epithelium.
1. That which covers the pharyngeal part of the dorsum (**466**) is smooth and glistening. As has been seen (**463B**) it exhibits numerous low swellings due to the presence of collections of lymphoid tissue and its epithelium contains numerous taste buds.

EXTRINSIC MUSCLES OF LEFT HALF OF TONGUE: LATERAL VIEW

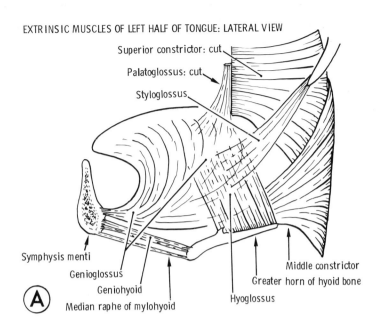

Superior constrictor: cut
Palatoglossus: cut
Styloglossus
Symphysis menti
Genioglossus
Geniohyoid
Median raphe of mylohyoid
Hyoglossus
Greater horn of hyoid bone
Middle constrictor

A

MOUTH & TONGUE: CORONAL SECTION: Dotted line represents mucous membrane

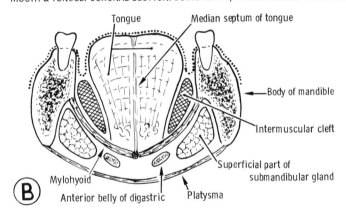

Tongue
Median septum of tongue
Body of mandible
Intermuscular cleft
Superficial part of submandibular gland
Mylohyoid
Anterior belly of digastric
Platysma

B

TONGUE & FLOOR OF MOUTH: SUPERIOR VIEW: Tongue turned upwards

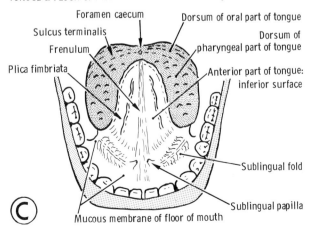

Foramen caecum
Sulcus terminalis
Frenulum
Plica fimbriata
Dorsum of oral part of tongue
Dorsum of pharyngeal part of tongue
Anterior part of tongue: inferior surface
Sublingual fold
Sublingual papilla
Mucous membrane of floor of mouth

C

467

Traced laterally it is continuous with the mucosa over the palatine tonsils and the lateral pharyngeal walls. Traced downwards it passes onto the epiglottis (**477A**).

2. In front of the sulcus terminalis, the mucous membrane on the dorsum and lateral margins of the oral part of the tongue appears dull and rough, owing to the presence of numerous surface papillae. The epithelium contains a large number of taste buds.

3. A short distance down the lateral aspect of the oral part of the tongue, the mucous membrane is reflected laterally to cover the alveolar process of the mandible, forming the gum (**467B**). This mucous membrane of the floor of the mouth forms a roof over an intermuscular cleft between the lateral aspect

of the tongue, and the mylohyoid and mandible (**467B**). The cleft will be seen later to contain a number of important structures.

4. On the conical anterior part of the oral region of the tongue, the inferior surface is covered by smooth, transparent mucous membrane, which exhibits a fringe-like plica fimbriata on either side of the midline (**467C**). Traced backwards, this area of mucous membrane turns first downwards and then forwards to the central part of the lower gum. This mucosa of the anterior part of the floor of the mouth roofs over the anteromedial end of the intermuscular cleft noted above and exhibits, as shown in **467C**, a median frenulum, paired sublingual papillae and paired sublingual folds.

STRUCTURES IN THE FLOOR OF THE MOUTH

The submandibular salivary gland

The submandibular gland is C-shaped, consisting of a large superficial part, and a small deep part which are continuous with each other at the posterior pole. The superficial part is triangular in coronal section (**467B**). Its medial surface rests on the outer surface of mylohyoid, and its lateral surface against the submandibular fossa on the deep aspect of the body of the mandible (**B, 439C**). Its inferior surface (**A, 467B**) extends from the inferior margin of the body of the mandible down to the digastric and stylohyoid muscles, and is covered by the investing layer of the deep cervical fascia and the superficial fascia, which here contains the facial vein (**A, 445B**) and the cervical branch of the facial nerve (**445A**).

The posterior pole of the gland curls medially round the posterior margin of mylohyoid and is in contact medially

with the middle constrictor muscle, and laterally with the insertion of medial pterygoid (**B**).

The deep part extends forwards into the intermuscular cleft of the mouth which has been noted (**471A**) between hyoglossus and mylohyoid. Here the mucous membrane of the floor of the mouth lies a short distance above it.

The gland has a particularly intimate relationship to the loop of the facial artery which is often partially embedded in its substance. It will be recalled that the artery exhibits a pronounced loop before it passes into the tissues of the face (**A, 453A**). The artery passes upwards and forwards on the medial aspect of the posterior pole, turns laterally, and thereafter runs downwards and forwards on the lateral aspect of the superficial part of the gland. It then turns round the inferior margin of the mandible just in front of masseter, where its pulse can be readily palpated against the bone, and ascends into the face (**A, B**).

SUBMANDIBULAR GLAND: SUPERFICIAL PART: Lateral view

Facial vein

Facial artery

Body of mandible

Masseter

Stylohyoid

Posterior belly of
digastric

Facial artery

Facial vein

Anterior
belly of digastric

Mylohyoid

Hyoglossus

Inferior surface of superficial part of
submandibular gland

A

SUBMANDIBULAR GLAND: SUPERFICIAL PART:

Medial view (mylohyoid removed)

Medial pterygoid

Deep surface of body of mandible

Mylohyoid line

Facial artery

Deep part of gland removed

Medial surface of superficial part of
submandibular gland

B

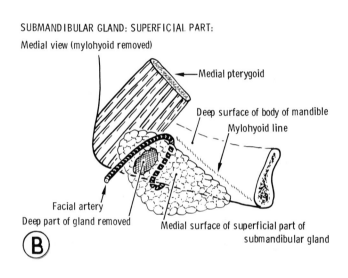

The submandibular duct

A single duct, which receives tributaries from all parts of the gland, arises from the anterior end of the deep part and runs forwards and medially in the intermuscular cleft, lying first on hyoglossus and subsequently on genioglossus (**A**). It opens into the cavity on the sublingual papilla, which has been observed already on the mucous membrane of the floor of the mouth close to the frenulum (**467C**).

The sublingual salivary gland

The sublingual gland, which is about the size and shape of an almond, is the smallest of the three main salivary glands. It lies in the anterior part of the intermuscular cleft of the mouth (**A**). Laterally, it lies against the sublingual fossa on the mandible (**439C**). Medially, it is separated from the genioglossus by the submandibular duct, and, as will be seen below, by the lingual nerve. Above it raises the sublingual fold on the mucous membrane of the floor of the mouth (**467C**), on which its multiple small ducts open into the oral cavity.

The lingual artery

The origin of the lingual artery from the external carotid, its characteristically looped course forwards on the middle constrictor muscle and its passage into the substance of the tongue deep to hyoglossus have been noted previously (**452, 463A**). Thereafter, the vessel runs upwards and forwards amongst the lingual muscles and continues along the inferior aspect of the tip of the tongue just deep to its mucous membrane (**B**). It supplies the tongue and the structures in the intermuscular cleft of the mouth and supplies small ascending branches to the palatine tonsil.

The nerves of the tongue and floor of the mouth

The glossopharyngeal nerve

Revise the course and branches of this nerve (**396, 411B, 451A**). Its terminal lingual branches run in close association with the styloglossus muscle through the middle triangular gap to the pharyngeal part of the tongue. It transmits general sensation and taste from the mucous membrane of the pharyngeal part of the tongue and from a narrow strip of the mucous membrane of the oral part in front of the sulcus terminalis.

The lingual nerve

Revise the course and fibre content of the lingual nerve in the infratemporal fossa. It enters the cavity of the mouth through the middle triangular gap and at that point consists of fibres of both general sensation and taste, and preganglionic parasympathetic fibres. In the mouth it lies first beneath the mucous membrane on the inner aspect of the gum below the third molar tooth (**463A**) where it may be affected by a local anaesthetic injected for dental procedures. The nerve then inclines downwards and forwards a short distance above the deep part of the submandibular gland within the intermuscular cleft of the mouth (**A, B**). Here it passes medial to the sublingual gland and hooks from lateral to medial beneath the submandibular duct. A spray of branches then spread to the mucous membrane of the tongue anterior to the glossopharyngeal area (see above) and to the mucous membrane of the floor of the mouth. The fibres which have their cell bodies in the trigeminal ganglion transmit general sensations from the region, while those which have their cell bodies in the genicular ganglion of the facial nerve and join the lingual through the chorda tympani transmit the sensation of taste.

The submandibular ganglion

This parasympathetic ganglion lies in the intermuscular cleft of the mouth between the lingual nerve and the deep part of the submandibular gland (**A, B**). It is joined by communicating branches to both these structures. The proximal communication with the lingual nerve carries all the preganglionic parasympathetic fibres which joined that nerve in the infratemporal fossa through the chorda tympani branch of the facial nerve (**457A**). After relay in the ganglion, postganglionic parasympathetic fibres leave the ganglion by two routes.

1. Many pass through the communications to the deep part of the submandibular gland and constitute the secretomotor supply to the whole of that gland.
2. The others pass into the lingual nerve through the distal of its two communications with the ganglion and, passing distally in the nerve, are distributed to the sublingual gland as its secretomotor supply.

STRUCTURES IN INTERMUSCULAR CLEFT: LATERAL VIEW:

Mylohyoid & body of mandible removed

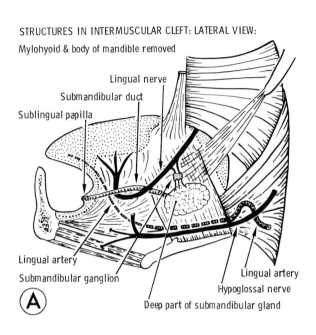

Lingual nerve

Submandibular duct

Sublingual papilla

Lingual artery

Submandibular ganglion

Lingual artery

Hypoglossal nerve

Deep part of submandibular gland

(A)

STRUCTURES IN INTERMUSCULAR CLEFT: As in 467 B

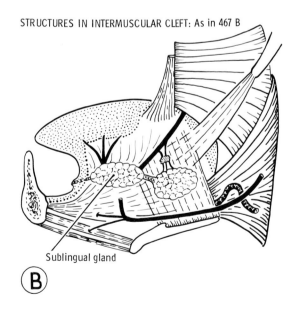

Sublingual gland

(B)

The hypoglossal nerve

Revise the early part of the course of the hypoglossal nerve (**396, 453A**) and recall that the fibres originating in the medulla are joined by fibres from the ventral ramus of the first cervical nerve just below the base of the skull. The nerve enters the intermuscular cleft of the mouth through the middle triangular gap in the pharynx lying on the outer surface of hyoglossus which separates it from the lingual artery (**471A, 471B**). It runs forwards on hyoglossus, below the deep part of the submandibular gland, and divides into its terminal branches on genioglossus (**471A**). It is the motor nerve to all the extrinsic and intrinsic muscles of the tongue except palatoglossus which, being also a muscle of the soft palate, receives its innervation from the pharyngeal branch of the vagus (**450**). Although geniohyoid has been treated as an extrinsic tongue muscle in this account, the branch of the hypoglossal nerve which supplies it is derived from the first cervical nerve.

THE LARYNX

The oral part of the pharynx is continuous below with a tube composed of the structures shown in **A**. The outer aspect of the region has been considered already (**448, 450**) and should be revised.

The more or less cylindrical larynx lies within this tube, close to its anterior wall, as shown diagrammatically in **B, C**. The lowest part of the larynx is formed by the ring of the cricoid cartilage and is continuous with the trachea, while its upper end is the obliquely disposed laryngeal inlet.

The remainder of the tube constitutes the laryngeal part of the pharynx from the level of the upper border of the anterior laryngeal wall to the upper end of the oesophagus. Note that it communicates with the larynx through the laryngeal inlet (**B**) and extends forwards on either side of the laryngeal wall forming the piriform fossae (**C**).

Observe the following structures which take part in the formation of the laryngeal wall.

The epiglottis

The epiglottis (**D, E**) is a thin, leaf-shaped plate of elastic cartilage with anterior and posterior surfaces. Its narrow inferior end is fixed in the angle between the laminae of the thyroid cartilage by the short fibres of the thyro-epiglottic ligament, while at a higher level its anterior surface is attached to the body of the hyoid bone by the longer hyo-epiglottic ligament. The long axis of the cartilage is consequently inclined upwards and backwards. Between the hyo-epiglottic and thyro-epiglottic ligaments the anterior surface of the epiglottis is separated from the thyroid cartilage and the thyrohyoid membrane by fatty areolar tissue. At a higher level the same surface is separated from the pharyngeal surface of the tongue by a deep recess.

The posterior surface of the cartilage is gently concave in both directions in its upper part but bulges backwards in the broad tubercle in its lower part.

At rest the free upper margin lies at the level of the body of the third cervical vertebra.

MEDIAN SECTION OF TUBE WHICH IS DIVIDED INTO LARYNX & PHARYNX

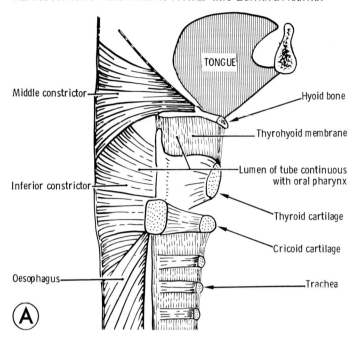

TONGUE

Middle constrictor

Inferior constrictor

Oesophagus

Hyoid bone

Thyrohyoid membrane

Lumen of tube continuous with oral pharynx

Thyroid cartilage

Cricoid cartilage

Trachea

A

LARYNX & PHARYNX: DIAGRAMMATIC MEDIAN SECTION

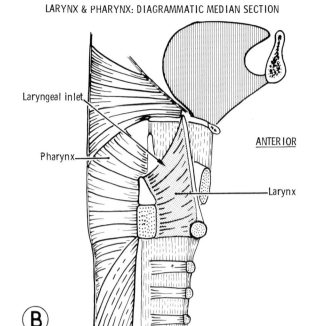

Laryngeal inlet

Pharynx

ANTERIOR

Larynx

B

LARYNX &|PHARYNX: DIAGRAMMATIC HORIZONTAL SECTION
ANTERIOR

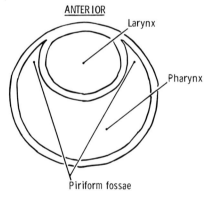

Larynx

Pharynx

Piriform fossae

C

EPIGLOTTIS: POSTERIOR ASPECT
SUPERIOR

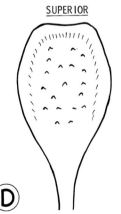

D

EPIGLOTTIS: MEDIAN SECTION

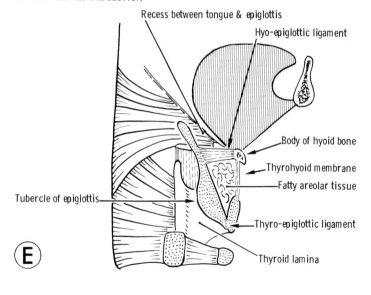

Recess between tongue & epiglottis

Hyo-epiglottic ligament

Body of hyoid bone

Thyrohyoid membrane

Fatty areolar tissue

Thyro-epiglottic ligament

Tubercle of epiglottis

Thyroid lamina

E

The arytenoid cartilages

The small paired arytenoid cartilages are situated one on either side of the midline. Each is conical in shape with a base, an apex and three surfaces (**A, B, C**). The base articulates with a facet on the upper surface of the cricoid lamina, forming a synovial crico-arytenoid joint which is enclosed by a delicate fibrous capsule. The apex is directed upwards, backwards and medially. The surfaces are posterior, medial and anterolateral, the latter facing obliquely in an upward, forward and lateral direction. Two of the angles between these surfaces are prolonged as slender processes, the anterior angle forming the vocal process (**A, B**) and the lateral angle the muscular process (**A, C**).

The quadrangular membranes

On each side the thin fibro-elastic quadrangular membrane (**B, C**) has a long anterior attachment to the lateral margin of the epiglottis and a short posterior attachment to the anterolateral surface of the corresponding arytenoid cartilage. Its free upper margin inclines steeply upwards and forwards and contains in its posterior part two small nodules of cartilage. The corniculate cartilage articulates with the apex of the arytenoid, while the cuneiform cartilage is situated a little further forwards. The horizontal lower free margin of the membrane is thickened and is called the vestibular ligament.

   Observe in **C** that on either side the outer surface of the quadrangular membrane is separated by a wedge-shaped recess of the pharynx from the thyroid lamina, the thyrohyoid membrane and the greater horn of the hyoid bone. This is the piriform fossa noted on the previous page.

The cricovocal membrane

The shape of this single fibro-elastic membrane, which is thicker than the quadrangular membrane, can be appreciated if it is visualised as a flat semilunar sheet which is bent into a U open backwards (**D**) as shown in **B**. Its lower margin is attached to the upper margin of the cricoid arch from one crico-arytenoid joint to the other. Its upper margin is attached posteriorly to the vocal processes of the two arytenoids, and in the midline to the inferior margin of the thyroid cartilage. Between these two attachments the margin is free and constitutes the vocal ligament which is separated from the vestibular ligament by an interval.

The transverse arytenoid muscle

This is a small intrinsic muscle (**C**) of the larynx which passes transversely from the posterior surface of one arytenoid to that of the other.

The walls of the larynx

The structures which form the walls of the larynx from above down can now be visualised in **B**.

1. The anterior wall is long, and consists of the epiglottis, the median part of the cricovocal membrane and the anterior part of the cricoid arch.
2. The posterior wall is much shorter and consists of the transverse arytenoid muscle and the cricoid lamina.
3. Each lateral wall contains the quadrangular membrane, the medial surface of the arytenoid cartilage, the cricovocal membrane and the lateral part of the cricoid arch. It is deficient between the vestibular and vocal ligaments.

LARYNX: MEDIAN SECTION

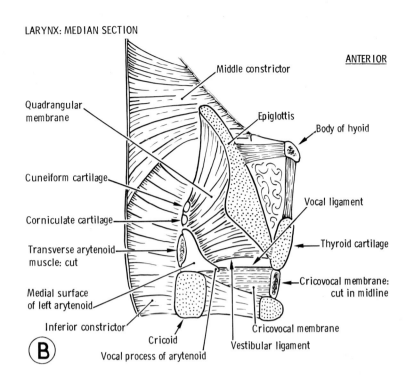

ANTERIOR

Middle constrictor

Quadrangular membrane

Epiglottis

Body of hyoid

Cuneiform cartilage

Corniculate cartilage

Vocal ligament

Transverse arytenoid muscle: cut

Thyroid cartilage

Medial surface of left arytenoid

Cricovocal membrane: cut in midline

Inferior constrictor

Cricovocal membrane

Cricoid

Vestibular ligament

Vocal process of arytenoid

B

CRICOID & ARYTENOID CARTILAGES: LATERAL VIEW

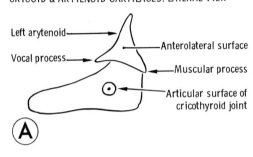

Left arytenoid

Anterolateral surface

Vocal process

Muscular process

Articular surface of cricothyroid joint

A

LARYNX: POSTERIOR VIEW: Lateral walls of pharynx turned aside

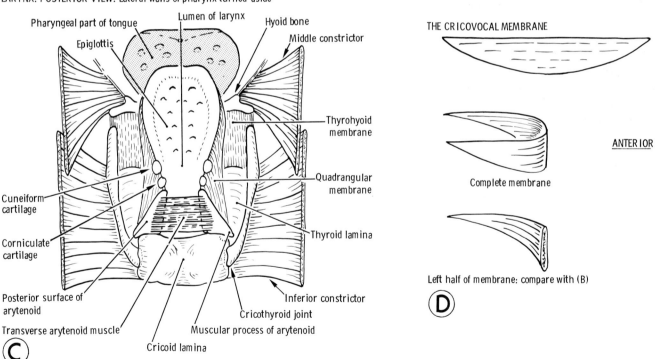

Pharyngeal part of tongue

Lumen of larynx

Hyoid bone

Epiglottis

Middle constrictor

Thyrohyoid membrane

Quadrangular membrane

Thyroid lamina

Cuneiform cartilage

Corniculate cartilage

Posterior surface of arytenoid

Inferior constrictor

Cricothyroid joint

Transverse arytenoid muscle

Muscular process of arytenoid

Cricoid lamina

C

THE CRICOVOCAL MEMBRANE

ANTERIOR

Complete membrane

Left half of membrane: compare with (B)

D

475

The mucous membrane of the larynx

Mucous membrane passes into the larynx through its inlet from the neighbouring regions. The mucosa of the laryngeal part of the pharynx which covers the posterior aspects of the cricoid lamina and the transverse arytenoid muscle turns forwards over the upper margin of that muscle and then descends on the posterior wall of the larynx (**A**). Mucosa passes downwards over the pharyngeal part of the tongue and after turning backwards on the upper surface of the hyo-epiglottic ligament ascends on the anterior surface of the epiglottis to its upper margin. It turns over this margin and descends on the anterior wall of the larynx (**A**). The recess between the tongue and the epiglottis is called the vallecula and is partially divided into two halves by a median fold of mucous membrane. The mucosa which lines the lateral wall of the laryngeal part of the pharynx passes forwards into the depth of the piriform fossa and then returns on the outer aspect of the quadrangular membrane (**C**). It eventually turns medially over the upper free margin of that membrane forming the ary-epiglottic mucosal fold. This extends from the upper part of the epiglottis to the apex of the corresponding arytenoid and exhibits in its lower part two elevations produced by the corniculate and cuneiform cartilages (**A**). Traced downwards this mucous membrane lines the components of the lateral wall of the larynx and bulges laterally through the gap between the quadrangular and cricovocal membranes to form a fusiform recess of the laryngeal cavity (**B**, **C**). This is the sinus of the larynx which is situated deep to the thyroid lamina and below the mucous membrane of the piriform fossa (**B**, **C**). From its anterior part a slender diverticulum called the saccule of the larynx passes upwards.

As the mucous membrane turns from the main laryngeal cavity into the sinus it is wrapped round the vestibular and vocal ligaments (**C**) forming two anteroposterior mucosal folds on each side (**A**). These are the vestibular and vocal folds.

The vocal folds, which are almost white in colour, extend, like the vocal ligaments which support them, from the angle of the thyroid cartilage to the vocal processes of the corresponding arytenoid cartilages. It is important to note (**C**) that they lie nearer the median plane than the vestibular folds so that they can be clearly seen when the larynx is examined from above with a laryngoscopic mirror.

Over both surfaces of the upper part of the epiglottis, the upper parts of the aryepiglottic folds, and the vocal folds, the membrane is of the stratified squamous type. All other areas of laryngeal mucous membrane are covered by ciliated columnar epithelium. All areas of laryngeal mucosa, except that over the free margin of the vocal folds, contain mucous glands, and these are particularly numerous in the saccule.

The cavity of the larynx

The cavity of the larynx may be divided into several named parts.

The vestibule extends from the laryngeal inlet to the level of the vestibular folds.

The middle part of the larynx is the segment between the levels of the vestibular and vocal folds which extends into the sinuses and saccules.

The rima glottidis is the part of the cavity which lies in the plane of the vocal folds (**D**). Its anterior part lies between the vocal folds and is consequently described as intermembranous. Its posterior or intercartilaginous part lies between the medial surfaces of the arytenoid cartilages and is limited behind by the transverse arytenoid muscle.

The infraglottic part of the cavity extends from the rima glottidis to the lower margin of the cricoid cartilage where it becomes continuous with the lumen of the trachea.

The joints of the larynx

The crico-arytenoid joints are small synovial articulations between the bases of the arytenoid cartilages and the upper surface of the cricoid lamina. They permit two types of movement (**E**). The arytenoid may rotate about a vertical central axis, rotation in one direction carrying the vocal process medially and the muscular process forwards, and in the other direction carrying the vocal process laterally and the muscular process backwards. Sliding movements in a transverse direction allow appreciable approximation or separation of the arytenoids. On the other hand the range of anteroposterior sliding of the arytenoids on the cricoid lamina is very limited.

MUCOUS MEMBRANE OF LARYNX & LARYNGEAL PART OF PHARYNX:
MEDIAN SECTION

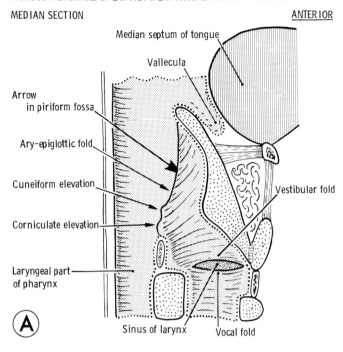

ANTERIOR

Median septum of tongue

Vallecula

Arrow in piriform fossa

Ary-epiglottic fold

Cuneiform elevation

Corniculate elevation

Laryngeal part of pharynx

Vestibular fold

Sinus of larynx   Vocal fold

A

LARYNX: LEFT LATERAL ASPECT

ANTERIOR

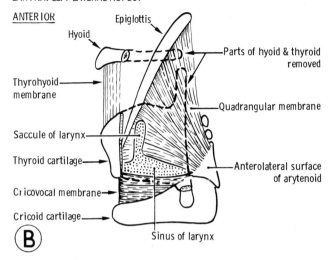

Hyoid   Epiglottis

Thyrohyoid membrane

Saccule of larynx

Thyroid cartilage

Cricovocal membrane

Cricoid cartilage

Parts of hyoid & thyroid removed

Quadrangular membrane

Anterolateral surface of arytenoid

Sinus of larynx

B

CORONAL SECTION OF LARYNX:

Lumen stippled, mucous membrane interrupted line

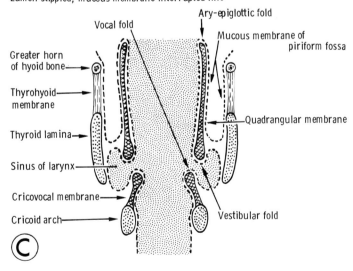

Vocal fold   Ary-epiglottic fold

Mucous membrane of piriform fossa

Greater horn of hyoid bone

Thyrohyoid membrane

Thyroid lamina

Sinus of larynx

Cricovocal membrane

Cricoid arch

Quadrangular membrane

Vestibular fold

C

THE RIMA GLOTTIDIS

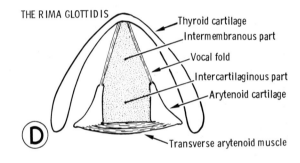

Thyroid cartilage

Intermembranous part

Vocal fold

Intercartilaginous part

Arytenoid cartilage

Transverse arytenoid muscle

D

MOVEMENTS OF CRICO-ARYTENOID JOINTS

Vocal process   Muscular process

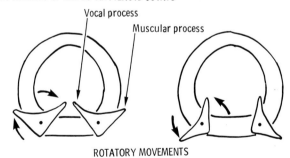

ROTATORY MOVEMENTS

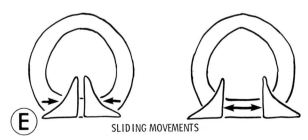

SLIDING MOVEMENTS

E

477

The cricothyroid joints are paired synovial joints formed by the articulation of the inferior horns of the thyroid cartilage with the posterior part of the cricoid arch (**A**). A common transverse axis of rotation passes through the two joints. The movements are primarily between the cricoid and thyroid. However, because of the restricted degree of anteroposterior movement possible at the crico-arytenoid joints, the arytenoid cartilages and the cricoid lamina move more or less as one, so that cricothyroid movements secondarily alter the relationship of the arytenoids to the thyroid. Thus approximation of the anterior parts of the cricoid and thyroid cartilages results in backward displacement of the arytenoid cartilages in relation to the thyroid cartilage and *vice versa*.

The muscles of the larynx

The shape of the rima glottidis, the tension in the vocal folds and the form of the laryngeal inlet are controlled by a number of small voluntary muscles. The transverse arytenoid is a single muscle, whereas all the others are paired.

Each cricothyroid muscle (**B**) has a C-shaped origin from the lamina and inferior horn of the thyroid cartilage (**446**). Its fibres converge downwards and forwards to be inserted into the lateral parts of the cricoid arch.

The single transverse arytenoid (**C, 475C**) passes across the midline from the posterior surface of one arytenoid to the posterior surface of the other.

Each posterior crico-arytenoid muscle (**C**) arises from the posterior surface of the cricoid lamina and converges upwards and laterally to the muscular process of the arytenoid.

Each lateral crico-arytenoid muscle (**D**) arises from the upper border of the lateral part of the cricoid arch and passes backwards and upwards to the muscular process of the arytenoid.

Each thyro-arytenoid muscle (**D**) arises from the lower half of the angle between the thyroid laminae and passes backwards as a flat sheet across the lateral aspect of the sinus of the larynx and the vocal ligament to the antero-lateral surface of the arytenoid.

Each ary-epiglottic muscle (**D**) arises from the apex of the arytenoid cartilage and passes forwards to the lateral margin of the upper part of the epiglottis. It lies in the ary-epiglottic fold (**477A**) in close relationship to the upper margin of the quadrangular membrane.

Changes in tension in the vocal folds

As in any stringed musical instrument, the pitch of the sound produced by vibration of the vocal folds varies with their tension. A high note is produced when the folds are tense and a low note when they are comparatively slack.

As the vocal ligament, which forms the foundation of the fold extends from the anterior part of the thyroid cartilage to the vocal process of the arytenoid (**A**), its tension depends on the distance between these cartilages which, as noted above, is controlled by movements at the cricothyroid joints.

Tension is increased by contraction of the cricothyroid muscle (**B**) which approximates the anterior parts of the thyroid and cricoid cartilages and, as a result, moves the arytenoid cartilages backwards in relation to the thyroid (**A**).

Tension is reduced by the thyro-arytenoid muscle (**D**) which moves the arytenoid forwards towards the thyroid and, as a result, separates the anterior parts of the cricoid and thyroid (**A**).

CRICOTHYROID MOVEMENTS

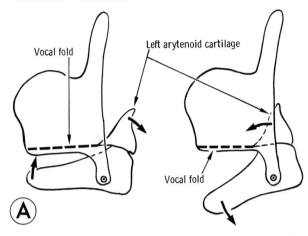

Vocal fold

Left arytenoid cartilage

Vocal fold

A

LARYNGEAL MUSCLES

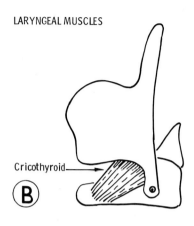

Cricothyroid

B

LARYNGEAL MUSCLES

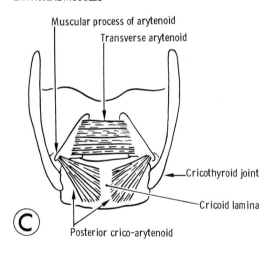

Muscular process of arytenoid

Transverse arytenoid

Cricothyroid joint

Cricoid lamina

Posterior crico-arytenoid

C

LARYNGEAL MUSCLES:

Interrupted line indicates part of left half of thyroid cartilage removed

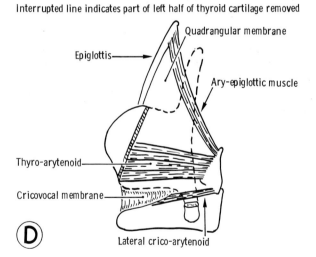

Quadrangular membrane

Epiglottis

Ary-epiglottic muscle

Thyro-arytenoid

Cricovocal membrane

Lateral crico-arytenoid

D

Changes in the form of the rima glottidis

1. In the resting form of the rima glottidis (**A**) the vocal folds are midway between their abducted (**B**) and adducted (**C**) positions. The intermembranous part is triangular and the intercartilaginous square.

2. During inspiration, the posterior crico-arytenoid muscles pull the muscular processes of the arytenoid cartilages backwards and medially. The resulting rotation of the arytenoids about their vertical axes carry the vocal processes laterally and thus abduct the vocal folds (**B**). The widening of the rima glottidis facilitates the entry of air into the lungs.

3. During phonation the rima glottidis is narrowed to a median chink so that the rate of air flow in expiration and the resulting vibrations of the vocal folds are maximal (**C**). The narrowing of the intercartilaginous part of the rima is caused by the transverse arytenoid muscle approximating the arytenoid cartilages. However, it will be evident in **C** that the forces exerted by the transverse arytenoid muscle on the arytenoids also have rotatory components, tending to carry the vocal processes laterally. These components are countered by the lateral crico-arytenoid muscles, which produce opposite rotatory forces by pulling the muscular processes forwards. In this way the vocal folds are held in a position of adduction. Very firm closure of the rima glottidis is an essential part of the act of coughing. The act begins with inspiration, which is due mainly to contraction of the diaphragm, and is associated with abduction of the vocal folds (**B**). The rima glottidis is then closed (**C**) and intrathoracic pressure is raised by contraction of the muscles of the abdominal wall. When pressure reaches a sufficient level the rima glottidis suddenly reopens and air is forced under pressure from the respiratory tract.

4. Although the cricothyroid muscles are not attached to the arytenoid cartilages they can nevertheless affect the shape of the rima glottidis. The tensile stresses which activity of the cricothyroid muscles create in the vocal folds (**478**) may be resolved into anteroposterior and transverse components (**D**). The transverse components approximate the two arytenoid cartilages and narrow the rima glottidis. This effect of the cricothyroid is not of great significance in the normal adduction of the vocal folds in phonation, but, as will be seen below, it is of great importance in some lesions of the laryngeal nerves.

The nerves of the larynx

The motor and sensory nerves to the larynx are branches of the vagus which have already been traced some distance along their courses.

The external laryngeal nerve (**450**) supplies only the cricothyroid muscle.

The internal laryngeal nerve (**450**) has been seen to pass deep to the thyrohyoid muscle and pierce the thyrohyoid membrane. It emerges beneath the mucous membrane which lines the piriform recess (**E**) and divides into a number of divergent branches. These branches are sensory to the pharyngeal mucous membrane which surrounds the laryngeal inlet, and the laryngeal mucous membrane which lines the vestibule, sinus and saccule.

The recurrent laryngeal nerves (**399B**) have already been traced from their origins to different symmetrical positions in the upper parts of the tracheo-oesophageal grooves. Here the nerves enter the laryngeal part of the pharnyx by passing deep to the lower margin of the inferior constrictor muscle, immediately behind the inferior horn of the thyroid cartilage (**E**).

Each nerve divides into a spray of branches. Many innervate all the laryngeal muscles except the cricothyroid, while others pierce the cricovocal membrane and transmit sensory impulses from the laryngeal mucous membrane below the vocal folds.

RESTING FORM OF RIMA GLOTTIDIS

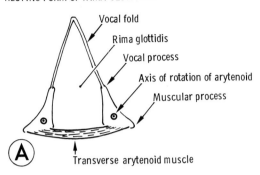

Vocal fold
Rima glottidis
Vocal process
Axis of rotation of arytenoid
Muscular process

A

Transverse arytenoid muscle

ABDUCTION OF VOCAL FOLDS: INSPIRATION

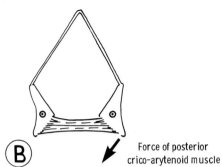

B

Force of posterior
crico-arytenoid muscle

ADDUCTION OF VOCAL FOLDS: PHONATION

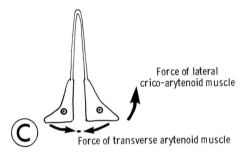

Force of lateral
crico-arytenoid muscle

C

Force of transverse arytenoid muscle

EFFECT OF CRICOTHYROID ON ARYTENOID CARTILAGE

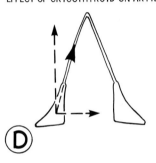

D

NERVES OF LARYNX

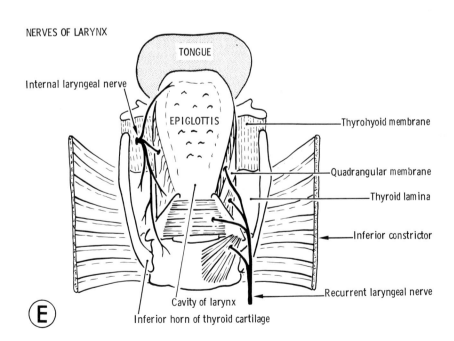

TONGUE

Internal laryngeal nerve

EPIGLOTTIS

Thyrohyoid membrane

Quadrangular membrane

Thyroid lamina

Inferior constrictor

Recurrent laryngeal nerve

E

Cavity of larynx

Inferior horn of thyroid cartilage

Some lesions of the laryngeal nerves

1. When the external laryngeal nerves are inoperative the cricothyroid muscles are paralysed and the vocal folds cannot be tensed. The voice is consequently deep and hoarse.
2. When one recurrent laryngeal nerve is inoperative the corresponding vocal fold is fixed close to the median plane by the cricothyroid muscle. In these circumstances the mobility of the normal fold allows the rima glottidis to be reduced to a median chink in phonation (**A**), or increased to half its normal maximum in inspiration (**B**). Neither activity is therefore seriously affected.
3. In a bilateral lesion of both recurrent laryngeal nerves adduction of both vocal folds by the cricothyroid muscles fixes the rima glottidis as a median chink (**A**) and phonation is not much affected. However the rima glottidis cannot be enlarged beyond the median chink conformation so that anything beyond slight exertion causes inspiratory embarrassment.
4. In concurrent lesions of the recurrent and external laryngeal nerves of the same side, the corresponding vocal fold is immobile in the 'cadaveric' position, midway between adduction and abduction (**C, D**). In these circumstances the normal vocal fold can be abducted to produce a wide rima glottidis in inspiration (**C**), and can also be adducted across the midline until it is closely parallel with the cadaveric fold in phonation (**D**). Thus, neither inspiration nor phonation is much affected by the lesion.

THE ACT OF SWALLOWING (DEGLUTITION)

1. After mastication of food has been completed, or immediately after fluid has been taken into the mouth, the root of the tongue is stabilised through fixation of the hyoid bone by the mylohyoid, geniohyoid, stylohyoid and digastric muscles. Synchronously, respiration is inhibited and remains so throughout the whole act of swallowing.
2. The intrinsic muscles of the stabilised tongue now produce a wave-like elevation of the dorsum of the oral part of the tongue against the hard palate. As the elevation travels backwards it pushes the food bolus or the fluid in advance of it into the oropharyngeal isthmus.
3. The isthmus is now narrowed by the displacement of its margins towards its centre, so that the bolus is squirted, rather like toothpaste, into the oropharynx. Because of their relationship to the medial pterygoid plates (**E**), the tensor palati muscles flatten the normally curved soft palate, displacing its central part downwards. The styloglossus muscles pull the posterior part of the tongue upwards and backwards. The palatoglossus muscles contribute to both the above movements and also draw the palatoglossal arches towards each other.
4. In the pharynx, the food or fluid is carried downwards partly by gravity and partly by a wave of contraction passing along the constrictor muscles. During its downward passage its diversion into neighbouring respiratory regions must be prevented.
5. Diversion into the nasopharynx is prevented by closure of the pharyngeal isthmus. The posterior margin of the soft palate is pulled upwards and backwards by the levator palati muscles, so that it makes contact with a ridge on the posterior pharyngeal wall raised by the middle fibres of the superior constrictor (palatopharyngeal sphincter).
6. Entry into the larynx is prevented in two ways. Much of the bolus, particularly if it is of fluid consistency, divides, as it leaves the tongue, into two streams which descend along the piriform recesses. Nevertheless, the laryngeal inlet is also actively closed. The longitudinal muscles of the pharynx (salpingopharyngeus, palatopharyngeus and stylopharyngeus) are all inserted in part into the posterior margin of the thyroid laminae (**463A**). Contraction of these muscles consequently produces the elevation of the thyroid cartilage which is always associated with swallowing, and secondarily elevates all the other skeletal elements, such as the epiglottis, which are attached to the thyroid. Forced upwards in this way, the upper part of the epiglottis impinges against the overlying pharyngeal part of the tongue, already pulled backwards by styloglossus. As a result the suprahyoid part of the epiglottis is bent backwards as a protective shelf over the laryngeal inlet (**F**). The deflection of the epiglottis is aided by contraction of the ary-epiglottic muscle which also reduces the transverse diameter of the inlet.

LESIONS OF LARYNGEAL NERVES: Interrupted lines represent median plane

RIGHT RECURRENT LARYNGEAL NERVE

RIGHT RECURRENT & EXTERNAL LARYNGEAL NERVES

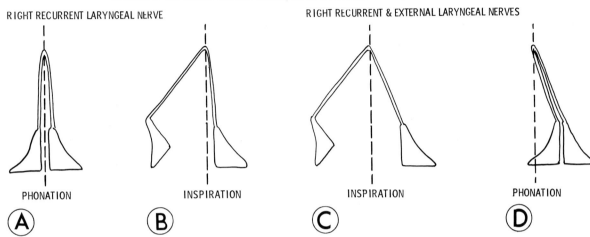

PHONATION

(A)

INSPIRATION

(B)

INSPIRATION

(C)

PHONATION

(D)

MEDIAN SECTION OF LARYNX: CLOSURE OF INLET IN SWALLOWING

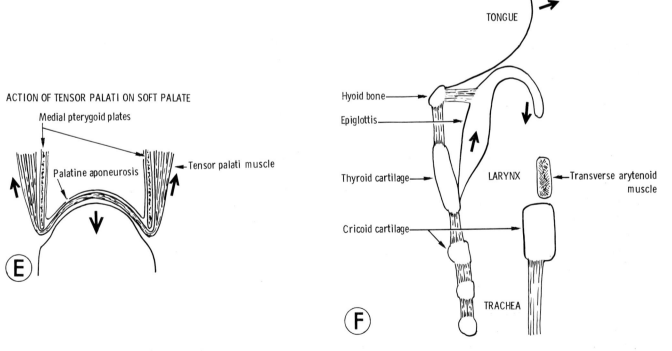

TONGUE

Hyoid bone

Epiglottis

Thyroid cartilage

LARYNX

Transverse arytenoid muscle

Cricoid cartilage

TRACHEA

(F)

ACTION OF TENSOR PALATI ON SOFT PALATE

Medial pterygoid plates

Palatine aponeurosis

Tensor palati muscle

(E)

THE THYROID GLAND

This is a large endocrine gland which is closely associated with the respiratory and digestive tracts in the lower part of the neck. It consists of paired conical lobes connected across the midline by an isthmus (**A**) and is enveloped by the pretracheal layer of the deep cervical fascia (**B**).

The lobes have pointed upper poles which lie just below and behind the oblique lines of the laminae of the thyroid cartilage, and blunt lower poles which are placed on either side of the fourth or fifth tracheal rings. Each lobe has superficial, medial and posterolateral surfaces (**B**), a continuous blunt posterior border (**C**), and a sharper anterior border which is interrupted by the continuity of the lobe and isthmus (**A**). The upper part of the medial surface lies against the inferior constrictor of the pharynx, the external laryngeal nerve intervening (**A**); its lower part is moulded against the lateral aspects of the trachea and oesophagus, and is closely related to the recurrent laryngeal nerve in the tracheo-oesophageal groove (**B**). The posterolateral surface rests against the carotid sheath, covering the common carotid artery and the medial part of the internal jugular vein (**A**, **B**). The superficial surface is covered by three of the strap-like infrahyoid muscles, the sternothyroid, sternohyoid and the superior belly of omohyoid (**B**).

The isthmus, which measures 1.25 cm from above down, joins the lower parts of the anterior border of the lobes, anterior to the second and third rings of the trachea (**A**). An additional lobe known as the pyramidal lobe not infrequently extends upwards from the isthmus towards the hyoid bone.

The pretracheal fascia is toughest where it binds the isthmus and the medial surfaces of the lobes of the gland to the trachea (**B**). Because of this firm adhesion, the thyroid gland always moves with the trachea. In particular, it ascends in the neck as the trachea is elevated with the laryngeal cartilages in swallowing.

The thyroid arteries

In the majority of individuals the gland is supplied by two arteries on each side. All supply branches to neighbouring structures as well as to the gland.

The superior thyroid artery (**A**, **C**) arises from the external carotid artery close to its origin and accompanies the external laryngeal nerve to the upper pole of the cor-responding thyroid lobe. Here it divides into an anterior branch, which passes along the anterior border of the lobe to the upper border of the isthmus, and a posterior branch, which runs along the posterior border.

The inferior thyroid artery has been considered earlier (**393A**) and should be revised. As it approaches the inferior pole of the thyroid lobe it divides into a cluster of branches. These usually pass in front of the recurrent laryngeal nerve but in some cases the nerve threads a course amongst them. Most of these branches enter the gland substance directly, but one passes upwards along the posterior border of the lobe and forms an anastomotic channel with the posterior branch of the superior artery (**C**). The channel lies between the surface of the gland and the pretracheal fascia.

The thyroidea ima is an additional unpaired artery which ascends to the isthmus from the brachiocephalic artery or the aortic arch in some individuals.

The thyroid veins

The veins of the gland drain into a profuse plexus on its surface. This plexus is drained by paired superior and middle thyroid veins into the internal jugular veins and a number of inferior thyroid veins which drain downwards in front of the trachea into the left brachiocephalic vein in the superior mediastinum (**A**).

The parathyroid glands

The four parathyroids are yellowish-brown ovoid bodies about 5 mm in diameter, two of which are usually situated on the posterior border of each lobe of the thyroid gland in close relation to the anastomotic arterial channel which joins the superior and inferior thyroid arteries.

The superior parathyroids are usually placed about the middle of the thyroid lobe and the inferior parathyroids near its inferior poles, but their positions and their number vary quite considerably.

Because the glands are developed from the endoderm of the third and fourth pharyngeal pouches, the superior parathyroids are sometimes called the parathyroids IV, and the inferior parathyroids the parathyroids III.

THYROID GLAND

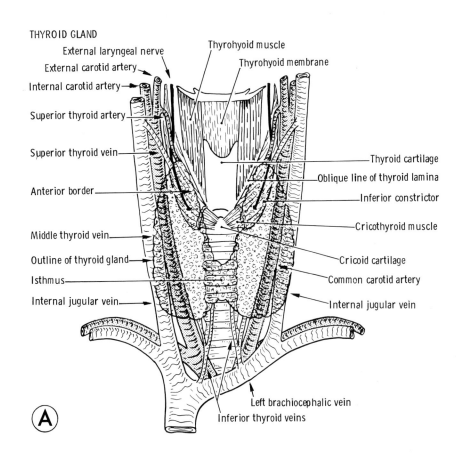

External laryngeal nerve
External carotid artery
Internal carotid artery
Superior thyroid artery
Superior thyroid vein
Anterior border
Middle thyroid vein
Outline of thyroid gland
Isthmus
Internal jugular vein

Thyrohyoid muscle
Thyrohyoid membrane

Thyroid cartilage
Oblique line of thyroid lamina
Inferior constrictor
Cricothyroid muscle
Cricoid cartilage
Common carotid artery
Internal jugular vein

Left brachiocephalic vein
Inferior thyroid veins

(A)

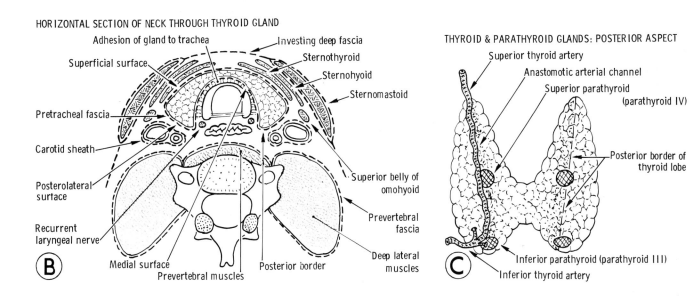

HORIZONTAL SECTION OF NECK THROUGH THYROID GLAND

Adhesion of gland to trachea
Superficial surface
Pretracheal fascia
Carotid sheath
Posterolateral surface
Recurrent laryngeal nerve

Investing deep fascia
Sternothyroid
Sternohyoid
Sternomastoid

Superior belly of omohyoid
Prevertebral fascia
Deep lateral muscles

Medial surface
Prevertebral muscles
Posterior border

(B)

THYROID & PARATHYROID GLANDS: POSTERIOR ASPECT

Superior thyroid artery
Anastomotic arterial channel
Superior parathyroid (parathyroid IV)
Posterior border of thyroid lobe
Inferior parathyroid (parathyroid III)
Inferior thyroid artery

(C)

485

THE INFRAHYOID MUSCLES

These are strap-like muscles most of which cover the superficial surfaces of the lobes of the thyroid gland (**485B**), and lie deep to the lower parts of the sternomastoid muscles and the investing layer of the deep cervical fascia. They are innervated by branches of the ansa cervicalis (**A**) which, it will be recalled, consists of fibres derived from the ventral rami of the upper three cervical nerves (**398**).

The thyrohyoid muscle has been considered previously (**446**).

The sternothyroid muscle passes downwards and somewhat medially, in line with the thyrohyoid, from the oblique line on the thyroid cartilage to the posterior aspect of the manubrium sterni (**A**).

The sternohyoid muscle is attached above to the body of the hyoid bone and passes downwards and somewhat laterally, superficial to thyrohyoid and sternothyroid. Below, it is attached to the posterior aspects of the medial end of the clavicle, the sternoclavicular joint and the manubrium sterni (**A**, **B**).

The omohyoid muscle consists of superior and inferior bellies joined at an angle by an intermediate tendon. The superior belly is attached to the hyoid bone at the junction of the body and greater horn and gradually diverges from the lateral border of sternohyoid (**A**). The intermediate tendon overlies the internal jugular vein (**A**) deep to sternomastoid (**B**) and is held in this position by a fascial loop attached to the clavicle.

The inferior belly has been considered already (**400**). Emerging from underneath the sternomastoid muscle, it passes laterally and downwards across the lower part of the posterior triangle of the neck superficial to the supraclavicular part of the brachial plexus (**401A**). It is attached to the superior border of the scapula close to the scapular notch.

The anterior jugular veins

These two veins begin by the confluence of small tributaries at the level of the hyoid bone and descend through the superficial fascia of the neck between the sternomastoid muscles (**401A**). A short distance above the manubrium sterni they pierce the investing layer of the cervical fascia and turn laterally between the sternohyoid and sternomastoid muscles (**A**, **B**). Reaching the posterior triangles they end by joining the terminal parts of the external jugular veins (**400**). In the lower part of the neck, where they turn laterally, the two anterior jugular veins are joined across the midline by an anastomotic channel called the jugular venous arch (**A**, **B**).

Tracheostomy

Tracheostomy is the insertion of a tube into the trachea to overcome an obstruction in the upper respiratory tract or to allow ventilation of the lungs by an anaesthetic apparatus over a prolonged period. Before the operation is begun, the anaesthetised patient's head is extended over a pillow placed behind the neck; this brings the trachea forwards and also upwards. The cricoid cartilage is identified and a transverse 5 cm incision made in the skin of the front of the neck about a fingerbreadth below it. The anterior jugular veins in the superficial fascia are displaced or ligated and divided. The platysma, deep cervical fascia and pretracheal fascia are divided in the midline. The sternothyroid muscles are deep to the deep fascia on each side of the midline and inferior thyroid veins also pass downwards in front of the trachea. A small window is then excised in the anterior wall of the trachea, including part of one of the rings, to allow the tracheostomy tube to be passed.

INFRAHYOID MUSCLES

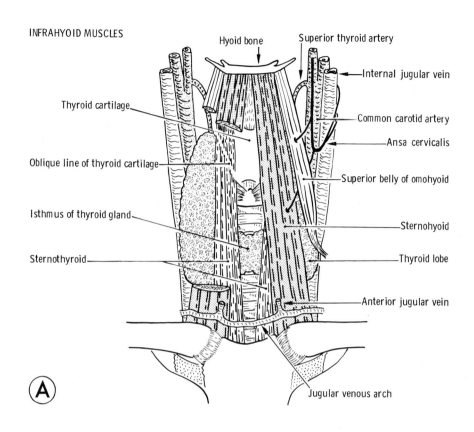

Hyoid bone

Superior thyroid artery

Internal jugular vein

Common carotid artery

Ansa cervicalis

Superior belly of omohyoid

Sternohyoid

Thyroid lobe

Anterior jugular vein

Thyroid cartilage

Oblique line of thyroid cartilage

Isthmus of thyroid gland

Sternothyroid

Jugular venous arch

(A)

INFRAHYOID REGION OF NECK: ANTERIOR ASPECT

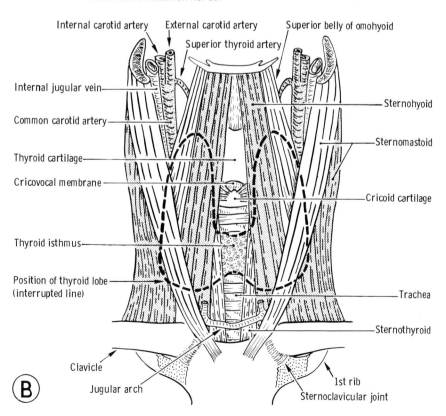

Internal carotid artery

External carotid artery

Superior thyroid artery

Superior belly of omohyoid

Internal jugular vein

Common carotid artery

Thyroid cartilage

Cricovocal membrane

Thyroid isthmus

Position of thyroid lobe (interrupted line)

Sternohyoid

Sternomastoid

Cricoid cartilage

Trachea

Sternothyroid

Clavicle

Jugular arch

1st rib

Sternoclavicular joint

(B)

LYMPHATIC DRAINAGE OF THE HEAD AND NECK

In this region the lymph nodes form groups, either in the superficial fascia or deep to the investing layer of the deep cervical fascia. The lymph flows in a downward direction into the deep nodes either directly or after passage through the superficial nodes. From the lower deep nodes the jugular lymph trunk, after a short course, joins the thoracic duct or the right lymphatic duct.

It should be noted that the names applied to some of these groups of nodes differ from those in standard usage which are given in brackets.

The deep nodes (A)

The internal jugular nodes (deep cervical nodes) form a long chain along the course of the internal jugular vein from the base of the skull to the root of the neck. The chain may be artificially divided into upper and lower parts.

Most of the lower nodes are deep to the lower half of the sternomastoid though some encroach beyond the posterior border of that muscle into the posterior triangle of the neck.

The jugulo-omohyoid node (**A**), which belongs to this group, lies on the vein just above the intermediate tendon of the omohyoid muscle.

The upper nodes lie anterior to sternomastoid but the highest members of the chain are deeply situated medial to the parotid gland and the styloid process.

The jugulodigastric node or nodes (**A**) occupy the lower angle between the internal jugular vein and the posterior belly of the digastric muscle.

Other groups of deep nodes lie at some distance from the internal jugular chain but drain into it.

The retropharyngeal nodes are situated a short distance below the base of the skull between the prevertebral layer of deep cervical fascia and a layer of fascia which covers the posterior wall of the nasopharynx (**B**). The two layers of fascia are only loosely connected by areolar tissue throughout the length of the neck. Consequently, if an abscess develops as a result of inflammation of the retropharyngeal nodes, it can spread downwards, stripping the pharynx from the prevertebral muscles, and even reach the superior mediastinum.

The submandibular nodes lie on the outer surfaces of mylohyoid and hyoglossus between the body of the mandible and the digastric muscle (**A**). They are always closely related to the submandibular salivary gland (**468**) and are often embedded within its substance.

The laryngeal and tracheal nodes are scattered over the anterior and lateral aspects of the larynx, trachea and oesophagus (**A**), deep to the infrahyoid group of muscles.

The superficial nodes (C)

Observe the positions and names of the superficial groups of lymph nodes in **C**.

The submental nodes lie in the midline below the symphysis menti.

The external jugular nodes (superficial cervical nodes) are disposed along the course of the external jugular vein.

The anterior jugular nodes (anterior cervical nodes) lie along the course of the anterior jugular vein.

Lymph drainage of skin

The lymph from the skin of the head and neck is drained into the lower two-thirds of the internal jugular group of nodes either directly or, more commonly, after passing through the neighbouring superficial group of nodes.

Lymph drainage of midline viscera

The lymph from the midline viscera of the head and neck drains into the internal jugular nodes, usually after passing through other deep cervical nodes or the submental nodes which belong to the superficial group.

1. The central part of the lower lip, the central part of the lower gum and the lower incisor teeth, the anterior part of the floor of the mouth and the tip of the tongue, drain through the submental nodes into the internal jugular group.
2. The lips, the cheeks, the gums and teeth, the anterior part of the nose, and the floor of the mouth except the parts associated with the submental nodes (see above) drain through the submandibular nodes into the internal jugular group.
3. The anterior two-thirds of the tongue, except the tip, drain through the submandibular nodes into the internal jugular group, particularly the jugulo-omohyoid node.
4. The posterior third of the tongue, the oropharynx and the palatine tonsil drain directly into the internal jugular group, particularly the jugulodigastric nodes.
5. The posterior part of the nose, the paranasal air sinuses, the nasopharynx and nasopharyngeal tonsil and the palate drain through the retropharyngeal nodes into the internal jugular group.
6. The laryngeal part of the pharynx, the larynx and the cervical parts of the oesophagus and trachea drain through the laryngeal and tracheal nodes into the internal jugular group.

DEEP CERVICAL GROUPS OF LYMPH NODES

(sternomastoid & mandibular ramus in outline)

LYMPHATICS OF HEAD & NECK: SUPERFICIAL GROUPS OF NODES

Retropharyngeal nodes

Jugulodigastric node

Internal jugular vein

Submandibular nodes

Laryngeal nodes

Jugulo-omohyoid node

Tracheal nodes

(A)

Buccal nodes

Submental nodes

Anterior jugular nodes

Anterior jugular vein

Occipital nodes

Mastoid nodes

Parotid nodes

Outline of sternomastoid

External jugular vein

External jugular nodes

Outline of trapezius

Clavicle

(C)

UPPER PART OF NECK: HORIZONTAL SECTION

NASOPHARYNX

Fascia on pharyngeal wall

Internal carotid artery

Retropharyngeal nodes

Internal jugular vein

Prevertebral muscles

Prevertebral fascia

Atlas

(B)

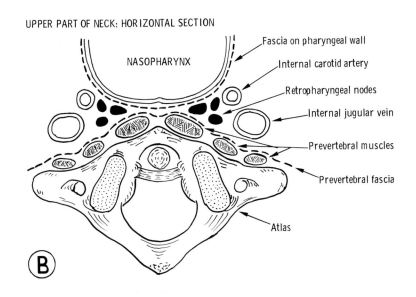

489

CHAPTER 7

The upper limb

INTRODUCTION

The upper limb is connected to the axial skeleton through the shoulder girdle. As has been seen (**384**) this consists, on either side, of the clavicle and scapula joined to each other at the acromioclavicular joint. The clavicle articulates with the thoracic cage at the synovial sternoclavicular joint. On the other hand, the scapula does not articulate directly with the axial skeleton, but lies against the posterolateral aspect of the upper half of the chest wall, and is attached to the axial skeleton only by muscles. The upper limb itself consists of three articulating segments, namely, the arm containing the humerus, the forearm containing the radius and ulna, and the hand. The arm articulates with the shoulder girdle at the shoulder joint, the arm and forearm are separated by the elbow joint and the forearm and hand by the wrist joint. Notice the different colloquial and anatomical uses of the term 'arm'.

Although the upper and lower limbs exhibit many structural similarities, their functions are distinct. In contrast to the rigidity and supportive role of the foot, the hand is essentially manipulative in function and is capable of a wide range of different movements of both delicacy and power. Moreover, because the hand must be capable of operating in a great variety of positions in relation to the trunk, the rest of the upper limb has a much greater mobility than the lower limb. Thus the shoulder girdle is movable on the thoracic cage, the shoulder joint has a greater range of movement than any other joint in the body, and the axial orientation of the hand can be varied by rotation of the forearm bones on each other.

The nerves of the upper limb are derived almost entirely from the brachial plexus (**389C, 389D**) while the vessels of the part are branches and tributaries of the subclavian vessels (**391A**). The plexus and vessels converge on the upper limb from the lower part of the neck and the thoracic inlet and should be revised at this time.

THE SHOULDER GIRDLE

The bones and joints of the shoulder girdle have already been considered (**380–384**). They should now be revised (**A, B**). Recall that, at rest, the superior angle of the scapula is normally level with the spine of the second thoracic vertebra and the inferior angle with the spine of the seventh thoracic vertebra. Also that the clavicle lies more or less horizontally and, by its strut-like action on the acromion process, holds the lateral border and angle of the scapula away from the chest wall so that the glenoid fossa faces laterally, forwards and upwards.

The muscles and fascia connecting the shoulder girdle to the axial skeleton

The trapezius and levator scapulae have been considered previously (**399C, 391A**). They should now be revised (**C**).

The serratus anterior (**A, B**) is a large flat muscle closely applied to the lateral aspect of the rib cage. It arises by digitations from the upper eight ribs, midway between their angles and costochondral junctions, its lower four slips interdigitating with the upper five digitations of the external oblique muscle of the abdominal wall (**209A**). The fibres pass backwards and upwards and are inserted into the medial border of the scapula. It is functionally significant (see below) that, whereas the upper three digitations are spread along most of the medial border, the lower five converge like a fan on the inferior angle (**507A**).

The rhomboid muscle is a flat quadrilateral sheet which is often separated by a narrow interval into upper and lower parts. The muscle arises from the spines of the lower cervical and upper thoracic vertebrae and passes downwards and laterally between erector spinae (**387A**) and trapezius to the medial border of the scapula between its spine and inferior angle (**B**).

The pectoralis minor is a fan-shaped muscle which passes upwards and somewhat laterally from the third, fourth and fifth ribs, near their costochondral junctions, to the horizontal part of the coracoid process of the scapula (**D**).

The subclavius is small and extends laterally from its origin on the upper surface of the first costochondral junction to the grooved inferior aspect of the middle third of the clavicle.

The clavipectoral fascia (**D**) is a strong fibrous sheet which occupies the interval between pectoralis minor and subclavius. Medially it blends with the first and second external intercostal membranes (**125B**), while laterally it is attached to the conoid part of the coracoclavicular ligament (**383E**).

SERRATUS ANTERIOR

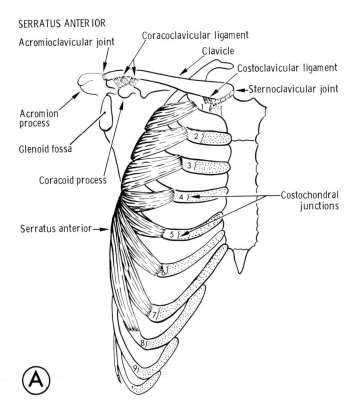

- Acromioclavicular joint
- Coracoclavicular ligament
- Clavicle
- Costoclavicular ligament
- Sternoclavicular joint
- Acromion process
- Glenoid fossa
- Coracoid process
- Costochondral junctions
- Serratus anterior

(A)

THE RHOMBOID MUSCLES

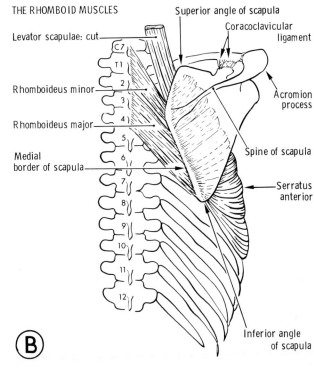

- Levator scapulae: cut
- Superior angle of scapula
- Coracoclavicular ligament
- Rhomboideus minor
- Rhomboideus major
- Medial border of scapula
- Acromion process
- Spine of scapula
- Serratus anterior
- Inferior angle of scapula

(B)

TRAPEZIUS MUSCLE

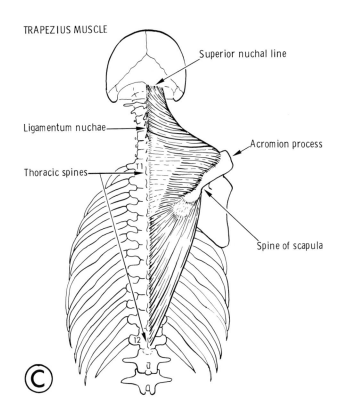

- Superior nuchal line
- Ligamentum nuchae
- Thoracic spines
- Acromion process
- Spine of scapula

(C)

PECTORALIS MINOR & CLAVIPECTORAL FASCIA

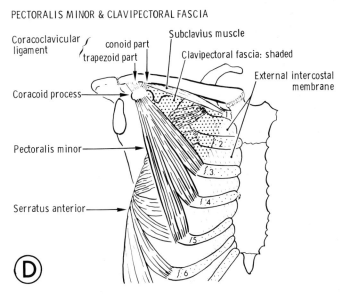

- Coracoclavicular ligament
- conoid part
- trapezoid part
- Subclavius muscle
- Clavipectoral fascia: shaded
- External intercostal membrane
- Coracoid process
- Pectoralis minor
- Serratus anterior

(D)

The movements of the shoulder girdle

The essential parts of these movements are various displacements of the scapula on the rib cage, but these are inevitably associated with changes in the position of the clavicle by virtue of movements at the acromioclavicular (**383E**) and sternoclavicular (**381F**) joints. Movements at the acromioclavicular joint are small and allow alterations in the angulation between the scapula and clavicle. Most movements at the sternoclavicular joint occur around an axis formed by the attachment of the clavicle to the first costochondral junction by the costoclavicular ligament (**B, 381F**) so that, except in the case of rotation of the bone around its long axis, the medial and lateral ends of the clavicle move in opposite directions.

The six cardinal movements of the scapula on the chest wall are elevation, depression, forward displacement (protraction), backwards displacement (retraction) and rotation such that the inferior angle of the bone moves forwards or backwards.

It is important to appreciate that several of these scapular movements are essential concomitants of certain movements of the upper limb at the shoulder joint, and that some of them cannot, in fact, be voluntarily executed in the absence of the corresponding shoulder joint movements.

The movements are produced in the main by the muscles which extend to the scapula from the axial skeleton (see above). Acting individually, nearly all these muscles would produce more than one of the several scapular displacements, as is shown diagrammatically in **A**. Consequently, each cardinal movement of the scapula is usually produced by two of these muscles acting in concert so that the opposing and unwanted moieties of their actions cancel one another out.

In protraction, although the medial border of the scapula follows the curvature of the rib cage, the acromion process and lateral border of the scapula move forwards round a path of more open curvature, of which the clavicle forms the radius (**B**). Consequently, the power of the force on the glenoid fossa is exerted almost directly forwards. This is of functional importance because protraction of the scapula is an inherent part of all forward pushing or punching movements and provides much of the power of these actions.

Protraction is produced by the combined actions of pectoralis minor (**A1**) and serratus anterior (**A2**), the potential rotatory effects of the two muscles cancelling each other.

Retraction of the scapula braces the shoulder backwards and medially. The medial border of the bone follows the curvature of the chest wall while the lateral border follows the arc traced by the lateral end of the clavicle, so that the glenoid fossa comes to face more laterally than it does in the position of rest. The movement is motivated by the trapezius (**A4**) and the rhomboid muscles (**A3**), the potential rotatory effects of the two muscles again cancelling out.

Elevation, or shrugging of the shoulders is produced by levator scapulae (**A5**) which does not have a significant rotatory effect on the scapula.

Depression of the scapula may be effected in three ways.

It may be an active movement produced by two large muscles, the pectoralis major (**501D**) and the latissimus dorsi (**501C**). It is to be noted that both these are inserted into the upper part of the humerus so that the force they exert on the scapula is an indirect one transmitted through the ligaments of the shoulder joint.

More frequently, it is largely or wholly a passive movement caused by the weight of the upper limb acting on the scapula.

Thirdly, the scapula may be forced downwards and medially by a fall of the point of the shoulder. In these circumstances the direction of the force may tear the coracoclavicular ligament and the fibrous capsule of the acromioclavicular joint (**493A**) so that the acromion process is noticeably displaced beneath the lateral end of the clavicle (step deformity).

Rotation of the scapula on the chest wall so that its inferior angle moves forwards, turns the glenoid fossa in an upward direction, and is associated with rotation of the clavicle around its long axis at the sternoclavicular joint. This scapular movement is an essential component of the movement of raising the upper limb above the head and it will be described in that context later (**503E**). The scapula is moved by the simultaneous actions of trapezius (**A4**) and serratus anterior (**A2**), the potential retracting and protracting effects of these muscles cancelling each other.

Rotation of the scapula in the opposite direction, which is also of course associated with axial rotation of the clavicle, is often a passive movement, occurring automatically as the raised upper limb returns to the side. But if the downward movement of the arm is used to raise the body, as it often is in gymnastics, this displacement of the scapula is produced actively by the combined actions of pectoralis minor (**A1**) and the rhomboids (**A3**), the potential protracting and retracting effects of these muscles again cancelling out.

ACTIONS OF MUSCLES ON SCAPULA (The forces exerted by individual muscles are shown by interrupted arrows, and the resulting displacements of the scapula by solid arrows)

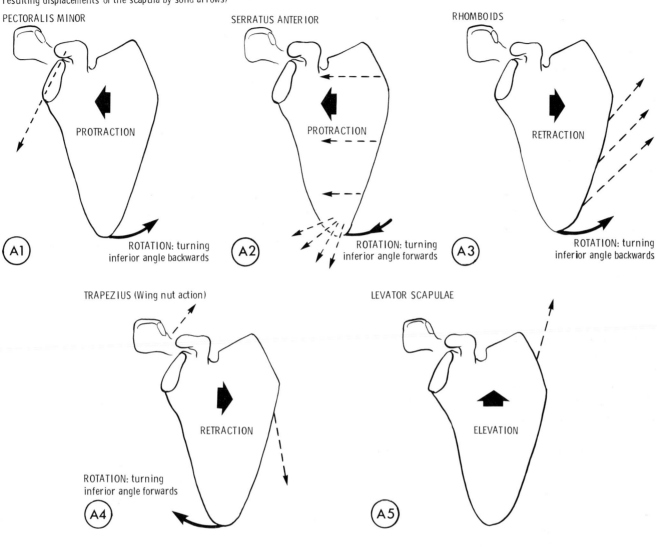

PECTORALIS MINOR

PROTRACTION

ROTATION: turning inferior angle backwards

(A1)

SERRATUS ANTERIOR

PROTRACTION

ROTATION: turning inferior angle forwards

(A2)

RHOMBOIDS

RETRACTION

ROTATION: turning inferior angle backwards

(A3)

TRAPEZIUS (Wing nut action)

RETRACTION

ROTATION: turning inferior angle forwards

(A4)

LEVATOR SCAPULAE

ELEVATION

(A5)

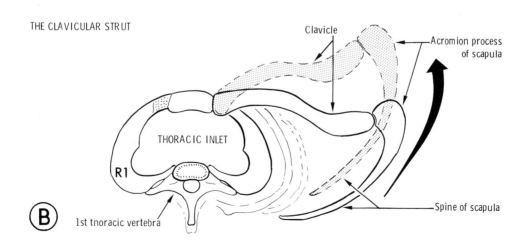

THE CLAVICULAR STRUT

Clavicle

Acromion process of scapula

THORACIC INLET

R1

Spine of scapula

1st thoracic vertebra

(B)

THE SHOULDER REGION

The upper part of the humerus

Examine this part of the humerus in **A** and **B**. Note particularly the following features.

1. The hemispherical head of the bone is angulated on the shaft, so that when the arm is by the side it faces upwards, medially and backwards. The surface of the head is completely covered by hyaline cartilage.
2. At the upper end of the shaft and lateral to the head two tubercles are separated by a deep longitudinal groove. The lesser tubercle is directed forwards and exhibits a smooth impression which corresponds to the area of insertion of a tendon (**A**). The greater tubercle is directed laterally and backwards and is marked by three tendon impressions on its upper and posterior aspects (**A, B**). The groove which separates the tubercles is situated on the anterolateral aspect of the shaft and is named the intertubercular sulcus (**A**).
3. The prominent rough area at about the middle of the lateral aspect of the shaft is named the deltoid tuberosity after the large deltoid muscle which is inserted into it (see below).
4. Rather more than the upper half of the posterior aspect of the shaft is crossed obliquely from its medial to its lateral side by a wide shallow groove which passes below and behind the deltoid tuberosity (**B**). It is known as the sulcus for the radial nerve (or the spiral groove).
5. From an anatomical point of view the neck of the humerus is the slight constriction demarcating the head of the bone from the upper end of the shaft including the tubercles (**A, B**). On the other hand the narrowest part of the upper end of the bone, which is important clinically as the site of most fractures in this region, is situated immediately below the tubercles and is commonly described as the surgical neck (**A, B**).
6. The growth cartilage, at which longitudinal growth of the upper end of the humerus occurs, lies a little above the surgical neck so that the proximal epiphysis of the bone includes the greater parts of both tubercles as well as the head (**D**). Secondary centres appear in the head during the first year, in the greater tubercle during the second and in the lesser tubercle during the fifth. Although initially separate, these three centres coalesce at about the sixth year (**C**), and fuse with the shaft at about 20.

The shoulder joint

The articular surfaces of this large synovial joint lie on the scapula and humerus. The proximal surface is the shallow glenoid fossa of the scapula, deepened and extended by the fibrocartilaginous glenoid labrum (**E**). The ring-like labrum is triangular in cross section and its deep aspect is attached to the bone around the margins of the fossa (**F**). The distal articular surface covers the head of the humerus (**A, B**). It is considerably more extensive than the proximal, so that when the arm is by the side only its lower half or so is in contact with the scapula (**499C**).

The fibrous capsule is attached proximally to the peripheral margin of the glenoid labrum and the adjacent bone (**E**). Observe that this line of attachment skirts above both the supraglenoid and infraglenoid tubercles so that the former area of bone is within the joint cavity while the latter is outside it. Distally, the capsule is attached to the superior, anterior and posterior aspects of the anatomical neck of the humerus, while below it is attached to the shaft of the bone some 1 cm below the articular cartilage (**D**). Note the relationship of the distal capsular attachment to the peripheral margin of the proximal humeral growth plate (**D**). As a consequence of this relationship, the medial part of the growth plate is intracapsular.

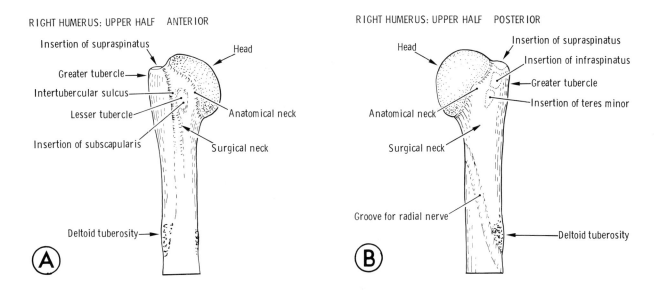

RIGHT HUMERUS: UPPER HALF   ANTERIOR

Insertion of supraspinatus
Greater tubercle
Intertubercular sulcus
Lesser tubercle
Insertion of subscapularis
Deltoid tuberosity

Head
Anatomical neck
Surgical neck

A

RIGHT HUMERUS: UPPER HALF   POSTERIOR

Head
Anatomical neck
Surgical neck
Groove for radial nerve

Insertion of supraspinatus
Insertion of infraspinatus
Greater tubercle
Insertion of teres minor
Deltoid tuberosity

B

RADIOGRAPH: PROXIMAL END OF ADOLESCENT HUMERUS

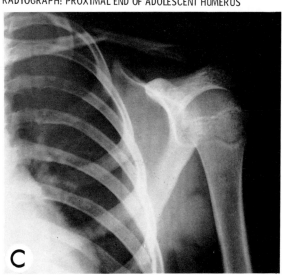

C

RIGHT HUMERUS: UPPER END
ANTERIOR ASPECT

Greater tubercle
Lesser tubercle
Cartilaginous growth plate

Articular surface of head
Distal attachment of fibrous capsule of shoulder joint

D

RIGHT SHOULDER JOINT: Anterolateral aspect of scapula

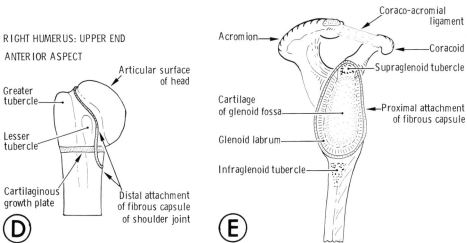

Acromion
Cartilage of glenoid fossa
Glenoid labrum
Infraglenoid tubercle

Coraco-acromial ligament
Coracoid
Supraglenoid tubercle
Proximal attachment of fibrous capsule

E

SHOULDER JOINT: HORIZONTAL SECTION
OF PROXIMAL ARTICULAR SURFACE

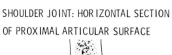
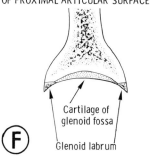

Cartilage of glenoid fossa
Glenoid labrum

F

497

The capsular fibres run a spiral course between scapula and humerus (**A**) so that they tighten as the shaft of the humerus is moved backwards (extension) and becomes slack as the bone is carried forwards (flexion). Note, by moving your own shoulder joint, how extension is consequently limited at less than 90° while flexion is free through a range of 180°.

The tendons of a number of scapulo-humeral muscles, known as the rotator-cuff muscles, are applied to the upper, anterior and posterior aspects of the capsule and project many of their deeper fibres into its substance (**A**). These aspects of the capsule may therefore be maintained in a taut condition in all positions of the joint. Projection of tendinous fibres does not occur into the inferior aspect of the capsule and so this part of the capsule is comparatively unsupported.

There are usually two openings in the fibrous capsule, one in its anterior part (**A**) and one in its superior part at the upper end of the intertubercular sulcus.

The coraco-acromial ligament is a triangular, approximately horizontal structure which is attached to the horizontal part of the coracoid process and the tip of the acromion process (**A, B**). It lies above the upper part of the fibrous capsule of the shoulder and is separated from it by a number of structures (see below). It cannot be regarded as a ligament of the shoulder joint. On the other hand, it is involved in the mechanics of that joint to the extent that it counteracts the upward displacement of the humeral head which the shallowness of the glenoid fossa and the laxity of the capsule of the shoulder joint tend to permit.

The long head of the biceps muscle (one of the muscles in the anterior compartment of the arm) has an intra-articular tendinous origin from the supraglenoid tubercle and the uppermost part of the glenoid labrum (**A**). It passes laterally through the cavity of the shoulder joint, above the head of the humerus (**C**). Emerging through the superior opening in the capsule, it descends along the intertubercular sulcus before giving way to muscle fibres (**B**).

The synovial membrane lines the deep aspect of the fibrous capsule. Observe the following features of the membrane.

1. It covers the medial aspect of the humeral shaft between the articular cartilage and the inferior attachment of the capsule (**C**).
2. It invests the intra-articular part of the tendon of the long head of the biceps (**C**).
3. It is evaginated through the superior capsular opening and forms a double tube around the biceps tendon as it descends through the upper half of the intertubercular sulcus (**C**).
4. It is also evaginated through the anterior capsular opening to form the subscapular bursa (**B**).

The movements at the shoulder joint will be discussed later (**502**).

The muscles of the shoulder joint

Functionally these muscles fall into two groups. Those of one group are comparatively small and their tendons of insertion lie close to, or even in, the substance of the fibrous capsule. They are thus unable to exert any very significant movements at the shoulder joint. On the contrary, they are mainly concerned in maintaining the humeral head in the glenoid fossa, thus stabilising the joint during movements produced by other muscles. They may be called the stabilising group. The second group consists of much larger muscles whose tendons of insertion lie at a greater distance from the joint. They are consequently capable of producing powerful joint movements and may be described collectively as the effector group.

The stabilising muscles

The rotator-cuff muscles is the collective name commonly given to four small muscles called supraspinatus, infraspinatus, teres minor and subscapularis. All arise on the scapula and are inserted into the tendon impressions on the greater or lesser tubercles of the humerus (**B**). Observe the attachments and positions of these muscles in **D** and **E** and note the following facts.

1. The tendon of subscapularis is separated from the front of the shoulder joint by the subscapular bursa which, as has been seen (**B**), communicates with the joint cavity. One anterior approach to the joint at operation is through this bursa after division of the subscapularis tendon near its insertion.
2. The tendon of supraspinatus is intimately incorporated into the upper part of the fibrous capsule of the shoulder joint. Here it may rupture following a slow degenerative process or as the result of trauma.
3. As it runs laterally, the tendon of supraspinatus passes below the acromion process and the coraco-acromial ligament, but is separated from these structures by the large subacromial bursa (**B**).
4. This bursa does not communicate with the cavity of the shoulder joint as long as the supraspinatus tendon is intact, but, as will be seen later, extends for some distance deep to the deltoid muscle (**503B**).
5. The infraspinatus and teres minor cross the posterior aspect of the capsule of the shoulder.
6. None of the rotator-cuff muscles is related to the inferior aspect of the fibrous capsule, which is consequently comparatively unprotected (**A**). Dislocation of the shoulder joint may occur when abduction of the joint forces the head of the humerus against and through this unprotected part of the capsule.

RIGHT SHOULDER JOINT: SECTION AT RIGHT ANGLES TO SCAPULAR PLANE

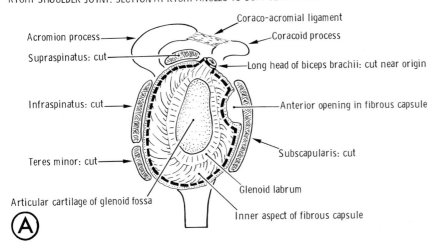

Acromion process

Coraco-acromial ligament

Coracoid process

Supraspinatus: cut

Long head of biceps brachii: cut near origin

Infraspinatus: cut

Anterior opening in fibrous capsule

Teres minor: cut

Subscapularis: cut

Articular cartilage of glenoid fossa

Glenoid labrum

Inner aspect of fibrous capsule

(A)

SHOULDER JOINT: SECTION IN SCAPULAR PLANE

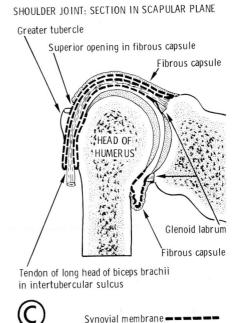

Greater tubercle

Superior opening in fibrous capsule

Fibrous capsule

HEAD OF HUMERUS

Glenoid labrum

Fibrous capsule

Tendon of long head of biceps brachii in intertubercular sulcus

(C)

Synovial membrane ▬ ▬ ▬ ▬ ▬

RIGHT SHOULDER JOINT: ANTEROLATERAL ASPECT

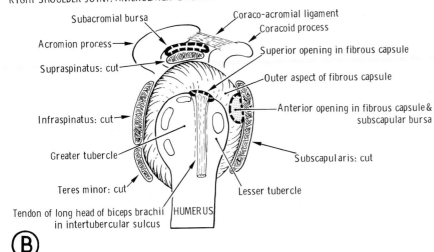

Subacromial bursa

Coraco-acromial ligament

Coracoid process

Acromion process

Superior opening in fibrous capsule

Supraspinatus: cut

Outer aspect of fibrous capsule

Infraspinatus: cut

Anterior opening in fibrous capsule & subscapular bursa

Greater tubercle

Teres minor: cut

Subscapularis: cut

Lesser tubercle

Tendon of long head of biceps brachii in intertubercular sulcus

HUMERUS

(B)

ORIGINS & INSERTIONS OF SHOULDER MUSCLES: ANTEROMEDIAL ASPECT

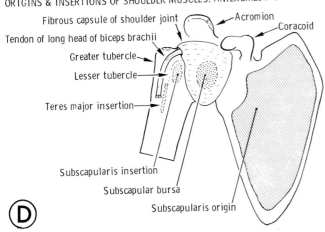

Fibrous capsule of shoulder joint

Acromion

Coracoid

Tendon of long head of biceps brachii

Greater tubercle

Lesser tubercle

Teres major insertion

Subscapularis insertion

Subscapular bursa

Subscapularis origin

(D)

ORIGINS & INSERTIONS OF SHOULDER MUSCLES: POSTEROLATERAL ASPECT

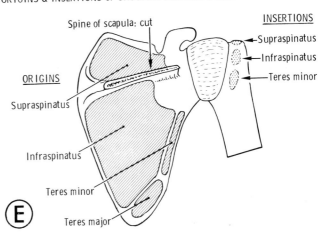

Spine of scapula: cut

INSERTIONS

Supraspinatus

Infraspinatus

Teres minor

ORIGINS

Supraspinatus

Infraspinatus

Teres minor

Teres major

(E)

499

The tendon of the long head of the biceps brachii has been described already in relation to the shoulder joint (**499C**). The biceps muscle is mainly concerned in producing movements of the forearm. However, it is evident from its relationship to the shoulder joint that the tendon of the long head is one of the several factors which help to control any tendency to upward displacement of the humeral head from the glenoid fossa.

The effector muscles

The form and position of the muscles of this group will be described here. Their actions will be considered in the succeeding section dealing with the movements of the arm on the trunk.

The long head of the triceps muscle has an extracapsular tendinous origin from the infraglenoid tubercle of the scapula (**A, B**). It passes downwards and laterally, in front of teres minor, below and at some distance from the shoulder joint (**A**). In the posterior compartment of the arm it fuses with two other heads which arise from the humeral shaft and are not therefore mechanically associated with the shoulder. As will be seen later the whole muscle is inserted into the proximal end of the ulna and acts mainly on the elbow joint.

Teres major arises from the lower third of the lateral border of the scapula and runs laterally, upwards and somewhat forwards (**A, B**). It passes in front of the long head of triceps and at some distance from the inferior aspect of the shoulder joint, to be inserted by a flat tendon into the medial lip of the intertubercular sulcus on the anterior aspect of the humerus (**B**). Note the different inclinations of teres major and minor and their different relationships to the long head of triceps.

Latissimus dorsi is a large flat triangular muscle, most of which lies on the posterior aspect of the trunk (**C**). It arises from the posterior lamina of the thoracolumbar fascia, by which it is attached to the vertebral spines below the mid-thoracic region and the posterior part of the iliac crest. Its upper horizontal fibres are covered by the lower fibres of trapezius (**C**) and pass over the inferior angle of the scapula,

while its lower oblique fibres overlap the posterior digitations of the external oblique muscle (**C**). Converging upwards and laterally the muscle twists round the lateral border of teres major so that its original posterior surface comes to face anteriorly (**B**). Its broad flat tendon covers most of the anterior surface of teres major and is inserted in front of that muscle into the floor of the intertubercular sulcus on the humerus.

The short head of biceps brachii (**D, E**), unlike the long head, is entirely outside the shoulder joint. From its origin on the tip of the coracoid process of the scapula, it passes downwards and laterally, in front of the tendons of subscapularis, teres major and latissimus dorsi. In the arm it lies along the medial side of the long head as that structure emerges from the intertubercular sulcus.

Coracobrachialis is a small and slender muscle which arises in common with the previous muscle and runs along its medial side to be inserted into the middle of the medial aspect of the humerus opposite the deltoid tuberosity (**D**).

Pectoralis major is a large, thick, powerful muscle which covers the greater part of the anterior chest wall. Its fibres arise from a number of structures (**D, E**).

1. The anterior aspect of the medial half of the clavicle.
2. The anterior aspects of the manubrium and body of the sternum.
3. The upper six costal cartilages.
4. The aponeurotic anterior wall of the upper part of the rectus sheath.

The fibres of the muscle converge laterally, the clavicular fibres being commonly demarcated from the sternocostal fibres by a narrow sulcus, and are inserted by a broad tendon into the lateral lip of the intertubercular sulcus (**D**) on the humerus.

Observe from the muscle outline shown in **E** the numerous structures which lie deep to it. It is in close contact with subclavius, the clavipectoral fascia, pectoralis minor, coracobrachialis and the two heads of biceps, but is separated from the muscles visible between pectoralis minor and coracobrachialis by a wide tissue space, the axilla (see below.)

MUSCLES OF THE SHOULDER JOINT: POSTEROLATERAL ASPECT

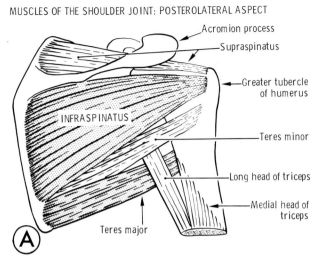

Acromion process
Supraspinatus
Greater tubercle of humerus
INFRASPINATUS
Teres minor
Long head of triceps
Medial head of triceps
Teres major
(A)

MUSCLES OF THE SHOULDER JOINT: ANTEROMEDIAL ASPECT

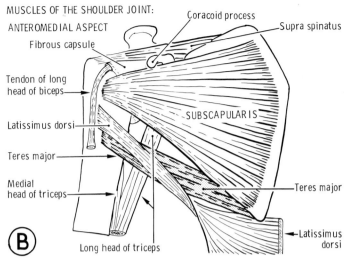

Coracoid process
Supra spinatus
Fibrous capsule
Tendon of long head of biceps
SUBSCAPULARIS
Latissimus dorsi
Teres major
Medial head of triceps
Teres major
Latissimus dorsi
Long head of triceps
(B)

MUSCLES OF SHOULDER JOINT: POSTERIOR ASPECT

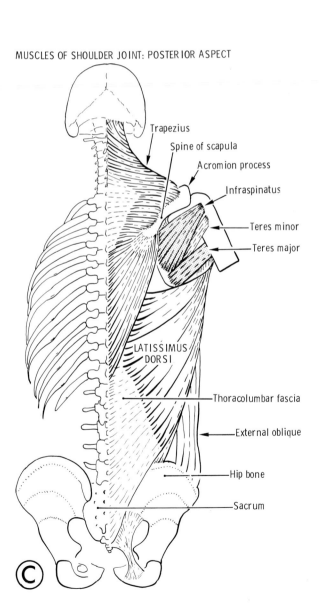

Trapezius
Spine of scapula
Acromion process
Infraspinatus
Teres minor
Teres major
LATISSIMUS DORSI
Thoracolumbar fascia
External oblique
Hip bone
Sacrum
(C)

MUSCLES OF SHOULDER: PECTORALIS MAJOR

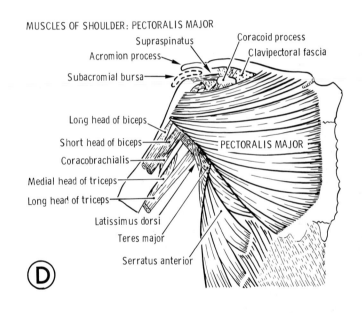

Supraspinatus
Coracoid process
Acromion process
Clavipectoral fascia
Subacromial bursa
Long head of biceps
Short head of biceps
Coracobrachialis
PECTORALIS MAJOR
Medial head of triceps
Long head of triceps
Latissimus dorsi
Teres major
Serratus anterior
(D)

MUSCLES OF SHOULDER (Interrupted line shows outline of pectoralis major)

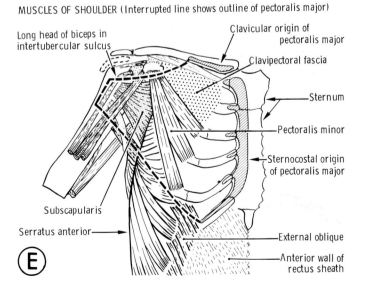

Long head of biceps in intertubercular sulcus
Clavicular origin of pectoralis major
Clavipectoral fascia
Sternum
Pectoralis minor
Sternocostal origin of pectoralis major
Subscapularis
Serratus anterior
External oblique
Anterior wall of rectus sheath
(E)

Deltoid is a large, thick muscle which covers the anterior upper and posterior aspects of the shoulder joint (**A, B**) and produces the smoothly rounded contour of the normal shoulder. It has a continuous C-shaped origin from the anterior aspect of the lateral third of the clavicle, the lateral margin of the acromion process and the lower lip of the crest of the scapular spine. Its fibres converge laterally and then downwards and are inserted into the deltoid tuberosity on the humerus (**A**).

The anterior margin of the muscle is separated from the upper margin of pectoralis major by the deltopectoral cleft, the upper part of which overlies the clavipectoral fascia.

It is important to be able to visualise the structures which lie deep to the deltoid. These relationships can be observed in **B**, in which the muscle is shown in outline.

Movements of the arm on the trunk

The greater part of these movements occur at the shoulder joint and are produced by the effector muscles of that joint, which have been described above. However, it is important to appreciate that all movements of the arm at the shoulder joint involve stabilisation of that articulation by the stabilising group of shoulder muscles, and that some are always associated with simultaneous displacements of the scapula and clavicle on the chest wall.

At most joints it is customary to regard flexion and extension as movements in a sagittal plane and abduction and adduction as movements in a coronal plane. However, at the shoulder joint the proximal articular surface faces forwards and laterally (and upwards), in a direction which conforms to the oblique plane in which the scapula lies on the chest wall (**C**). Consequently, although the arm can certainly be moved in both sagittal and coronal planes, it is usual to regard abduction and adduction as movements of the arm in the scapular plane, and flexion and extension as movements in an orthogonal plane.

Nevertheless, confusion does sometimes arise particularly in relation to abduction and flexion. This can be avoided if more fully explanatory, although more cumbersome terms are used, such as abduction in the scapular plane, abduction in a coronal plane, flexion at right angles to the scapular plane and flexion in a sagittal plane (**C**).

Rotation of the arm around the long axis of the humerus occurs purely at the shoulder joint. It is most easily appreciated if the hinge-like elbow joint is bent to a right angle and the forearm is used as a pointer which indicates the direction in which the anterior aspect of the arm is facing. Thus, starting with the arm by the side and the

forearm directed forwards, medial rotation displaces the anterior aspect of the arm medially and carries the forearm across the trunk, whereas lateral rotation displaces the anterior aspect of the arm laterally and carries the forearm as far as the scapular plane. It should be noted, however, that the directions of displacement of the anterior aspect of the arm during rotation depend on the position of the arm when rotation takes place. Thus if the arm is abducted from the side and the elbow bent it will be observed that the anterior aspect of the arm turns downwards in medial rotation and upwards in lateral rotation.

Medial rotation of the arm is produced by muscles which cross the anterior aspect of the shoulder joint and the upper end of the humerus. These are pectoralis major, latissimus dorsi, teres major, the anterior fibres of deltoid and, to a lesser extent, subscapularis. Lateral rotation is a much weaker movement and is produced by the posterior fibres of deltoid, teres minor and infraspinatus.

Extension of the arm at right angles to the scapular plane occurs entirely at the shoulder joint and carries the arm backwards and laterally. Observe on your own body that the movement is sharply limited after a range of about 90°. This is due to the fact that extension progressively increases the spiral twist of the fibres of the capsule of the shoulder joint until they arrest the movement (**D**). The movement is produced by latissimus dorsi and the posterior fibres of deltoid, the rotatory effects of these two muscles on the humerus (see above) cancelling out.

Flexion of the arm at right angles to the scapular plane occurs entirely at the shoulder joint and unlike extension which is limited at about 90° it can be continued through an arc of 180° until the arm is orientated vertically upwards (**E**). The reason for the greater range of this movement is that, whereas extension progressively tightens the spirally disposed fibres of the joint capsule of the shoulder joint, flexion unwinds the fibres and slackens the capsule. The movement is motivated by the clavicular fibres of pectoralis major and the anterior fibres of deltoid and it is consequently associated with some degree of medial rotation of the arm.

Flexion of the arm in a sagittal plane is an important movement, because, carried through a range of 90° it provides much of the force produced by all punching and pushing actions. The movement is produced at the shoulder joint by the clavicular fibres of pectoralis major and the anterior fibres of deltoid. On the other hand, as has been noted previously, much of the forward force of such a punch or push is derived from protraction of the scapula by the combined actions of serratus anterior and pectoralis minor (**495A1, 495A2**).

SHOULDER MUSCLES: FROM ABOVE

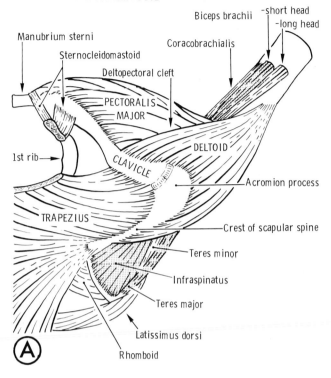

Manubrium sterni
Sternocleidomastoid
Deltopectoral cleft
Biceps brachii
—short head
—long head
Coracobrachialis
PECTORALIS MAJOR
DELTOID
1st rib
CLAVICLE
Acromion process
TRAPEZIUS
Crest of scapular spine
Teres minor
Infraspinatus
Teres major
Latissimus dorsi
Rhomboid

(A)

SHOULDER MUSCLES (Interrupted line shows outline of deltoid)

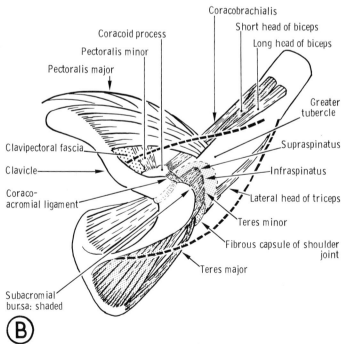

Coracobrachialis
Coracoid process
Short head of biceps
Pectoralis minor
Long head of biceps
Pectoralis major
Greater tubercle
Clavipectoral fascia
Supraspinatus
Clavicle
Infraspinatus
Coraco-acromial ligament
Lateral head of triceps
Teres minor
Fibrous capsule of shoulder joint
Teres major
Subacromial bursa: shaded

(B)

MOVEMENTS AT SHOULDER JOINT

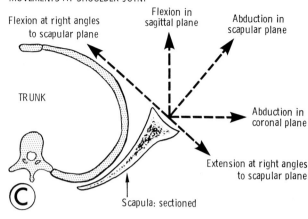

Flexion at right angles to scapular plane
Flexion in sagittal plane
Abduction in scapular plane
TRUNK
Abduction in coronal plane
Extension at right angles to scapular plane
Scapula: sectioned

(C)

EXTENSION OF RIGHT SHOULDER JOINT AT RIGHT ANGLES TO SCAPULAR PLANE

(Size of fibrous capsule is exaggerated)

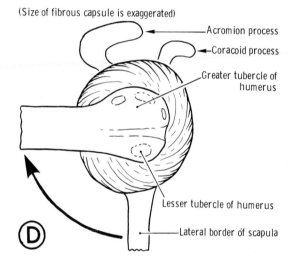

Acromion process
Coracoid process
Greater tubercle of humerus
Lesser tubercle of humerus
Lateral border of scapula

(D)

FLEXION OF RIGHT SHOULDER JOINT AT RIGHT ANGLES TO SCAPULAR PLANE

(Size of fibrous capsule is exaggerated)

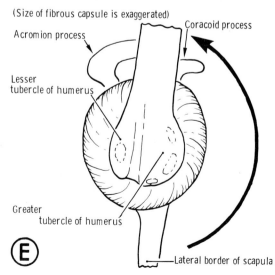

Acromion process
Coracoid process
Lesser tubercle of humerus
Greater tubercle of humerus
Lateral border of scapula

(E)

Abduction of the arm in the scapular plane carries the arm forwards and laterally and then upwards through a range of 180°. If the movement is carried out on your own body with the elbow bent, it will be observed that in contrast to abduction in the coronal plane (see below) it involves no rotation of the arm around its long axis. The movement can be considered as three simultaneously occurring components.

1. Supraspinatus exerts two effects on the shoulder joint. It acts with the other stabilising muscles (**498**) to maintain the head of the humerus in the glenoid fossa and also produces some measure of abduction of the shoulder.
2. Deltoid is the main abductor of the shoulder joint, moving the arm through a range of about 100° (**A**, **B**). However, it cannot produce this movement in the absence of the stabilising and abducting actions of supraspinatus described above. The reason is that, when the arm is by the side the fibres of deltoid run parallel to the shaft of the humerus, and unless the head of the bone is fixed, their contraction only serves to pull the humerus longitudinally upwards.
3. Abduction of the arm additional to that occurring at the shoulder joint is achieved by rotation of the scapula so that the inferior angle is displaced forwards and the glenoid fossa is tilted upwards (**A**, **B**). This movement is produced by the combined actions of serratus anterior and trapezius (**495A2**, **495A4**). It should be noted that such abduction of

the arm by scapular rotation can take place in the absence of abduction at the shoulder joint. Thus, if the supraspinatus tendon is ruptured and the deltoid is consequently ineffectual (see above), abduction of the arm to the extent of about 60° may still be achieved (**C**).

Abduction of the arm in a coronal plane is similar in most respects to abduction in the scapular plane, involving the same muscles which produce abduction at the shoulder joint and rotation of the scapula on the chest wall. But in one respect the two movements are different. It has been seen that abduction in the scapular plane does not involve rotation of the humerus, but if abduction in the coronal plane is carried out with the elbow flexed and the forearm directed forwards it will be found that the movement is abruptly limited at about 110°. If the humerus is then laterally rotated so that the forearm, as a pointer, is directed vertically upwards, the abduction movement will continue fluently to 180°. The reason for this phenomenon is still not certain and the matter will not be discussed further here.

Adduction of the arm may occur either in the scapular or the coronal plane. The mechanism is simply the reverse of that involved in abduction. It is often a passive movement produced by the force of gravity. If it is an active movement, adduction of the shoulder joint is produced by pectoralis major, latissimus dorsi and the long head of triceps, while the inferior angle of the scapula is rotated backwards by pectoralis minor and rhomboid.

THE AXILLA

The axilla or armpit is a conical tissue-space situated between the lateral aspect of the chest wall medially, and the shoulder joint and the upper end of the humerus laterally (**D**). The long axis of the space extends obliquely, from below, upwards and medially.

The following general features of the axilla in **D** and in the horizontal section **E** should be noted.

1. The space has extensive anterior, medial and posterior walls and a narrow lateral wall (**E**).
2. The narrow uppermost part of the space, called the apex of the axilla (**D**) is bounded by three bones, namely, the upper border of the scapula, the outer border of the first rib and the posterior aspect of the

middle third of the clavicle. These bones form the upper limits of the posterior, middle and anterior axillary walls respectively.
3. Through its apex the axilla is continuous with the lower part of the neck and the region of the thoracic inlet (**D**).
4. The axilla becomes very narrow anteriorly and posteriorly as the anterior and posterior walls approach the medial wall (**D**).
5. The base of the axilla faces downwards and laterally and it is evident that its size varies with the degree of abduction of the arm (**D**).

ABDUCTION OF ARM IN SCAPULAR PLANE (Posterior view)

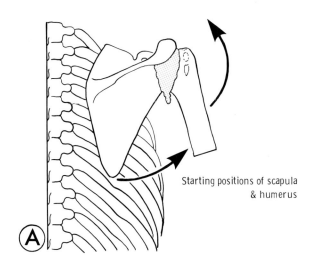

Starting positions of scapula & humerus

Ⓐ

ABDUCTION OF ARM IN SCAPULAR PLANE

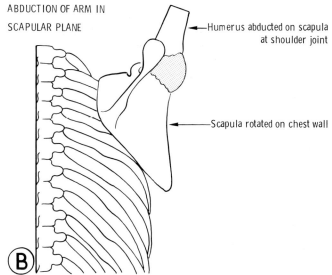

Humerus abducted on scapula at shoulder joint

Scapula rotated on chest wall

Ⓑ

ABDUCTION OF ARM IN SCAPULAR PLANE
(After rupture of supraspinatus tendon)

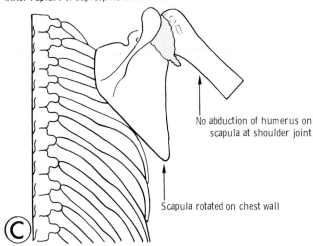

No abduction of humerus on scapula at shoulder joint

Scapula rotated on chest wall

Ⓒ

OUTLINE OF AXILLA

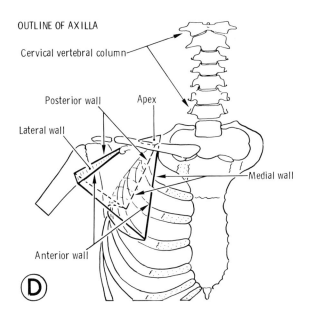

Cervical vertebral column

Posterior wall   Apex

Lateral wall

Medial wall

Anterior wall

Ⓓ

HORIZONTAL SECTION OF AXILLA

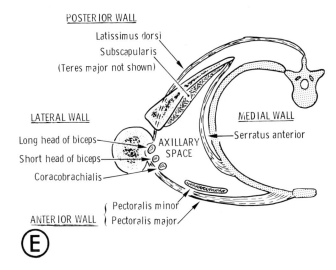

POSTERIOR WALL
Latissimus dorsi
Subscapularis
(Teres major not shown)

LATERAL WALL
Long head of biceps
Short head of biceps
Coracobrachialis

AXILLARY SPACE

MEDIAL WALL
Serratus anterior

ANTERIOR WALL
{ Pectoralis minor
{ Pectoralis major

Ⓔ

505

6. The axilla contains the neurovascular bundle of the upper limb and the axillary lymph nodes, embedded in abundant fatty areolar tissue.

The neurovascular bundle consists of the axillary artery and vein and the cords (**389**) and many of the branches of the brachial plexus, bound closely together by a downward extension of the fascial axillary sheath (**392**). In the axilla the bundle runs from the apex along the lateral wall, in close contact with the structures which form the convergent anterior and posterior walls.

The walls of the axilla

The medial wall is convex laterally and is formed by the outer surface of serratus anterior (**A**).

The posterior wall (**B**) consists of subscapularis, teres major and the tendon of latissimus dorsi, but on a more posterior plane it is contributed to by the long head of triceps and teres minor (**501A**).

The intermuscular cleft between subscapularis and teres minor above and teres major and latissimus dorsi below is limited laterally by the surgical neck of the humerus. The cleft is divided into two parts by the long head of triceps as that muscle passes between teres major and teres minor. The lateral part is the quadrangular space and the medial the triangular space. Learn their boundaries by study of **B**, in which the size of the spaces is exaggerated. These spaces allow the passage of certain vessels and nerves from the axilla through its posterior wall to the structures they supply.

The anterior wall is somewhat shorter than the posterior and consists of two layers. The deep layer is formed by subclavius, pectoralis minor and the clavipectoral fascia (**C**). Most of the vessels and nerves leaving the axilla through its anterior wall pass through this fascia. The superficial layer consists of pectoralis major and to a lesser extent the most anterior fibres of origin of deltoid (**D**).

The narrow lateral wall, as has been noted, lies between the convergent anterior and posterior walls. It is formed by the intertubercular sulcus of the humerus, coracobrachialis and both heads of biceps brachii (**B**).

The base of the axilla is formed by skin and the thick axillary fascia. At its margins this fascia becomes continuous with the deep fascia associated with the other four walls. When the upper limb is by the side, the axillary fascia is lax, and consequently the axillary contents are always palpated by the clinician with the limb in that position. Observe on your own body that, when the limb is abducted, the fascia becomes taut and concave, so that the lower margins of the muscular anterior and posterior axillary walls stand out as blunt ridges known as the anterior and posterior axillary folds (**E**). Vertical lines projected downwards from these folds are called anterior and posterior axillary lines, while a vertical line midway between these is known as the midaxillary line. These lines are used clinically in making the surface markings of certain structures in the thorax and upper abdomen.

AXILLA: MEDIAL WALL

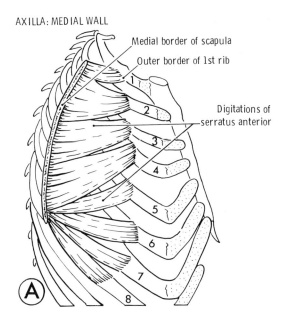

Medial border of scapula
Outer border of 1st rib
Digitations of serratus anterior

1
2
3
4
5
6
7
8

A

AXILLA: POSTERIOR & LATERAL WALLS (Viewed in posterolateral direction & spaces exaggerated)

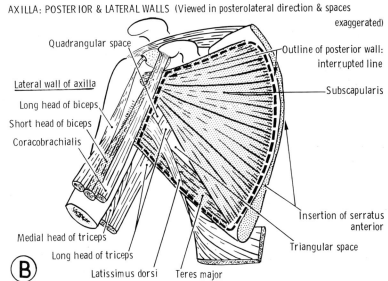

Quadrangular space
Outline of posterior wall: interrupted line
Subscapularis

Lateral wall of axilla
Long head of biceps
Short head of biceps
Coracobrachialis

Insertion of serratus anterior

Medial head of triceps
Long head of triceps
Triangular space
Latissimus dorsi
Teres major

B

AXILLA: DEEP LAYER OF ANTERIOR WALL

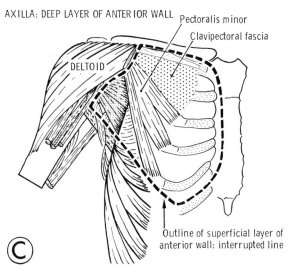

Pectoralis minor
Clavipectoral fascia
DELTOID

Outline of superficial layer of anterior wall: interrupted line

C

AXILLARY FOLDS

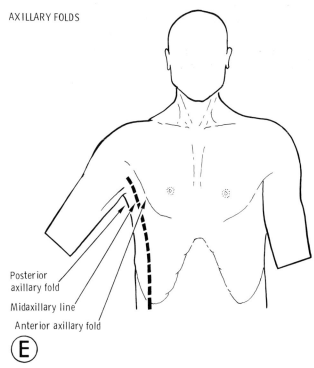

Posterior axillary fold
Midaxillary line
Anterior axillary fold

E

AXILLA: SUPERFICIAL LAYER OF ANTERIOR WALL (Outlined by interrupted line)

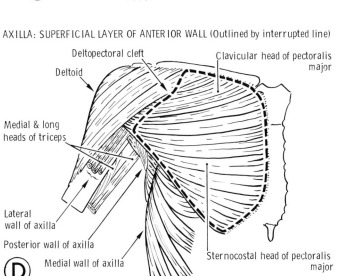

Deltopectoral cleft
Clavicular head of pectoralis major
Deltoid

Medial & long heads of triceps

Lateral wall of axilla
Posterior wall of axilla
Medial wall of axilla

Sternocostal head of pectoralis major

D

The blood vessels in the axilla

The axillary artery

This vessel is a direct continuation of the subclavian artery (**391A**) where it crosses the outer border of the first rib, which, it will be recalled, is one of the boundaries of the axillary apex (**A**). Visualise its relationship to the muscles and fascia of the anterior, posterior and lateral axillary walls (**A**). Its relationship to pectoralis minor is used to divide the artery into three parts lying above, behind and below the muscle. It gives off numerous branches, three of which are important. Two of these are associated with the anterior axillary wall and one with the posterior.

The thoraco-acromial artery arises from the second part and, curling round the medial border of pectoralis minor, pierces the clavipectoral fascia to be distributed to pectoralis major and deltoid (**A**). Its terminal twigs reach the superficial fascia of the anterior thoracic wall.

The lateral thoracic artery also arises from the second part of the axillary but curls downwards round the lateral border of pectoralis minor (**A**). It supplies branches to both pectoral muscles, and to the superficial fascia on the anterior thoracic wall, including the breast, and the upper part of the abdominal wall.

The subscapular artery is a large vessel arising from the third part of the axillary. It runs down the posterior axillary wall, along the cleft between subscapularis and teres major, and supplies large branches to the muscles on both aspects of the scapula.

These branches of the axillary artery are involved in anastomoses with other vessels in two main regions. These may be of importance in establishing a collateral circulation if blood flow through the distal part of the subclavian artery, or the proximal part of the axillary, is obstructed.

1. The scapular anastomosis is formed in the muscles around the scapula by the capillaries of the subscapular artery and the suprascapular and transverse cervical branches of the thyrocervical trunk (**C**) which, it will be recalled, arises from the first part of the subclavian artery in the root of the neck.
2. In the pectoral muscles and in the superficial fascia of the anterior chest wall, the thoraco-acromial and lateral thoracic arteries anastomose with perforating branches which spring from the internal thoracic branch of the first part of the subclavian artery (**A**) and run forwards through the anterior ends of the upper six intercostal spaces. All these vessels are larger in the female, particularly during and after pregnancy, because of the presence of the mammary gland within this area of superficial fascia.

The axillary vein

Note first that in the arm the brachial artery, the downward continuation of the axillary, is accompanied by venae comitantes (**A**), while two large veins extend upwards in the superficial fascia, the cephalic vein on the anterolateral aspect and the basilic vein on the anteromedial aspect (**B**). The upper part of the cephalic vein runs along the deltopectoral cleft and enters the axilla by piercing the clavipectoral fascia a short distance below the clavicle (**A**). The basilic vein pierces the deep fascia about halfway up the arm (**B**) and enters the lower part of the axilla in company with the brachial artery and its venae comitantes (**A**).

The axillary vein begins as a continuation of the basilic vein in front of the lower border of subscapularis (**A**) and runs through the axilla on the medial side of the axillary artery to the axillary apex, where it becomes the subclavian vein. It receives tributaries corresponding to the branches of the artery and the venae comitantes of the brachial artery which run for a short distance into the axilla. Near its termination it is joined by the cephalic vein.

The nerves in the axilla

Recall that the intercostobrachial nerve, which is the lateral cutaneous branch of the second intercostal nerve, emerges from the lateral part of the second intercostal space, and crosses the axilla to reach the skin on the medial side of the upper arm (**D**).

All the many other nerves associated with the axilla are parts or branches of the brachial plexus and it is consequently advisable to revise the general form of the plexus (**389**). The proximal or supraclavicular part of the plexus, that is the roots, trunks and divisions, lies in the posterior triangle of the neck and has been considered already (**401A**). The cords and most of the branches lie below the clavicle, in the axilla. Two branches of the supraclavicular part innervate axillary structures.

The long thoracic nerve (C5, 6, 7)

This nerve arises from the upper three roots of the plexus and descends behind the proximal part of the plexus and the axillary vessels to reach the medial axillary wall. It runs vertically downwards on that wall giving branches to each digitation of serratus anterior.

The suprascapular nerve (C5, 6)

This is a large branch of the upper trunk of the plexus which runs laterally across the posterior triangle of the neck above the rest of the plexus, so that it is the first element of the plexus seen by a surgeon approaching it from above (**D**). The nerve disappears deep to trapezius and passes through the suprascapular notch onto the posterior aspect of the scapula (**C**). From there it gives branches to supraspinatus, infraspinatus and the shoulder joint.

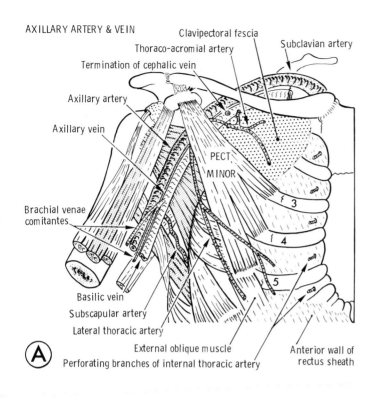

AXILLARY ARTERY & VEIN

- Clavipectoral fascia
- Thoraco-acromial artery
- Termination of cephalic vein
- Subclavian artery
- Axillary artery
- Axillary vein
- PECT. MINOR
- Brachial venae comitantes
- Basilic vein
- Subscapular artery
- Lateral thoracic artery
- External oblique muscle
- Perforating branches of internal thoracic artery
- Anterior wall of rectus sheath

Ⓐ

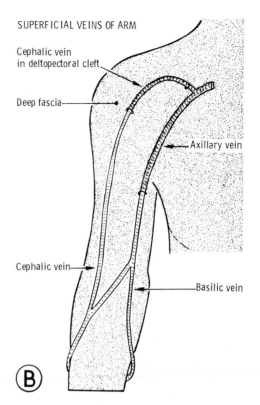

SUPERFICIAL VEINS OF ARM

- Cephalic vein in deltopectoral cleft
- Deep fascia
- Axillary vein
- Cephalic vein
- Basilic vein

Ⓑ

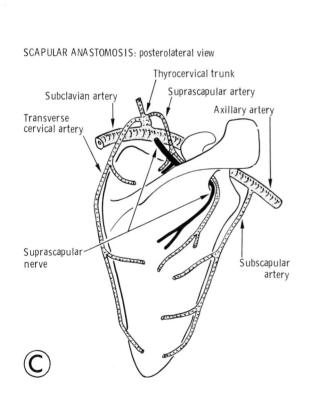

SCAPULAR ANASTOMOSIS: posterolateral view

- Thyrocervical trunk
- Suprascapular artery
- Subclavian artery
- Axillary artery
- Transverse cervical artery
- Suprascapular nerve
- Subscapular artery

Ⓒ

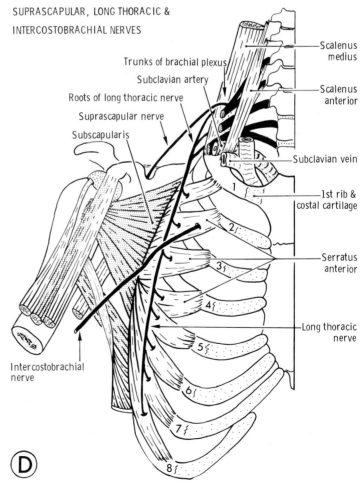

SUPRASCAPULAR, LONG THORACIC & INTERCOSTOBRACHIAL NERVES

- Trunks of brachial plexus
- Subclavian artery
- Roots of long thoracic nerve
- Suprascapular nerve
- Subscapularis
- Scalenus medius
- Scalenus anterior
- Subclavian vein
- 1st rib & costal cartilage
- Serratus anterior
- Long thoracic nerve
- Intercostobrachial nerve

Ⓓ

The cords of the brachial plexus

These lie in the upper half of the axilla in close association with its lateral wall. Near the apex, the lateral and posterior cords are above and lateral to the first part of the axillary artery and the medial cord behind it (**A**). These relationships gradually change as the structures pass laterally and downwards behind the clavipectoral fascia, until behind pectoralis minor the relations of the three cords to the artery are those indicated by their names. The posterior cord is between the artery and subscapularis, the lateral cord between the artery and the coracoid process and the medial cord between the artery and the axillary vein. At or about the lateral border of pectoralis minor, the cords end by dividing into terminal branches.

It can be observed from their mode of formation (**389C**) that the lateral cord contains fibres from C5, 6 and 7, the posterior cord fibres from C5, 6, 7, 8 and T1 and the medial cord fibres from C8 and T1. It must, however, be appreciated that all the branches of a cord do not necessarily contain fibres from all the available segments.

The lateral pectoral nerve (C5, 6, 7)

This arises from the lateral cord just beyond its commencement, and passes forwards through the clavipectoral fascia to reach and supply the upper part of pectoralis major (**A**).

The musculocutaneous nerve (C5, 6, 7)

This is one terminal branch of the lateral cord. At first it is situated between the lateral wall of the axilla and the axillary artery (**A**). It leaves the axilla by passing downwards and laterally through the substance of coracobrachialis which it supplies.

The medial pectoral nerve (C8, T1)

This nerve takes origin from the proximal part of the medial cord and passes forwards between the axillary artery and vein into pectoralis minor which it supplies. Many of its branches continue through that muscle and supply the lower part of pectoralis major.

The medial cutaneous nerve of the arm (T1)

Arises near the end of the medial cord. It runs downwards and laterally in front of the axillary vein and in the lower part of the axilla forms a loop with the intercostobrachial nerve (**A**). From this loop fine branches pierce the deep fascia and supply the skin of the base of the axilla and the medial aspect of the arm nearly as far as the elbow (**D**).

The medial cutaneous nerve of the forearm (C8, T1)

Arises distal to the previous nerve from the medial cord and runs through the lower part of the axilla between the axillary artery and vein (**A**).

The ulnar nerve (C8, T1)

This large and important nerve arises from the medial cord close to the previous branch and follows it into the arm.

The median nerve (C6, 7, 8 and T1)

This large nerve is formed on the lateral aspect of the axillary artery, in the lower part of the axilla, by the union of two branches of the brachial plexus.

The lateral root (C6, 7) is a terminal branch of the lateral cord which continues in the line of that cord between the axillary artery and the musculocutaneous nerve (**A**).

The medial root (C8, T1) is a terminal branch of the medial cord. From its origin on the medial side of the axillary artery, it crosses obliquely in front of that vessel to its lateral side, where it joins the lateral root to form the definitive median nerve. This nerve then passes distally into the arm lying between the axillary artery and the coracobrachialis.

The upper subscapular (C5, 6), thoracodorsal (C6, 7, 8) and lower subscapular (C5, 6) nerves

These three nerves arise in that order from the posterior cord as it lies between the axillary artery and subscapularis. They run downwards on the posterior wall of the axilla (**B**). The subscapular nerves supply subscapularis and teres major, while the thoracodorsal nerve supplies the whole of latissimus dorsi.

The axillary (circumflex) nerve (C5, 6)

One of the terminal branches of the posterior cord, this nerve initially continues in the line of the posterior cord lying on subscapularis and behind the axillary artery and the radial nerve. It then turns backwards through the quadrangular space in the posterior wall of the axilla, the postion and boundaries of which should be revised (**B**). Just beyond the space the nerve divides into anterior and posterior branches (**C**). The anterior branch winds round the posterior and lateral aspects of the surgical neck of the humerus. It lies on the deep surface of deltoid and supplies that muscle. The posterior branch supplies teres minor and, piercing the deep fascia at the posterior border of deltoid, sweeps forwards across that muscle as *the upper lateral cutaneous nerve of the arm* (**511C**). This innervates an area of

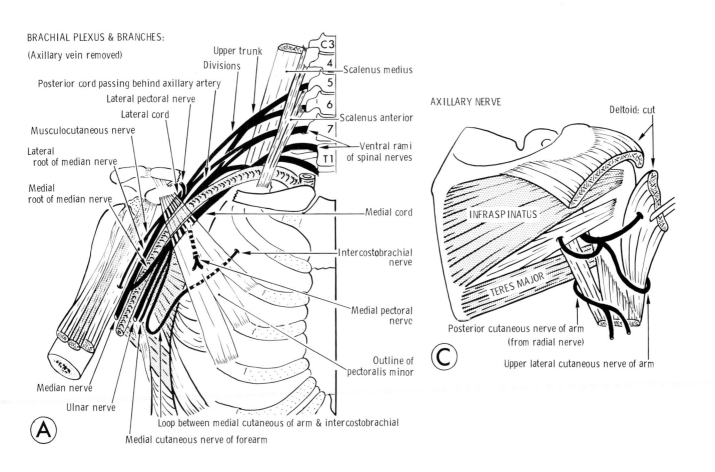

BRACHIAL PLEXUS & BRANCHES:
(Axillary vein removed)

Upper trunk

Divisions

Posterior cord passing behind axillary artery

Lateral pectoral nerve

Lateral cord

Musculocutaneous nerve

Lateral root of median nerve

Medial root of median nerve

C3

4 — Scalenus medius

5

6 — Scalenus anterior

7

T1 — Ventral rami of spinal nerves

Medial cord

Intercostobrachial nerve

Medial pectoral nerve

Outline of pectoralis minor

Median nerve

Ulnar nerve

Loop between medial cutaneous of arm & intercostobrachial

Medial cutaneous nerve of forearm

(A)

AXILLARY NERVE

Deltoid: cut

INFRASPINATUS

TERES MAJOR

Posterior cutaneous nerve of arm (from radial nerve)

Upper lateral cutaneous nerve of arm

(C)

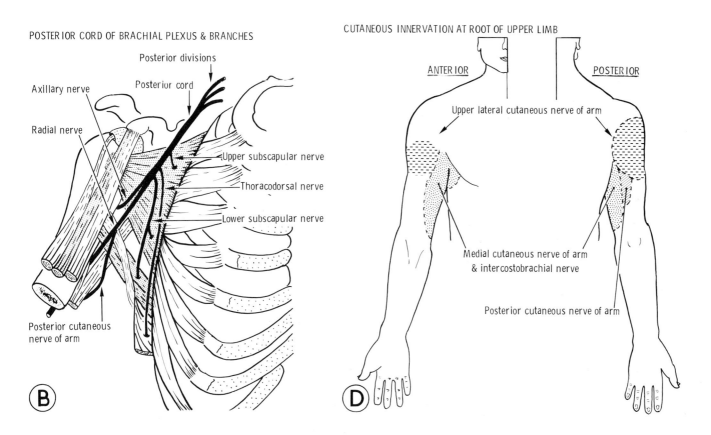

POSTERIOR CORD OF BRACHIAL PLEXUS & BRANCHES

Posterior divisions

Posterior cord

Axillary nerve

Radial nerve

Upper subscapular nerve

Thoracodorsal nerve

Lower subscapular nerve

Posterior cutaneous nerve of arm

(B)

CUTANEOUS INNERVATION AT ROOT OF UPPER LIMB

ANTERIOR   POSTERIOR

Upper lateral cutaneous nerve of arm

Medial cutaneous nerve of arm & intercostobrachial nerve

Posterior cutaneous nerve of arm

(D)

skin over the lower half of deltoid (**511D**). Note that the skin over the upper half of deltoid is innervated by C4 fibres through the lateral supraclavicular nerve, which is a branch of the cervical plexus.

The axillary nerve is prone to injury in the region of the quadrangular space when the head of the humerus is forced through the inferior part of the capsule of the shoulder joint, in dislocations produced by abduction of the upper limb (**570**). The clinical results of such an injury are paralysis of the deltoid and skin anaesthesia over its lower part.

The radial nerve (C5, 6, 7, 8, T1)

This is the continuation of the posterior cord beyond the origin of the axillary nerve. In the axilla it is placed behind the axillary artery and in front of the axillary nerve, teres major and latissimus dorsi (**511B**). Leaving the axilla at the lower border of teres major, it inclines downwards and backwards through the interval between the long and medial heads of triceps, and comes to lie on the oblique groove already noted (**497B**) on the back of the humerus.

Although the majority of the branches of this long nerve arise in the arm and forearm its first branch is given off in the axilla.

The posterior cutaneous nerve of the arm winds backwards round the medial side of the long head of triceps to supply a small skin area on the posterior aspect of the arm at the level of the insertion of deltoid (**511D**).

The axillary lymph nodes

A large number of lymph nodes lie amongst the fatty areolar tissue in the axilla (**A**). They receive lymph from the whole of the upper limb, and from the skin and superficial fascia of all aspects of the trunk from the level of the clavicle to that of the umbilicus. The latter level is a lymphatic watershed, for the superficial vessels below it drain downwards to the inguinal nodes in the proximal part of the lower limb.

It is convenient to divide the axillary nodes into groups according to their position.

1. The pectoral group lie on the anterior axillary wall along the course of the lateral thoracic vessels. Their afferents sweep round the lower border of pectoralis major from the skin and superficial fascia on the anterior aspect of the trunk including the mammary gland.
2. The subscapular group are situated on the posterior axillary wall along the course of the subscapular vessels. Their afferents curl round the lateral border of latissimus dorsi from the skin and superficial fascia on the posterior aspect of the trunk.

3. The lateral group are placed on the lateral wall of the axilla along the course of the axillary vessels. They receive all the lymph vessels from the upper limb except a few which accompany the terminal part of the cephalic vein.
4. The central group lie in the central part of the axilla and receive afferents from the three preceding groups.
5. The infraclavicular nodes are not, strictly speaking, in the axilla, but it is nevertheless convenient to consider them with the axillary nodes. They lie in the upper part of the deltopectoral cleft, close to the terminal part of the cephalic vein and superficial to the clavipectoral fascia. Their afferents are derived from the upper limb and from the upper part of the anterior chest wall, including the upper part of the mammary gland.
6. The apical group are situated near the apex of the axilla around the uppermost parts of the axillary vessels. They receive afferents from the pectoral, subscapular and lateral axillary nodes, either directly or through the central group, and from the infraclavicular group through the clavipectoral fascia.

The apical axillary nodes drain into the subclavian trunk, which opens into the venous blood stream in the angle between the subclavian and internal jugular veins either directly or through the thoracic duct (on the left side) or right lymphatic trunk (on the right side).

Palpation of the shoulder and axilla

A number of bony features can be palpated in these regions (**B, C**).

1. The clavicle and the acromion process and crest of the spine of the scapula are readily palpable through the skin.
2. The lower parts of the medial and lateral borders of the scapula and the inferior angle of the bone are less easily felt through the muscles which overlie them.
3. Through the upper part of the thick deltoid, when it is relaxed, the greater and lesser tubercles of the humerus and the tip of the coracoid process of the scapula can be located but not clearly delineated. Examine these features on your own body and note that the lesser tubercle and the coracoid process, which are both directed forwards, can be differentiated in cases of doubt by the fact that the tubercle moves when the humerus is rotated whereas the coracoid process remains stationary.
4. As has been noted the contents of the axilla, such as the lymph nodes, are examined clinically when the arm is by the side, because with the limb in that position the axillary fascia is lax.

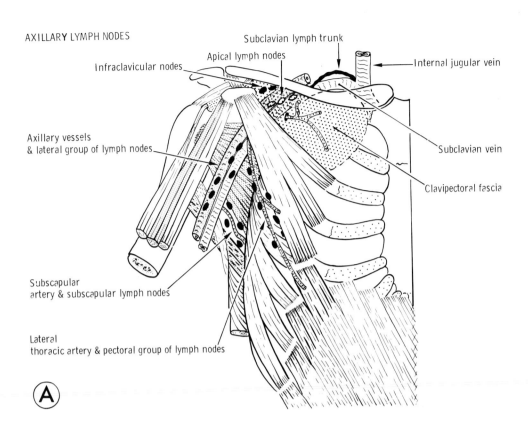

AXILLARY LYMPH NODES

Infraclavicular nodes

Apical lymph nodes

Subclavian lymph trunk

Internal jugular vein

Axillary vessels
& lateral group of lymph nodes

Subclavian vein

Clavipectoral fascia

Subscapular
artery & subscapular lymph nodes

Lateral
thoracic artery & pectoral group of lymph nodes

(A)

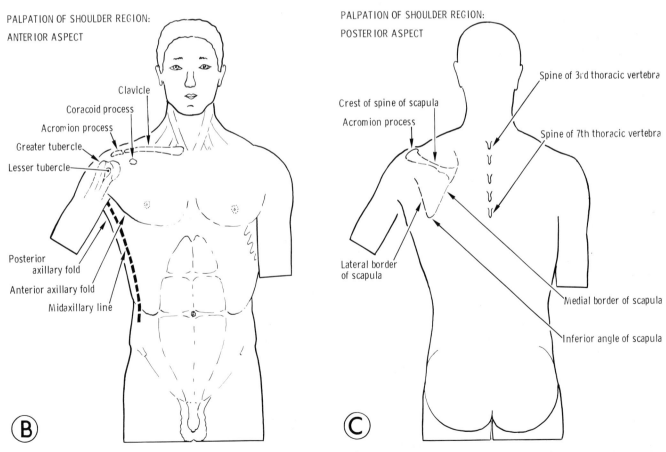

PALPATION OF SHOULDER REGION:
ANTERIOR ASPECT

Clavicle

Coracoid process

Acromion process

Greater tubercle

Lesser tubercle

Posterior
axillary fold

Anterior axillary fold

Midaxillary line

(B)

PALPATION OF SHOULDER REGION:
POSTERIOR ASPECT

Spine of 3rd thoracic vertebra

Crest of spine of scapula

Acromion process

Spine of 7th thoracic vertebra

Lateral border
of scapula

Medial border of scapula

Inferior angle of scapula

(C)

THE BREAST (MAMMARY GLAND)

Consideration of the breast has been delayed until this time because its lymphatic drainage, which is one of its most important features for the clinician, passes predominantly to the axillary nodes.

In the male the glands are rudimentary throughout life. In the female they become apparent at puberty and undergo further development in the later months of pregnancy and during lactation.

The glandular tissue of the adult female breast (**A**) is embedded in the superficial fascia, where it is intermingled with adipose and fibrous tissue. Particularly in the upper part of the breast, many of the fibrous septa reach the skin and constitute suspensory ligaments. The twenty or so lactiferous ducts open through separate minute orifices on the summit of the nipple, a cylindrical prominence projecting from a little below the centre of the anterior surface of the breast. The nipple is surrounded by the areola, a circular zone of skin which is pink in nulliparous women, but becomes pigmented during pregnancy and retains this darker colour thereafter.

The base of the gland extends from the second to the sixth rib in the lateral plane (**217D**). At the level of the fourth costal cartilage its medial part reaches the lateral margin of the sternum while its lateral part curls round the lateral margin of pectoralis major onto the axillary fascia as far as the midaxillary line (the axillary tail of the breast). The base thus rests on the deep fascia covering pectoralis major, part of serratus anterior, part of the axillary fascia and the uppermost part of the anterior wall of the sheath of the rectus abdominis muscle. Between the base of the breast and these areas of deep fascia, is a zone of loose areolar tissue which is sometimes described as the retro-mammary space.

In clinical examination of the breast radiographs of the region are sometimes taken using very low-dose X-rays. These are known as mammograms (**B**). They give an indication of the outline of the glandular tissue and blood vessels, and may disclose distortion of the normal pattern by disease processes, especially carcinoma.

The blood supply of the female breast is derived from the perforating branches of the internal thoracic artery, the pectoral branches of the thoraco-acromial artery, and the lateral thoracic artery (**C**). The venous drainage is through the corresponding veins and is of importance since malignant disease of the breast often spreads along these vessels.

The lymphatic drainage is of paramount importance in a consideration of the breast because it is through lymphatic vessels that most of the spread from a primary malignant focus in that structure occurs. The lymph vessels originate in the fibrous septa which penetrate amongst the lobules of glandular tissue and the lactiferous ducts. The vessels normally pass in a number of directions to different groups of lymph nodes (**D**).

1. The major route, constituting about 75% of the total lymph drainage, is laterally. The vessels turn round the lateral border of the pectoralis major in the axillary tail of the breast and pierce the axillary fascia to reach the pectoral group of the axillary nodes. The route continues beyond these nodes to the central and lateral axillary nodes and eventually to the apical group and the subclavian trunk. Despite previous teaching it is now appreciated that, before reaching the axilla, these vessels run in the breast tissue itself and not in the deep fascia on the muscles underlying it.
2. From the medial part of the breast, vessels pierce the pectoralis major and follow the perforating branches of the internal thoracic artery to the parasternal chain of nodes which drain upwards into the broncho-mediastinal trunk.
3. From the upper part of the gland a few vessels pass to the infraclavicular nodes, whose efferents pass through the apical axillary nodes to the subclavian trunk.
4. Lymph vessels from the lower part of the gland pass over the costal margin and, after piercing the anterior wall of the rectus sheath, communicate with intra-abdominal lymph vessels.
5. Although the above are the normal routes of lymphatic drainage of the breast, their vessels anastomose with vessels in neighbouring areas, and if the nodes on these primary routes become blocked by metastasising malignant cells the lymph from the breast may be diverted through these anastomoses. Spread may then occur in neighbouring areas such as the opposite breast, through vessels which cross the midline in front of the sternum, or in the upper abdomen by retrograde spread along the parasternal chain and diaphragmatic lymph nodes (**305A**).

THE BREAST

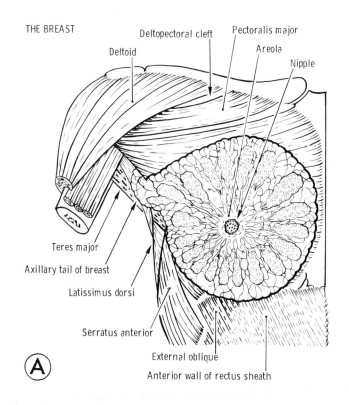

Deltoid
Deltopectoral cleft
Pectoralis major
Areola
Nipple
Teres major
Axillary tail of breast
Latissimus dorsi
Serratus anterior
External oblique
Anterior wall of rectus sheath

(A)

MAMMOGRAM

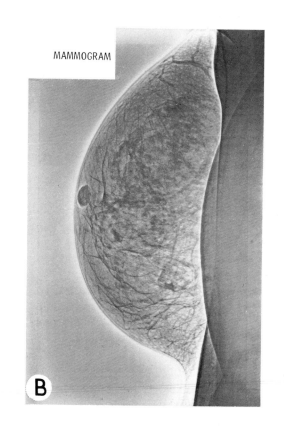

(B)

THE BREAST: BLOOD SUPPLY

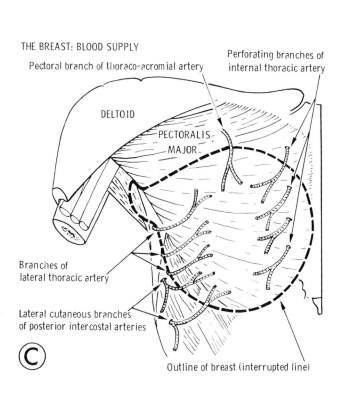

Pectoral branch of thoraco-acromial artery
Perforating branches of internal thoracic artery
DELTOID
PECTORALIS MAJOR
Branches of lateral thoracic artery
Lateral cutaneous branches of posterior intercostal arteries
Outline of breast (interrupted line)

(C)

THE BREAST: LYMPHATIC DRAINAGE

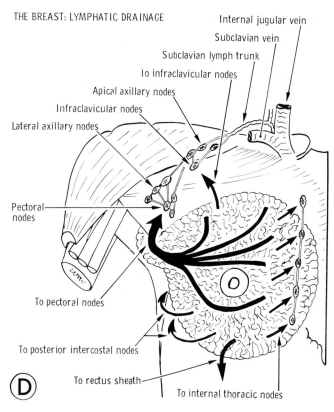

Internal jugular vein
Subclavian vein
Subclavian lymph trunk
To infraclavicular nodes
Apical axillary nodes
Infraclavicular nodes
Lateral axillary nodes
Pectoral nodes
To pectoral nodes
To posterior intercostal nodes
To rectus sheath
To internal thoracic nodes

(D)

THE ARM AND FOREARM

The bones and joints

The distal half of the humerus

1. The distal half of the shaft of the humerus is triangular in cross section with anteromedial, anterolateral and posterior surfaces (**C**). The anterior border is rounded. The medial and lateral borders are sharp ridges known as the medial and lateral supracondylar ridges (**A, B, C**). They become indistinct in the upper half of the bone.
2. The distal end of the bone is expanded transversely. Note the terminations of the medial supracondylar ridge in the large non-articular medial epicondyle, and the lateral supracondylar ridge in the much smaller non-articular lateral epicondyle (**A, B**).
3. Observe that the continuous distal articular surface is divided by a groove into the trochlea medially and the smaller capitulum laterally (**A**). The pulley-shaped trochlea extends over the anterior, distal, and posterior aspects of the bone, and is related above to the coronoid fossa on the anterior aspect of the shaft and the olecranon fossa on the posterior aspect (**A, B**). The medial lip of the surface is much more prominent than the lateral. The capitulum is part of a sphere and is confined to the anterior and distal aspects of the bone. It is related above to the shallow radial fossa on the anterior aspect of humerus (**A**).
4. When the lower end of the humerus is in the coronal plane the head of the humerus faces medially and backwards so that the shaft of the bone can be regarded as being twisted.

The radius

The radius is the lateral bone of the forearm. Observe its several parts in **D, E**.

1. The head is anular, with a gently concave proximal surface and a circular peripheral surface, both entirely covered by a continuous layer of articular cartilage.
2. The tuberosity is large and prominent and projects from the medial aspect of the shaft just below the neck.
3. The shaft below the tuberosity is gently bowed laterally. It has anterior, posterior and interosseous borders which are separated by anterior, posterior and lateral surfaces. In its lower half the shaft is distinctly triangular in cross section (**F**) and the lateral surface is confined to the lateral aspect (**D, E, F**). In its upper half the anterior and posterior borders sweep upwards and medially across the corresponding aspects of the bone to join the interosseous border below the tuberosity. As a result, the anterior and posterior surfaces become progressively narrower while the lateral surface expands into a triangular area covering the anterior, lateral and posterior aspects of the shaft (**D, E, F**).
4. The distal end of the radius is wider than the shaft and quadrangular in cross section owing to the expansion of the interosseous border into an additional medial surface called the ulnar notch (**E, F**). This is concave from before backwards and is covered by articular cartilage. The lateral part of the bone is continued below the level of the rest of the lower end as the styloid process (**D, E**). The anterior surface is smooth and featureless (**D**), whereas the posterior surface is marked by a number of longitudinal elevations and grooves (**E**). The most prominent of these are the dorsal tubercle which is easily palpable in the living subject and the narrow groove which lies to its medial side. The distal surface is smooth and quadrangular (**519D**). It is covered by articular cartilage which extends over the medial surface of the styloid process but is separated from that lining the ulnar notch by a narrow non-articular strip of bone.

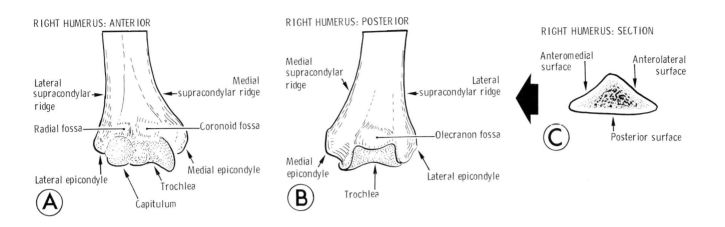

RIGHT HUMERUS: ANTERIOR

Lateral supracondylar ridge
Medial supracondylar ridge
Radial fossa
Coronoid fossa
Lateral epicondyle
Medial epicondyle
Trochlea
Capitulum

A

RIGHT HUMERUS: POSTERIOR

Medial supracondylar ridge
Lateral supracondylar ridge
Olecranon fossa
Medial epicondyle
Lateral epicondyle
Trochlea

B

RIGHT HUMERUS: SECTION

Anteromedial surface
Anterolateral surface
Posterior surface

C

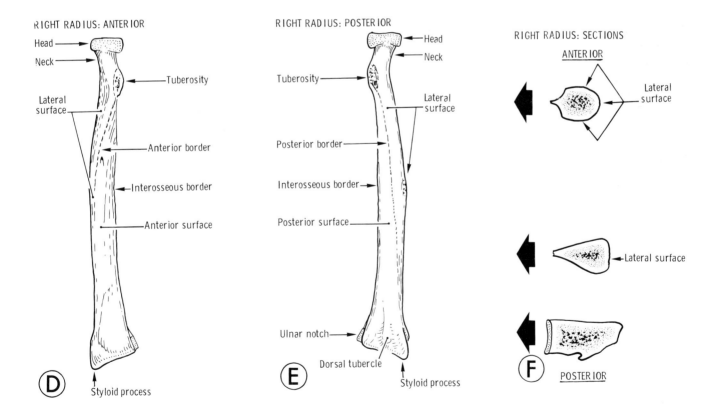

RIGHT RADIUS: ANTERIOR

Head
Neck
Tuberosity
Lateral surface
Anterior border
Interosseous border
Anterior surface
Styloid process

D

RIGHT RADIUS: POSTERIOR

Head
Neck
Tuberosity
Lateral surface
Posterior border
Interosseous border
Posterior surface
Ulnar notch
Dorsal tubercle
Styloid process

E

RIGHT RADIUS: SECTIONS

ANTERIOR

Lateral surface

Lateral surface

POSTERIOR

F

517

The ulna

The ulna is the medial of the forearm bones. It consists of an expanded proximal part, a shaft which narrows in a proximo-distal direction, and a slightly expanded distal part. Observe the features of the bone in **A, B, C**.

1. The proximal part of the ulna consists of two bony projections. The massive olecranon process extends proximally in line with the shaft and is bent slightly forwards at its free end; it has a proximal surface of appreciable size. The smaller beak-like coronoid process projects forwards just below the olecranon and presents a rough triangular anterior surface.
2. The pulley-shaped trochlear notch is formed by the anterior aspect of the olecranon and the proximal surface of the coronoid processes, and is lined by articular cartilage.
3. This cartilage is continuous onto an oval concave impression on the lateral aspect of the coronoid process (**C**) called the radial notch.
4. The central part of the shaft is triangular in section exhibiting a sharp interosseous (lateral) border and rounded anterior and posterior borders separated by anterior, medial, and posterior surfaces.
5. Observe the extensions of these borders and surfaces onto the proximal end of the bone. The interosseous border divides into two ridges which bound the shallow triangular supinator fossa. This is limited above by the radial notch (**C**). The anterior border blends with the medial edge of the coronoid process. The posterior border expands into a long triangular surface which extends to the upper end of the olecranon. This is a subcutaneous bone surface which can be readily felt through the skin (**B**). The anterior surface ends as the lower limit of the coronoid process (**A**), the medial surface extends proximally over the medial aspects of the coronoid and olecranon processes (**A, B**), and the posterior surface extends behind the supinator fossa onto the posterolateral aspect of the olecranon (**B, C**).
6. Traced downwards, the borders and surfaces become indistinct in the lower quarter of the shaft which is approximately circular in cross section.
7. The distal end of the ulna consists of the head and the styloid process. The head has a distal surface which is covered by cartilage (**D**) and a peripheral surface which is cartilage covered on its lateral and anterior aspects (**A, C**). Note that the heads of the radius and ulna are at the opposite ends of these two bones. The styloid process projects distally from the posteromedial aspect of the head (**B**) and is separated from it by a longitudinal groove posteriorly and a rough pit distally (**D**). Palpate the styloid processes of the radius and ulna on your own limb and note that

the radial process extends further distally than the ulnar. This relationship may be disturbed in fractures of the lower end of the radius with impaction of the fragments (Colles fracture).

Ossification of the humerus, radius and ulna

1. Ossification of the proximal end of the humerus has been considered earlier (**496**). It should be revised now in **E**.
2. Ossification of the lower end of the humerus occurs in a cartilaginous epiphysis which at birth includes both epicondyles, the trochlea and the capitulum (**F**). During childhood, however, a spicule of diaphyseal bone extends downwards and separates the cartilaginous medial epicondyle from the rest of the epiphysis (**G**). Separate secondary centres appear in the capitulum and lateral part of the trochlea at 1 year, in the medial part of the trochlea at 9 and in the lateral epicondyle at 12 (**G**). These coalesce at puberty and unite with the shaft at the comparatively early age of about 15. Another secondary centre appears in the medial epicondyle at 5 years but this does not unite with the shaft until about 20 (**G**). Thus in adolescence it is not unusual, in a radiograph of the elbow, to see the medial epicondyle separate from the shaft although the rest of the lower end and shaft have consolidated. This appearance must not be mistaken for a fracture.
3. The positions of proximal and distal growth plates in the developing radius are shown in **H**. The proximal epiphysis, which is practically coextensive with the head of the bone, is ossified from a single secondary centre which appears at 5 years and joins the shaft at about 15. The distal epiphysis, which includes the styloid process, the dorsal tubercle and the ulnar notch, is ossified from a secondary centre which forms at 1 year and unites with the shaft at about 18. A traction epiphysis is often associated with the radial tuberosity.
4. The growth plates of the ulna are shown in **J**. The proximal epiphysis, which is no more than a thin flake on the upper surface of the olecranon, begins to ossify at about 10 years and unites with the shaft at about 15. In the distal epiphysis, ossification starts at 5 years and fusion of diaphysis and epiphysis occurs at about 18.
5. In each of the bones considered above, the rate of longitudinal bone growth is about four times greater at the growth plates distant from the elbow than at the plates near the elbow. This is in contrast to the conditions in the lower limb where the greatest growth rates occur in the growth plates near the knee joint.

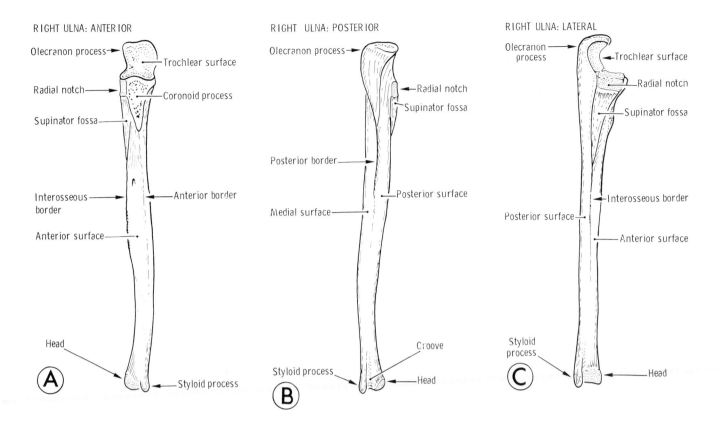

RIGHT ULNA: ANTERIOR

Olecranon process
Trochlear surface
Radial notch
Coronoid process
Supinator fossa
Interosseous border
Anterior border
Anterior surface
Head
Styloid process

A

RIGHT ULNA: POSTERIOR

Olecranon process
Radial notch
Supinator fossa
Posterior border
Posterior surface
Medial surface
Groove
Styloid process
Head

B

RIGHT ULNA: LATERAL

Olecranon process
Trochlear surface
Radial notch
Supinator fossa
Interosseous border
Posterior surface
Anterior surface
Styloid process
Head

C

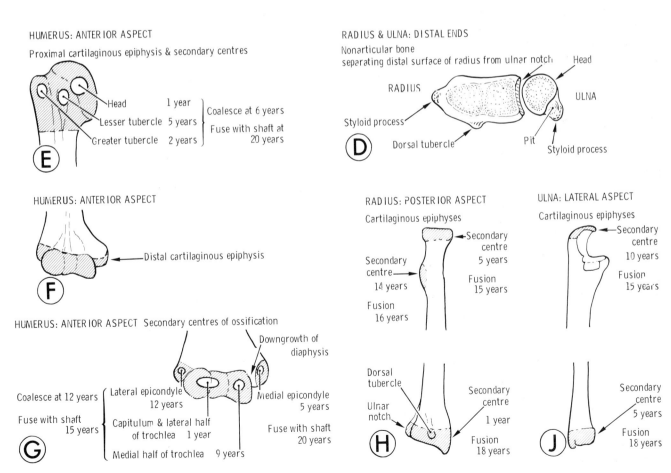

HUMERUS: ANTERIOR ASPECT

Proximal cartilaginous epiphysis & secondary centres

Head   1 year
Lesser tubercle 5 years   Coalesce at 6 years
Greater tubercle 2 years   Fuse with shaft at 20 years

E

RADIUS & ULNA: DISTAL ENDS

Nonarticular bone separating distal surface of radius from ulnar notch
Head
RADIUS
ULNA
Styloid process
Dorsal tubercle
Pit
Styloid process

D

HUMERUS: ANTERIOR ASPECT

Distal cartilaginous epiphysis

F

HUMERUS: ANTERIOR ASPECT   Secondary centres of ossification

Downgrowth of diaphysis
Coalesce at 12 years   Lateral epicondyle 12 years   Medial epicondyle 5 years
Fuse with shaft 15 years Capitulum & lateral half of trochlea 1 year
                          Medial half of trochlea 9 years   Fuse with shaft 20 years

G

RADIUS: POSTERIOR ASPECT

Cartilaginous epiphyses

Secondary centre 5 years
Secondary centre 14 years
Fusion 15 years
Fusion 16 years

Dorsal tubercle
Ulnar notch
Secondary centre 1 year
Fusion 18 years

H

ULNA: LATERAL ASPECT

Cartilaginous epiphyses

Secondary centre 10 years
Fusion 15 years

Secondary centre 5 years
Fusion 18 years

J

Moreover union of diaphysis and epiphyses occurs at about 15 years in the growth plates near the elbow whereas in those distant from the elbow fusion is delayed until 18 to 20 years.

6. The elongation of the forearm bones deserves special consideration. It is evident that, whereas the proximal growth plate of the radius contributes to the elongation of the radial shaft between the elbow and wrist, the proximal plate of the ulna is so placed that it cannot contribute to the elongation of that bone between the same levels. Consequently there is a gradual change in the relationship of the ulnar and radial diaphyses during the growth period.

The radio-ulnar joints

The superior radio-ulnar joint is a synovial joint of pivot type (**A, B, C, D**) whose synovial cavity is directly continuous proximally with that of the elbow joint.

The cartilage-covered peripheral surface of the head of the radius forms one articular surface. The other, which surrounds it, is formed in part by the cartilage lining the radial notch on the ulna and in part by the deep surface of the band-like anular ligament, which is attached to the anterior and posterior margins of the notch (**C**).

Synovial membrane extends downwards for a short distance from the lower margin of this outer articular surface and is then reflected upwards over the neck of the radius to the margin of the inner articular surface (**A, D**). It is supported only by loose areolar tissue because any more inextensible tissue would restrict rotation of the head of the radius within its osteoligamentous ring (see below).

The radio-ulnar interosseous membrane is a sheet of collagenous fibres which extends between the interosseous borders of the forearm bones (**A, B**). In general its fibres are directed distally and medially from radius to ulna. Below, the membrane reaches the upper limits of the ulnar notch on the radius and the lateral aspect of the head of the ulna (see below). Above, the membrane has a free margin which passes between the lower limit of the radial tuberosity and the lower angle of the supinator fossa on the ulna. At these points the interosseous borders of both bones end as distinct features (**A**).

The membrane is regarded by some as constituting a syndesmosis and may be called the middle radio-ulnar joint.

The inferior radio-ulnar joint involves a flat triangular plate of fibrocartilage, which has an apical attachment to the pit between the distal surface of the head of the ulna and the ulnar styloid, and a basal attachment to the non-articular strip of bone which separates the cartilage-covered distal surface of the radius and the ulnar notch (**A, F**).

In a coronal section along the long axis of the forearm bones, the cavity of the synovial inferior radio-ulnar joint is L-shaped (**E**). One articular surface consists of the cartilage which covers the distal anterior and lateral aspects of the head of the ulna (**A, F**). The other is formed by the cartilage lining the ulnar notch on the radius, and the upper surface of the triangular fibrocartilage. The joint cavity is enclosed by a fibrous capsule attached to the margins of the articular surfaces including the fibrocartilage.

Radio-ulnar movements

In the forearm the radius may be displaced in relation to the ulna and it is evident that such displacements necessarily involve simultaneous movements at both proximal and distal radio-ulnar joints about a common axis of rotation. This axis extends through the centre of the head of the radius and the attachment of the triangular fibrocartilage to the distal end of the ulna (**A, B**). Movements at the proximal joint are simple rotations of the radial head within the circle formed by the radial notch and the anular ligament. In those at the distal joint the ulnar notch on the radius moves medially or laterally around the facet on the anterolateral aspect of the peripheral surface of the head of the ulna, while the triangular fibrocartilage glides correspondingly on the facet on the distal surface of the ulna (**F**). Because, as will be seen below (**539F**), the proximal bones of the hand (the carpal bones) articulate with the distal surfaces of the radius and the triangular fibrocartilage, the hand moves with the radius in radio-ulnar displacements.

Observe in your own limb as it hangs vertically downwards, that radio-ulnar movement in one direction carries the distal end of the radius plus the hand across the anterior aspect of the distal end of the ulna to its medial side so that the palm of the hand faces backwards. The head of the radius remains on the lateral side of the ulna (**B, F**). This movement is described as pronation. Movement in the opposite direction carries the distal end of the radius plus the hand to the lateral side of the ulna and turns the palm of the hand forwards. The head of the radius again remains lateral to the ulna (**A, F**). This movement is called supination.

When the elbow is flexed, rotation of the hand is due entirely to radio-ulnar movements and the range between full pronation and full supination is about 140° (**F**). When the elbow is extended, a considerably greater rotation of the hand becomes possible when radio-ulnar movements are combined with appropriate rotations of the humerus at the shoulder joint.

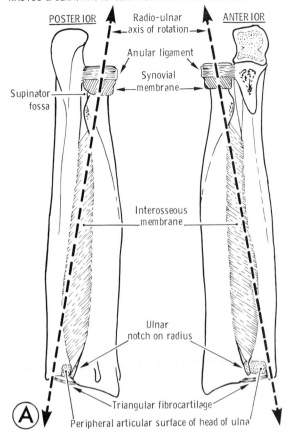

POSTERIOR

Radio-ulnar axis of rotation

ANTERIOR

Anular ligament

Synovial membrane

Supinator fossa

Interosseous membrane

Ulnar notch on radius

Triangular fibrocartilage

Peripheral articular surface of head of ulna

(A)

RADIUS & ULNA:
RADIO-ULNAR JOINTS IN PRONATION

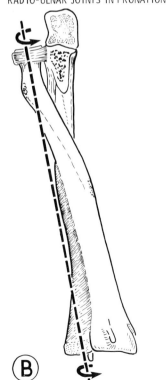

(B)

SUPERIOR RADIO-ULNAR JOINT Transverse section: superior view

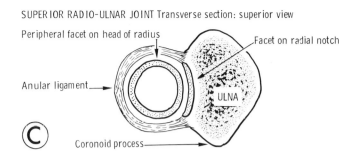

Peripheral facet on head of radius

Facet on radial notch

Anular ligament

ULNA

Coronoid process

(C)

SUPERIOR RADIO-ULNAR JOINT Coronal section: anterior view

Capitular articular facet

Trochlear articular facet

Anular ligament

Facet on radial notch

Peripheral facet on head of radius

Synovial membrane

RADIUS

ULNA

(D)

INFERIOR RADIO-ULNAR JOINT Coronal section: anterior view

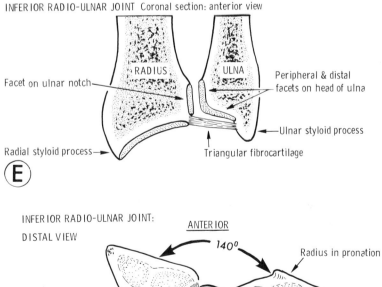

RADIUS

ULNA

Facet on ulnar notch

Peripheral & distal facets on head of ulna

Ulnar styloid process

Radial styloid process

Triangular fibrocartilage

(E)

INFERIOR RADIO-ULNAR JOINT:
DISTAL VIEW

ANTERIOR

140°

Radius in pronation

Radius in supination

Triangular fibrocartilage

Ulnar styloid process

Distal articular surface of head of ulna

POSTERIOR

(F)

It is helpful to note that, when the elbow is flexed, the application of the terms pronation and supination to the positions of the hand produced by radio-ulnar movements corresponds to the use of the terms prone and supine to describe the body lying face down and face up.

The elbow joint

This is a complex synovial hinge joint, at which the humerus articulates with both the radius and ulna, and the synovial cavity is continuous with that of the proximal radio-ulnar joint.

The articular surfaces are the humeral trochlea, which is paired with the trochlear notch on the ulna, and the humeral capitulum, which is apposed to the facet on the proximal surface of the head of the radius (**A, B, C**).

The fibrous capsule is comparatively thin, except for its medial and lateral parts, which are considerably thicker and constitute the ulnar and radial collateral ligaments (**A**).

Observe the attachments of the fibrous capsule in **A, B, C, D**.

Proximally, the radial, coronoid and olecranon fossae on the humerus are intracapsular, whereas the medial and lateral epicondyles of the humerus are extracapsular and give attachment to the collateral ligaments.

Distally, the capsule is attached to the margins of the trochlear notch on the ulna except where it is continuous with the radial notch, and to the whole of the outer aspect of the anular ligament. Thus the fibrous capsule has no attachment to the radius.

The synovial membrane lines the deep aspect of the fibrous capsule and covers all the intracapsular areas of bone which are not covered by articular cartilage including the olecranon, coronoid and radial fossae (**A, B, C**). It is absent over the deep surface of the anular ligament but, as has been noted previously, it extends from the lower margins of the anular ligament and the radial notch on the ulna onto the neck of the radius, where it is reflected upwards to the margin of the peripheral facet on the radial head (**A, C**).

The movements of the joint are flexion and extension around an axis of rotation passing through the medial and lateral humeral epicondyles.

Extension is limited abruptly at 180° by the olecranon coming into contact with the olecranon fossa on the humerus. Flexion is limited less abruptly by apposition of the anterior aspects of the arm and forearm. In this position the coronoid process of the ulna and the anterior margin of the radial head lie in, but do not completely fill, the coronoid and radial fossae on the humerus.

It should be noted that, when the elbow is extended and the forearm supinated, the long axes of the arm and forearm form an angle of about 160° open laterally. This is known as the 'carrying angle' because it is supposed to facilitate the carrying of a bucket or similar object. If the supinated forearm is flexed on the humerus at the elbow, the angle disappears so that the forearm bones and humerus become aligned and the hand lies in front of shoulder joint. The reason is that the axis of rotation of the elbow joint bisects the carrying angle and is thus slightly oblique to the long axes of both arm and supinated forearm. The carrying angle also disappears if the extended forearm is pronated, because this movement alters the position of the long axis of the forearm.

Additional note of radio-ulnar movements

Although in pronation and supination the ulna does not rotate in relation to the humerus, whereas the radius does, this does not mean that the head of the ulna is stationary in space in all radio-ulnar movements. Indeed if the elbow is flexed to a right angle, pronation and supination will usually be found to involve practically equal side-to-side displacement of the distal ends of both forearm bones. And as a result the hand, moving with the forearm bones, then rotates around its own long axis without being displaced medially or laterally. This is an important advantage in the manipulation of an instrument such as a screwdriver.

The cause of these medial and lateral displacements of the distal end of the ulna appears to be the unconscious combination of axial rotation of the humerus at the shoulder joint with radio-ulnar movements. In pronation the humerus undergoes slight lateral rotation so that the distal end of the ulna is displaced laterally while the distal end of the radius moves around it, while in supination slight medial rotation of the humerus carries the distal end of the ulna medially as the radius moves round it.

The anatomical position of the upper limb

Because of the changes in the orientation of the forearm and hand produced by radio-ulnar movements it is particularly necessary in the upper limb to define, albeit arbitrarily, a standard position which forms the basis of anatomical description of its structure. The standard position is one in which the body is erect, the upper limb is by the side and the forearm is supinated. In this position the forearm bones lie side by side with the radius laterally and the ulna medially, the forearm has anterior and posterior surfaces and the palm is the anterior surface of the hand.

CORONAL SECTION OF ELBOW JOINT:

Synovial membrane indicated by interrupted lines

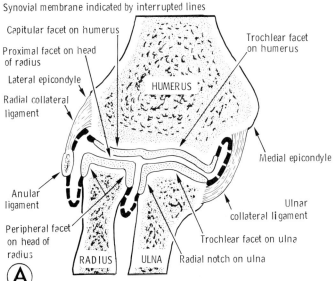

Capitular facet on humerus

Proximal facet on head of radius

Lateral epicondyle

Radial collateral ligament

HUMERUS

Trochlear facet on humerus

Medial epicondyle

Ulnar collateral ligament

Anular ligament

Peripheral facet on head of radius

RADIUS   ULNA

Trochlear facet on ulna

Radial notch on ulna

(A)

ELBOW JOINT: ANTERIOR ASPECT

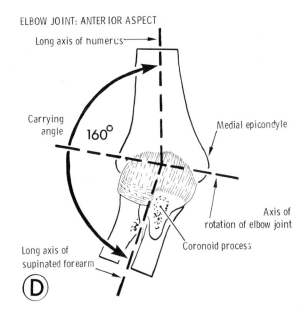

Long axis of humerus

Carrying angle

160°

Medial epicondyle

Axis of rotation of elbow joint

Coronoid process

Long axis of supinated forearm

(D)

SAGITTAL SECTION THROUGH HUMERO-ULNAR PART OF ELBOW JOINT

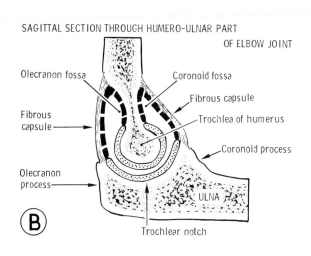

Olecranon fossa

Coronoid fossa

Fibrous capsule

Trochlea of humerus

Coronoid process

Fibrous capsule

Olecranon process

ULNA

Trochlear notch

(B)

SAGITTAL SECTION THROUGH HUMERO-RADIAL PART OF ELBOW JOINT

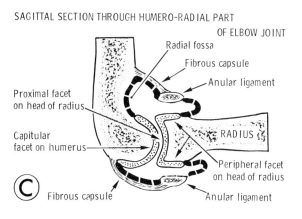

Radial fossa

Fibrous capsule

Anular ligament

Proximal facet on head of radius

Capitular facet on humerus

RADIUS

Peripheral facet on head of radius

Fibrous capsule

Anular ligament

(C)

RADIO-ULNAR SUPINATION: ELBOW FLEXED
(Medial rotation of humerus)

RADIO-ULNAR PRONATION: ELBOW FLEXED
(Lateral rotation of humerus)

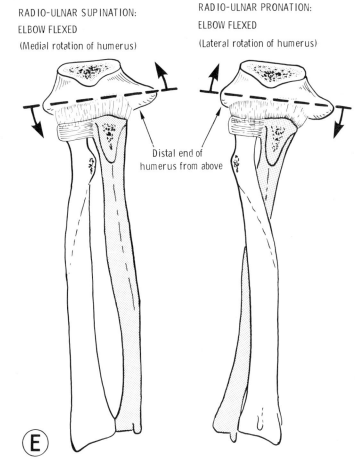

Distal end of humerus from above

(E)

Palpable bony points in the arm and forearm

Palpate on your own limb the following bony features (**A**).

1. On the humerus, the deltoid tuberosity can usually be made out through the fibres of insertion of deltoid. The medial and lateral epicondyles are clearly palpable and the corresponding supracondylar ridges can be traced proximally for a short distance. The lower part of the capitulum can be felt just below and medial to the lateral epicondyle when the elbow is flexed.
2. In the case of the radius, the posterior aspect of the head can be felt through the anular ligament, while at the distal end of the bone the dorsal tubercle and the styloid process are palpable.
3. On the ulna, the subcutaneous posterior surface of the olecranon and the whole of the posterior border of the shaft are very evident through the skin. At the distal end of the bone the rounded posterior surface of the head, the styloid process and the groove between these two features can be easily felt.

The muscles and fascia of the arm

The muscles of this region are enclosed by a tube of deep fascia which is continuous above with the axillary fascia and the deep fascia covering the shoulder muscles, and below with the deep fascia of the forearm.

The lower half of the tube is divided into anterior and posterior compartments by the attachment of medial and lateral intermuscular septa to the medial and lateral supracondylar ridges and epicondyles of the humerus (**E**). In the upper half of the arm the septa become indistinct.

Coracobrachialis (**B**, **C**) has been considered in the section on the axilla and should be revised (**500**).

Brachialis is a muscle of considerable bulk lying largely in the anterior compartment of the arm. It arises from the anteromedial and anterolateral surfaces of the lower half of the humerus between the levels of the deltoid tuberosity and the proximal attachment of the fibrous capsule of the elbow joint (**B**). It passes in front of the elbow joint and is inserted by a thick tendon into the rough anterior aspect of the coronoid process of the ulna (**C**). Its sole action is flexion of the elbow joint.

Biceps brachii arises by long and short tendinous heads which have been considered already and should now be revised (**500**). The two tendons, with that of the long head lying lateral to that of the short head, pass from the axilla into the anterior aspect of the arm between the tendons of pectoralis major and latissimus dorsi (**C**). Here they form separate muscle bellies which descend first between coracobrachialis and deltoid, and then anterior to brachialis in the anterior compartment of the arm. The bellies fuse in the lower part of the arm. Soon thereafter the muscle fibres join a strong tendon which diverges to the lateral margin of brachialis and inclines distally and backwards across the elbow joint to its insertion into the posterior aspect of the radial tuberosity (**C**). The tendon is separated from the summit and anterior aspect of the tuberosity by a bursa. Opposite the bend of the elbow the medial side of the tendon gives off the broad bicipital aponeurosis (**C**), which crosses the brachial artery (**533B**) and blends with the deep fascia of the forearm.

Apart from its stabilising effect on the shoulder joint (**499C**) the biceps produces two powerful movements. It flexes the elbow joint and, by virtue of its insertion into the posterior aspect of the radial tuberosity, it rotates the radius into the position of supination. It is to be noted, however, that biceps can supinate the forearm only when the elbow is flexed (**D**). If that joint is extended the biceps tendon is more or less aligned with the radius and is unable to produce a rotatory couple.

The triceps is a large and powerful muscle which occupies the posterior aspect and posterior compartment of the arm. As its name indicates it arises as three separate heads (**E**). The medial head arises from the posterior aspect of the shaft of the humerus between the lower lip of the groove for the radial nerve and the olecranon fossa. The lateral head has a linear origin from the upper lip of the groove for the radial nerve between the insertions of teres minor and deltoid. It descends superficial to the lateral part of the medial head (**F**). The origin of the long head and its passage into the posterior aspect of the arm between teres minor and teres major should be revised (**500**). Its muscle fibres pass down the back of the arm, medial to the lateral head and superficial to the medial part of the medial head (**F**). The three heads join a common tendon which is inserted into the upper surface of the olecranon process (**F**).

The muscle is the great extensor of the elbow joint. Its long head also acts as an adductor of the shoulder joint, a movement which is, of course, usually produced passively by gravity.

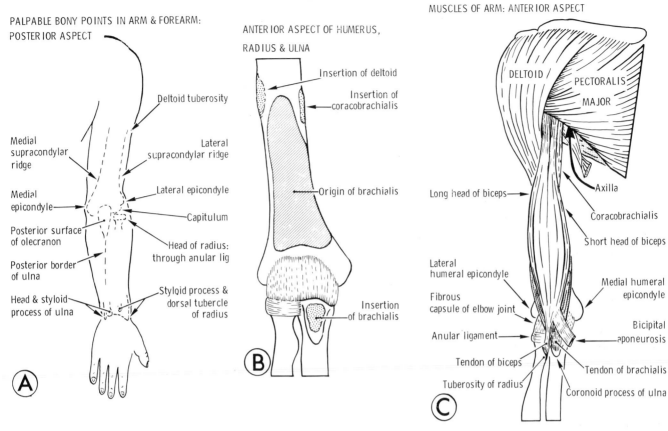

PALPABLE BONY POINTS IN ARM & FOREARM:
POSTERIOR ASPECT

- Deltoid tuberosity
- Medial supracondylar ridge
- Lateral supracondylar ridge
- Medial epicondyle
- Lateral epicondyle
- Capitulum
- Posterior surface of olecranon
- Head of radius: through anular lig
- Posterior border of ulna
- Head & styloid process of ulna
- Styloid process & dorsal tubercle of radius

(A)

ANTERIOR ASPECT OF HUMERUS,
RADIUS & ULNA

- Insertion of deltoid
- Insertion of coracobrachialis
- Origin of brachialis
- Insertion of brachialis

(B)

MUSCLES OF ARM: ANTERIOR ASPECT

- DELTOID
- PECTORALIS MAJOR
- Long head of biceps
- Axilla
- Coracobrachialis
- Short head of biceps
- Lateral humeral epicondyle
- Medial humeral epicondyle
- Fibrous capsule of elbow joint
- Bicipital aponeurosis
- Anular ligament
- Tendon of biceps
- Tendon of brachialis
- Tuberosity of radius
- Coronoid process of ulna

(C)

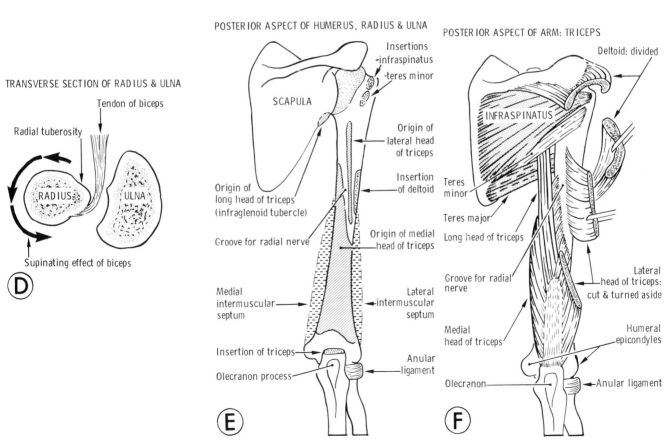

TRANSVERSE SECTION OF RADIUS & ULNA

- Tendon of biceps
- Radial tuberosity
- RADIUS
- ULNA
- Supinating effect of biceps

(D)

POSTERIOR ASPECT OF HUMERUS, RADIUS & ULNA

- Insertions -infraspinatus -teres minor
- SCAPULA
- Origin of lateral head of triceps
- Insertion of deltoid
- Origin of long head of triceps (infraglenoid tubercle)
- Groove for radial nerve
- Origin of medial head of triceps
- Medial intermuscular septum
- Lateral intermuscular septum
- Insertion of triceps
- Anular ligament
- Olecranon process

(E)

POSTERIOR ASPECT OF ARM: TRICEPS

- Deltoid: divided
- INFRASPINATUS
- Teres minor
- Teres major
- Long head of triceps
- Groove for radial nerve
- Lateral head of triceps: cut & turned aside
- Medial head of triceps
- Humeral epicondyles
- Olecranon
- Anular ligament

(F)

525

The muscles and fascia of the forearm

A tube of deep fascia surrounds the muscles of the region. It is firmly attached to the posterior aspect of the olecranon process and the posterior border of the shaft of the ulna, but elsewhere its deep surface gives rise to many of the fibres of the superficial muscles. Proximally, it is continuous with the deep fascia of the arm, while distally it is continuous with two retinacula which will be described later.

Some of the forearm muscles are inserted into the forearm bones and these are described completely in this section. However, the majority of the muscles in this region send their tendons into the hand. In this section these will be traced only as far as the distal part of the forearm.

The muscles may be divided into anterior and posterior groups. The anterior group consists of superficial, middle and deep layers and the posterior group of superficial and deep layers.

The deep layer of anterior muscles

Pronator quadratus is a quadrilateral muscle which arises from the medial and anterior aspects of the distal quarter or so of the ulnar shaft and is inserted into a corresponding extent of the anterior surface of the radial shaft (**A**). It is the strongest pronator of the radio-ulnar joints.

Flexor digitorum profundus arises from the anterior and medial surfaces of the shaft of the ulna, between the coronoid process and pronator quadratus, and from the medial half of the anterior aspect of the adjacent part of the interosseous membrane (**B**). The bulky muscle belly gives way to four tendons which are destined for the four medial fingers and pass distally across the anterior aspect of pronator quadratus (**A, D**).

Flexor pollicis longus is somewhat smaller than the preceding muscle. It arises from the anterior surface of the radius, between the levels of the radial tuberosity and pronator quadratus, and from the adjacent part of the anterior aspect of the interosseous membrane. Its single tendon, which ultimately passes to the thumb, runs distally across pronator quadratus, lying just lateral to the four tendons of flexor digitorum profundus (**A, D**).

The middle layer of anterior muscles

The flexor digitorum superficialis is a large muscle which arises by two separate heads. The humero-ulnar head runs distally from the medial humeral epicondyle, the medial side of the coronoid process of the ulna, and the fibrous capsule of the elbow joint between these bony points. The radial head is a thin sheet of oblique fibres which arises from the upper half of the anterior border of the radius and runs downwards and medially to join the rest of the muscle (**C**).

The muscle covers the anterior, but not the medial, aspect of flexor digitorum profundus, and the anterior aspect of the upper two-thirds of flexor pollicis longus.

In the lower part of the forearm it gives off four tendons, which are destined for the four medial fingers and pass distally, anterior to those of the flexor digitorum profundus and medial to that of flexor pollicis longus. In contrast to the four tendons of the profundus muscle, which all lie in the same plane, those of the superficialis muscle are arranged as an anterior pair for the middle and ring fingers and a posterior pair for the index and little fingers (**D**).

The superficial layer of anterior muscles

These muscles arise as two unequal groups on the medial and lateral sides of the elbow region.

The larger medial group consists of pronator teres, flexor carpi radialis, palmaris longus (in most individuals) and flexor carpi ulnaris, from the lateral to the medial side. The lateral group is formed by brachioradialis alone.

Pronator teres arises as separate superficial and deep heads from the lowest part of the medial supracondylar ridge of the humerus and the medial side of the coronoid process of the ulna respectively. The heads fuse as they pass distally and laterally across the forearm, distal to supinator and superficial to the radial origin of flexor digitorum superficialis. The muscle is inserted into the middle of the lateral surface of the radius (**E, F**). As its name indicates it acts with pronator quadratus (see above) to pronate the forearm.

Flexor carpi radialis and palmaris longus arise from the anterior aspect of the medial humeral epicondyle and pass distally along the middle of the anterior aspect of the forearm lying superficial to flexor digitorum superficialis. Both muscles form single tendons about halfway down the forearm (**E**).

Flexor carpi ulnaris has two origins which are connected by a fibrous arch. The humeral fibres arise from the medial epicondyle and the ulnar fibres from an aponeurosis attached to the medial aspect of the olecranon and the upper two-thirds of the posterior border of the shaft of the ulna. The muscle passes distally along the medial margin of the forearm, lying superficial to the flexor digitorum profundus and pronator quadratus, and becomes tendinous just above the wrist (**E**).

Brachioradialis arises from the middle third of the lateral supracondylar ridge of the humerus. Its fusiform muscle belly descends over the fibres of insertion of supinator and pronator teres and gives way to a flat tendon. This runs distally on the lateral surface of the radius and is inserted into the distal part of that surface just above the styloid process (**F**).

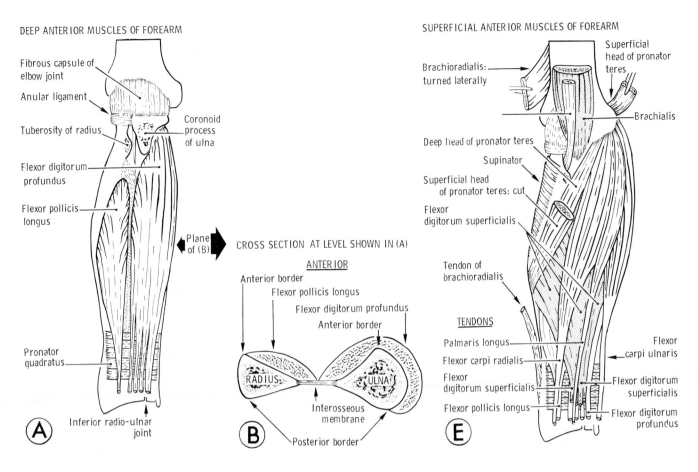

DEEP ANTERIOR MUSCLES OF FOREARM

Fibrous capsule of elbow joint

Anular ligament

Tuberosity of radius

Coronoid process of ulna

Flexor digitorum profundus

Flexor pollicis longus

Pronator quadratus

Plane of (B)

Inferior radio-ulnar joint

(A)

CROSS SECTION AT LEVEL SHOWN IN (A)

ANTERIOR

Anterior border

Flexor pollicis longus

Flexor digitorum profundus

Anterior border

RADIUS

ULNA

Interosseous membrane

Posterior border

(B)

SUPERFICIAL ANTERIOR MUSCLES OF FOREARM

Brachioradialis: turned laterally

Superficial head of pronator teres

Brachialis

Deep head of pronator teres

Supinator

Superficial head of pronator teres: cut

Flexor digitorum superficialis

Tendon of brachioradialis

TENDONS

Palmaris longus

Flexor carpi radialis

Flexor digitorum superficialis

Flexor pollicis longus

Flexor carpi ulnaris

Flexor digitorum superficialis

Flexor digitorum profundus

(E)

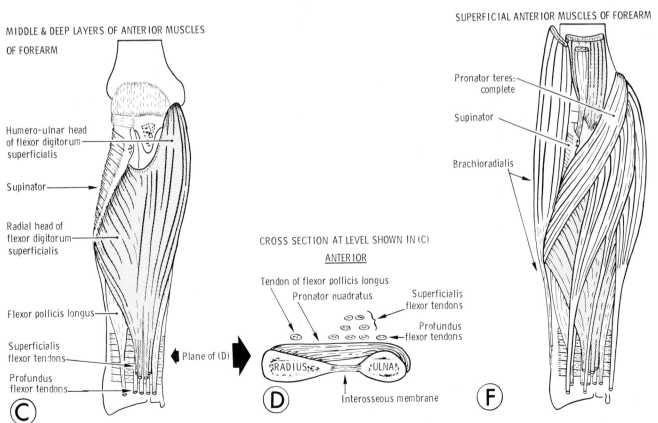

MIDDLE & DEEP LAYERS OF ANTERIOR MUSCLES OF FOREARM

Humero-ulnar head of flexor digitorum superficialis

Supinator

Radial head of flexor digitorum superficialis

Flexor pollicis longus

Superficialis flexor tendons

Profundus flexor tendons

(C)

CROSS SECTION AT LEVEL SHOWN IN (C)

ANTERIOR

Tendon of flexor pollicis longus

Pronator quadratus

Superficialis flexor tendons

Profundus flexor tendons

RADIUS

ULNA

Plane of (D)

Interosseous membrane

(D)

SUPERFICIAL ANTERIOR MUSCLES OF FOREARM

Pronator teres: complete

Supinator

Brachioradialis

(F)

Examine the positions of the tendons of the anterior muscles of the forearm immediately above the wrist in **A** and in your own forearm. When the hand is flexed on the supinated forearm, the slender tendon of palmaris longus stands out prominently beneath the skin at the middle of the anterior aspect of the forearm. The tendon of flexor carpi radialis, though not so prominent, can be seen as a ridge about 1 cm to its lateral side, while the tendon of flexor carpi ulnaris can be felt, but not usually seen, some 3 cm to its medial side. On deeper planes the tendons of flexor digitorum superficialis lie in the interval between palmaris longus and flexor carpi ulnaris, and the tendon of flexor pollicis longus in that between palmaris longus and flexor carpi radialis.

The cubital fossa

This is a triangular intermuscular depression in front of the elbow (**527E, 527F**). Its base is taken as a line joining the medial and lateral epicondyles of the humerus, and its medial and lateral boundaries are formed by the adjacent edges of pronator teres and brachioradialis respectively. Above, its floor consists of brachialis with the tendon of biceps brachii on its anterolateral side, while below it is formed by the anterior aspect of supinator.

The deep posterior muscles

Supinator has a continuous origin from the supinator crest and fossa of the ulna, from the back of the anular ligament and from the radial collateral ligament of the elbow joint and the lateral humeral epicondyle (**B**). Its fibres sweep laterally and then forwards round the shaft of the radius and are inserted into the upper third of its lateral surface. It is important to recall (**517D**) that this part of the lateral surface of the radius is extensive and triangular and lies on the anterior and posterior, as well as the lateral, aspects of the bone.

The muscle is a strong supinator of the radio-ulnar joints, acting in concert with biceps brachii when the elbow is flexed.

The other deep posterior muscles arise from the posterior surfaces of the radius, the ulna and the interosseous membrane below the level of supinator. Note their names and origins in **B**. Traced distally, each of these muscles forms a slender tendon (**C**). These run with a lateral inclination to the distal end of the radius where they establish the following relationships.

The extensor indicis and extensor pollicis longus tendons lie on the posterior surface of distal end of the radius to the medial side of the dorsal tubercle.

The abductor pollicis longus and extensor pollicis brevis tendons emerge from their originally deep plane by passing between two of the superficial posterior muscles, extensor carpi radialis brevis and extensor digitorum (**D**). Thereafter they curl forwards and distally to lie on the lowest part of the lateral surface of the radius superficial to the insertion of brachioradialis.

The superficial posterior muscles

Observe the names and positions of these muscles in **D** and note that, apart from anconeus, all are inserted in the hand.

Anconeus is a small triangular muscle situated behind the elbow joint (**C**). Its fibres arise from the posterior aspect of the lateral humeral epicondyle and diverge downwards and laterally across the posterior aspects of the anular ligament and supinator to the lateral aspect of the olecranon process of the ulna. It assists triceps in extension of the elbow.

Extensor carpi ulnaris arises from the lateral humeral epicondyle and, passing distally just lateral to the posterior border of the ulna, becomes tendinous in the distal part of the forearm (**D**).

Extensor digitorum arises in common with the preceding muscle and lies lateral to it (**D**). Its large muscle belly passes distally, superficial to the deep posterior muscles. The medial fibres separate from the rest as the extensor digiti minimi which becomes tendinous in the lower part of the forearm. The rest of the muscle gives rise to four tendons for the medial four fingers.

Extensor carpi radialis brevis arises in common with the preceding muscle and lies lateral to it (**D**). It passes distally along the lateral aspect of the radius and becomes tendinous in the middle of the forearm. The tendon winds backwards onto the posterior surface of the radial shaft being crossed obliquely by the muscle bellies of abductor pollicis longus above and the extensor pollicis brevis below (**D**).

Extensor carpi radialis longus takes origin above the lateral humeral epicondyle from the lower third or so of the lateral supracondylar ridge (**D**). It passes distally between extensor carpi radialis brevis and brachioradialis along the lateral aspect of the forearm and its tendon follows that of the brevis muscle onto the posterior aspect of the radius.

Examine the positions of the tendons of the posterior muscles in a plane just above the wrist joint in **E**.

CROSS SECTION THROUGH TENDONS IN LOWEST PART
OF ANTERIOR COMPARTMENT OF FOREARM

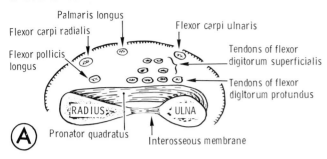

Palmaris longus
Flexor carpi radialis
Flexor carpi ulnaris
Flexor pollicis longus
Tendons of flexor digitorum superficialis
Tendons of flexor digitorum profundus
RADIUS
ULNA
Pronator quadratus
Interosseous membrane
(A)

POSTERIOR ASPECT OF FOREARM: DEEP MUSCLES:

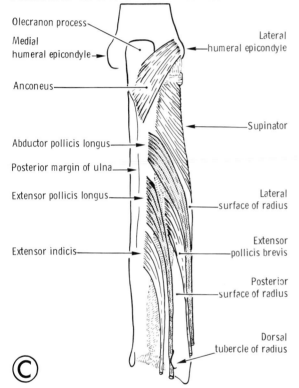

Olecranon process
Medial humeral epicondyle
Lateral humeral epicondyle
Anconeus
Supinator
Abductor pollicis longus
Posterior margin of ulna
Extensor pollicis longus
Lateral surface of radius
Extensor indicis
Extensor pollicis brevis
Posterior surface of radius
Dorsal tubercle of radius
(C)

TENDONS OF POSTERIOR MUSCLES AT DISTAL END OF FOREARM

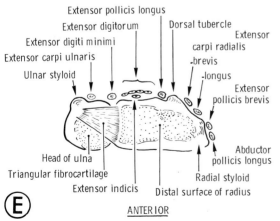

Extensor pollicis longus
Extensor digitorum
Dorsal tubercle
Extensor digiti minimi
Extensor carpi radialis
Extensor carpi ulnaris
brevis
Ulnar styloid
longus
Extensor pollicis brevis
Head of ulna
Triangular fibrocartilage
Abductor pollicis longus
Extensor indicis
Radial styloid
Distal surface of radius
(E)
ANTERIOR

POSTERIOR ASPECT OF FOREARM: DEEP MUSCLES:

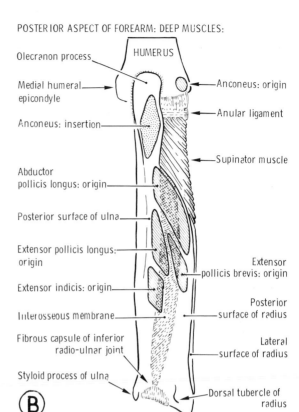

Olecranon process
HUMERUS
Medial humeral epicondyle
Anconeus: origin
Anular ligament
Anconeus: insertion
Supinator muscle
Abductor pollicis longus: origin
Posterior surface of ulna
Extensor pollicis longus: origin
Extensor pollicis brevis: origin
Extensor indicis: origin
Interosseous membrane
Posterior surface of radius
Fibrous capsule of inferior radio-ulnar joint
Lateral surface of radius
Styloid process of ulna
Dorsal tubercle of radius
(B)

POSTERIOR ASPECT OF FOREARM: SUPERFICIAL MUSCLES:

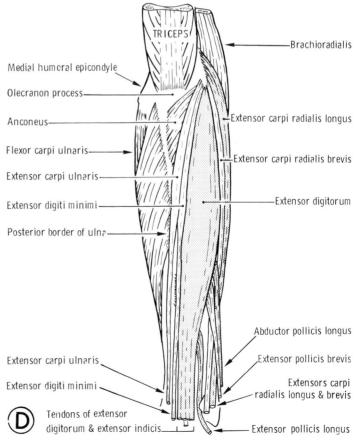

TRICEPS
Brachioradialis
Medial humeral epicondyle
Olecranon process
Anconeus
Extensor carpi radialis longus
Flexor carpi ulnaris
Extensor carpi radialis brevis
Extensor carpi ulnaris
Extensor digiti minimi
Extensor digitorum
Posterior border of ulna
Abductor pollicis longus
Extensor carpi ulnaris
Extensor pollicis brevis
Extensor digiti minimi
Extensors carpi radialis longus & brevis
Tendons of extensor digitorum & extensor indicis
Extensor pollicis longus
(D)

It should be noted that the tendons are in fact covered here by the extensor retinaculum. The retinaculum and its relationship to the tendons will be considered later.

Note the following points in **529E**.

1. Extensor carpi ulnaris lies most medially in the dorsal groove between the head and styloid process of the ulna.
2. Extensor digiti minimi overlies the posterior aspect of the inferior radio-ulnar joint.
3. The four tendons of extensor digitorum, with the tendon of extensor indicis deep to them and that of extensor pollicis longus on their lateral side, pass over the posterior surface of the distal end of the radius medial to the dorsal tubercle.
4. Extensor carpi radialis brevis with extensor carpi radialis longus, which is lateral to it, lie on the posterior surface of the distal end of the radius lateral to the dorsal tubercle.
5. Abductor pollicis longus, and extensor pollicis brevis immediately behind it, are situated on the lateral surface of the distal end of the radius.

The superficial veins of the arm and forearm

Although the superficial fascia of these regions receives numerous arterial twigs from the deep arteries, the main vessels are large veins which communicate at a number of points through the deep fascia with the venae comitantes of the deep arteries.

The pattern of the superficial veins is variable, but usually there are two large vessels which are interconnected, particularly in the forearm. These arise from a superficial venous network which permeates the superficial fascia on the posterior aspect of the hand (**A**). The vessels of this network are fairly large and have a general longitudinal orientation. They are usually clearly visible through the thin overlying skin and so are used for the injection of intravenous anaesthetics.

Most of the superficial veins can be examined in your own limb if the blood flow through them is obstructed by compression of the upper part of the arm.

The cephalic vein

This vessel begins at the radial side of the superficial venous network on the posterior aspect of the hand (**A**). Running proximally in the superficial fascia, it winds forwards round the radial side of the forearm to its anterior aspect and ascends until it overlies the lateral part of the cubital fossa. Still in the superficial fascia, it runs upwards overlying the lateral border of biceps brachii until it pierces the deep fascia just below the anterior axillary fold. It then continues upwards and medially in the deltopectoral cleft to a point a little below the clavicle. There, as has been seen previously (**509A**), it turns backwards, pierces the clavipectoral fascia and ends by joining the axillary vein.

The basilic vein

The basilic vein begins at the ulnar side of the same venous network which forms the origin of the cephalic (**A**). Passing proximally in the superficial fascia, it winds round the ulnar border of the forearm to its anterior aspect and comes to overlie the medial part of the cubital fossa. Thereafter it ascends in line with the medial border of biceps brachii until it pierces the deep fascia about half way up the arm, and becomes immediately related to the brachial artery and its venae comitantes. It runs proximally with these vessels, and in front of the lower border of teres major continues as the axillary vein.

The median cubital vein

This is a short vessel which runs medially and upwards from the cephalic to the basilic vein and overlies the upper part of the cubital fossa (**A**). This vein is used in clinical practice for the withdrawal of blood, and sometimes to insert a cannula for certain investigatory procedures.

The lymphatics of the arm and forearm

In the upper limb the great majority of lymphatic vessels are derived from the skin or the synovial membranes of joints. The latter group follow the courses of the deep arteries (see below) to the lateral axillary lymph nodes (**513A**). Those from the skin become aggregated into two groups which accompany the cephalic and basilic veins (**B**).

Of those following the cephalic vein, the majority diverge medially in the upper part of the arm and pierce the axillary fascia to end in the lateral axillary nodes, but a few continue with the vein and reach the infraclavicular nodes on the clavipectoral fascia (**513A**). The efferents from these nodes pierce the fascia and join the apical axillary nodes.

Of those which follow the basilic vein, some are interrupted by one or two supratrochlear nodes which lie in the superficial fascia just above the medial humeral epicondyle. Thereafter some of the vessels pierce the deep fascia with the basilic vein while others continue upwards in the superficial fascia and enter the axilla through the axillary fascia. All run to the lateral axillary nodes.

SUPERFICIAL VEINS OF UPPER LIMB: RIGHT

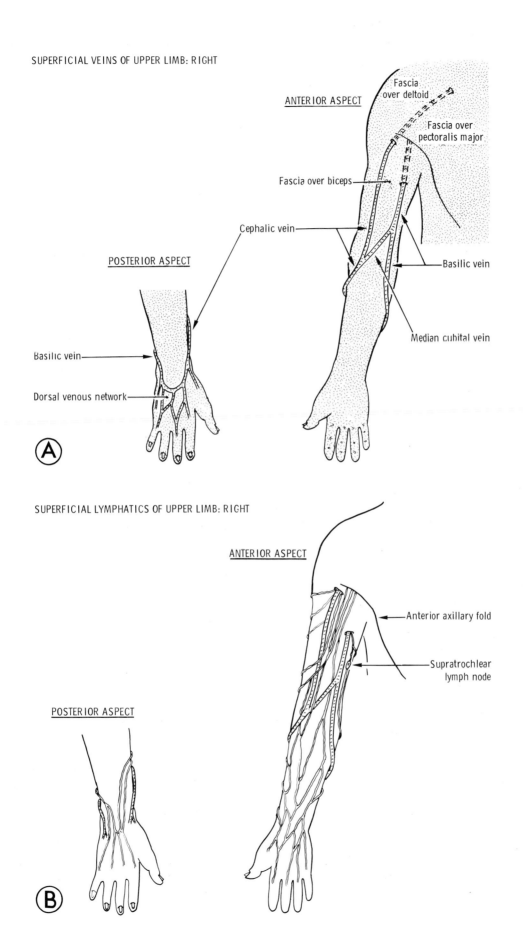

ANTERIOR ASPECT

Fascia over deltoid

Fascia over pectoralis major

Fascia over biceps

Cephalic vein

Basilic vein

Median cubital vein

POSTERIOR ASPECT

Basilic vein

Dorsal venous network

Ⓐ

SUPERFICIAL LYMPHATICS OF UPPER LIMB: RIGHT

ANTERIOR ASPECT

Anterior axillary fold

Supratrochlear lymph node

POSTERIOR ASPECT

Ⓑ

The deep blood vessels of the arm and forearm

The brachial artery

The brachial artery begins as the continuation of the axillary artery in front of the lower margin of the tendon of teres major (**A**). It ends in the cubital fossa just medial to the neck of the radius by dividing into ulnar and radial arteries (**B**). In the upper half of the arm it lies medial to the shaft of the humerus and is related to the long head of triceps posteriorly and coracobrachialis laterally (**A**). In the lower half of the arm it gradually deviates laterally in front of the humerus and lies on the anterior surface of brachialis along the medial margin of biceps brachii (**B**). Throughout its course it is just deep to the deep fascia of the arm and forearm, including the bicipital aponeurosis, and its pulsations are consequently palpable throughout its length.

The artery gives off a number of branches in the arm. It is unnecessary to learn the names and positions of these vessels, but the following general features should be noted.

1. They supply muscles on both the anterior and posterior aspects of the arm.
2. Many of them run in close association with major nerves.
3. The general direction of most is distal towards the elbow where they form a considerable anastomosis with proximally directed branches of the radial and ulnar arteries.

The ulnar and radial arteries

These are formed by the bifurcation of the brachial artery in the lower angle of the cubital fossa, and diverge respectively to the medial and lateral borders of the anterior compartment of the forearm. The muscular relations of the divergent parts of the two arteries are evident in **C** and **D**.

In the lower two-thirds of the forearm both arteries run longitudinally. The ulnar is at first deep to the anterior margin of flexor carpi ulnaris (**D**), but later it is superficially placed between the tendon of that muscle and those of flexor digitorum superficialis (**E**). The radial is at first overlapped by the anterior border of brachioradialis (**D**) but as that muscle narrows to its tendon of insertion the artery comes to lie immediately beneath the deep fascia on the lateral side of the tendon of flexor carpi radialis (**E**). Distal to pronator quadratus the radial artery lies directly on the anterior surface of the lower end of the radius (**E**). The ease with which the vessel can be gently compressed against the bone makes this an ideal situation for the assessment of the character and rapidity of a patient's pulse. The student should palpate his own radial pulse in the position described.

The positions of the ulnar and radial arteries and their relationships to the anterior tendons in the lowest part of the forearm are shown in **E**.

Both arteries give off recurrent branches which anastomose around the elbow with descending branches of the brachial artery, and numerous twigs which supply the anterior muscles of the forearm. Only one of these several branches deserves individual consideration. *The common interosseous artery* arises close to the origin of the ulnar and, after a short course, bifurcates over the upper border of the interosseous membrane into anterior and posterior interosseous arteries (**C**). The former runs distally between the deep anterior muscles. The latter appears in the posterior compartment between supinator and abductor pollicis longus and runs distally amongst the posterior muscles of the forearm.

Venae comitantes accompany the brachial, ulnar and radial arteries throughout their courses. Note that in the upper limb the main arteries are accompanied by venae comitantes as far as the axilla, whereas in the lower limb (**342**) the venae comitantes, characteristic of the distal part of the limb, are replaced by single large veins above the level of the knee joint.

ANTERIOR ASPECT OF UPPER PART OF RIGHT ARM: BRACHIAL ARTERY

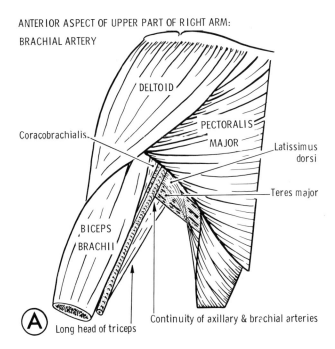

DELTOID

PECTORALIS MAJOR

Coracobrachialis

Latissimus dorsi

Teres major

BICEPS BRACHII

Continuity of axillary & brachial arteries

Long head of triceps

(A)

ANTERIOR ASPECT OF RIGHT FOREARM: ULNAR & RADIAL ARTERIES

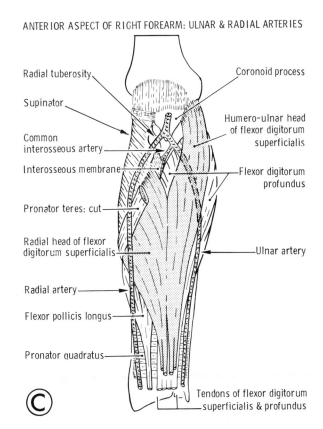

Radial tuberosity

Supinator

Common interosseous artery

Interosseous membrane

Pronator teres: cut

Radial head of flexor digitorum superficialis

Radial artery

Flexor pollicis longus

Pronator quadratus

Coronoid process

Humero-ulnar head of flexor digitorum superficialis

Flexor digitorum profundus

Ulnar artery

Tendons of flexor digitorum superficialis & profundus

(C)

RIGHT CUBITAL FOSSA: BRACHIAL ARTERY

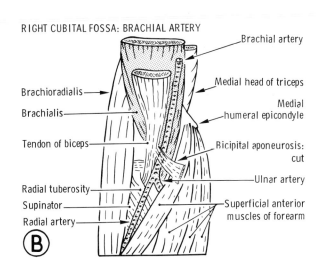

Brachial artery

Medial head of triceps

Medial humeral epicondyle

Bicipital aponeurosis: cut

Ulnar artery

Superficial anterior muscles of forearm

Brachioradialis

Brachialis

Tendon of biceps

Radial tuberosity

Supinator

Radial artery

(B)

ANTERIOR ASPECT OF RIGHT FOREARM: ULNAR & RADIAL ARTERIES

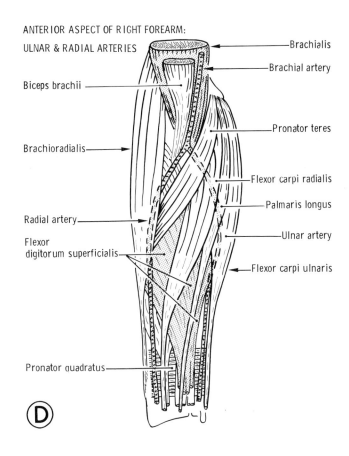

Brachialis

Brachial artery

Biceps brachii

Pronator teres

Brachioradialis

Flexor carpi radialis

Palmaris longus

Radial artery

Ulnar artery

Flexor digitorum superficialis

Flexor carpi ulnaris

Pronator quadratus

(D)

CROSS SECTION OF TENDONS & ARTERIES IN DISTAL PART OF ANTERIOR COMPARTMENT OF FOREARM

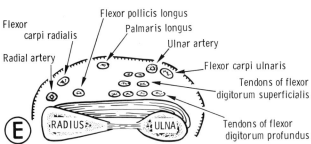

Flexor carpi radialis

Flexor pollicis longus

Palmaris longus

Ulnar artery

Radial artery

Flexor carpi ulnaris

Tendons of flexor digitorum superficialis

Tendons of flexor digitorum profundus

RADIUS

ULNA

(E)

The nerves of the arm and forearm

The nerves which supply the arm, forearm and hand arise from the cords of the brachial plexus in the axilla where they have been studied already.

The musculocutaneous nerve

It has been noted that this nerve passes through coracobrachialis as it leaves the axilla (**511A**). Leaving the lateral side of the muscle it passes downwards and laterally through the anterior compartment of the arm between biceps brachii and brachialis supplying both. It emerges from between the lateral borders of these two muscles at the level of the elbow joint (**A**) and, piercing the deep fascia, changes its name.

The lateral cutaneous nerve of the forearm follows the cephalic vein fairly closely and supplies the area of skin shown in **C**.

The medial cutaneous nerve of the forearm

Leaving the axilla (**511A**) this nerve runs distally between the brachial artery and the basilic vein (**A**). It pierces the deep fascia with that vein (**531A**) and follows it closely to supply the skin area indicated in **C**.

The median nerve in the arm

As has been observed earlier (**511A**), the median nerve enters the arm from the axilla on the lateral side of the brachial artery, between it and coracobrachialis. As it descends, it crosses anterior to the artery and enters the cubital fossa on its medial side lying on brachialis. In the fossa both artery and nerve are crossed by the bicipital aponeurosis.

The nerve has no branches in the arm.

The ulnar nerve in the arm

In the axilla or upper arm, the ulnar nerve is usually joined by a branch from the lateral cord or the lateral root of the median nerve carrying fibres from the seventh cervical segment which are destined mainly for skin in the regions of the hand and digits. Thus as the nerve enters the arm the segmental origin of its fibres is C7, 8, T1.

In the upper half of the arm the nerve is situated between the brachial artery and the basilic vein and in front of the long head of triceps (**A**). It then inclines backwards through the medial intermuscular septum, and runs distally on the anterior surface of the medial head of triceps in the posterior compartment of the arm. At the elbow it lies on a groove on the posterior aspect of the medial humeral epicondyle (**B**) where it is readily palpable as a thick movable cord. The nerve has no branches in the arm.

The radial nerve in the arm

Leaving the axilla, the nerve inclines downwards and backwards, between the head of triceps and the medial aspect of the shaft of the humerus, and then winds obliquely round the posterior aspect of the bone in a shallow groove (**B**). In the groove it lies above the origin of the medial head of triceps and below the origin of the lateral head whose descending fibres cover it and hide it from view.

Reaching the lateral side of the arm, it pierces the lateral intermuscular septum and descends in the anterior compartment of the arm (**A**) in the deep intermuscular cleft between brachioradialis and extensor carpi radialis longus laterally and brachialis medially. In front of the lateral epicondyle of the humerus it ends by dividing into two terminal branches which continue into the forearm (see below).

Unlike the median and ulnar nerves the radial gives off numerous branches before reaching the level of the elbow.

1. The posterior cutaneous nerve of the arm arising in the axilla has been noted already (**C, 511B**).
2. Motor branches to the long and medial heads of triceps (C7, 8) arise beyond teres major but before the nerve has entered its groove on the humerus.
3. Motor branches to the lateral and medial head of triceps and anconeus (C7, 8) arise in the upper part of the groove.
4. The lower lateral cutaneous nerve of the arm (C5, 6) arises just before the radial nerve pierces the lateral intermuscular septum (**B**). Observe its area of distribution in **C**.
5. The posterior cutaneous nerve of the forearm (C6, 7) arises at about the same point (**B**) and is distributed to the area shown in **C**.
6. Motor branches also arise in the anterior compartment of the arm, and supply the brachioradialis muscle (C5, 6) and the extensor carpi radialis longus (C7, 8).

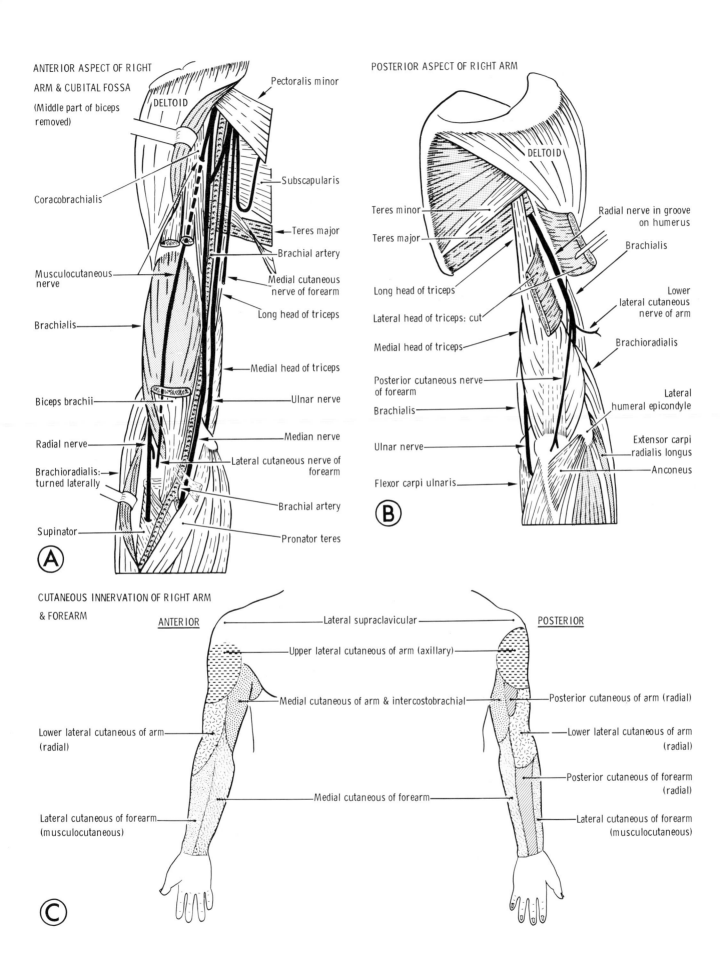

ANTERIOR ASPECT OF RIGHT ARM & CUBITAL FOSSA
(Middle part of biceps removed)

DELTOID

Pectoralis minor

Coracobrachialis

Musculocutaneous nerve

Brachialis

Biceps brachii

Radial nerve

Brachioradialis: turned laterally

Supinator

Ⓐ

Subscapularis

Teres major

Brachial artery

Medial cutaneous nerve of forearm

Long head of triceps

Medial head of triceps

Ulnar nerve

Median nerve

Lateral cutaneous nerve of forearm

Brachial artery

Pronator teres

POSTERIOR ASPECT OF RIGHT ARM

DELTOID

Teres minor

Teres major

Long head of triceps

Lateral head of triceps: cut

Medial head of triceps

Posterior cutaneous nerve of forearm

Brachialis

Ulnar nerve

Flexor carpi ulnaris

Ⓑ

Radial nerve in groove on humerus

Brachialis

Lower lateral cutaneous nerve of arm

Brachioradialis

Lateral humeral epicondyle

Extensor carpi radialis longus

Anconeus

CUTANEOUS INNERVATION OF RIGHT ARM & FOREARM

ANTERIOR

POSTERIOR

Lateral supraclavicular

Upper lateral cutaneous of arm (axillary)

Medial cutaneous of arm & intercostobrachial

Lower lateral cutaneous of arm (radial)

Posterior cutaneous of arm (radial)

Lower lateral cutaneous of arm (radial)

Medial cutaneous of forearm

Posterior cutaneous of forearm (radial)

Lateral cutaneous of forearm (musculocutaneous)

Lateral cutaneous of forearm (musculocutaneous)

Ⓒ

535

The median nerve in the forearm

In the forearm the nerve passes between the superficial and deep heads of pronator teres (**A**). At the same point it crosses the ulnar artery from medial to lateral side, the deep head of pronator teres intervening. The nerve continues distally in a central position in the forearm, lying between flexor digitorum superficialis and profundus. Above the wrist it becomes more superficial and lies amongst the tendons of the anterior forearm muscles, the positions of which should be revised (**B, D**). It is situated between the tendons of flexor digitorum superficialis and the tendon of flexor pollicis longus, deep to the interval between the readily palpable tendons of palmaris longus and flexor carpi radialis. These relationships are very important because of the frequency of incised wounds in the region. The subsequent course of the nerve in the hand will be described later (**565A**).

In the proximal part of the forearm it gives off numerous muscular branches which supply all the anterior group of muscles except brachioradialis, which is supplied by the radial nerve, and flexor carpi ulnaris and the medial half of flexor digitorum profundus, both of which are supplied by the ulnar nerve (see below). The fibres supplied by the median nerve to the forearm muscles are derived almost entirely from C7 and 8.

The ulnar nerve in the forearm

The ulnar nerve enters the forearm by passing under the fibrous arch joining the humeral and ulnar origins of flexor carpi ulnaris (**C**), and descends between that muscle and the medial half of flexor digitorum profundus (**A, B**). At about the junction of the proximal and middle thirds of the forearm it comes into relation with the medial side of the ulnar artery and maintains that relationship into the hand (**A**). As the flexor carpi ulnaris narrows into its tendon in the lower part of the forearm, the nerve and artery appear at its lateral margin (**B**) where their superficial position makes them especially prone to injury in incised wounds in the region of the wrist (**D**).

In the upper part of the forearm the nerve supplies flexor carpi ulnaris and the medial half of flexor digitorum profundus (C8), between which it lies. Note the double innervation of the profundus muscle from both median and ulnar nerves. Some 5 cm above the wrist the nerve gives off a dorsal cutaneous branch (C6, 7) which winds medially and distally round the ulna deep to flexor carpi ulnaris (**A**) to its distribution to skin on the posterior aspects of the hand and digits (**565D**).

The radial nerve in the forearm

While the nerve lies in front of the lateral humeral epicondyle, between brachialis medially and brachioradialis and extensor carpi radialis longus laterally, it divides into superficial and deep terminal branches (**A**).

The deep terminal branch (C7, 8) is almost entirely distributed to muscles. Close to its origin it gives a branch to extensor carpi radialis brevis, and then winds obliquely backwards and distally round the upper part of the shaft of the radius, embedded in the substance of supinator which it innervates (**A, C**). Emerging from supinator it divides into branches which supply all the rest of the superficial and deep posterior muscles of the forearm.

The superficial terminal branch (C7, 8), in contrast to the deep branch, is a cutaneous nerve which supplies some of the skin over the hand and digits (**565D**) but gives off no branches to the skin of the forearm. In the upper two-thirds of the forearm it runs distally lying successively on supinator, pronator teres, the radial head of flexor digitorum superficialis and flexor pollicis longus (**A**). It gradually comes into association with the radial artery, which approaches it from the medial side, and is overlapped by brachioradialis (**B**). In the lower third of the forearm it parts company with the artery, and inclines backwards deep to the tendon of brachioradialis (**B**).

ANTERIOR ASPECT OF RIGHT FOREARM: NERVES

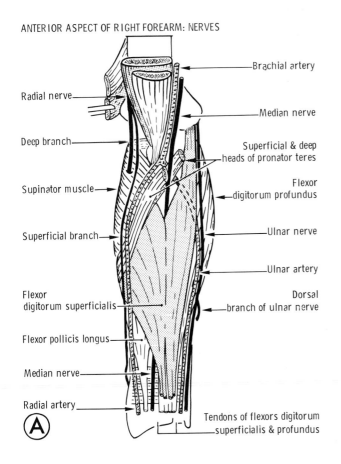

- Radial nerve
- Deep branch
- Supinator muscle
- Superficial branch
- Flexor digitorum superficialis
- Flexor pollicis longus
- Median nerve
- Radial artery

- Brachial artery
- Median nerve
- Superficial & deep heads of pronator teres
- Flexor digitorum profundus
- Ulnar nerve
- Ulnar artery
- Dorsal branch of ulnar nerve
- Tendons of flexors digitorum superficialis & profundus

(A)

ANTERIOR ASPECT OF RIGHT FOREARM: NERVES

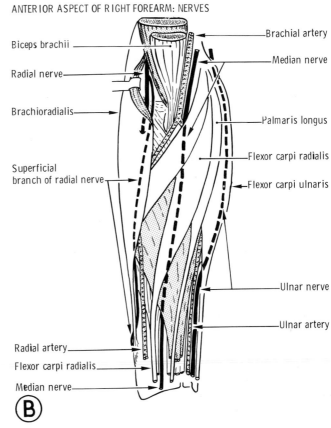

- Biceps brachii
- Radial nerve
- Brachioradialis
- Superficial branch of radial nerve
- Radial artery
- Flexor carpi radialis
- Median nerve

- Brachial artery
- Median nerve
- Palmaris longus
- Flexor carpi radialis
- Flexor carpi ulnaris
- Ulnar nerve
- Ulnar artery

(B)

POSTERIOR ASPECT OF RIGHT FOREARM: NERVES

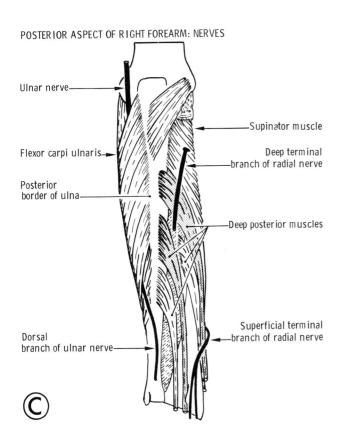

- Ulnar nerve
- Flexor carpi ulnaris
- Posterior border of ulna
- Dorsal branch of ulnar nerve

- Supinator muscle
- Deep terminal branch of radial nerve
- Deep posterior muscles
- Superficial terminal branch of radial nerve

(C)

TENDONS, ARTERIES & NERVES AT LEVEL OF DISTAL ENDS OF RADIUS & ULNA

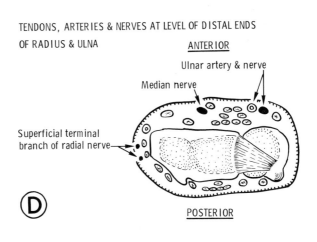

ANTERIOR

- Ulnar artery & nerve
- Median nerve
- Superficial terminal branch of radial nerve

POSTERIOR

(D)

THE HAND

It should be recalled (**522**) that in its standard anatomical position the hand has palmar (anterior) and dorsal (posterior) surfaces and medial (ulnar) and lateral (radial) borders.

The hand has five digits. Coloquially, one differentiates the thumb from the four fingers but, despite its obvious differences from the other digits, anatomically the thumb is regarded as the first of five fingers numbered from lateral to medial side, so that the third finger is called the middle finger. Of the other fingers the second is often called the index finger because it is used in pointing, while for obvious reasons the fourth and fifth fingers are often called the ring finger and the little finger respectively. In clinical practice it is safer to name the digits than to number them, to avoid risk of confusion.

The bones and joints of the hand

The bones of the hand are arranged in three groups (**A**).

1. Proximally, the carpus consists of eight small irregular carpal bones.
2. The five metacarpals are longitudinally orientated, miniature long bones lying distal to the carpus. They are numbered 1–5 from the lateral to the medial side.
3. The phalanges are also miniature long bones. They form the skeletons of the digits, two being present in the thumb (proximal and distal) and three in each of the fingers (proximal middle and distal).

The carpus

The carpal bones which comprise the carpus are arranged in proximal and distal rows containing four bones each. Observe the names and positions of the bones in **B** and **C**. The dorsal aspect of the carpus (**C**) is gently convex from side to side and has no prominent features. The palmar aspect (**B**) is concave and exhibits the features listed below.

1. The scaphoid lies at the lateral end of the proximal row. The distal and lateral part of its palmar surface is in the form of a rounded prominence, called the tubercle. It may be noted here that in about 15% of individuals the small arteries which supply the scaphoid all enter the bone through foramina on its distal part (**D**). If such a scaphoid is fractured across its waist, the blood supply to the proximal fragment is cut off and that fragment may undergo avascular necrosis.
2. The pisiform, which is about the size of a pea, has all the characteristics of a sesamoid bone. It lies in the substance of the tendon of flexor carpi ulnaris (**527E**) but articulates by its deep surface with the palmar aspect of the triquetrum (**B**).
3. The hamate, at the medial end of the distal row of the carpus, is characterised by a process which arises from the distal part of its palmar surface and is known as the hook of the hamate (**B**). The process is spatulate and concave on its lateral surface.
4. The trapezium lies at the lateral end of the distal row of the carpus. Its palmar surface is crossed by a prominent longitudinal ridge which is limited on its medial side by a deep groove (**B**).

The carpal bones are involved in two major articulations.

The radiocarpal (wrist) joint

The articular surfaces both consist of a number of elements. The proximal surface, which is gently concave from side to side, is formed by the continuous area of cartilage covering the distal surface of the radius and the medial aspect of its styloid process, and the distal surface of the fibrocartilaginous radio-ulnar articular disc which separates the radiocarpal from the inferior radio-ulnar joint. The distal surface consists of the convex cartilaginous facets on the proximal aspects of the scaphoid, lunate, and triquetrum and the interosseous ligaments which intervene between them (**B, C, F**). As a whole it is convex from side to side and from before backwards. Note that in the neutral position of the joint the lunate articulates with both the radius and the articular disc.

The fibrous capsule, which is lined by synoval membrane, is a thick sleeve of interlacing fibres attached to the margins of the articular surfaces.

The midcarpal joint

The distal row of carpal bones are united by interosseous ligaments attached to the distal parts of their contiguous surfaces (**F**).

The midcarpal joint has an extensive, irregular, cartilage-lined cavity which separates the distal carpal bones from the triquetrum, lunate and scaphoid and sends cleft-like recesses between the components of both rows as far as the proximal and distal intercarpal ligaments (**F**).

This cavity is enclosed by a feltwork of collagen fibres which is attached to the nonarticular aspects of all the carpal bones except the pisiform.

BONES OF HAND

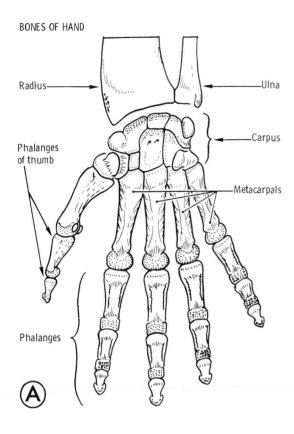

Radius

Ulna

Carpus

Phalanges of thumb

Metacarpals

Phalanges

(A)

CARPUS & METACARPUS: ANTERIOR ASPECT

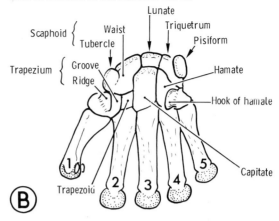

Scaphoid { Waist
           Tubercle

Lunate

Triquetrum

Pisiform

Trapezium { Groove
            Ridge

Hamate

Hook of hamate

Trapezoid

Capitate

(B)   1   2   3   4   5

CARPUS & METACARPUS: POSTERIOR ASPECT

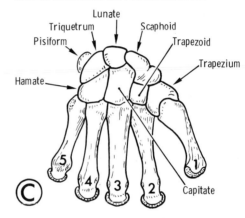

Triquetrum

Lunate

Scaphoid

Pisiform

Trapezoid

Hamate

Trapezium

(C)   5   4   3   2   1

Capitate

RIGHT SCAPHOID: ANTERIOR ASPECT

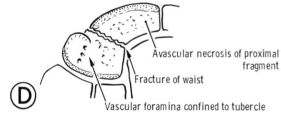

Avascular necrosis of proximal fragment

Fracture of waist

Vascular foramina confined to tubercle

(D)

RIGHT RADIOCARPAL JOINT: PROXIMAL ARTICULAR SURFACE

POSTERIOR

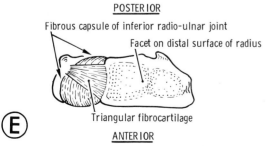

Fibrous capsule of inferior radio-ulnar joint

Facet on distal surface of radius

Triangular fibrocartilage

(E)

ANTERIOR

CORONAL SECTION OF CARPUS & ADJACENT BONES

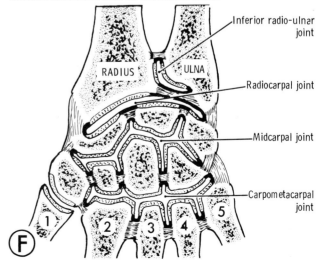

RADIUS   ULNA

Inferior radio-ulnar joint

Radiocarpal joint

Midcarpal joint

Carpometacarpal joint

(F)   1   2   3   4   5

Movements between the hand and forearm

All the movements between the hand and the forearm have components which occur at both the radiocarpal and midcarpal joints.

1. *Flexion*, in which the palm of the hand is moved towards the anterior aspect of the forearm, has a range of about 90° (**A**). Its major component occurs at the midcarpal joint.
2. *Extension* has a smaller range of about 45°, but most of this occurs at the radiocarpal joint (**B**).
3. *Adduction* (ulnar deviation) carries the hand medially in relationship to the long axis of the forearm. It has a range of about 60° and is predominantly a radiocarpal movement (**C**). In full adduction the lunate articulates solely with the radius instead of both the radius and the triangular fibrocartilage (**539F**).
4. *Abduction* (radial deviation) is a much smaller movement with a range of only about 10–15° (**D**). It occurs almost entirely at the midcarpal joint.

The metacarpal bones 2–5

These bones are all of similar form. Each has a shaft with a slightly concave palmar surface, an expanded ovoid distal end called the head, and a rather less expanded, oblong, proximal end called the base (**E**).

The heads carry cartilage facets which are convex from side to side and from before backwards. The facets are longer sagittally than coronally and although they cover the palmar and distal aspects they extend only marginally onto the sides and dorsal aspects (**E, F, G**).

The bases carry more or less plane cartilage facets on their opposed and proximal surfaces (**E, 539F**).

Collectively these metacarpals lie on a curved plane which is concave from side to side towards the palm (**F**). The long axes of the facets on their heads are radially related to that curvature, so that when the fingers are bent individually their tips all meet the palm within a small area. This fact can be confirmed on your own hand.

The carpometacarpal joints 2–5

An irregular synovial joint cavity separates the bases of metacarpals 2–5 both from one another and from the distal

aspects of the hamate, capitate, and trapezoid and a small area on the medial aspect of the trapezium (**539F**).

The articulation is strengthened by a number of short interosseous ligaments and enclosed by a general fibrous capsule which is continuous with that of the midcarpal joint.

Comparatively little movement occurs at these joints. Passive displacement of the metacarpal heads in your own hand will show that metacarpal 5 is the most mobile, while metacarpals 2 and 3 are the least mobile.

The first metacarpal

This bone differs from the other metacarpals which have been considered above in a number of ways.

1. The bone may be regarded as being rotated through 90° around its long axis compared to the other metacarpals (**F, G**). Despite this, it is convenient to keep to the same terminology for its various aspects as that used in the other metacarpals, even though some of the terms become directionally inappropriate. Thus, in its position of rest, the palmar aspect of the bone faces in a medial direction, parallel to the plane of the rest of the palm while the dorsal aspect faces laterally. The medial and lateral aspects of the bone face backwards and forwards respectively, both in directions at right angles to the palm.
2. The shaft is shorter and thicker than those of the other metacarpals.
3. The articular surface on the head is wider mediolaterally, and shorter from its palmar to its dorsal margin, than the corresponding surface on the other metacarpals (**F**).
4. The base carries a single cartilage facet which articulates solely with the trapezium. Its shape will be described in the next section (**G**).

The first carpometacarpal joint

From the point of view of the normal activities of everyday life, this small synovial joint between the trapezium and the base of the first metacarpal is one of the most important in the body, because it allows the palmar aspect of the thumb to be opposed to the palmar aspect of the other digits.

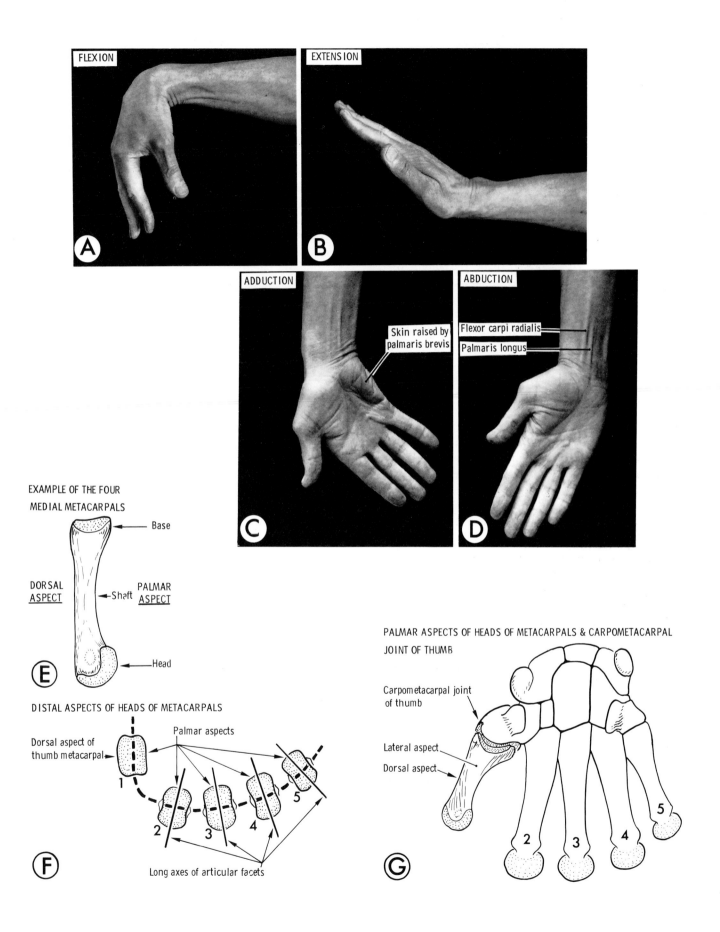

FLEXION

EXTENSION

ADDUCTION

Skin raised by palmaris brevis

ABDUCTION

Flexor carpi radialis

Palmaris longus

A

B

C

D

EXAMPLE OF THE FOUR
MEDIAL METACARPALS

Base

DORSAL
ASPECT

Shaft

PALMAR
ASPECT

Head

E

DISTAL ASPECTS OF HEADS OF METACARPALS

Palmar aspects

Dorsal aspect of
thumb metacarpal

1

2

3

4

5

Long axes of articular facets

F

PALMAR ASPECTS OF HEADS OF METACARPALS & CARPOMETACARPAL
JOINT OF THUMB

Carpometacarpal joint
of thumb

Lateral aspect

Dorsal aspect

2

3

4

5

G

The articular surfaces are saddle-shaped (sellar) in an approximately reciprocal fashion (**A**, **B**). That on the proximal surface of the base of the metacarpal is convex in a plane at right angles to that of the palm, that is, sagittally (**C**), and concave parallel to the plane of the palm, that is, coronally (**D**). Conversely the distal surfaces of the trapezium is concave sagittally (**C**) and convex coronally (**D**). Thus the metacarpal surface can be regarded as a rounded ridge whose long axis is concave and parallel to the plane of the palm, while the surface on the trapezium can be regarded as a groove whose long axis is convex and again parallel to the plane of the palm. When the surfaces are in contact the ridge lies in the groove (**A**, **B**).

It is important to appreciate two other features of the articular surfaces. In a coronal plane the length of the proximal surface is considerably greater than that of the distal surface (**D**). Also the surfaces are not perfectly congruent with one another either coronally or sagittally (**C**, **D**). Consequently, they are in contact over a comparatively small area and elsewhere are separated by wedge-shaped spaces occupied by synovial fluid.

The ligamentous apparatus of the joint consists of a loose sleeve-like fibrous capsule attached to the margins of the articular surfaces, and two additional ligaments which are partially blended with the capsule. The palmar oblique ligament is attached to the upper, medial corner of the palmar surface of the trapezium (**A**) and winds obliquely round the palmar aspect of the joint to reach the medial aspect of the metacarpal base (**A**, **B**). The dorsal oblique ligament arises from the upper lateral corner of the dorsal aspect of the trapezium, and passes across the joint to be attached close to the attachment of the previous ligament on the medial aspect of the metacarpal base (**B**).

The movements at the first carpometacarpal joint are considerably more extensive than those which are possible at the other carpometacarpal joints (see above).

1. Because of the incongruity of its articular surfaces and the laxity of its fibrous capsule the first metacarpal can rotate about its own long axis. Rotation such that its palmar surface is turned towards the rest of the palm is medial rotation (**B**), whereas rotation in the opposite direction is lateral rotation (**A**). Although rotation can be produced passively as an isolated movement (most simply by bending the thumb and using its phalanges as a lever) active rotation occurs only in combination with other movements at the primary joint.
2. Movement of the metacarpal in a medial direction across the palm of the hand involves the ridge on its base gliding in a medial direction along the groove on the trapezium (**B**). This movement is invariably associated with medial rotation (**B**), so that as the metacarpal moves across the palm its palmar aspect is simultaneously turned towards, that is opposed to, the palm. Consequently the complete movement is called opposition. The constant association of medial rotation with medial displacement of the metacarpal is due to the fact that as the metacarpal base glides medially on the trapezium, the dorsal oblique ligament tightens and restrains movement of the medial aspect of the metacarpal whereas no comparable restraint is exerted on the lateral aspect of the bone (**B**).
3. Similarly lateral movement of the metacarpal in the plane of the palm is always associated with lateral rotation. This results from tightening of the palmar oblique ligament (**A**) which restrains displacement of the medial aspect of the metacarpal while no restraint is exerted on the lateral aspect of the bone. The complete movement, involving lateral displacement and lateral rotation of the first metacarpal is known as reposition.
4. In abduction, the first metacarpal moves anteriorly at right angles to the plane of the palm, while in adduction the movement is in the opposite direction. Both movements involve displacement of the sagittal convexity of the metacarpal articular surface upon the sagittal concavity on the trapezium (**C**) and neither is necessarily associated with rotation.

The phalanges

Of the three phalanges in each of the four medial fingers the proximal is the longest and the distal the shortest. Each has a shaft, a head and a base. Both the heads and bases of the proximal and middle phalanges are articular. The distal phalanx has an articular base, but its head is nonarticular and bears a roughened tuberosity on its palmar aspect to which the connective tissue of the finger tip is attached.

The thumb has only two phalanges, of which the proximal is longer than the distal. In general form and in the character of their articular surfaces they closely resemble the proximal and distal phalanges of the fingers.

The articular surfaces on the phalanges will be described in the succeeding sections in relation to the joints in which they are involved.

FIRST CARPOMETACARPAL JOINT: PALMAR ASPECT:
MOVEMENT OF REPOSITION

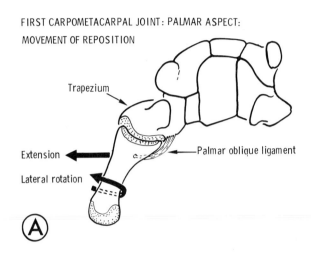

Trapezium

Extension

Lateral rotation

Palmar oblique ligament

(A)

FIRST CARPOMETACARPAL JOINT: DORSAL ASPECT:
MOVEMENT OF OPPOSITION

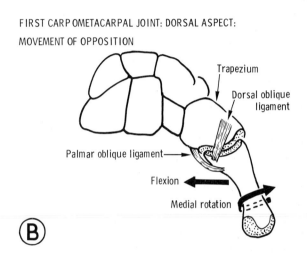

Trapezium

Dorsal oblique
ligament

Palmar oblique ligament

Flexion

Medial rotation

(B)

FIRST CARPOMETACARPAL JOINT:
SAGITTAL SECTION

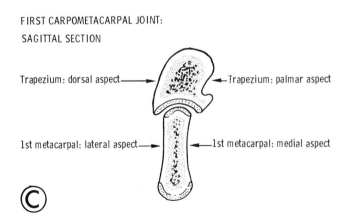

Trapezium: dorsal aspect

Trapezium: palmar aspect

1st metacarpal: lateral aspect

1st metacarpal: medial aspect

(C)

FIRST CARPOMETACARPAL JOINT:
CORONAL SECTION

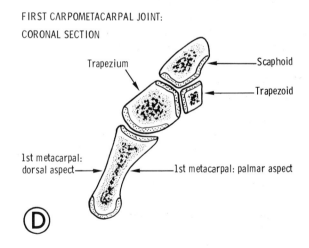

Trapezium

Scaphoid

Trapezoid

1st metacarpal:
dorsal aspect

1st metacarpal: palmar aspect

(D)

The metacarpophalangeal joints 2–5

These four joints are similar both in form and in function.

The cartilaginous articular surfaces at each joint are a cup-shaped facet on the base of the proximal phalanx and a more extensive convex surface which, it will be recalled, covers the distal and palmar aspects of the metacarpal head but extends to a much lesser extent onto the sides and dorsal aspect (**541E**).

The ligamentous apparatus at each joint consists of three components.

1. A fibrous capsule which is attached to the margins of the articular surfaces (**B**). The capsule is thin dorsally and on the lateral and medial sides, but its palmar part consists of a thick fibrocartilaginous plaque, which articulates with the palmar aspect of the proximal articular surface when the joint is extended (**A**).
2. Cord-like collateral ligaments lie on the medial and lateral aspects of each joint (**B, C**). They are attached proximally to the posterior part of the metacarpal head and pass obliquely across the joint to blend with the distal attachment of the palmar part of the fibrous capsule.
3. The deep transverse metacarpal ligament is a common ligament of the four joints (**D, E**). It joins the palmar aspect of their fibrous capsules to one another and severely restricts separation of the corresponding metacarpals.

The movements of the proximal phalanges on the meta-carpals at these joints are those of flexion, extension, abduction and adduction. Circumduction is a combination of these four movements. Note the following features of the four primary movements.

1. In full flexion the proximal phalanx is at right angles to the metacarpal whereas in full extension the two bones are in alignment or a little beyond that position (**B, C**). Both movements are limited by tension in the appropriate parts of the fibrous capsule.
2. In some descriptions abduction and adduction are related to the long axis of the third metacarpal. This has the disadvantage that side to side movements of the third digit must then be described as abduction in both directions. It seems preferable to hold to the practice observed in other parts of the body and call medial displacement of any of the fingers adduction and lateral displacement abduction.

3. Because the proximal attachments of the collateral ligaments lie dorsal to the transverse axes of rotation of flexion-extension movements (**B**), these ligaments are lax in extension and taut in flexion (**B, C**). Observe in your own hand, that as a result, although adduction-abduction movements have a small but appreciable range when the metacarpophalangeal joints are extended, the same movements cannot be produced at all when the joints are flexed.

The metacarpophalangeal joint of the thumb

The form of this joint is essentially similar to that of the metacarpophalangeal joints of the fingers. However it does differ from these joints in certain aspects.

1. The thick palmar aspect of its fibrous capsule contains medial and lateral sesamoid bones (**D, E**). These are associated, as will be seen later, with the tendons of some of the short muscles of the thumb and articulate by their deep surfaces with the palmar aspect of the articular surface on the head of the metacarpal.
2. In conformity with the comparatively wide range of movement which occurs between the first metacarpal and the trapezium, the deep transverse metacarpal ligament, which joins the other metacarpophalangeal joints to one another, does not extend to the corresponding joint of the thumb (**D, E**).
3. Because of the unique orientation of the first carpometacarpal joint (**542**), flexion and extension movements at the metacarpophalangeal joint of the thumb occur parallel to the plane of the palm.
4. Although in full extension the metacarpal and proximal phalanx are aligned, flexion at the joint has a range only about 50° compared with the 90° of movement possible in the other fingers.
5. Because the articular surfaces of the joint are wider in the mediolateral direction than in the dorsopalmar, abduction-adduction movements are negligible.

The interphalangeal joints

The proximal and distal interphalangeal joints of the fingers and the single interphalangeal joint of the thumb are all similar in structure and function (**F**).

METACARPOPHALANGEAL JOINTS 2 - 5 : FROM LATERAL SIDE

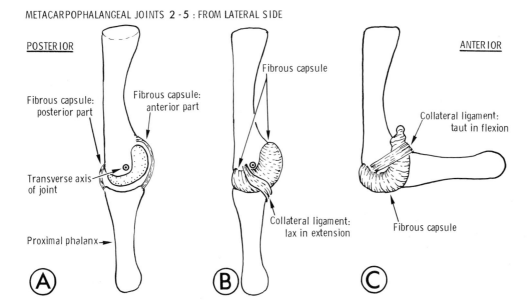

POSTERIOR

Fibrous capsule: posterior part

Fibrous capsule: anterior part

Transverse axis of joint

Proximal phalanx →

Ⓐ

Fibrous capsule

Collateral ligament: lax in extension

Ⓑ

ANTERIOR

Collateral ligament: taut in flexion

Fibrous capsule

Ⓒ

METACARPOPHALANGEAL JOINTS:
PALMAR ASPECT

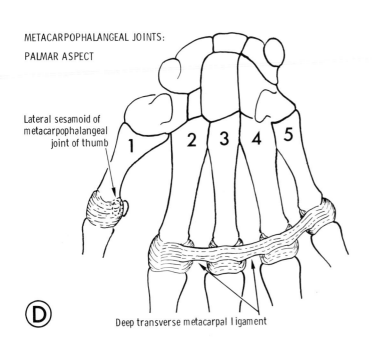

Lateral sesamoid of metacarpophalangeal joint of thumb

1 2 3 4 5

Ⓓ

Deep transverse metacarpal ligament

METACARPOPHALANGEAL JOINTS: TRANSVERSE SECTION

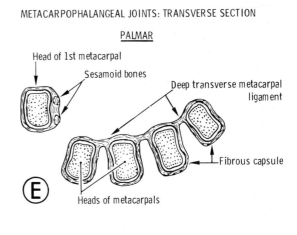

PALMAR

Head of 1st metacarpal

Sesamoid bones

Deep transverse metacarpal ligament

Fibrous capsule

Ⓔ

Heads of metacarpals

INTERPHALANGEAL JOINT

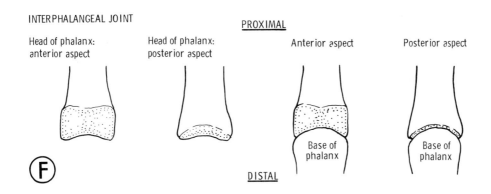

Head of phalanx: anterior aspect

Head of phalanx: posterior aspect

PROXIMAL

Anterior aspect

Posterior aspect

Base of phalanx

Base of phalanx

Ⓕ

DISTAL

The proximal articular surfaces which extend over the distal and palmar surfaces of the head of a phalanx are pulley-shaped in a dorsopalmar direction. The distal surfaces are reciprocally shaped but are much shorter from before backwards. Each joint is enclosed by a fibrous capsule and equipped on its medial and lateral aspects with collateral ligaments similar to those of the metacarpophalangeal joints.

As would be expected from the shape of their articular surfaces, movement at these joints is virtually restricted to flexion and extension. In the case of the thumb these movements occur parallel to the plane of the palm. At all the joints full extension brings the respective phalanges more or less into alignment whereas full flexion involves an angulation of approximately 90°.

Ossification of the bones of the hand

The carpus, at the time of birth, is entirely cartilaginous. After birth a single centre of ossification appears in each carpal unit, and spreads slowly so that the carpal bones reach their definitive size at about 20 years. The dates at which these primary centres appear vary somewhat in different individuals, particularly in the case of the pisiform, but the dates shown in **A** are average values.

The metacarpals and phalanges are miniature long bones. In each bone the shaft is ossified from a primary centre which appears in the third month of intra-uterine life. This bony shaft elongates and, at birth, is continuous at both ends with cartilaginous epiphyses. At about this time the primary ossification of the shaft proceeds through the epiphysis at one end, leaving in most instances a thin layer of articular cartilage, and elongation of the shaft at that end then ceases. The cartilaginous epiphysis at the other end of the bone persists and is ossified by a secondary centre of ossification which appears at about 2 years. The resulting bony epiphysis remains separated from the diaphysis by a cartilaginous growth plate, at which elongation of the diaphysis continues until about 16 years. Then the growth plate is obliterated and longitudinal growth of the bone ceases.

Thus, in contrast to most long bones, postnatal elongation of the metacarpals and phalanges occurs at one end only.

In all the phalanges the single bony epiphysis and its associated single growth plate are situated at the proximal end of the bone. On the other hand it is most important to note that in the metacarpals the bony epiphysis and growth plate lie at the proximal end of the first metacarpal but at the distal ends of the other four.

The fibrous structures of the hand and wrist

The regions of the hand and wrist contain a number of purely fibrous structures. Several of these are retaining structures which prevent displacement of long tendons away from the joints they pass over on their way to their insertions.

The extensor retinaculum is a broad thickened zone in the deep fascia which extends obliquely across the posterior aspect of the wrist from the distal part of the anterior margin of the radius to the ulnar styloid and the medial aspect of the triquetrum (**B**). Its deep surface is attached at intervals to the radius and ulna. These attachments divide the space deep to the retinaculum into six compartments, one on the lateral aspect of the radius, three on the posterior aspect of that bone, one behind the inferior radio-ulnar joint and one between the head of the ulna and the ulnar styloid (**C**). Through these compartments the long tendons of the posterior muscles of the forearm pass distally on to the dorsum of the hand.

The flexor retinaculum is a broad, thick band of connective tissue which extends transversely across the palmar concavity of both rows of carpal bones (**D**), converting that concavity into the carpal tunnel (**E**). Unlike that on the extensor aspect, this retinaculum has no direct connection with the forearm bones. It is attached on the medial side to the lateral aspect of the pisiform and the hook of the hamate. On the lateral side it splits into superficial and deep lamellae. The superficial part attaches to the tubercle of the scaphoid and the ridge on the trapezium. The deep part attaches to the medial lip of the groove on the trapezium so that the two lamellae and the bony groove form the walls of a subsidiary lateral compartment of the carpal tunnel (**E**).

The superficial surface of the retinaculum is fused, on the lateral side, to the deep fascia of the forearm. Centrally it is continuous with both the tendon of palmaris longus and the overlying deep fascia. Towards the medial side it is separated from the deep fascia by an interval which allows the ulnar vessels and nerve to pass into the hand, superficial to the retinaculum, but deep to the deep fascia (see below).

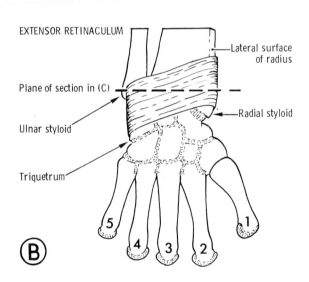

OSSIFICATION OF HAND:
Secondary ossification hatched

4th year
3rd year
5th year
10th year
1st year

1 2 3 4 5

(A)

FLEXOR RETINACULUM

Radiocarpal joint
Tuberosity of scaphoid
Ridge of trapezium

Plane of section in (E)
Pisiform
Hook of hamate

1 2 3 4 5

(D)

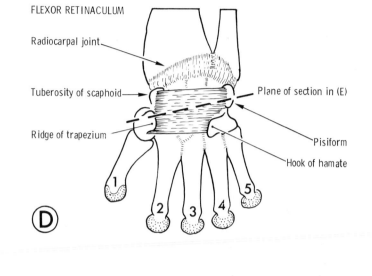

EXTENSOR RETINACULUM

Lateral surface of radius
Plane of section in (C)
Radial styloid
Ulnar styloid
Triquetrum

5 4 3 2 1

(B)

FLEXOR RETINACULUM:
TRANSVERSE SECTION ALONG PLANE SHOWN IN (D)

ANTERIOR

Palmaris longus tendon
Deep fascia
Pisiform

Trapezium { - ridge
            - groove

Carpal tunnel:
- subsidiary compartment
- main compartment

Scaphoid
Capitate
Hamate
Triquetrum

(E)

POSTERIOR

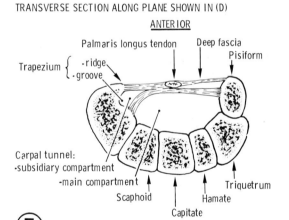

EXTENSOR RETINACULUM:
TRANSVERSE SECTION ALONG PLANE SHOWN IN (B)

POSTERIOR

Root of ulnar styloid

Lateral surface of radius

Interosseous membrane

(C)

ANTERIOR

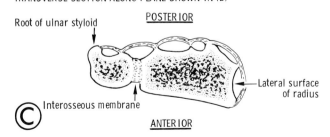

547

The fibrous flexor sheaths are five osteo-aponeurotic canals on the palmar aspects of the five fingers (**A**) which extend in each case from the distal end of the metacarpal shaft to the middle of the shaft of the distal phalanx. The dorsal wall of a sheath is formed by the palmar aspects of the phalanges, the fibrous capsules of the metacarpophalangeal and interphalangeal joints (**A**, **C**). The palmar and side walls consist of transversely orientated collagenous fibres which are stronger over the phalanges than over the joints.

The palmar aponeurosis is the name given to the deep fascia which covers the palm of the hand. However, in this description the term will be restricted to the central triangular part of that fascia which is quite distinct in appearance and structure to the parts lying lateral and medial to it.

Using this terminology the palmar aponeurosis is a thick, dense, triangular plaque of deep fascia which covers and protects the central part of the palm (**B**). Its superficial surface is intimately attached to the skin, which consequently cannot be moved over the underlying structures, as is possible in most regions of the body. This immobility of the skin obviously increases the security of the grip.

Proximally, the apex of the aponeurosis is attached to the central part of the superficial surface of the flexor retinaculum where it is continuous with the tendon of palmaris longus. Distally, its base divides into four digitations, one for each of the four medial fingers. Each digitation then divides into two processes which embrace the proximal end of the corresponding fibrous flexor sheath (**B**, **C**) and flare out to become attached to the sides of both the proximal and middle phalanges (**B**). Because of the extent of these attachments, the not uncommon condition of pathological contracture of the palmar aponeurosis (Dupuytren's con-tracture) causes flexion deformity of both the metacarpophalangeal and the proximal interphalangeal joints, but not of the distal interphalangeal joints.

The superficial transverse metacarpal ligament (**B**, **C**) is a broad band which joins the digitations of the palmar aponeurosis and the palmar aspects of the fibrous flexor sheaths of the medial four fingers to one another. Like the deep transverse metacarpal ligament (**545D**) it does not extend between the index finger and the thumb. Between the fingers, the superficial and deep transverse metacarpal ligaments are separated by three spaces known as lumbrical canals (**C**).

The palmar spaces are three regions of the palm lying in front of the interosseous muscles and fascia (see below) which are isolated from one another by two thin fascial septa (**D**). The medial septum passes from the medial margin of the palmar aponeurosis to the shaft of the fifth metacarpal. The lateral septum arises from the lateral margin of the palmar aponeurosis and follows a sinuous course, first dorsally, then medially, and then dorsally again to be attached to the shaft of the third metacarpal. The three regions or 'spaces' so demarcated are called, from the lateral to the medial side, the thenar, middle palmar and hypothenar spaces. Infections in the palm tend to be restricted to one or other of these regions by the fascial planes.

The middle palmar space (**E**) is continuous proximally through the main compartment of the carpal tunnel with the anterior compartment of the forearm, into which an abscess in the space may spread. Distally, it is continuous with the three lumbrical canals, through which an abscess within it may be drained.

THE FIBROUS FLEXOR SHEATHS

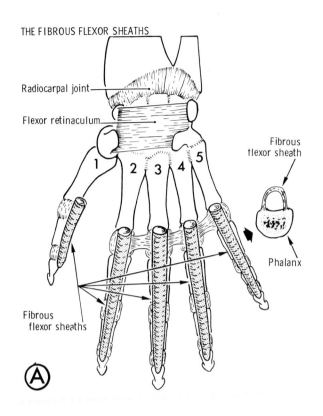

Radiocarpal joint

Flexor retinaculum

1 2 3 4 5

Fibrous flexor sheath

Phalanx

Fibrous flexor sheaths

PALMAR APONEUROSIS

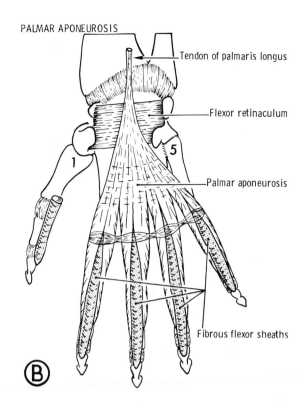

Tendon of palmaris longus

Flexor retinaculum

1 5

Palmar aponeurosis

Fibrous flexor sheaths

SCHEMATIC TRANSVERSE SECTION THROUGH METACARPOPHALANGEAL JOINTS

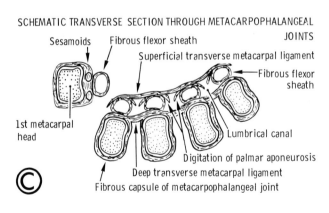

Sesamoids

Fibrous flexor sheath

Superficial transverse metacarpal ligament

Fibrous flexor sheath

1st metacarpal head

Lumbrical canal

Digitation of palmar aponeurosis

Deep transverse metacarpal ligament

Fibrous capsule of metacarpophalangeal joint

TRANSVERSE SECTION THROUGH HAND: PALMAR SPACES

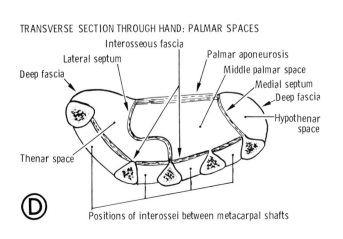

Interosseous fascia

Lateral septum

Deep fascia

Palmar aponeurosis

Middle palmar space

Medial septum

Deep fascia

Hypothenar space

Thenar space

Positions of interossei between metacarpal shafts

MIDDLE PALMAR SPACE

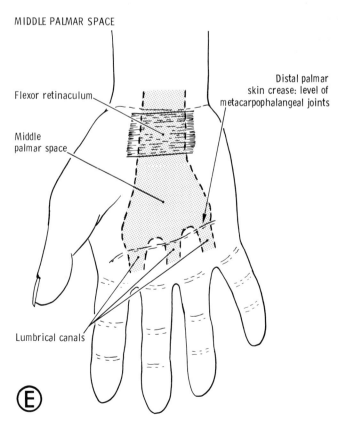

Flexor retinaculum

Middle palmar space

Distal palmar skin crease: level of metacarpophalangeal joints

Lumbrical canals

The muscles and tendons of the hand

These muscles and tendons will be described as a number of functional groups.

The interosseous muscles

The four bipennate dorsal interossei are shown in **A** and the four unipennate palmar interossei in **B**. The members of each group are numbered one to four from the lateral to the medial side. Observe the following features of these muscles.

1. Both groups are symmetrically disposed about the long axis of the third digit. As they pass distally the tendons of the dorsal muscles incline towards that axis (**A**) and those of the palmar muscles away from it (**B**).
2. The tendons of all the interossei, except the first palmar and dorsal muscles, pass dorsal to the deep transverse metacarpal ligament between adjacent metacarpophalangeal joints.
3. The tendon of the first palmar interosseous is inserted (**B**) through the medial sesamoid of the thumb (**549C**) into the proximal phalanx, and is a flexor of the first metacarpophalangeal joint.
4. The tendons of all the other interossei are inserted into the dorsal digital expansions which cover the dorsal aspects of the proximal phalanges of the medial four fingers. Work out from **A** and **B** which interossei join each of the four expansions.
5. The dorsal digital expansions cannot be considered at this time but their structure and the actions of the interossei and other muscles inserted into them will be discussed later (**556**).
6. All the interossei are covered on their palmar aspects by the thin interosseous fascia which forms the dorsal walls of the palmar spaces (**549D**).

The muscles acting on the radiocarpal and midcarpal joints

The dispositions of these muscles in the forearm have already been considered (**526, 528**). Now trace these tendons into the hand noting their insertions and their relationships to the flexor and extensor retinacula.

The tendon of flexor carpi ulnaris is primarily inserted into the pisiform but is projected through the pisohamate and pisometacarpal ligaments to the hook of the hamate and the base of the fifth metacarpal (**C**). Note that it does not pass beneath the flexor retinaculum.

The tendon of palmaris longus, as has been noted, is attached to the superficial surface of the flexor retinaculum (**C**), where it is continuous with the apex of the palmar aponeurosis.

The tendon of flexor carpi radialis passes through the subsidiary lateral compartment of the flexor retinaculum lying in the groove on the trapezium (**E**). The tendon then splits into two parts which are inserted into the bases of the second and third metacarpals (**C**).

The tendon of extensor carpi ulnaris passes through the most medial compartment of extensor retinaculum (**F**) and is inserted into the base of the fifth metacarpal (**D**).

The tendons of extensor carpi radialis longus and brevis pass through that compartment of the extensor retinaculum which is situated on the most lateral part of the dorsal surface of the radius, the longus tendon lying lateral to the brevis (**F**). Beyond the retinaculum the longus tendon is inserted into the base of the second metacarpal and the brevis tendon into the base of the third metacarpal (**D**).

All these muscles are prime movers of the radiocarpal and midcarpal joints (**539F**). The flexor muscles plus palmaris longus produce flexion of the hand on the forearm, while the extensor muscles produce extension. Adduction of the hand is effected by the combined actions of the ulnar flexor and extensor and abduction by the combined actions of the radial flexor and extensors.

Observe in your own hand that flexion of the fingers is more complete when the hand is partially extended on the forearm than when it is fully flexed. Consequently, when an object is gripped by flexion of the fingers, the position of the hand is fixed in partial extension by the synergic activity of all the above muscles.

The long and short muscles of the thumb

The tendon of abductor pollicis longus (**529D**) passes from the forearm through the compartment of the extensor retinaculum which lies on the lateral surface of the radius. It then continues distally, lateral to, but separate from, the lateral aspects of the radiocarpal and midcarpal joints, and is inserted into the lateral side of the base of the first metacarpal (**C, D**).

The tendon of extensor pollicis brevis accompanies the previous tendon as far as the first metacarpal, then crosses the dorsal aspect of the corresponding metacarpophalangeal joint to be inserted into the base of the proximal phalanx of the thumb.

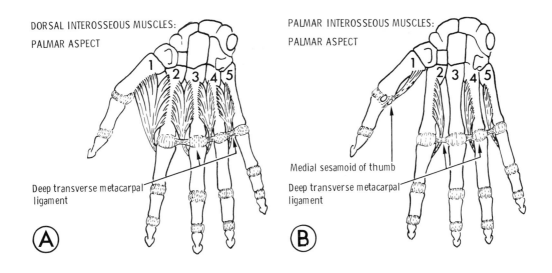

DORSAL INTEROSSEOUS MUSCLES:
PALMAR ASPECT

Deep transverse metacarpal
ligament

Ⓐ

PALMAR INTEROSSEOUS MUSCLES:
PALMAR ASPECT

Medial sesamoid of thumb

Deep transverse metacarpal
ligament

Ⓑ

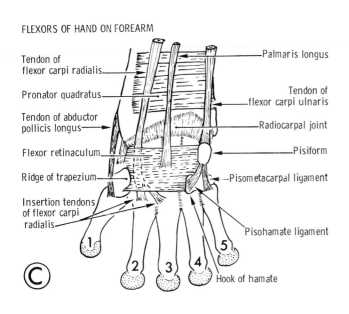

FLEXORS OF HAND ON FOREARM

Tendon of
flexor carpi radialis

Pronator quadratus

Tendon of abductor
pollicis longus

Flexor retinaculum

Ridge of trapezium

Insertion tendons
of flexor carpi
radialis

Palmaris longus

Tendon of
flexor carpi ulnaris

Radiocarpal joint

Pisiform

Pisometacarpal ligament

Pisohamate ligament

Hook of hamate

Ⓒ

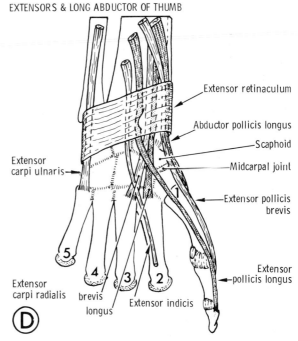

EXTENSORS OF HAND ON FOREARM:
EXTENSORS & LONG ABDUCTOR OF THUMB

Extensor retinaculum

Abductor pollicis longus

Scaphoid

Midcarpal joint

Extensor pollicis
brevis

Extensor
pollicis longus

Extensor
carpi ulnaris

Extensor
carpi radialis

brevis

longus

Extensor indicis

Ⓓ

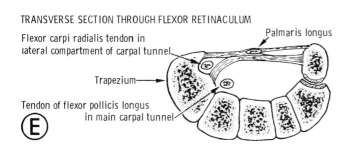

TRANSVERSE SECTION THROUGH FLEXOR RETINACULUM

Flexor carpi radialis tendon in
lateral compartment of carpal tunnel

Palmaris longus

Trapezium

Tendon of flexor pollicis longus
in main carpal tunnel

Ⓔ

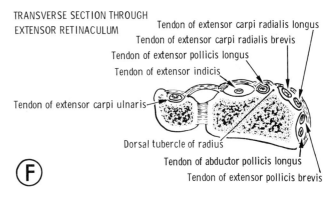

TRANSVERSE SECTION THROUGH
EXTENSOR RETINACULUM

Tendon of extensor carpi radialis longus

Tendon of extensor carpi radialis brevis

Tendon of extensor pollicis longus

Tendon of extensor indicis

Tendon of extensor carpi ulnaris

Dorsal tubercle of radius

Tendon of abductor pollicis longus

Tendon of extensor pollicis brevis

Ⓕ

The tendon of extensor pollicis longus (**551F**) leaves the forearm through the compartment of the extensor retinaculum on the medial side of the dorsal tubercle of the radius. It then passes obliquely in a distal and lateral direction, crossing the tendons of extensor carpi radialis longus and brevis and converging on the tendon of extensor pollicis brevis. Having crossed the dorsal aspects of the metacarpophalangeal and interphalangeal joints of the thumb, it is inserted into the base of the distal phalanx.

Observe in your own hand that, when the thumb is extended, its two extensor tendons stand out prominently under the skin, and outline a triangular depression known, traditionally, as the anatomical snuff box. The two radial carpal extensor tendons and the scaphoid bone lie in the floor of this depression (**551D**).

The adductor pollicis muscle is confined to the hand and arises by transverse and oblique heads (**A, B**). The former arises from the palmar aspect of the third metacarpal and its fibres converge in a lateral direction. The latter arises from the bases of the central metacarpals and the central distal carpal bones and passes distally and laterally. The two heads, which lie across the palmar aspects of the interossei of the first and second intermetacarpal spaces, are inserted, together with the first palmar interosseous, through the medial sesamoid of the first metacarpophalangeal joint, into the medial side of the proximal phalanx of the thumb.

The tendon of flexor pollicis longus passes into the palm through the lateral part of the main carpal tunnel (**551E**). Turning somewhat laterally it runs along the palmar aspect of the first metacarpal, lying in front of the adductor pollicis muscle, and enters the fibrous flexor sheath of the thumb (**A**). It is inserted into the base of the distal phalanx.

The opponens pollicis muscle, like the adductor pollicis and the two succeeding muscles, is confined to the hand. It arises from the lateral and distal corner of the flexor retinaculum, and passes obliquely across the tendon of flexor pollicis longus to be inserted into the whole length of the lateral aspect of the first metacarpal (**A**).

The flexor pollicis brevis muscle arises close to the opponens pollicis, runs anterior to the tendon of flexor pollicis longus and is inserted through the lateral sesamoid of the first metacarpophalangeal joint into the radial side of the proximal phalanx of the thumb (**B**).

The abductor pollicis brevis muscle arises from the proximal and lateral corner of the flexor retinaculum. It passes distally superficial to the opponens pollicis and is inserted with the flexor pollicis brevis into the lateral side of the base of the proximal phalanx of the thumb (**B**).

The thenar eminence is the name applied to the rounded elevation over the lateral and proximal corner of the palm which is produced by opponens pollicis, flexor pollicis brevis and abductor pollicis brevis. These three small muscles together with the adductor pollicis and the tendon of flexor pollicis longus occupy the thenar space of the palm (**249D**).

The actions of the muscles of the thumb, and the first palmar and dorsal interossei which are also attached to the bones of the thumb, are complicated by the fact that most cross more than one of the three joints in that digit. In the following description the actions of the muscles will be considered in relation to movements of the thumb as a whole, rather than in relation to isolated movements of individual joints.

1. *Opposition*, in which the thumb is carried across the palm and opposed to the other fingers (**C**), is the most common and most useful movement of the thumb. It is employed in such activities as gripping an object such as a cricket ball, picking up a small object between finger and thumb, and writing. It usually involves a) opposition at the first carpometacarpal joint (opponens pollicis), b) flexion at the metacarpophalangeal joint (the first palmar interosseous, flexor pollicis brevis and abductor pollicis brevis) and c) flexion at the interphalangeal joint (flexor pollicis longus).
2. *Reposition*, in which the thumb is moved laterally and backwards into the plane of the palm (**D**), is a much less common activity, but when it does occur it usually involves a) reposition at the carpometacarpal joint (abductor pollicis longus, extensor pollicis longus and extensor pollicis brevis) b) extension at the metacarpophalangeal joint (extensor pollicis longus and brevis) and c) extension at the interphalangeal joint (extensor pollicis longus).
3. *Adduction*, in which the thumb is carried backwards at right angles to the palm (**E**), occurs purely at the carpometacarpal joint. It is produced by adductor pollicis, the lateral head of the first dorsal interosseous and, because of the oblique course of its tendon, the extensor pollicis longus. Carry out this movement forcibly in your own hand and observe on the dorsum of the hand the taut tendon of extensor pollicis longus and the firm swelling between the first and second metacarpals caused by contraction of the first dorsal interosseous.
4. *Abduction*, in which the thumb is carried forwards at right angles to the palm (**F**), also occurs purely at the carpometacarpal joint. It is produced by abductor pollicis longus and brevis.

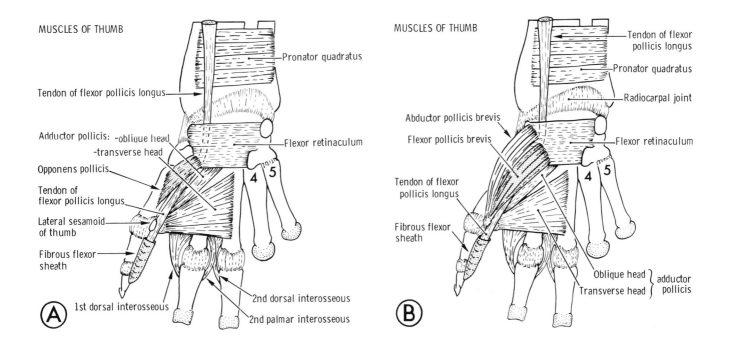

MUSCLES OF THUMB

Pronator quadratus

Tendon of flexor pollicis longus

Adductor pollicis: -oblique head
-transverse head

Opponens pollicis

Tendon of
flexor pollicis longus

Lateral sesamoid
of thumb

Fibrous flexor
sheath

Flexor retinaculum

4 5

1st dorsal interosseous

2nd dorsal interosseous

2nd palmar interosseous

(A)

MUSCLES OF THUMB

Tendon of flexor
pollicis longus

Pronator quadratus

Radiocarpal joint

Abductor pollicis brevis

Flexor pollicis brevis

Tendon of flexor
pollicis longus

Fibrous flexor
sheath

Flexor retinaculum

4 5

Oblique head } adductor
Transverse head } pollicis

(B)

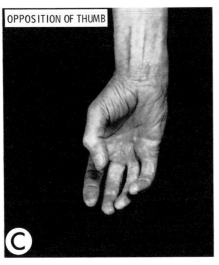

OPPOSITION OF THUMB

(C)

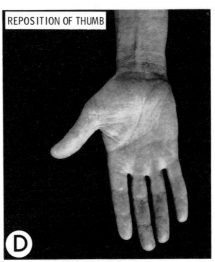

REPOSITION OF THUMB

(D)

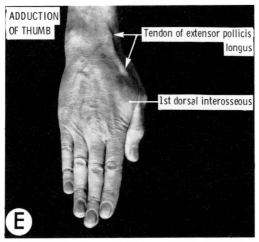

ADDUCTION
OF THUMB

Tendon of extensor pollicis
longus

1st dorsal interosseous

(E)

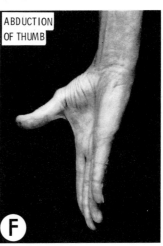

ABDUCTION
OF THUMB

(F)

The hypothenar muscles

These are a group of small muscles which occupy the hypothenar space of the palm. It should be noted that the names of some of them are not in keeping with their actions in man.

Opponens digiti minimi (**A**) arises from the distal, medial part of the flexor retinaculum and is inserted into the whole of the ulnar margin of the fifth metacarpal. As the geometry of the intermetacarpal and carpometacarpal joints of this bone severely restrict any rotatory movement, the effect of contraction of the muscle is to flex the metacarpal on the carpus. Observe in your own hand that the lateral rotation of the little finger which would result from any true voluntary opposition of the fifth metacarpal is impossible.

The flexor digiti minimi brevis arises from the distal medial part of the flexor retinaculum and the *abductor digiti minimi* from the proximal medial part of that structure (**B**). The two muscles converge to a common tendinous insertion into the medial side of the proximal phalanx of the little finger and into the medial side of its dorsal digital expansion (**557D**). The two muscles together are perhaps best regarded as being comparable to an additional dorsal interosseous muscle which flexes and adducts the metacarpophalangeal joint and has additional effects (**556**) through the dorsal digital expansion on the interphalangeal joints (**558**).

Palmaris brevis arises from the medial margin of the proximal part of the palmar aponeurosis and passes medially through the superficial fascia to be inserted into the skin at the medial margin of the palm. Contraction of the muscle elevates this area of skin and so deepens the concavity of the palm as when the palm is cupped to scoop up water.

The long flexor tendons of the medial four fingers

The four tendons of flexor digitorum profundus, which have already been described in the forearm (**527A & D**), pass into the hand through the posterior part of the main compartment of the carpal tunnel (**C**). They then diverge through the middle palmar space (**A, D**) dorsal to the tendons of flexor digitorum superficialis and in front of the interosseous fascia and adductor pollicis. Leaving the palm, they pass along the fibrous flexor sheaths of the medial four fingers (**E, F**) and are inserted into the bases of the distal phalanges.

The lumbrical muscles are four small muscles which arise in the palm from the tendons of flexor digitorum profundus and are numbered from lateral to medial (**A**). The first and second are unipennate and arise from the radial sides of the corresponding profundus tendons. The third and fourth are bipennate and arise from two adjacent profundus tendons. The tendon of the first muscle passes across the lateral aspect of the second metacarpophalangeal joint, while the other three pass through the three lumbrical canals (**549C**) so that they are separated from the tendons of the interossei by the deep transverse metacarpal ligament (**E**). The tendons then turn dorsally and medially and join the lateral edges of the dorsal digital expansions of the medial four digits (**557C, 557D**).

The four tendons of flexor digitorum superficialis pass through the main compartment of the carpal tunnel (**C**) anterior to those of flexor digitorum profundus. Diverging through the middle palmar space, deep to the palmar aponeurosis (**B**), the tendons enter the fibrous flexor sheaths of the four medial fingers on the palmar aspects of the tendons of the profundus muscle (**E, F**). Over the proximal phalanges each superficialis tendon divides into two parts which pass round the sides of the profundus tendon and re-unite dorsal to it before inserting into the middle phalanx (**F**).

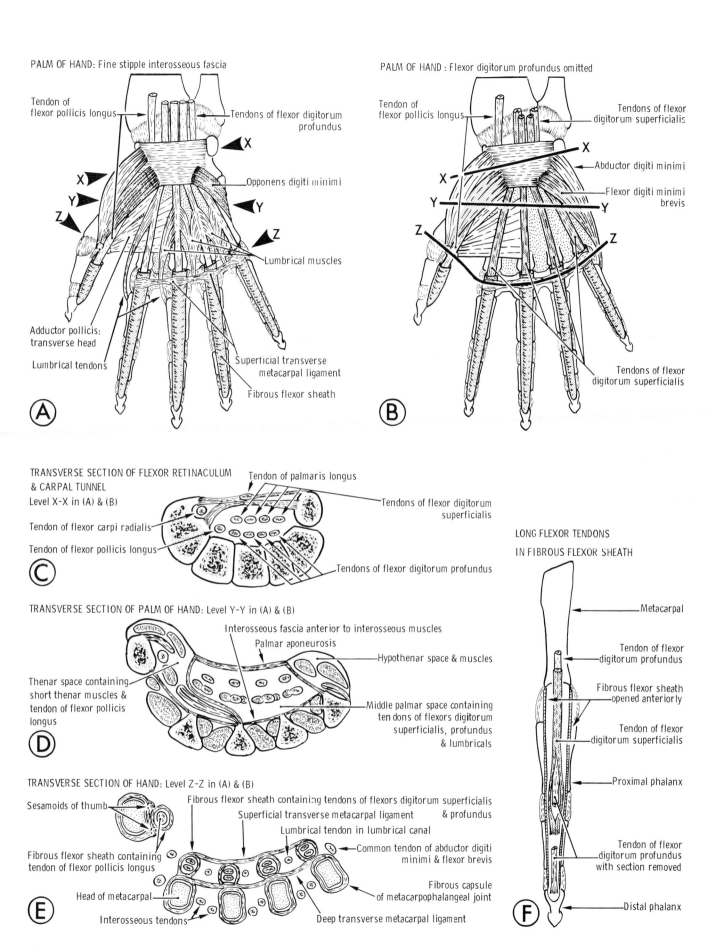

PALM OF HAND: Fine stipple interosseous fascia

Tendon of flexor pollicis longus

Tendons of flexor digitorum profundus

Opponens digiti minimi

Lumbrical muscles

Adductor pollicis: transverse head

Lumbrical tendons

Superficial transverse metacarpal ligament

Fibrous flexor sheath

Ⓐ

PALM OF HAND: Flexor digitorum profundus omitted

Tendon of flexor pollicis longus

Tendons of flexor digitorum superficialis

Abductor digiti minimi

Flexor digiti minimi brevis

Tendons of flexor digitorum superficialis

Ⓑ

TRANSVERSE SECTION OF FLEXOR RETINACULUM & CARPAL TUNNEL
Level X-X in (A) & (B)

Tendon of palmaris longus

Tendons of flexor digitorum superficialis

Tendon of flexor carpi radialis

Tendon of flexor pollicis longus

Tendons of flexor digitorum profundus

Ⓒ

TRANSVERSE SECTION OF PALM OF HAND: Level Y-Y in (A) & (B)

Interosseous fascia anterior to interosseous muscles

Palmar aponeurosis

Hypothenar space & muscles

Thenar space containing short thenar muscles & tendon of flexor pollicis longus

Middle palmar space containing tendons of flexors digitorum superficialis, profundus & lumbricals

Ⓓ

TRANSVERSE SECTION OF HAND: Level Z-Z in (A) & (B)

Sesamoids of thumb

Fibrous flexor sheath containing tendons of flexors digitorum superficialis & profundus

Superficial transverse metacarpal ligament

Lumbrical tendon in lumbrical canal

Common tendon of abductor digiti minimi & flexor brevis

Fibrous flexor sheath containing tendon of flexor pollicis longus

Fibrous capsule of metacarpophalangeal joint

Head of metacarpal

Interosseous tendons

Deep transverse metacarpal ligament

Ⓔ

LONG FLEXOR TENDONS
IN FIBROUS FLEXOR SHEATH

Metacarpal

Tendon of flexor digitorum profundus

Fibrous flexor sheath opened anteriorly

Tendon of flexor digitorum superficialis

Proximal phalanx

Tendon of flexor digitorum profundus with section removed

Distal phalanx

Ⓕ

The long extensor tendons of the medial four fingers

Observe in your own hand that full extension of one finger while the others are fully flexed is possible only in the index and little fingers. The individuality of the index finger is necessary for pointing, while the similar individuality of the little finger has been explained on the grounds that it facilitates cleaning out the external acoustic meatus! It will be seen below that in conformity with this functional arrangement, the extensor digitorum muscle gives tendons to each of the four medial fingers, while the index and little fingers each have an additional extensor muscle.

The four tendons of extensor digitorum pass side by side through a compartment of the extensor retinaculum which lies on the dorsal aspect of the lower end of the radius to the medial side of the dorsal tubercle (**A, 529E**). They then diverge across the dorsum of the hand, where they are usually joined to one another by three fibrous inter-tendinous connections (**A**), and reach the dorsal digital expansions (see below) on the medial four fingers.

The tendon of extensor indicis passes, deep to the four tendons of extensor digitorum, through the same compart-ment of the extensor retinaculum. It then passes across the dorsal aspect of the hand on the medial side of the most lateral tendon of extensor digitorum (**A**), and fuses with that tendon in the dorsal digital expansion on the index finger.

The tendon of extensor digiti minimi passes through its own compartment of the extensor retinaculum on the posterior aspect of the inferior radio-ulnar joint. On the dorsum of the hand it runs medial to the medial tendon of extensor digitorum (**A**) and the two tendons join the dorsal digital expansion on the little finger.

The dorsal digital expansions of the medial four fingers

Each expansion is a thin aponeurotic sheet of elongated triangular shape with a distal apex and a proximal base (**B**). It overlies the dorsal aspects of the bones and joints of the corresponding finger. The expansion is firmly attached to the bases of the three phalanges but elsewhere it is loosely attached and can move on the underlying structures. The base of the expansion is displaced distally in relation to the bones of the fingers when the finger joints are flexed (**F**) and proximally when the same joints are extended (**E**). The extremities of the base of the expansion, which may be called the basal processes, curl forwards round the meta-carpophalangeal joint (**E, F**), and are firmly attached to the fibrous capsule and the deep transverse metacarpal liga-ment. The firm attachment of these processes imposes a limit on the range through which the base of expansion can be proximally displaced (**E**).

The long extensor tendon or tendons of each finger are incorporated into the corresponding digital expansion at the centre of its base (**C, D**). The deep fibres of the tendon are attached to the base of the proximal phalanx. The superficial fibres divide over the proximal phalanx into a central and two marginal bands which lie in the substance of the expansion (**C, D**). The central band is attached to the base of the middle phalanx while the marginal bands re-unite and are inserted into the base of the distal phalanx.

The tendons of either one or two short muscles of the fingers join both margins of the expansion just distal to the basal processes. The short muscles which join the expan-sion on the middle finger are shown in **C** and from the previous descriptions of the interosseous (**551A, 551B**) and lumbrical muscles (**555A**) it is easy for the student to work out which short muscles are attached to the expansions on the index and ring fingers. In the case of the little finger expansion (**D**), the medial margin is formed by the fused tendons of the abductor and the short flexor instead of by an interosseous muscle.

On either side the fibres of these tendons diverge through the substance of the expansion as three projections (**C**).

1. The most proximal group run transversely and, joining the corresponding fibres from the other margin of the expansion, form a sling over the dorsum of the proximal phalanx.
2. A second projection blends with the central band of the superficial fibres of the long extensor tendon and are thus inserted into the base of the middle phalanx.
3. A third blends with the corresponding marginal band of the long extensor tendon and are thereby inserted into the base of the distal phalanx.

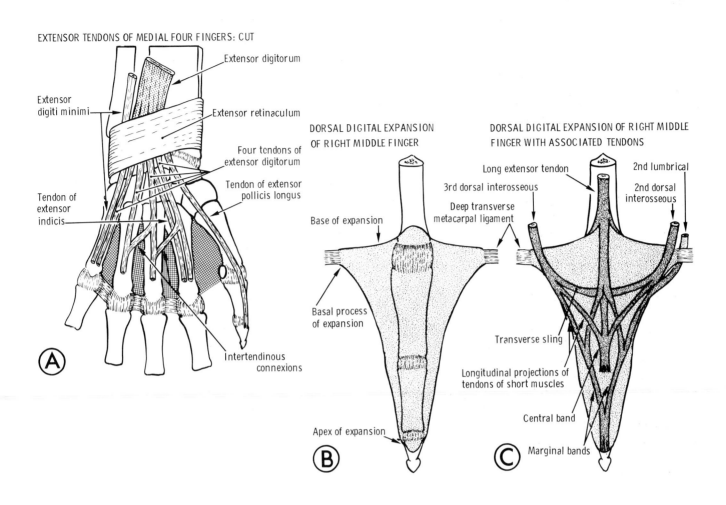

EXTENSOR TENDONS OF MEDIAL FOUR FINGERS: CUT

Extensor digiti minimi

Extensor digitorum

Extensor retinaculum

Four tendons of extensor digitorum

Tendon of extensor pollicis longus

Tendon of extensor indicis

Intertendinous connexions

(A)

DORSAL DIGITAL EXPANSION OF RIGHT MIDDLE FINGER

Base of expansion

Basal process of expansion

Apex of expansion

(B)

DORSAL DIGITAL EXPANSION OF RIGHT MIDDLE FINGER WITH ASSOCIATED TENDONS

Long extensor tendon

3rd dorsal interosseous

Deep transverse metacarpal ligament

2nd lumbrical

2nd dorsal interosseous

Transverse sling

Longitudinal projections of tendons of short muscles

Central band

Marginal bands

(C)

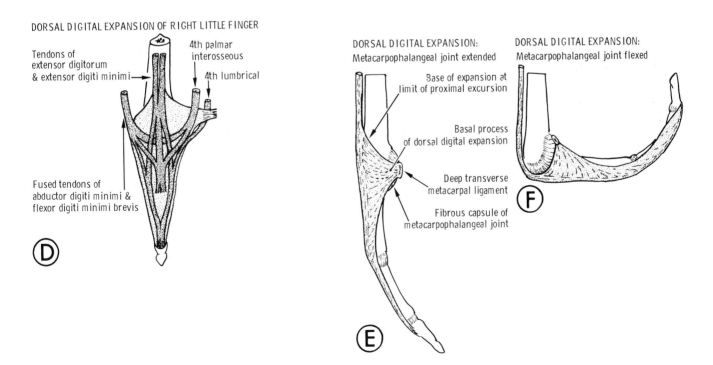

DORSAL DIGITAL EXPANSION OF RIGHT LITTLE FINGER

Tendons of extensor digitorum & extensor digiti minimi

4th palmar interosseous

4th lumbrical

Fused tendons of abductor digiti minimi & flexor digiti minimi brevis

(D)

DORSAL DIGITAL EXPANSION: Metacarpophalangeal joint extended

Base of expansion at limit of proximal excursion

Basal process of dorsal digital expansion

Deep transverse metacarpal ligament

Fibrous capsule of metacarpophalangeal joint

(E)

DORSAL DIGITAL EXPANSION: Metacarpophalangeal joint flexed

(F)

The movements of the medial four fingers

Three groups of muscles are concerned in movements of these fingers. These are the long flexors (flexor digitorum profundus and superficialis (**527A, 527C**), the short muscles (the interosseous except the first palmar, the lumbricals and the abductor and short flexor of the little finger (**551, 555**)) and the long extensors (extensor digitorum, extensor indicis and extensor digiti minimi (**557A**)).

Adduction and abduction of the fingers on their metacarpals (**544**) are produced by those short muscles which are inserted into the medial and lateral margins of the dorsal digital expansions (**556**). It will be recalled that in this text, in contrast to general practice, adduction refers to medial movement of a finger and abduction to lateral movement (**544**) and that both movements become severely restricted when flexion tightens the collateral ligaments of the metacarpophalangeal joints (**557E, 557F**).

Flexion of a finger occurs at three joint levels. The distal and proximal interphalangeal joints are flexed by flexor digitorum profundus and superficialis respectively. The main flexors of the metacarpophalangeal joint are the short muscles. These pass in front of the transverse axis of the joint and exert a force on the dorsum of the proximal phalanges through the transverse sling which they form in the dorsal digital (**A**) expansion.

Extension of a finger involves the long extensor and the short muscles both of which are incorporated into the dorsal digital expansion of the digit.

1. Extension at the metacarpophalangeal joint is produced solely by the deep fibres of the long extensor tendon inserted into the base of the proximal phalanx.
2. The superficial fibres of the long extensors, through their projections in the dorsal expansion, can extend both interphalangeal joints. However, full extension of these joints is only possible when the metacarpophalangeal joint is flexed (**B**), for in those circumstances a considerable proximal displacement of the base of the expansion is possible (**557E, 557F**). When the metacarpophalangeal joint is extended (**C**) proximal displacement of the base of the expansion is limited when the interphalangeal joints are only partially extended.
3. The short muscles' tendons are connected, within the dorsal expansion, to the central and marginal bands of the superficial fibres of the long extensor tendon. When the metacarpophalangeal joint is flexed, the short muscles are already fully shortened and cannot therefore exert the tension through their projections which would be necessary to extend the interphalangeal joints (**A**). On the other hand, extension at the metacarpophalangeal joint stretches the short muscles and they can then contract sufficiently to extend the interphalangeal joints fully (**D**).
4. Thus in the normal hand extension of a finger at the metacarpophalangeal joint is produced only by the long extensor or extensors of that digit. Extension at the interphalangeal joints is produced by the long extensor alone when the metacarpophalangeal joint is flexed, but to a progressively increasing degree by the short muscles as the metacarpophalangeal joint is progressively extended.
5. If the short muscles of a finger are paralysed as in simultaneous lesions of the median and ulnar nerves, the long extensors, in the absence of antagonistic tone in the short muscles, hyperextend the metacarpophalangeal joint. Furthermore because of the failure of the short muscles to exert longitudinal tension in the dorsal digital expansion, the long extensor can only partially extend the interphalangeal joints (**E**). This produces the claw-like position of the finger characteristic of this double nerve lesion.
6. If the long extensors are paralysed as in a lesion of the radial nerve or its deep branch, the interphalangeal joints can still be fully extended by the short muscles provided that the metacarpophalangeal joint is passively fixed in full extension (**D**).

The synovial sheaths of the hand

As the long tendons which move the fingers and thumb pass beneath the several retaining bands which hold them in place, they are protected from the effects of friction by enclosure in synovial sheaths.

The synovial sheaths of the extensor tendons line the several compartments beneath the extensor retinaculum. Examine these sheaths in **F** and note that, while three contain single tendons, the other three enclose groups of tendons, namely, the four tendons of extensor digitorum and that of extensor indicis, the tendons of extensor carpi radialis longus and brevis and the tendons of abductor pollicis longus and extensor pollicis brevis. The sheaths extend less than 1 cm proximal to the retinaculum and as far as the bases of the metacarpals in a distal direction. It is to be noted that, unlike the flexor tendons, the extensor tendons have no synovial sheaths in the fingers.

FLEXION OF METACARPOPHALANGEAL JOINT
BY SHORT MUSCLES

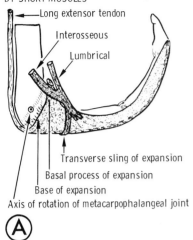

Long extensor tendon
Interosseous
Lumbrical
Transverse sling of expansion
Basal process of expansion
Base of expansion
Axis of rotation of metacarpophalangeal joint

(A)

EXTENSION OF INTERPHALANGEAL JOINTS
BY LONG EXTENSORS

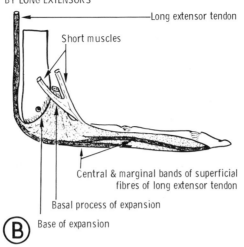

Long extensor tendon
Short muscles
Central & marginal bands of superficial
fibres of long extensor tendon
Basal process of expansion
Base of expansion

(B)

EXTENSION OF METACARPOPHALANGEAL
JOINT BY LONG EXTENSORS

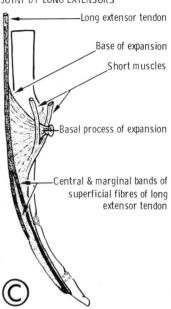

Long extensor tendon
Base of expansion
Short muscles
Basal process of expansion
Central & marginal bands of
superficial fibres of long
extensor tendon

(C)

EXTENSION OF INTERPHALANGEAL
JOINTS BY SHORT MUSCLES

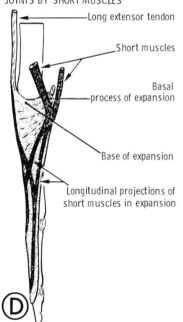

Long extensor tendon
Short muscles
Basal process of expansion
Base of expansion
Longitudinal projections of
short muscles in expansion

(D)

EXTENSION OF FINGER BY LONG
EXTENSOR: SHORT MUSCLES PARALYSED

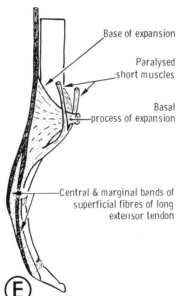

Base of expansion
Paralysed short muscles
Basal process of expansion
Central & marginal bands of
superficial fibres of long
extensor tendon

(E)

SYNOVIAL SHEATHS OF RIGHT EXTENSOR TENDONS

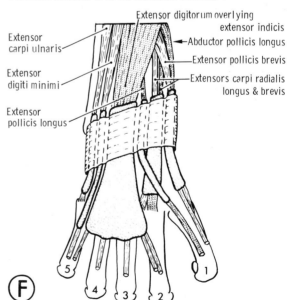

Extensor digitorum overlying
extensor indicis
Extensor carpi ulnaris
Extensor digiti minimi
Extensor pollicis longus
Abductor pollicis longus
Extensor pollicis brevis
Extensors carpi radialis
longus & brevis

5 4 3 2 1

(F)

The synovial sheaths of the carpal tunnel are associated with the flexor tendons which pass beneath the flexor retinaculum (**B**). Each extends for 2–3 cm into the forearm (**A**).

1. One sheath encloses the tendon of flexor carpi radialis as it passes through the subsidiary lateral compartment of the carpal tunnel to its insertion into the bases of the second and third metacarpals (**A, B**).

2. Another encloses the tendon of flexor pollicis longus as it traverses the lateral part of the main compartment of the carpal tunnel (**B**). The same sheath continues to surround the tendon as it passes along the palmar aspect of the first metacarpal and thereafter through the fibrous flexor sheath of the thumb to its insertion into the distal phalanx. The whole long sheath is often called the radial bursa (**A**).

3. In the main compartment of the carpal tunnel the tendons of flexor digitorum profundus and superficialis invaginate a large common sheath from the lateral side (**B**). A diverticulum protrudes from the medial part of the sheath for a variable distance between the superficial and deep tendons. The sheath continues distal to the retinaculum into the middle palmar space of the hand, enclosing the same tendons and also the proximal parts of the lumbrical muscles (**A**). The greater part of the sheath, which is associated with flexor tendons to the index, middle and ring fingers, ends at about the middle of the metacarpal bones. On the other hand the medial part, which is associated with the flexor tendons of the little finger, is continuous with the digital synovial sheath (see below) of that digit (**A**). The long sheath resulting from this continuity is often known as the ulnar bursa. In many individuals a narrow communication exists between the radial and ulnar bursae in the carpal tunnel.

The digital synovial sheaths enclose the long flexor tendons within the fibrous flexor sheaths (**555E**) of the medial four fingers (**A**). Those of the index, middle and ring fingers extend beyond the fibrous flexor sheaths for 1 cm or so into the palm, but are discontinuous with the ulnar bursa. On the other hand, as has been noted, the digital sheath of the little finger is part of the ulnar bursa and is thus continuous with the common flexor sheath in the carpal tunnel. The superficialis and profundus tendons in each sheath are completely invested by separate visceral layers of synovial membrane (**C**). In this isolated situation

they receive their blood supplies through vessels which run through narrow synovial tubes connecting the parietal to the two visceral layers of the sheath (**C**). These vascular connections are known as vincula.

Penetrating wounds of the fingers or palm may carry infection into the digital synovial sheaths or the radial or ulnar bursae, throughout which the inflammatory process spreads rapidly. The greater danger of such infections is that, by causing thrombosis of the vessels in the vincula, they may cause death of tendons within their sheaths, and adhesion of the tendon remnants to the parietal synovial membrane, with resultant loss of movement.

The arteries of the hand

The hand is supplied by the radial and ulnar arteries which have already been described in the forearm (**532**). In the hand these arteries or their branches join end to end without the intervention of capillary plexuses to form three arterial arches from which digital arteries supply the fingers including the thumb. Two features of these arches will be evident from their mode of formation. First, division of such an arch causes arterial bleeding from both cut ends so that control of haemorrhage may require ligature of both ends. Secondly the arches have no exact limits.

The dorsal carpal arch which is small compared to the two palmar arches extends more or less transversely across the dorsum of the carpus, deep to the long extensor tendons as they emerge from the extensor retinaculum (**563C**).

The superficial palmar arch passes across the palm along a course which is convex distally and reaches the level of the distal margin of the thenar eminence of the extended thumb (**563B**). It is deep to the palmar aponeurosis and the palmaris brevis muscle and superficial to the long flexor tendons of the medial four fingers the lumbricals and the synovial ulnar bursa.

The deep palmar arch follows a course across the palm and is situated 1 cm proximal to the superficial arch (**563A**). The vessel lies on the palmar aspects of the second, third and fourth metacarpals and their associated interossei, and passes between the transverse and oblique heads of adductor pollicis. It is dorsal to the long flexor tendons of the fingers and the ulnar synovial bursa (**563B**).

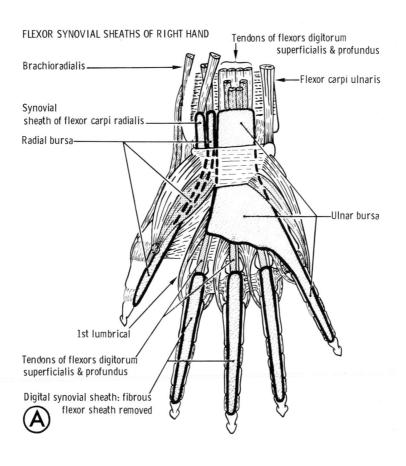

FLEXOR SYNOVIAL SHEATHS OF RIGHT HAND

Brachioradialis

Tendons of flexors digitorum superficialis & profundus

Synovial sheath of flexor carpi radialis

Flexor carpi ulnaris

Radial bursa

Ulnar bursa

1st lumbrical

Tendons of flexors digitorum superficialis & profundus

Digital synovial sheath: fibrous flexor sheath removed

(A)

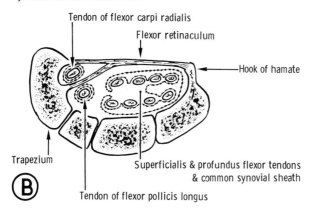

SYNOVIAL SHEATHS IN CARPAL TUNNEL:
Synovial membrane dotted lines

Tendon of flexor carpi radialis

Flexor retinaculum

Hook of hamate

Trapezium

Superficialis & profundus flexor tendons & common synovial sheath

Tendon of flexor pollicis longus

(B)

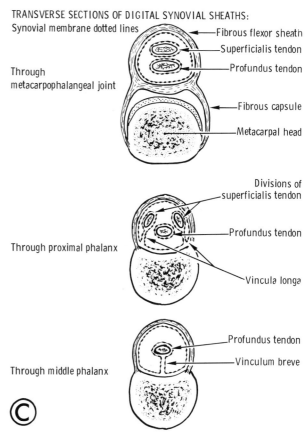

TRANSVERSE SECTIONS OF DIGITAL SYNOVIAL SHEATHS:
Synovial membrane dotted lines

Fibrous flexor sheath

Superficialis tendon

Profundus tendon

Through metacarpophalangeal joint

Fibrous capsule

Metacarpal head

Divisions of superficialis tendon

Profundus tendon

Through proximal phalanx

Vincula longa

Profundus tendon

Vinculum breve

Through middle phalanx

(C)

561

The radial artery

As has been seen (**533D**), in the distal part of the forearm this vessel lies on the anterior surface of the radius lateral to the tendon of flexor carpi radialis which is palpable and usually visible. Immediately distal to the radius the artery turns backwards (**A**) between the lateral aspect of the radiocarpal joint and the tendons of abductor pollicis longus and extensor pollicis brevis. It then passes distally on the dorsal aspects of the scaphoid and trapezium in the floor of the anatomical snuff box and is crossed obliquely by the tendon of extensor pollicis longus (**B**). A short distance beyond this tendon the artery turns forwards, through the first intermetacarpal space and between the two heads of the first dorsal interosseous muscle, to reach the palm of the hand. Here it joins the lateral end of the deep palmar arch (**A**).

The superficial palmar branch arises from the radial artery while it is still on the anterior aspect of the radius and runs distally through the muscles of the thenar eminence to join the lateral end of the superficial palmar arch (**B**).

The dorsal carpal branch arises from the radial artery while it is in the anatomical snuff box and immediately turns medially to join the dorsal carpal arch (**C**).

The ulnar artery

It will be recalled (**533D**) that at the distal end of the forearm, this artery is situated beneath the deep fascia on the lateral side of the tendon of flexor carpi ulnaris (**A, B**). It continues into the hand superficial to the flexor retinaculum and lateral to the pisiform bone and becomes the major tributary of the superficial palmar arch (**B**).

The dorsal carpal branch takes origin from the artery a short distance proximal to the pisiform and the flexor retinaculum. It winds backwards between the medial aspect of the radiocarpal joint and the tendons of flexor and extensor carpi ulnaris, and becomes continuous with the dorsal carpal arch (**A, B, C**).

The deep palmar branch arises superficial to the flexor retinaculum and passes deeply, first in a medial direction through the hypothenar muscles and then distally on the medial side of the hook of the hamate. At the distal border of the hook it becomes continuous with the deep palmar arch (**A**).

The digital arteries

Longitudinal vessels run distally from the three arterial arches described above. After being linked to one another in a complex fashion, these vessels pass onto the sides of the digits as palmar and dorsal digital arteries. The dorsal arteries are small and extend only as far as the proximal interphalangeal joints. The palmar arteries are larger and supply the whole of the palmar aspects of the digits and the distal parts of their dorsal aspects.

The venous drainage of the hand

Both sides of each digit are drained by dorsal and palmar digital veins. The dorsal veins join the dorsal venous network on the dorsum of the hand (**531A**) which in turn gives rise proximally to the basilic and cephalic veins. The palmar digital veins also drain predominantly into the dorsal plexus through vessels which pass dorsally between the metacarpophalangeal joints, but they are also in communication with a finer venous network lying between the palmar aponeurosis and the overlying skin.

The vessels of the palm are drained into the venae comitantes of the two palmar arches which become continuous medially and laterally with the ulnar and radial venae comitantes.

The innervation of the hand

The structures of the hand are innervated by the ulnar and median nerves and the superficial branch of the radial nerve. The courses of these nerves in the forearm (**536**) should be revised.

The superficial branch of the radial nerve

The nerve parts company from the radial artery in the distal part of the forearm and winds backwards deep to the brachioradialis tendon (**537B**). It then pierces the deep fascia a short distance above the wrist (**D**) and divides into four dorsal digital branches. These are usually distributed to the area shown in (**D, E**) but in some individuals they also supply the adjacent halves of the dorsal aspects of the middle and ring fingers.

Note the following points.

1. The radial nerve supplies none of the short muscles of the hand. In particular, it does not supply any of the dorsal interosseous muscles.
2. Although the nerve is distributed largely to the dorsum of the hand, some twigs curl round the lateral border of the thumb and supply the skin over the lateral part of the thenar eminence (**E**).
3. The digital nerves do not extend as far as the regions around the nail beds, which are supplied by palmar digital branches of the median nerve (**565D**).
4. Several of the branches of the nerve can be palpated as narrow cords over the tendon of extensor pollicis longus when the thumb is actively extended (**D**).

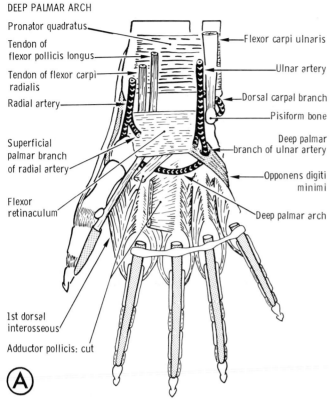

DEEP PALMAR ARCH

- Pronator quadratus
- Tendon of flexor pollicis longus
- Tendon of flexor carpi radialis
- Radial artery
- Superficial palmar branch of radial artery
- Flexor retinaculum
- 1st dorsal interosseous
- Adductor pollicis: cut

- Flexor carpi ulnaris
- Ulnar artery
- Dorsal carpal branch
- Pisiform bone
- Deep palmar branch of ulnar artery
- Opponens digiti minimi
- Deep palmar arch

(A)

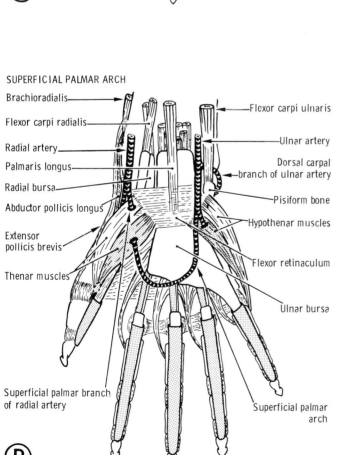

SUPERFICIAL PALMAR ARCH

- Brachioradialis
- Flexor carpi radialis
- Radial artery
- Palmaris longus
- Radial bursa
- Abductor pollicis longus
- Extensor pollicis brevis
- Thenar muscles
- Superficial palmar branch of radial artery

- Flexor carpi ulnaris
- Ulnar artery
- Dorsal carpal branch of ulnar artery
- Pisiform bone
- Hypothenar muscles
- Flexor retinaculum
- Ulnar bursa
- Superficial palmar arch

(B)

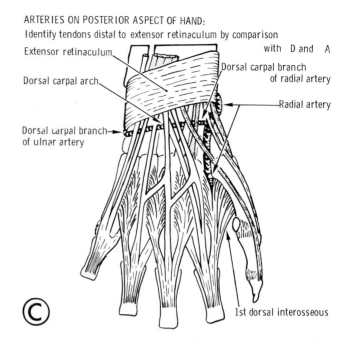

ARTERIES ON POSTERIOR ASPECT OF HAND:
Identify tendons distal to extensor retinaculum by comparison
with D and A

- Extensor retinaculum
- Dorsal carpal arch
- Dorsal carpal branch of ulnar artery
- Dorsal carpal branch of radial artery
- Radial artery
- 1st dorsal interosseous

(C)

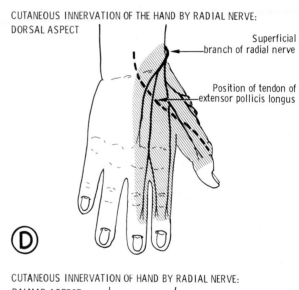

CUTANEOUS INNERVATION OF THE HAND BY RADIAL NERVE:
DORSAL ASPECT

- Superficial branch of radial nerve
- Position of tendon of extensor pollicis longus

(D)

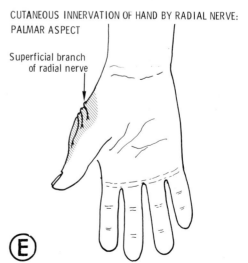

CUTANEOUS INNERVATION OF HAND BY RADIAL NERVE:
PALMAR ASPECT

- Superficial branch of radial nerve

(E)

The median nerve in the hand

Leaving the forearm (**A**), the nerve passes deep to the centre of the flexor retinaculum, lying in the main compartment of the carpal tunnel on the palmar aspect of the tendons of flexor digitorum superficialis and their common synovial sheath (**C**). Note the slight change in the relationship of the nerve to the tendons between the levels of **A** and **C**. Emerging from the carpal tunnel, the nerve divides abruptly into its terminal branches (**A**).

The palmar cutaneous branch arises just above the flexor retinaculum and pierces the deep fascia to the lateral side of the tendon of palmaris longus (**A**). Thereafter it runs distally, supplying the area of skin shown in **E**.

The main motor branch separates from the parent nerve at the distal border of the flexor retinaculum and turns proximally into the short muscles of the thenar eminence (**A**). It may supply all these muscles, namely, opponens pollicis, abductor pollicis brevis and flexor pollicis brevis, but it is to be noted that in a large proportion of the population the last muscle is wholly or partly innervated by the deep branch of the ulnar nerve.

The five palmar digital branches which originate at the distal border of the flexor retinaculum are distributed in the manner shown in **A**. Observe in **E** and **D** the area of skin which these nerves supply, particularly their distribution of dorsal twigs to the region of the nail beds and note their following features.

1. In the palm they run distally deep to the superficial palmar arch.
2. Further distally they incline forwards, so that in the fingers they lie in front of the palmar digital arteries.
3. The nerves which are directed to the clefts between the second, third, and fourth digits pass from the palm to the fingers through the corresponding lumbrical canals (**549C**) in front of the lumbrical tendons.
4. The two nerves which pass to the lateral side of the index finger and to the cleft between the index and middle fingers supply motor branches to the first and second lumbrical muscles.

The ulnar nerve in the hand

The ulnar nerve passes into the hand superficial to the flexor retinaculum, lying between the ulnar artery and the pisiform bone and deep to the deep fascia and palmaris brevis muscle (**A, B, C**). Opposite the interval between the pisiform and the hook of the hamate it ends by dividing into superficial and deep branches.

The dorsal branch arises from the ulnar nerve some 5 cm above the wrist (**A, 537A**). Passing deep to the tendon of flexor carpi ulnaris it winds backwards round the lower end of the ulna and pierces the deep fascia to supply the area of skin shown in **D**. Note that usually the distributions of the dorsal branch of the ulnar and the superficial branch of the radial nerve on the dorsum of the hand are more or less symmetrical, though variations are not uncommon. Observe also that neither nerve supplies the distal parts of the fingers.

The palmar cutaneous branch of the ulnar nerve, which arises proximal to the flexor retinaculum, pierces the deep fascia and runs distally (**A**) to supply the area of skin shown in **E**.

The superficial terminal branch of the ulnar nerve (**A**) supplies the palmaris brevis muscle and continues distally into the palm as two palmar digital branches. Observe the distribution of the latter nerves in **E** and **D**, particularly the distribution of dorsal twigs to the regions of the nail beds, and note the following features.

1. Like the palmar digital branches of the median nerve, those of the ulnar nerve lie in front of corresponding arteries in the fingers.
2. Unlike the palmar digital branches of the median nerve, they do not supply any lumbrical muscles.
3. The nerve passing to the cleft between the ring and little fingers traverses the corresponding lumbrical canal.
4. The adjacent palmar digital branches of the ulnar and median nerves are joined by a connecting loop (**A**).
5. The symmetry of the cutaneous distributions of the ulnar and radial nerves on the dorsum of the hand is not present in the distributions of the ulnar and median nerves on the palmar aspect. Here the median nerve supplies the palmar aspects of three and a half fingers and the ulnar the palmar aspects of one and a half.

The deep terminal branch of the ulnar nerve accompanies the deep branch of the corresponding artery and the deep palmar arch across the palm of the hand. Follow its course in **B**. It passes deeply through the origins of the hypothenar muscles and turns round the distal border of the hook of the hamate. It then runs laterally between the interossei and the long flexor tendons of the medial four fingers and between the two heads of adductor pollicis, to the interval between the first and second metacarpals.

This is the main motor nerve to the short muscles of the hand, supplying the hypothenar muscles, all the interossei, adductor pollicis, the medial two lumbricals, and in most individuals innervating wholly or in part the flexor pollicis brevis. Contrast this with the distribution of the median nerve to the abductor pollicis brevis, opponens pollicis and the lateral two lumbricals, and the purely cutaneous distribution in the hand of the radial nerve.

NERVES OF PALM: Identify unlabelled structures by comparison with B

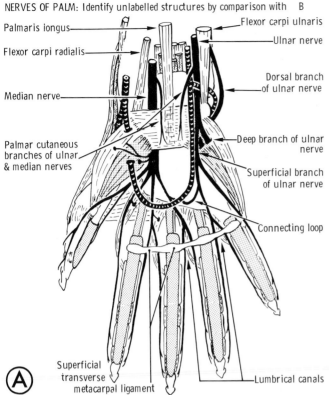

Palmaris longus

Flexor carpi radialis

Median nerve

Palmar cutaneous branches of ulnar & median nerves

Flexor carpi ulnaris

Ulnar nerve

Dorsal branch of ulnar nerve

Deep branch of ulnar nerve

Superficial branch of ulnar nerve

Connecting loop

Superficial transverse metacarpal ligament

Lumbrical canals

Ⓐ

FLEXOR RETINACULUM: Synovial membrane dotted lines

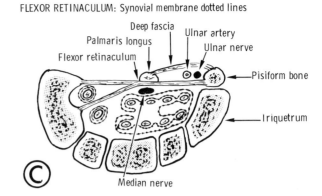

Deep fascia

Palmaris longus

Flexor retinaculum

Ulnar artery

Ulnar nerve

Pisiform bone

Triquetrum

Median nerve

Ⓒ

CUTANEOUS INNERVATION OF HAND: DORSAL ASPECT

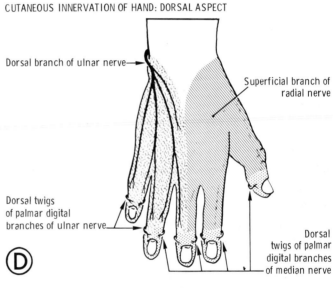

Dorsal branch of ulnar nerve

Superficial branch of radial nerve

Dorsal twigs of palmar digital branches of ulnar nerve

Dorsal twigs of palmar digital branches of median nerve

Ⓓ

DEEP BRANCH OF ULNAR NERVE:
Identify unlabelled structures by comparison with   A

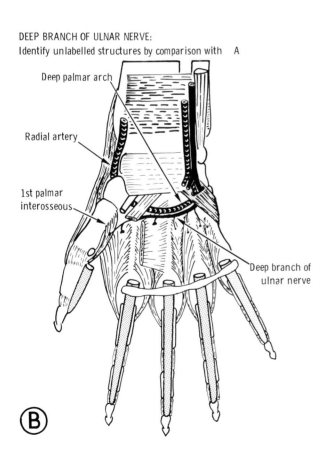

Deep palmar arch

Radial artery

1st palmar interosseous

Deep branch of ulnar nerve

Ⓑ

CUTANEOUS INNERVATION OF HAND: PALMAR ASPECT

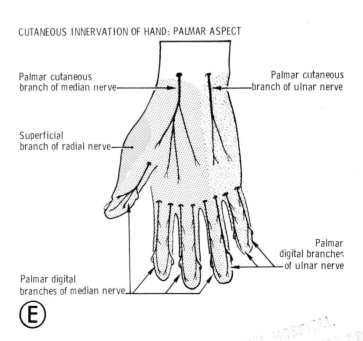

Palmar cutaneous branch of median nerve

Palmar cutaneous branch of ulnar nerve

Superficial branch of radial nerve

Palmar digital branches of ulnar nerve

Palmar digital branches of median nerve

Ⓔ

565

THE AUTONOMIC NERVE SUPPLY TO THE UPPER LIMB

The autonomic supply to the upper limb consists solely of two-neuron sympathetic pathways which innervate the involuntary muscle in the walls of its blood vessels and the sweat glands of the covering skin.

The preganglionic fibres arise from nerve cells in the lateral cell column of the central grey matter of the spinal cord, from the third to the sixth thoracic segments inclusive. Passing by way of the corresponding spinal nerves and their white rami communicantes, the fibres reach the corresponding ganglia on the sympathetic trunk. In the trunk the majority ascend to higher levels and synapse with postganglionic neurons in the upper three thoracic ganglia and the middle and inferior cervical ganglia (**A**).

These postganglionic fibres leave the sympathetic ganglia in which they arise in two ways.

1. Direct vascular branches pass from the upper three thoracic ganglia on to the wall of the subclavian artery and form a peri-arterial plexus on that vessel and the axillary artery.

2. Grey rami communicantes pass from the middle cervical ganglion to the ventral rami of C5 and 6, from the inferior cervical ganglion to the ventral rami of C7 and 8 and from the first thoracic ganglion to the ventral ramus of T1. These postganglionic fibres run through the brachial plexus and eventually enter all of its branches. The fibres in the cutaneous branches innervate sweat glands and superficial vessels. The major deep arteries of the limb below the junction of the axillary and brachial receive their sympathetic supply through small twigs from the nerves which lie adjacent to them. Thus the brachial artery is innervated from the median nerve, the radial artery from the superficial branch of the radial nerve and the ulnar artery and the deep palmar arch from the ulnar nerve.

Sympathetic denervation of the upper limb is sometimes employed to alleviate the symptoms of Raynaud's disease, a condition in which spasm of the arteries is brought on by emotion or cold. It has been recognised for many years that interruption of the postganglionic neurons by removal of ganglia from the sympathetic trunk or by stripping the adventitial coat from the major blood vessels results, within a short time, in an increased susceptibility of the structures supplied to circulating adrenaline, and consequently in a recurrence of symptoms. Denervation is therefore usually achieved by division of the third thoracic white ramus and the sympathetic trunk between the third and fourth thoracic ganglia (**B**). This interrupts all the preganglionic fibres concerned in the innervation of the upper limb. On the other hand, it does not affect the preganglionic fibres which join the sympathetic trunk through the first and second thoracic white rami and are concerned in the sympathetic innervation of most of the structures in the head and neck, particularly the eye.

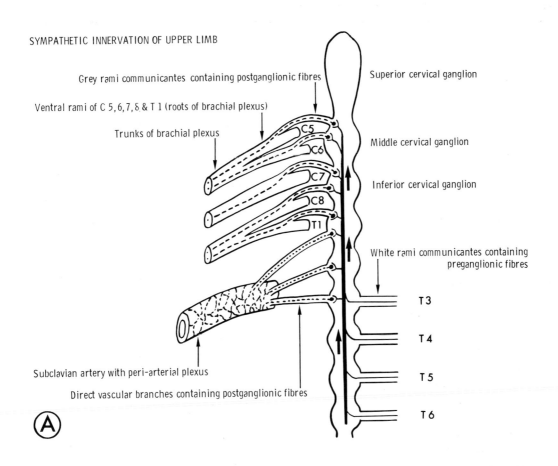

SYMPATHETIC INNERVATION OF UPPER LIMB

Grey rami communicantes containing postganglionic fibres

Ventral rami of C 5,6,7,8 & T 1 (roots of brachial plexus)

Trunks of brachial plexus

Subclavian artery with peri-arterial plexus

Direct vascular branches containing postganglionic fibres

Superior cervical ganglion

Middle cervical ganglion

Inferior cervical ganglion

White rami communicantes containing preganglionic fibres

C5
C6
C7
C8
T1

T 3
T 4
T 5
T 6

Ⓐ

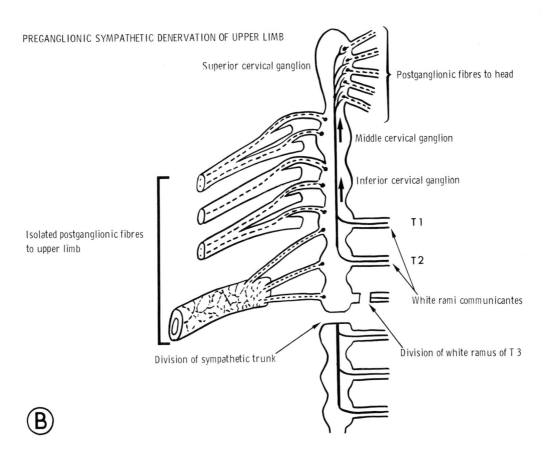

PREGANGLIONIC SYMPATHETIC DENERVATION OF UPPER LIMB

Superior cervical ganglion

Isolated postganglionic fibres to upper limb

Division of sympathetic trunk

Postganglionic fibres to head

Middle cervical ganglion

Inferior cervical ganglion

T 1

T 2

White rami communicantes

Division of white ramus of T 3

Ⓑ

567

SEGMENTAL INNERVATION OF THE UPPER LIMB

Motor innervation

With the exception of trapezius, which is supplied by the spinal part of the accessory nerve, and levator scapulae, which is supplied from the cervical plexus (**391A**), all the muscles of the upper limb are innervated through the ventral rami of the spinal nerves which take part in the formation of the brachial plexus, that is usually from C5 to T1 inclusive. Each muscle receives nerve fibres from a number of spinal segments but, because the muscles always act in groups to produce specific joint movements, it is of more practical value to know the segments which are associated with these movements than those concerned in the innervation of individual muscles.

The table below, which is worth learning by heart, shows the predominant spinal segments which motivate joint movements in the upper limb. In nearly all cases other segments are also concerned but to a minor and clinically unimportant degree. It should be noted that the short muscles of the hand which take part in movements of the digits are innervated mostly from T1.

C5 and 6	Abduction of the shoulder
	Lateral rotation of the shoulder
	Flexion of the elbow
	Supination of the forearm
C7 and 8	Adduction of the shoulder
	Medial rotation of the shoulder
	Extension of the elbow
	Pronation of the forearm
	Both flexion and extension of the wrist
C8 and T1	Movements of the digits

Cutaneous innervation

The diagrams **A** and **B** show the skin areas predominantly innervated by the segments of the spinal cord from C4 to T2 inclusive. Note particularly the following features.

1. The dispositions and extents of the ventral and dorsal axial lines which demarcate adjacent skin areas not innervated from consecutive spinal segments.
2. There is considerable overlap in the distribution of nerve fibres from adjacent spinal segments. Thus the total area on the anterior aspect of the limb to which C5 fibres are distributed (**C**) is considerably larger than the area predominantly innervated by C5 fibres (**A**).
3. With the exception of C4 and T2, the skin areas supplied by ventral rami are not continuous with skin areas supplied by the numerically corresponding dorsal rami (**B**).
4. Successive spinal segments from C4–T2 are associated with skin areas which are situated in order down the lateral aspect of the limb and up its medial aspect (**A, B**).
5. On both the palmar and dorsal aspects of the hand the skin is innervated by C6, C7 and C8 in that order from lateral to medial side (**A, B**).
6. Although no muscles of the upper limb are innervated by T2, an appreciable area of skin is supplied from that spinal segment.

It is difficult to memorise the pattern of segmental cutaneous innervation shown in **A** and **B** and it is perhaps more useful to know localities which are associated with each of the relevant spinal segments. Such localities are circled in **A** and listed in the table below.

C4 over the acromion process of the scapula
C5 over the insertion of deltoid
C6 the skin of the thumb
C7 the skin of the middle finger
C8 the skin of the little finger
T1 over the medial aspect of the elbow
T2 at the junction of the medial aspect of the arm and the floor of the axilla.

PREDOMINANT SEGMENTAL CUTANEOUS INNERVATION OF
ANTERIOR ASPECT OF UPPER LIMB

PREDOMINANT SEGMENTAL CUTANEOUS INNERVATION OF DORSAL
ASPECT OF UPPER LIMB:

Shaded areas dorsal rami,
clear areas ventral rami

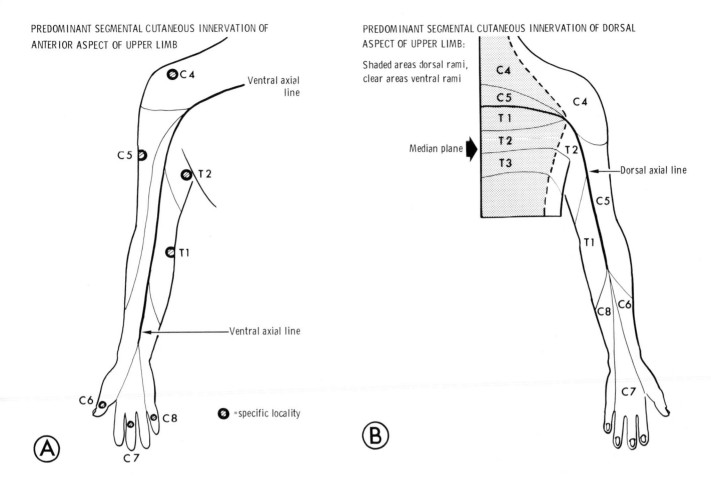

SHADED AREA IS TOTAL VENTRAL AREA
FROM WHICH SENSORY IMPULSES
PASS TO C 5 SEGMENT

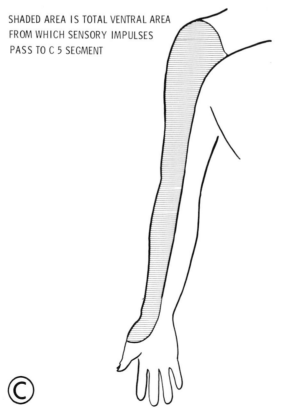

NERVE INJURIES IN THE UPPER LIMB

Certain nerves are particularly prone to injury and these injuries tend to occur at certain specific sites.

Lesions of the upper trunk of the brachial plexus affect all the C5 and C6 fibres passing to the limb. Reference to the segmental innervation of movements (**568**) will show that, if the lesion is complete, abduction and lateral rotation of the shoulder, flexion of the elbow and supination of the forearm will be paralysed. Owing to gravity and the unopposed actions of normal muscles, the limb consequently hangs by the side, the shoulder is medially rotated, the forearm pronated and the elbow extended. In addition a variable extent of the skin area innervated by C5 and 6 (**569A, 569B**) will be anaesthetic.

Lesions of the lower trunk of the plexus are frequently incomplete and due to friction between the trunk and the subclavian groove on the first rib. The C8 and T1 fibres to the limb are affected. This gives rise to weakness in the movements of the fingers, wasting of the small muscles of the hand, and paraesthesia or anaesthesia along the medial border of the forearm and hand (**569A, 569B**).

The axillary nerve (**511C**) may be injured as it passes through the quandrangular space in the posterior wall of the axilla by fractures of the surgical neck of the humerus or dislocation of the shoulder joint. Abduction of the shoulder cannot be carried out because of paralysis of the deltoid, and the skin over the lower part of the deltoid, supplied by the upper lateral cutaneous nerve of the arm (**511D**) is anaesthetic.

The radial nerve is prone to injury at a number of levels and progressively more of the total distribution of the nerve is spared the lower the site of the lesion.

1. Prolonged pressure on the lateral wall of the axilla by a crutch or by the arm hanging over the back of a chair (**B1**) may cause temporary paralysis of all the muscles supplied by the nerve and temporary anaesthesia of all the skin areas it innervates (**535C, 563D**).
2. In injuries caused by fractures of the humeral shaft about the middle of the groove for the radial nerve (**B2**) the skin supplied by the posterior cutaneous nerve of the arm, and the triceps muscle, are spared.
3. In injuries caused by fractures of the upper end of the shaft of the radius (**B3**) there is no skin loss. On the other hand, owing to paralysis of the posterior muscles of the forearm, supination is weak and the

wrist and metacarpophalangeal joints cannot be extended (drop wrist). The interphalangeal joints *can* be extended by the interossei and lumbricals, provided the metacarpophalangeal joints are passively extended (**558**).

Lesions of the median nerve are most commonly due to an incised wound on the anterior aspect of the wrist. The anterior muscles of the forearm are not affected unless their tendons are divided by the same wound. In the hand sensory loss occurs over the greater part of the median nerve area shown in **565D, 565E**. Muscle paralysis is usually confined to opponens pollicis, abductor pollicis brevis and the lateral two lumbricals, and does not produce a serious functional loss. At rest the first metacarpal lies in reposition (**553D**). Active opposition of the thumb is weak but not impossible because provided the first metacarpal is pulled medially across the palm of the hand by intact muscles such as flexor pollicis brevis and adductor pollicis, the rotation of the bone characteristic of opposition is produced automatically by the oblique ligaments of the first carpometacarpal joint (**543**).

Compression of the median nerve as it passes beneath the flexor retinaculum may cause pain in the sensory distribution of the nerve in the fingers, but not in the hand, and wasting of the thenar eminence (carpal tunnel syndrome).

A lesion of the ulnar nerve occurs most commonly behind the medial humeral epicondyle. At this level the lesion affects all the sensory and motor branches of the nerve. The nerve may also be injured by an incised wound on the anterior aspect of the wrist. This usually spares the dorsal branch of the nerve but causes sensory loss in the skin area supplied by the palmar cutaneous and palmar digital branches (**565E**). The most important muscle paralysis is that of all the interossei, the medial two lumbricals and the hypothenar muscles and a resulting inability to flex the metacarpophalangeal joints and extend the interphalangeal joints (**559E**) in the medial four fingers. As a result, in the medial four fingers side to side movements are lost, and the metacarpophalangeal joints are hyperextended and the interphalangeal joints partially flexed (claw hand). The simultaneous paralysis of adductor pollicis considerably weakens adduction of the thumb so that a piece of paper cannot be firmly held between the adjacent sides of the thumb and index fingers.

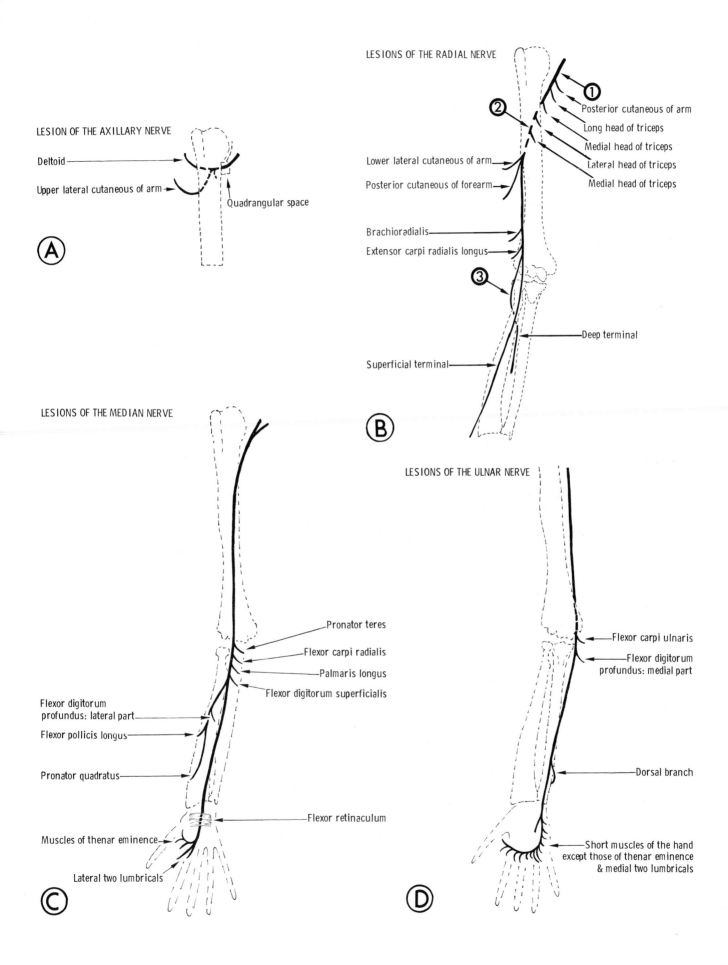

LESION OF THE AXILLARY NERVE

Deltoid

Upper lateral cutaneous of arm

Quadrangular space

Ⓐ

LESIONS OF THE RADIAL NERVE

① Posterior cutaneous of arm
Long head of triceps
② Medial head of triceps
Lateral head of triceps
Medial head of triceps

Lower lateral cutaneous of arm
Posterior cutaneous of forearm

Brachioradialis
Extensor carpi radialis longus

③
Deep terminal

Superficial terminal

Ⓑ

LESIONS OF THE MEDIAN NERVE

Pronator teres
Flexor carpi radialis
Palmaris longus
Flexor digitorum superficialis

Flexor digitorum profundus: lateral part
Flexor pollicis longus

Pronator quadratus

Flexor retinaculum

Muscles of thenar eminence

Lateral two lumbricals

Ⓒ

LESIONS OF THE ULNAR NERVE

Flexor carpi ulnaris
Flexor digitorum profundus: medial part

Dorsal branch

Short muscles of the hand except those of thenar eminence & medial two lumbricals

Ⓓ

INDEX